Macrosocial Determinants of Population Health

Sandro Galea

Macrosocial Determinants of Population Health

With 31 Illustrations

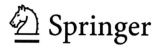
Springer

Sandro Galea
Department of Epidemiology
School of Public Health
University of Michigan
Ann Arbor, MI 48104-2548
USA
sgalea@umich.edu

ISBN: 978-0-387-70811-9   e-ISBN: 978-0-387-70812-6

Library of Congress Control Number: 2007926435

Printed on acid-free paper.

9 8 7 6 5 4 3 2 1

springer.com

Acknowledgements

I am grateful to all the authors who have contributed chapters to this book. I have learned a tremendous amount from them, both through our discussions as this book was taking shape and through reading the chapters themselves. I would like to thank my students in EPID 617 at the University of Michigan School of Public Health. This work was both inspired and shaped by discussions with many graduate students in the class. I am indebted to my colleagues at the Center for Social Epidemiology and Population Health at the University of Michigan, particularly Dr George Kaplan, Dr Ana Diez Roux, and Dr Allison Aiello. Our ongoing conversations about the social production of health has contributed immeasurably to my evolving thoughts about the role of macrosocial determinants of population health. I owe a debt of gratitude to Dr David Vlahov, who has long nurtured my evolution in scientific thinking, and to Dr Adam Karpati, with whom I learned social epidemiology and who has had a profound influence on my thinking about issues covered in this book. I am grateful to several reviewers who put tremendous time and energy into offering suggestions both to me and to the chapter authors that helped improve the work presented here. I am particularly indebted to Ms Sara Putnam who was an invaluable editorial partner in many aspects of this book's preparation. This book would not have been possible without the editorial assistance of Ms Katy Wortman who has shown dedication to this work that is above and beyond the call of duty. Finally, I owe my spouse, Dr Margaret Kruk, a debt of gratitude for her patience and forbearance with this and many other aspects of my work. This book is dedicated, as always, to Margaret, Oliver Luke, and Isabel Tess.

Sandro Galea

Contents

Contributors

Obijiofor Aginam, Department of Law, Carleton University, Ottawa, Ontario, Canada

Jennifer Ahern, Division of Epidemiology, University of California Berkeley, School of Public Health, Berkeley, California; Center for Social Epidemiology and Population Health, Department of Epidemiology, University of Michigan School of Public Health, Ann Arbor, Michigan

Jerry Avorn, Division of Pharmacoepidemiology and Pharmacoeconomics, Brigham and Women's Hospital, Harvard Medical School, Boston, Massachusetts

David M. Bishai, Department of Population, Family, and Reproductive Health, Johns Hopkins Bloomberg School of Public Health, Baltimore, Maryland

Tim Bruckner, Division of Epidemiology, University of California Berkeley, School of Public Health, Berkeley, California

Martin Caraher, Centre for Food Policy, City University, London, United Kingdom

Roy Carr-Hill, Centre for Health Economics, University of York, York, United Kingdom

Ralph Catalano, Division of Community Health and Human Development, University of California Berkeley, School of Public Health, Berkeley, California

Steven Cummins, Department of Geography, Queen Mary University of London, London, United Kingdom

Sarah Curtis, Department of Geography, University of Durham, Durham, United Kingdom

Kristie L. Ebi, E.S.S., L.C.C., Alexandria, Virginia

Richard M. Eckersley, National Centre for Epidemiology and Population Health, Australian National University, Canberra, Australia

Lia S. Florey, Center for Social Epidemiology and Population Health, University of Michigan School of Public Health, Ann Arbor, Michigan

Nicholas Freudenberg, Program in Urban Public Health, Hunter College School of Health Sciences, City University of New York, New York, New York.

Sandro Galea, Center for Social Epidemiology and Population Health, Department of Epidemiology, University of Michigan School of Public Health, Ann Arbor, Michigan; Department of Epidemiology, Mailman School of Public Health, Columbia University, New York, New York; Center for Urban Epidemiologic Studies, New York Academy of Medicine, New York, New York

M. Maria Glymour, Department of Epidemiology, Mailman School of Public Health, Columbia University, New York, New York

Jay S. Kaufman, Carolina Population Center and Department of Epidemiology, University of North Carolina School of Public Health, Chapel Hill, North Carolina

Ichiro Kawachi, Department of Society, Human Development, and Health, Harvard School of Public Health, Boston, Massachusetts

Aaron S. Kesselheim, Division of Pharmacoepidemiology and Pharmacoeconomics, Brigham and Women's Hospital, Harvard Medical School, Boston, Massachusetts

Emily Z. Kontos, Department of Society, Human Development, and Health, Harvard School of Public Health, Boston, Massachusetts

Yung-Ting Kung, Department of Population, Family, and Reproductive Health, Johns Hopkins Bloomberg School of Public Health, Baltimore, Maryland

Sana Loue, Department of Epidemiology and Biostatistics, School of Medicine at Case Western Reserve University, Cleveland, Ohio

Siobhan C. Maty, School of Community Health, College of Urban and Public Affairs, Portland State University, Portland, Oregon

Danielle C. Ompad, Center for Urban Epidemiologic Studies, New York Academy of Medicine, New York, New York

Marie S. O'Neill, Departments of Epidemiology and Environmental Health Sciences, University of Michigan School of Public Health, Ann Arbor, Michigan

Theresa L. Osypuk, Department of Epidemiology, University of Michigan School of Public Health, Ann Arbor, Michigan

Sara Putnam, Center for Urban Epidemiologic Studies, New York Academy of Medicine, New York, New York

Shoba Ramanadhan, Department of Society, Human Development, and Health, Harvard School of Public Health, Boston, Massachusetts

Jan C. Semenza, School of Community Health, College of Urban and Public Affairs, Portland State University, Portland, Oregon

S. V. Subramanian, Department of Society, Human Development, and Health, Harvard School of Public Health, Boston, Massachusetts

K. Viswanath, Department of Society, Human Development, and Health, Harvard School of Public Health, and Division of Population Sciences, Dana Farber Cancer Institute, Boston, Massachusetts

David Vlahov, Center for Urban Epidemiologic Studies, New York Academy of Medicine, New York, New York

Howard Waitzkin, Departments of Sociology, Family and Community Medicine, and Internal Medicine, University of New Mexico, Albuquerque, New Mexico

Mark L. Wilson, Global Health Program and Department of Epidemiology, University of Michigan School of Public Health, Ann Arbor, Michigan

Introduction

Chapter 1
The Role of Macrosocial Determinants in Shaping the Health of Populations

Sandro Galea and Sara Putnam

1. Introduction

The roots of epidemiology, coincident with the origin of public health, lie in exploring how social conditions may influence health and how these conditions may be manipulated so as to improve the health of populations (Mc Leod, 2000; Halliday, 2000; Hamlin & Sheard, 1998). However, in the last half century, with the advent of antibiotics as treatments for infectious diseases, the shift from infectious disease to chronic disease considerations, and the focus on genetic determination of disease, epidemiologic inquiry has grown increasingly concerned not with the social determination of population health, but rather with the individual exposures or characteristics that influence individual risk of health and disease (March & Susser, 2006). It is the central tenet of this book that social factors that lie beyond the individual and that affect whole populations, factors that we term "macrosocial", should remain central in our thinking about the production of health and disease, and that public health research and practice would be well served by an improved understanding of how these macrosocial factors shape population health. Setting the stage for the chapters to follow, in this introductory chapter we explore the challenges faced by most current inquiry concerned with the determination of health and argue that epidemiologic inquiry about macrosocial factors can help improve our understanding of population health and potentially guide the development of more effective public health interventions.

We note that this introduction, and this book, adopt very much an "epidemiologic" perspective. We mean this to refer to a central concern with the determination of health and disease and to inquiry aimed at understanding those factors that may influence health. Although the field formally constituted as "epidemiology" today is certainly most concerned with these questions, we do not mean to endorse an exclusive reliance on the methods of epidemiology and certainly do not intend to exclude the role of other disciplinary perspectives. As the chapters in this book amply illustrate, we suggest that disciplines such as economics, sociology, and health policy, among many others, play a central role in our understanding of the determination of health and of how those interested in the health of populations may fruitfully identify areas of intervention that can improve health.

2. Understanding the Determination
of Health and Disease

The epidemiologic approach typically begins with interest in a particular disease or health indicator (e.g., diabetes or lung cancer). Concurrent with the identification of a disease, we rely on theory and prior research to identify a particular factor that may be associated with the disease. This factor is generally an individual "exposure" (e.g., a gene or mutation) or behavior (e.g., smoking). A study is then designed to determine whether there is an association between the particular factor of interest and the health outcome; once data is collected, statistical methods are employed to measure the association of interest while taking into account other possible alternate explanations.

If a rigorous epidemiologic study demonstrates an association that is biologically plausible and replicable in subsequent studies, we may venture to consider the factor in question a "cause" of disease and recommend an intervention to alter or eliminate this stated cause. Given that most modern epidemiologic research is concerned with individual behaviors or exposures, the recommended interventions are typically behavioral (e.g., smoking cessation) or pharmacologic (e.g., developing a drug to lower high cholesterol levels). This approach has arguably contributed to some of the most compelling public health success stories of the past half-century, including the identification of smoking as a risk factor for lung cancer and cardiovascular disease and low maternal folic acid intake as a risk factor for neonatal neural tube defect.

Nevertheless, there are clear conceptual and practical limitations to this dominant epidemiologic paradigm. A significant limitation is that the principal empiric tools for considering associations within study samples are best for research at the population level. Typical epidemiologic etiologic analysis calculates population rates and risk of disease and then estimates the relative rates and risks of disease in the presence and absence of a particular "exposure" of interest. While these absolute and relative rates and risks that are used to determine association are adequate representations of population-level disease occurrence, they tell us very little about individual risk of disease (Kleinbaum, Kupper, & Morgenstern, 1982; Rockhill, 2005). Statistical associations at the population level may be inconsistent with mechanisms (e.g., biological processes) occurring within individuals. This tension between epidemiologic methods of inference and individual risk is an intractable feature of epidemiologic inference based on population summary estimates and has contributed to three serious challenges facing public health inquiry today.

First, as originally and most forcefully articulated by Geoffrey Rose (1985), there are clear limitations of the epidemiologic approach in informing our understanding of the determination of individual health. Rose noted that many of our attempts to improve health are aimed at improving the health of persons at the tail end of a distribution of risk. For example, all medical screening for risk factors essentially aims to identify and intervene with "high risk" persons. There is no attempt to reduce risk in the rest of the population, which is considered to be at "low risk" (or at least not at "high risk"). This approach might well be rational if (a) we could identify who is likely to develop disease simply by assessing their disease risk and (b) risk were binary, i.e., either present or absent. However, the first of these requisite conditions is false since our available methods of assessing where an individual sits on a risk distribution tell us little about individual likelihood of a particular disease (Pepe, Janes, Longton, Leisenring, & Newcomb, 2004; Wald, Hackshaw, & Frost, 1999). The second of these conditions is also false since ultimately exposure to risk factors is more likely continuous, and arbitrary cutoffs define and determine "high" vs. "low risks". Populations characterized by levels of risk that are just below the "high risk" cutoff are likely at much greater risk of an adverse health condition than are populations whose risk is much lower than the cutoff, though both would be identified as "low risk".

Second, an increasingly worrisome practical limitation is the preponderance of epidemiologic scrutiny focusing on the pursuit of single risk factors for disease in individuals. It is well established that with very few exceptions disease causation is multifactorial. However, our persistent epidemiologic focus on identifying single risk factors for individual disease has contributed to conflicting results from state-of-the-science studies that explore one particular aspect of causation while neglecting others. Unfortunately, the ever-changing catalog of risk and protective factors for disease documented in epidemiologic studies (e.g., the recent very public debate about the role of postmenopausal estrogen therapy) has occasioned substantial public confusion about the methods and conclusions of epidemiology and suggests that the quest for individual risks of individual disease may well be a reductionistic approach that has outlived its usefulness. In addition, as etiologic inquiry has become progressively more concerned with individual disease determination, this inquiry has also increasingly focused on determinants of disease that are, at least for the foreseeable future, immutable. The study of factors that predispose individuals to risk has increasingly involved genetic factors, molecular markers, and exposure to behaviors and environmental toxins that are not readily alterable. Despite several scientists' brash promises of genetic interventions (Varmus, 2006) and the dedication of enormous financial resources to genetic inquiry, thus far there has been little evidence that genetic manipulation is a realistic near-future goal.

Third, and relatedly, both the above limitations have contributed to a rather poor record of epidemiology and public health in eliciting genuine behavior changes that "address" the burden of individual risk behaviors. The past few decades offer several examples of behavior change interventions that were demonstrably efficacious in small and well-controlled trials but not effective when applied in the general population. For example, although several epidemiologic studies show that sexual behavior contributes to risk of sexually transmitted diseases (Kaestle, Halpern, Miller, & Ford, 2005), and controlled trials have achieved changes in sexual practices (DiClemente & Wingood, 1995), sexual risk behavior remains notoriously difficult to influence at the population level (Lyles et al., 2006; Herbst et al., 2006; Herbst et al., 2005). Comparably, the recent obesity epidemic has made it all too clear that simply demonstrating associations between greater weight and disease (demonstrated in countless epidemiologic studies during the past twenty years) is not sufficient for improving dietary habits, particularly when individual dietary habits are constrained by lack of healthy food options or safe places to exercise (Fitzgibbon & Stolley, 2004).

Particularly in the instance of enjoyable behaviors, appeals based on epidemiologic observations hold very little sway. This, of course, is not surprising given that epidemiologic studies frequently provide conflicting evidence and focus on factors which are indeed difficult to change. In addition, epidemiologic studies all too often suggest that changing single risk factors may be all important for disease prevention. However, the epidemiologic equating of being in the tail end of the risk distribution with "risk" means that persons with a particular "risk factor" may well not develop disease and others without may well indeed do so, which flies in the face of the notion of multifactorial disease causation that is intuitively and readily understood by the general public. Ultimately, these limitations "stack the deck" against epidemiologically-informed recommendations that put the onus of change only on individuals and promote goals that are, in a practical sense, unattainable. Nothing short of a colossal effort, or a dramatically terrifying disease, is required to change individual behavior. It is worth remembering that only after decades of public health effort in the Western world have population smoking rates decreased, and it took the definitive infectious disease of our time, HIV/AIDS, to change population sexual risk behaviors.

3. The Emergence of Social Epidemiology

A growing appreciation of the limitations of the individualization of epidemiologic thinking, coupled with a genuine abiding interest within public health in understanding the role that social factors play in determining health and disease, have contributed to a tremendous surge during the past fifteen years in research that takes a "social epidemiologic" approach (Kaplan, 2004). Social epidemiology emerged first from proponents of social medicine, who argued for greater consideration of social factors in disease determination (Galdston, 1947; Krieger, 2001) and subsequently went on to develop and implement studies on such social factors as gender (Perry, 1998), race/ethnicity (Baltrus, Lynch, Everson-Rose, Raghunathan, Kaplan, 2005) discrimination (Krieger, 2000; Williams, 1999), occupational conditions (Lallukka et al., 2006), socioeconomic status (Kanjilal et al., 2006) and education (Jacobsen & Thelle, 1988). Several books and papers considering social epidemiology as a discrete entity have traced its development (Berkman & Kawachi, 2000; Honjo, 2004; Krieger, 2001; Oakes & Kaufman, 2006), reviewed its methods (Berkman & Kawachi, 2000; Oakes & Kaufman, 2006) and examined the role of social factors as determinants of health (Marmot & Wilkinson, 2006). Formalizing the study of social factors within epidemiology has provided epidemiologists with an opportunity to reintroduce what likely should never have been absent from epidemiology's domain.

This essay, and this book, clearly and explicitly are informed by a social epidemiologic perspective and a concern with social factors that influence health. However, we propose that social epidemiology as currently understood and implemented falls short of its promise. As social epidemiology has fought for legitimacy within epidemiology and public health, epidemiologists interested in social determination have published studies with increasing methodologic sophistication, including studies that mimic mainstream epidemiologic publications and methods. Therefore, studies have used ever more complex statistical techniques to examine how factors such as gender, race/ethnicity, income, and so forth may come to contribute to individual risk of disease. While this has achieved the goal of establishing social epidemiology's intellectual bona fides within the epidemiologic and public health research and practice community, social epidemiology has not done much better than other risk factor epidemiology in expanding beyond the individual-level risk of disease or in offering practicable insights. This is frequently discussed in the literature as a challenge inherent in the study of immutable social factors, such as race/ethnicity (Berkman, 2004; Bhopal, 1997).

It should be clear from our discussion here that we do not think that this challenge is unique to social epidemiology, but is rather a function of the larger problems that face epidemiology (i.e., the impracticality of evaluating individual risk factors using population based measures, the immutability of individual-level risk factors, and the attempt to isolate single causes of individual disease when the nature of causation is inherently much more complicated). However, we suggest that social epidemiology can do better and consider questions and adopt methods that overcome some of the key challenges facing epidemiologic inquiry today. Indeed, social epidemiology presents an opportunity to address both conceptual and practical limitations of an individual risk perspective and to suggest new and dynamic areas of inquiry. In particular, we argue that this can be achieved by the adoption of a population-level approach to examining the distal social factors and processes that influence health.

4. A Population Health Strategy

Margaret Thatcher famously suggested that "there is no such thing as society. There are [just] individual men and women". Our central premise is that the health of populations is as much derived from the connections between individuals and the social factors or processes to which a given population is exposed as it is a function of the aggregate persons within that population. We use the term "population health" to refer to the health of whole groups of persons, be they groups within neighborhoods, occupational class, or other levels of aggregation. Therefore, populations are not simply the sum of their individual parts, and subsequently, population health is not simply the sum of individual health. A corollary is that an individual, if she were part of another population, might have a rather different health profile, and a population (e.g., a neighborhood), if comprised of alternate individuals and characterized by dissimilar local circumstances, might then have rather different population health.

If we accept the notion that population health is worthy of inquiry, we can then imagine solutions to the practical problems facing epidemiology. First, it follows that the epidemiologic methods that are better suited to population-level inference can be applied fruitfully to the study and improvement of population health (Rose, 1985). Second, group-level observations are not informed by the particular multifactorial causation of disease in a given individual and a population strategy avoids the flawed quest to identify single modifiable risk factors that provide (false) promises of improvement in individual risk of disease. Third, and centrally, a population strategy recognizes that population health is our ultimate goal and avoids futile attempts to change the behavior of individuals. Rather, a population strategy aims to improve population health generally, to shift the population disease curve by influencing the overall risk a population faces. From a very pragmatic point of view, this approach sidesteps the challenges discussed earlier that result in limited effectiveness of widespread attempts at individual behavior change. Therefore, a population approach might involve banning the use of escalators, increasing the likelihood that all able population members walk up an extra flight or two of stairs on a regular basis. This would be associated with lower risk of living a sedentary life for the whole population and therefore lower population rates of heart disease. Insofar as it is the aim of public health to improve the health of whole populations, the approach we propose here is congruent with this goal.

Importantly, we note that the improvement of population health is not at odds with the practical desire of improving the health of individuals. Rather, this conception suggests that individual health is so inextricably linked to the populations to which individuals belong that to think of ways only to improve individual health is ultimately a fallacy and a Sisyphean effort, a doomed and impractical attempt at improving health.

Clearly, different moral philosophical perspectives might find this perspective more, or less, appealing. A utilitarian might find the notion of populations as an undifferentiated grouping of individuals (each of whom, implicitly, are equally worthwhile) discomfiting, while this approach may be more congruent with a perspective that is primarily informed by considerations of social justice. Our argument is based strictly on an empiric conceptual and practical rationale; while we do think that there is ample philosophical reason to further buttress this argument, particularly with reference to health equity, a full discussion of the moral implications of a population health approach to epidemiologic thinking is beyond the scope of this brief introduction. We refer the reader to other published works for more on this issue (Bodenheimer, 2005; Brock, 1998; Edney, 2006; Kawachi, Kennedy, & Wilkinson, 1999; Menzel, 2003; Peter, 2001; Popay, 2006).

5. Macrosocial Determinants of Population Health

Thus, we suggest that social epidemiology can provide a conceptual lens and empiric methods for evaluating macrosocial determinants of population health. "Macrosocial" here refers to factors, such as culture, political systems, economics, and processes of migration or urbanization (all featured as chapter topics in this book), that are beyond the individual and are explicitly a function of population systems. Taking this perspective, social epidemiology would seek to understand the interconnections between and among the individuals that make up these systems and how these macrosocial factors shape the health of populations. Applying new epidemiologic methods and discipline to the study of macrosocial factors would serve to bring epidemiology back to the core concern that has long motivated public health, that is, discovering how we can improve social structures and circumstances to improve the health of populations.

Identifying macrosocial processes that influence population health can provide opportunities for interventions that influence the population distribution of risk and improve the health of whole populations, avoiding the "high risk" intervention trap into which much of our current individual risk thinking leads us. Improvements in motor vehicle safety, workplace safety, and family planning, as well as introduction of safer and healthier foods, were all recently suggested as among the greatest public health achievements of the twentieth century (Centers for Disease Control and Prevention, 1999), and all result from macrosocial interventions aimed at reducing population-level risk. An explicit focus on the macrosocial factors that underlie population health in the near future may permit us to identify, and effectively intervene on, the key determinants of population health of the twenty first century.

6. Conclusion and a Way Forward

A refocus of social epidemiologic methods and approaches to thinking about macrosocial determination of population health will not be easy. There are three likely key limitations to achieving such an end. First, with few exceptions, thinking about macrosocial factors as determinants of population health today is far from the core concern of most health researchers, including epidemiologists. Therefore, such a paradigm shift will require a substantial intellectual investment on our parts and will undoubtedly stretch our imaginations and practical capacities. Second, social epidemiologic methods are still nascent, and there is no question that a systematic consideration of macrosocial determinants of population health will require the refinement of our current methods, the development of new methods, and the judicious and careful interpretation of results from our studies. Researchers who are interested in the macrosocial determination of population health will have to make unimpeachable efforts to draw objective inferences using methods that are as robust as possible. Third, there is little doubt that change in public health, as in all human endeavors, comes slowly. We recognize that the adoption of research questions such as the role of globalization in influencing population rates of heart disease is a substantial departure from the overwhelming majority of extant modern public health literature that influences and shapes the work we all do. In addition, given the importance of research funding in driving academic and public health inquiry, a conceptual shift predicated on thinking about the macrosocial determinants of population health would need to make substantial inroads into traditionally biomedical-oriented funding institutions to allow for the sustainable grounding of this work.

We have little doubt that with time researchers and public health practitioners will find suitable ingenuity and imagination to develop the field. In meeting all of these challenges, public health stands to benefit greatly from cross-disciplinary communication and collaboration. Insight from multiple disciplines, including economics, sociology, health policy, among many others, play a critical role in advancing understanding of population health and how to improve it. In the following sections, various authors will consider a range of macrosocial determinants that may influence population health, as well as key methodologic challenges this work faces today and in the future. Additionally, they will offer some insights into what the implications of considering macrosocial determinants might be for public health intervention. It is the intent of this book to provide a first step toward the systematic consideration of macrosocial determinants of population health. We hope that this work inspires theoretic and empiric innovation and investigation in this area.

References

Baltrus, P. T., Lynch, J. W., Everson-Rose, S., Raghunathan, T. E., & Kaplan, G. A. (2005). Race/ethnicity, life-course socioeconomic position, and body weight trajectories over 34 years: The Alameda County Study. *American Journal of Public Health, 95*(9), 1595–1601.

Bentham, J. (1967). *A fragment on government and an introduction to the principles of morals and legislation*. Oxford: Basil Blackwell.

Berkman, L. F. (2004). Introduction: Seeing the forest and the trees – from observation to experiments in social epidemiology. *Epidemiologic Reviews, 26*, 2–6.

Berkman, L.F., & Kawachi, I. (2000). *Social epidemiology*. New York: Oxford University Press.

Bhopal, R. (1997). Is research into ethnicity and health racist, unsound, or important science? *British Medical Journal, 314*(7096), 1751–1756.

Bodenheimer, T. (2005). The political divide in health care: A liberal perspective. *Health Affairs, 24*(6), 1426–1435.

Brock, D. W. (1998). Ethical issues in the development of summary measures of population health status. In M. J. Field & M. R. Gold (Eds.), *Summarizing population health: Directions for the development and application of population metrics*. Washington, DC: National Academy Press.

Centers for Disease Control and Prevention. (1999). Ten great public health achievements – United States, 1900–1999. *MMWR: Morbidity and Mortality Weekly Report, 48*(12), 241–3.

DiClemente, R. J., & Wingood, G. M. (1995). A randomized controlled trial of an HIV sexual risk-reduction intervention for young African-American women. *Journal of the American Medical Association, 274*(16), 1271–1276.

Edney, J. (2006). How capitalism threatens your health: A terrible weapon in the hands of the rich. *Counterpunch.* (April 3, 2006); http://www.counterpunch.org/edney04032006.html.

Fitzgibbon, M. L., & Stolley, M. R. (2004). Environmental changes may be needed for prevention of overweight in minority children. *Pediatric Annals, 33*(1), 45–49.

Galdston, I. (1947). *Social medicine: Its derivations and objectives.* New York: The Commonwealth Fund.

Halliday, S. (2000). William Farr: Campaigning statistician. *Journal of Medical Biography, 8*(4), 220–227.

Hamlin, C., & Sheard, S. (1998). Revolutions in public health: 1848, and 1998? *British Medical Journal, 317*(7158), 587–591.

Herbst, J. H., Sherba, R. T., Crepaz, N., Deluca, J. B., Zohrabyan, L., Stall, R. D., et al. (2005). A meta-analytic review of HIV behavioral interventions for reducing sexual risk behavior of men who have sex with men. *Journal of Acquired Immune Deficiency Syndromes, 39*(2), 228–241.

Herbst, J., Kay, L., Passin, W., Lyles, C., Crepaz, N., & Marin, B. (2007). A systematic review and meta-analysis of behavioral interventions to reduce HIV risk behaviors of hispanics in the United States and Puerto Rico. *AIDS and Behavior, 11*(1), 25–47.

Honjo, K. (2004). Social epidemiology: Definition, history, and research examples. *Environmental Health and Preventive Medicine, 9*(5), 193–199.

Jacobsen, B. K., & Thelle, D. S. (1988). Risk factors for coronary heart disease and level of education. *American Journal of Epidemiology, 127*(5), 923–932.

Kaestle, C. E., Halpern, C. T., Miller, W. C., & Ford, C. A. (2005). Young age at first sexual intercourse and sexually transmitted infections in adolescents and young adults. *American Journal of Epidemiology, 161*(8), 771–780.

Kanjilal, S., Gregg, E. W., Cheng, Y. J., Zhang, P., Nelson, D. E., Mensah, G., et al. (2006). Socioeconomic status and trends in disparities in 4 major risk factors for cardiovascular disease among US adults, 1971–2002. *Archives of Internal Medicine, 166*(21), 2348–2355.

Kaplan, G. A. (2004). What's wrong with social epidemiology, and how can we make it better? *Epidemiologic Reviews, 26,* 124–135.

Kawachi, I., Kennedy, B. P., & Wilkinson, R.G. (Eds.). (1999). *The society and population health reader.* New York: The New Press.

Kleinbaum, D. G., Kupper, L. L., & Morgenstern, H. (1982). *Epidemiologic research, principles and quantitative methods.* New York: John Wiley & Sons Inc.

Krieger, N. (2000). Discrimination and health. In L. Berkman & I. Kawachi (Eds.), *Social epidemiology.* New York: Oxford University Press.

Krieger, N. (2001). Theories for social epidemiology in the 21st century: An ecosocial perspective. *International Journal of Epidemiology, 30*(4), 668–677.

Lallukka, T., Martikainen, P., Reunanen, A., Roos, E., Sarlio-Lahteenkorva, S., & Lahelma, E. (2006). Associations between working conditions and angina pectoris symptoms among employed women. *Psychosomatic Medicine, 68*(2), 348–54.

Lyles, C. M., Kay, L. S., Crepaz, N., Herbst, J. H., Passin, W. F., Kim, A. S., et al. (2007). Best-evidence interventions: Findings from a systematic review of HIV behavioral interventions for US populations at high risk, 2000–2004. *American Journal of Public Health, 97*(1), 133–143.

March, D., & Susser, E. (2007). The eco- in eco-epidemiology. *International Journal of Epidemiology. 35*(6), 1379–1383.

Marmot, M., & Wilkinson, R. G. (2006). *Social determinants of health.* New York: Oxford University Press.

McLeod, K. S. (2000). Our sense of Snow: The myth of John Snow in medical geography. *Social Science & Medicine, 50*(7–8), 923–935.

Menzel, P. T. (2003). How compatible are liberty and equality in structuring a health care system? *The Journal of Medicine and Philosophy, 28*(3), 281–306.

Oakes, J. M., & Kaufman, J. S. (2006). *Methods in social epidemiology.* San Francisco: Jossey-Bass.

Pepe, M. S., Janes, H., Longton, G., Leisenring, W., & Newcomb, P. (2004). Limitations of the odds ratio in gauging the performance of a diagnostic, prognostic, or screening marker. *American Journal of Epidemiology, 159*(9), 882–890.

Perry, M. J. (1998). Gender, race and economic perspectives on the social epidemiology of HIV infection: Implications for intervention. *Journal of Primary Prevention, 19*(2), 97–104.

Peter, F. (2001). Health equity and social justice. *Journal of Applied Philosophy, 18*(2), 159–170.

Popay, J. (2006). Post positivist theory: Whose theory is it anyway? *Journal of Epidemiology and Community Health, 60,* 571–572.

Rockhill, B. (2005). Theorizing about causes at the individual level while estimating effects at the population level: Implications for prevention. *Epidemiology, 16*(1), 124–129.

Rose, G. (1985). Sick individuals and sick populations. *International Journal of Epidemiology, 14*(1), 32–38.

Thatcher, M. (1987). Aids, education and the year 2000. *Women's Own, 3,* 8–10.

Varmus, H. (2006). The new era in cancer research. *Science, 312*(5777), 1162–1165.

Wald, N., Hackshaw, A., & Frost, C. (1999). When can a risk factor be used as a worthwhile screening test? *British Medical Journal, 319*(7224), 1562–1565.

Williams, D. (1999). Race, socioeconomic status, and health: The added effects of racism and discrimination. *Annals of the New York Academy of Sciences, 896,* 173–88.

Section 1
Determinants

Chapter 2
Macrosocial Determinants of Population Health in the Context of Globalization

Lia S. Florey, Sandro Galea, and Mark L. Wilson

1. Introduction

We live in an increasingly interconnected world, as some like to say, a "global village." As in any village, social, economic and biophysical environments shape individual action and interaction, which, in turn, influence the quality of life and the health of inhabitants. Technology, information, media, food, goods and services, as well as environmental pollution and diseases are shared among villages, cities, countries and continents. Not only are these exchanges great in scope, but the magnitude and speed of interaction among individuals and populations is also increasing. For example, international trade grew 8.6% per year during the decade 1990–1999 (World Trade Organization, 2000a, b), with an estimated US$1.7 trillion in daily global trading (Lee, 2000). An estimated 760 million people traveled to international destinations in 2004 (World Trade Organization, 2005), and circumnavigation of the globe is now possible in a mere 36 hours (Smolinski, Hamburg, & Lederberg, 2003). Immigration contributes to global exchanges, with an estimated 175 million individuals spending at least one year in another country (United Nations, 2002). Additionally, approximately 17 million refugees and internally displaced persons migrate from their homes every year (United Nations High Commissioner for Refugees, 2004). These trends of growing interactions on the global scale shape the environments in which we live and which influence our well-being and our health.

The term globalization is used to denote these global trends in exchanges and interactions. Historically, globalization has been defined in economic terms as "the removal of tariff and non-tariff barriers to trade" (Weisbrot, Baker, Kraev, & Chen, 2002) or "the process whereby national and international policy-makers promote domestic deregulation and external liberalization" (Cornia, 2001). We argue, as have many before us, that globalization is comprised of much more than fiscal trends and policies. For the purposes of this review we use an expansive definition for which globalization consists of the "processes contributing to intensified human interaction in a wide range of spheres (that is, economic, political, social, environmental) and across three types of boundaries—spatial, temporal and cognitive—that have hitherto separated individuals and societies"

(Bettcher & Lee, 2002). Implicit in this definition is the ubiquity of globalization processes and the pervasiveness with which these processes affect human lives.

Although the existence of global influences on individuals and populations is clear, the effect of globalization on individual well-being and population health is not well established. Empirical evidence suggests both positive and negative effects of globalization on health, but there is no simple equation that can encapsulate how globalization may improve, or harm, population health. Instead it is likely that myriad processes comprise globalization, and each may influence the health of populations through multiple pathways. The challenge lies in elucidating the mechanisms by which globalization affects health. An understanding of these mechanisms will inform the decision-making process and enable implementation of policies that will mitigate the negative consequences of globalization and enhance its potential positive influences.

This chapter addresses an important gap in knowledge on the global context of population health by providing a conceptual framework from an epidemiologic perspective. The aim of this framework is to facilitate understanding of the complex relationships among globalization, macro-level determinants of health, and population health. The relationships between each component of the framework and population health will be briefly discussed followed by a presentation of potential mechanisms that may explain these associations. This chapter integrates current knowledge pertaining to the relationships of interest, generates hypotheses about mechanisms where current knowledge is scarce, and presents a brief discussion of methodological issues pertaining to epidemiologic studies of globalization and population health. We acknowledge that we approach this chapter as epidemiologists, building explicitly on epidemiologic multilevel thinking. We suspect that other disciplinary perspectives may approach the issue of globalization differently. We hope that our approach is illuminating, regardless of the reader's disciplinary orientation, and may engender discussion and debate that can bring about cross-disciplinary synthesis.

1.1. Framework

Globalization is characterized by a plethora of components that may influence health at the population level. We propose a framework that summarizes a few key characteristics of the global, national and community level environments that are associated with population health. This framework builds on previously published conceptual models (Huynen, Martens, & Hilderink, 2005; Labonte et al., 2002; Spiegel, Labonte, & Ostry, 2004; Woodward, Drager, Beaglehole, & Lipson, 2001) and on the broader literature examining the effects of contextual determinants on health (Galea, Freudenberg, & Vlahov, 2005; Galea, Rudenstine, & Vlahov, 2005; Kaplan, 1999; Link & Phelan, 1995).

Our framework (Figure 2.1) builds upon the emerging thinking about multiple "levels" of determination of population health (Kaplan, 1999) and suggests that three levels of variables may be considered central to the role played by globalization in population health. Global-level factors (including global trade, income distribution, population movement, global governance and communications) are

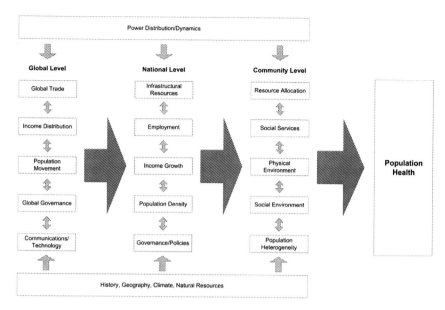

FIGURE 2.1. Conceptual framework summarizing how characteristics of the global, national and community-level environments may influence population health

conceptualized to shape national-level factors (infrastructural resources, employment, income growth, population density, and national governance). The national-level factors influence community-level factors (resource allocations, social services, physical environmental, social environment, and population heterogeneity). In turn, each of these elements are affected by global distributions and dynamics of power, as well as by underlying conditions such as history, climate, and geography that are represented by the horizontal rows at the top and the bottom of the model. Although this framework is designed to be hierarchical, with global-level factors influencing population health through the national and community-level factors, we recognize that there will be some direct effects between elements at any level of organization and health. Similarly, we consider that these associations could be bidirectional (a national-level factor may directly influence a global-level factor) as well as vertical (interrelationships among several components at the global level). The aim of this conceptual model, however, is to present the integral role of global-level processes in influencing population health as part of a multivariate, multilevel framework. This simplification of what is undoubtedly a far more complex web of associations is intended to clarify the current state of knowledge and help guide future research.

Although an unconventional approach, we begin by exploring the proximal relationships between community level factors and population health before approaching the more distal national-level and global-level factors (moving from right to left in Figure 2.1). This strategy allows clearer and more explicit development of the pathways through which globalization exerts influence on health and is compatible with clinical and epidemiologic approaches to health research.

2. Community-Level Processes

Despite extensive public health research focusing on the "community," a definition of this concept remains elusive. Considerable recent investigations have addressed "neighborhoods," while others have grouped people into census tracts or other administrative units. Such groupings may be convenient, affordable or otherwise useful for spatial analyses; however, they do not always carry social meaning for individuals. For purposes of this review, communities are defined as any sub-national aggregation that is socially meaningful to local residents.

As many scholars have noted, diverse aspects of community life that we characterized in Figure 2.1 play an enormous role in forming the health profiles of populations. These are the most proximal of the macro-level health determinants that are addressed in this chapter and should therefore affect population health indicators through the most direct pathways. Yet we recognize that multiple elements of communities may interact to shape health indicators through more complex, indirect pathways. The brief descriptions and examples presented below are not meant to be exhaustive, but rather to illustrate a few specific mechanisms whereby population health is affected by the environmental, social and political realities of communities.

2.1. Resource Allocation

Community allocation of resources affects population health through direct and indirect pathways. Directly, certain basic resources are necessary for the maintenance of body functions. Access to a sufficient quantity and quality of food is essential for proper nutrition. Malnutrition and undernutrition have severe consequences for growth and development of children (de Onis, Monteiro, Akre, & Glugston, 1993; Stevenson, Latham, & Ottesen, 2000; Weinreb et al., 2002), as well as for the functioning of the immune system and prevention of disease (Cunningham-Rundles, McNeeley, & Moon, 2005). Adequate nutrition requires either enough arable land for local food production or access to markets with imported food and income with which to purchase the food. Not only are the absolute quantities and costs of these resources in a community important, but the distribution of these resources also contributes to shaping health outcomes. For example, the availability and cost of fresh fruits and vegetables and the spatial patterns of supermarkets are strongly linked to the income and racial characteristics of neighborhoods in Detroit (Zenk et al., 2005; Zenk et al., 2006)

Similarly, the quantity and quality of a community's water supply is an important determinant of people's health (United Nations, 2005). Insufficient water sources may lead to insufficient food supplies due to lack of irrigation of crops. The economies of developing countries are highly dependent on agriculture, which generates 80% of export earnings; however, this important source of income requires almost 70% of the world's freshwater use (United Nations, 2005). In communities where potable water sources are far from residences, considerable time and energy is expended supplying households with water (Cosgrove & Rijsberman, 1998).

It has been estimated that 40 billion working hours are lost in Africa each year due to time spent transporting water, with the burden falling most heavily on women and children (United Nations, 2005). Poor quality water in conjunction with poor sanitation and hygiene is responsible for 1.6 million deaths per year due to diseases such as cholera, typhoid fever, trachoma, and schistosomiasis, to name a few (World Health Organization, 2004). Water can also be a source of toxicity. The well water consumed by 28–35 million Bangladeshi (United Nations, 2005) contains high levels of arsenic, causing skin lesions and various cancers (Smith, Lingas, & Rahman, 2000).

Shelter from the elements is another essential resource influenced by community-level factors. Good quality construction (Konradsen et al., 2003; Yé et al., 2006), and screened windows and doors (Lindsay, Emerson, & Charlwood, 2002) prevent spread of vector-born diseases such as malaria. Quality housing protects inhabitants from climate extremes (heat, cold, wet), which contribute to disease and mortality (Evans, Hyndman, Stewart-Brown, Smith, & Petersen, 2000; Gemmell, 2001; The Eurowinter Group, 1997). Insufficient physical space in a community may lead to overcrowded housing, which facilitates the spread of communicable diseases such as tuberculosis (Antunes & Waldman, 2001) and helminth infections (Carneiro, Cifuentes, Tellez-Rojo, & Romieu, 2002). Indoor air quality is another important characteristic of housing that can influence the risk of respiratory diseases (Bruce, Perez-Padilla, & Albalak, 2000).

In a similar manner, medications also are essential community resources. Insufficient or unreliable supplies of medications have serious health repercussions by contributing directly to morbidity and mortality as well as to drug resistance (Draper, Brubaker, Geser, Kilimali, & Wernsdorfer, 1985).

Aside from essential resources, communities also have differential access to goods that may be deleterious to health, such as tobacco, alcohol and narcotics. For example, neighborhoods in Baltimore, Maryland, comprised predominantly of African Americans have a higher density of alcohol distributing outlets than neighborhoods with different racial demographics (LaVeist & Wallace, 2000). Many other such directly detrimental social impacts exist at the community level.

Indirectly, the distribution, volatility, and cost of these resources in the community are likely to have effects on social interactions and behaviors which may shape population health (Gopalan, 2001). Food insecurity causes psychosocial stresses that are harmful to mental health and can increase susceptibility to other acute and chronic diseases (Weinreb et al., 2002). Residential crowding, resulting from limited access to housing or from prohibitory housing costs, also contributes to psychosocial stress in a community (Krieger & Higgins, 2002). Unequal access to basic resources such as food, water, housing and medical supplies may have repercussions for the entire community by decreasing social cohesion (Wakefield & Poland, 2005). Social cohesion and collective efficacy help to defend a community against crime and vandalism (Kawachi, Kennedy, Lochner, & Prothrow-Stith, 1997) and provide social resources that buffer the negative health effects of being resource deprived (Sampson, Raudenbush, & Earls, 1997) (see Section 2.4).

2.2. Social Services

Communities with local access to health care, emergency and security services, good educational opportunities and social support systems such as welfare and social security are more likely to have good health (Cheadle et al., 1991). Access to these social services increases opportunities to obtain necessary resources (discussed above) and provides a buffer against volatile economic situations. Important issues include presence of these services, physical proximity to communities, cost and distribution.

Mechanisms by which social services affect community health include the provision of basic human needs (e.g. food, shelter, medications) or the means by which people meet those needs (e.g. employment or supplementary income). For example, communities that lack access to good quality health services may have higher burdens of disease because sick individuals will delay seeking care or will turn to alternative options, such as traditional healers or self-treatment (Chen et al., 2004; Meerman et al., 2005). Delayed treatment can have serious health consequences. For example, Gambian children presenting with severe malaria were significantly more likely to have delayed seeking treatment by more than four days than were those presenting with mild malaria (Meerman et al., 2005). Furthermore, self-medication may encourage drug resistance, as has been observed with malaria (Evans et al., 2005). Because poor or nonexistent welfare services can lead to increased poverty, malnutrition, homelessness, and starvation (Marmot, 2002) as well as reduced access to good education, such services have long been considered a "fundamental" determinant of health (Adler & Newman, 2002; Adler & Ostrove, 1999; Link & Phelan, 1995). Education also may affect health by increasing knowledge of healthy behaviors and by increasing employment opportunities that provide income to meet basic health needs (Ross & Wu, 1995). Individuals with better education live longer and suffer less morbidity than do their more poorly educated counterparts (Bobak, Hertzman, Skodova, & Marmot, 1999; Hemingway, Shipley, Macfarlane, & Marmot, 2000; Lynch, Kaplan, Salonen, Cohen, & Salonen, 1995). Research by Winkleby and others (1992) revealed that even after controlling for the effects of income and occupation, education reduced risk of cardiovascular disease. Emergency services provide urgent care, which can lessen population morbidity and mortality. Security services such as fire fighting and policing help to deter crime and violence, which have serious implications for health. For example, the 1975 fiscal crisis in New York City led to a 20% reduction in the number of city police employees, which likely contributed to the homicide epidemic of the 1980s (Freudenberg, Fahs, Galea, & Greenberg, 2006).

2.3. Physical Environment

Environments have long been recognized to play an important role in population health, from the ancient Greek's association of malaria with swamps to the miasma theorists purporting that squalid living conditions caused illness. With the advent of germ theory and the advancement of modern epidemiologic methods and statistical tools, our understanding of relationships between environmental conditions and health outcomes has deepened. We now recognize that forces at many levels shape environments and associated diseases. Global climate patterns influence temperature, precipitation, and extreme weather events; accumulating evidence suggests that human behaviors, such as the expanding use of fossil fuels, are causing rapid changes in climate (Vitousek, Mooney, Lubchenco, & Melillo, 1997). Similarly, air and water pollution are affecting the quality of local, national and global environments and are shaped by human behaviors at each of these spatial/political scales. At the community level, environments are defined in part by physical conditions, which are affected by local, state or federal policies, such as zoning laws (Schilling & Linton, 2005), as well as by human behaviors and actions such as vandalism (Ross & Wu, 1995). The range of health indicators influenced by the built environment is vast and includes mental health (Weich et al., 2002), sexually transmitted infections (Cohen et al., 2000; Cohen, Mason et al., 2003), crime and violence (Newman, 1986; Sampson et al., 1997), substance abuse (Galea, Rudenstine et al., 2005), cardiovascular disease (Diez Roux, 2003) and physical activity (Frumkin, 2002), to name a few. Local environments, including homes and workplaces, may be sources of exposures to toxic substances, allergens or poor air quality (Bruce et al., 2000). Aspects of the outdoor environment are recognized as contributors to increased injury (Moore, Teixeira, & Shiell, 2006) or breeding of disease spreading vectors (McMichael et al., 1999; Moore, Gould, & Keary, 2002).

Community-level environmental characteristics and their potential health effects range in complexity and diversity. Climatic factors recently have drawn the attention of epidemiologists as measurement and analytic tools have improved. Greater climate extremes and global climate changes create or destroy microhabitats for many organisms that affect people's daily lives. Some changes may be beneficial, but most are expected to challenge efforts to improve health, particularly in developing countries. For example, insects that serve as vectors for various infectious diseases may become more abundant or widespread with global warming. One example is the possible increased range of malaria into previously uninfected highland regions (Bouma, Dye, & Van der Kaay, 1996; Loevinsohn, 1994; Zhou, Minakawa, Githeko, & Yan, 2004). Climate change, including extreme events, has been associated with other infectious diseases as well, such as cholera (Pascual, Rodo, Ellner, Colwell, & Bouma, 2000), cryptosporidiosis (Atherholt, LeChevallier, Norton, & Rosen, 1998), and other water-borne diseases (Curriero, Patz, Rose, & Lele, 2001).

Similarly, changes in precipitation and temperature may affect local agricultural yields, thereby affecting food availability with all of the accompanying health implications (Fischer, Shah , Tubiello, & van Velhuizen, 2005). As another example, temperature extremes may have direct effects on mortality, especially for poor, elderly or otherwise disadvantaged individuals. A heatwave in Chicago in July of 1995 resulted in 460 excess deaths that disproportionately affected African Americans and bed-ridden individuals (Semenza et al., 1996). In southern Chile, exposure to UV-B radiation due to the proximity to the Antarctic ozone hole has been linked to increased sunburn and photosensitivity (Abarca, Casiccia, & Zamorano, 2002), and increases in skin cancer rates have been predicted (Jones, 1987). Limiting outdoor activities might protect against these health risks, yet this may cause other morbidities, such as obesity and diabetes, due to decreased physical activity (Gracey, 2002; McMichael, 2000). Many health effects of the built environment are certainly mediated by forces of the social environment.

2.4. Social Environment

Environments are not only physical but are also social. Social environments shape our interactions, our beliefs and our behaviors, all of which have health effects. To complicate matters, social environments likely interact with physical environments in their relationships with population health.

Aspects of the social environment that are likely to influence human health include social disorganization, social resources (including support and capital), social contagion, spatial segregation and inequality. The theory of neighborhood social disorganization, arising from sociological research of urban Chicago in the 1940s, posits that social disorder is conducive to deviant behavior and crime (Shaw & McKay, 1942). This theory hypothesizes that social disorder originates from lack of social control, low density friendship networks, and lack of participation in local organizations (Sampson & Groves, 1989). More recent research has shown that communities with high social disorganization are more likely to suffer from violence, victimization and homicide (Sampson et al., 1997), as well as coronary heart disease (Sundquist et al., 2006). Social disorganization may arise from inequalities in levels of deprivation and lead to anomie, defined as strain caused by disparate levels of attainment within a community (Kawachi, Kennedy, & Wilkinson, 1999). Social strain not only encourages deviant behavior and crime (Agnew, 1992), but also has been shown to be associated with increased homicide and cardiovascular mortality (Cohen, Farley, & Mason, 2003). Social strain may also cause physiological stress responses, which have well established links with mental and physical health (Elliott, 2000; Latkin & Curry, 2003; Ross & Mirowsky, 2001).

Social resources, including social support and social capital, are recognized to provide better coping mechanisms for difficult situations and are therefore associated with better health (Kawachi & Berkman, 2001; McLeod & Kessler, 1990). Social capital is also likely to help buffer negative health effects of social disorder by providing economic and social support (Sampson et al., 1997). Negative associations have been found between social capital and mortality (Kawachi et al., 1997; Skrabski, Kopp, & Kawachi, 2004) and violent crime (Kennedy, Kawachi, Prothrow-Stith, Lochner, & Gupta, 1998) and positive associations between social capital and self-reported health (Subramanian, Kim, & Kawachi, 2002).

Social contagion, or social influence, is thought to affect health by the sharing of behaviors and attitudes among members of social networks, which can have both positive and negative health effects. These social norms are important in the transmission of infectious diseases, such as sexually-transmitted infections (STIs) and HIV (Pick & Obermeyer, 1996; Wellington, Ndowa, & Mbengeranwa, 1997), as well as in the spread of behaviors such as suicide (Phillips & Carstensen, 1986) and criminality (Jones & Jones, 1995).

2.5. Population Heterogeneity

The spatial distribution of racial and ethnic groups or groups of different socio-economic status may contribute to the determination of population health. From an economic viewpoint, segregation leads to homogeneity of resources, where those with low socio-economic position cannot access the resources that benefit more affluent individuals. Segregation by socio-demographic characteristics is known to accompany differential exposure to poor quality environments, including toxins, crime, violence, poverty and infectious diseases (Cohen, Mason et al., 2003). Poor, segregated populations have restricted access to health care services, shortages of health care providers and many under- or un-insured individuals (Mayberry, Mili, & Ofili, 2000). Finally, segregation and income inequality can cause both perceived and actual inequity, which erodes social trust and diminishes social capital with the resulting health effects as discussed above. This process may be enhanced by spatial proximity of the rich and the poor (Kaplan, Pamuk, Lynch, Cohen, & Balfour, 1996; Kawachi et al., 1997; Mayberry et al., 2000).

In contrast, spatial heterogeneity of socio-economic groups encourages diversity and allows an opportunity for resource sharing. Wealthier individuals may be encouraged to use their money and power to improve the access and distribution of resources needed for good health. This heterogeneity may also provide access to broader social networks, including positive role models and salubrious social norms. For example, unequal distribution of education in communities in New York City has been shown to have salutary effects for all residents, suggesting benefits of actions of highly educated individuals (Galea & Ahern, 2005). However, heterogeneous social environments may encourage social strain by providing images of unachievable aspirations to those with poor access to resources and few opportunities for advancement (Kawachi et al., 1999; Sampson & Groves, 1989).

3. National-Level Processes

A substantial amount of epidemiologic research has examined the role of globalization in shaping population health at the national level. Cross-national comparisons of health indicators have investigated the effects of national income (Dollar, 2001; Lynch, Smith, Kaplan, & House, 2000; Weisbrot et al., 2002), mode of governance (Navarro & Shi, 2001), and average educational attainment (Williamson & Boehmer, 1997), among others. We add to this body of literature by explicitly hypothesizing mechanisms through which aspects of nations may influence health and the extent to which this is mediated by the community-level determinants of health discussed above.

3.1. Infrastructural Resources

Availability of national resources and the distribution of those resources have great potential to influence population health. To the extent that money can finance infrastructural development, overall national income becomes an important element in this equation. National incomes are based on myriad factors, including exploitable natural resources, position in the global economy, import tax policies, and domestic tax policies. Income alone, however, does not equal infrastructure. National governments make choices about how income will be spent.

Explicit pathways through which national infrastructural resources may affect population health are many, making a thorough cataloguing beyond the scope of this chapter. We present a few examples for illustrative purposes.

Underinvestment in national health services can be manifest through scarce health clinics, hospitals or health providers, inadequate accessibility, or poor quality of available health services (Chen et al., 2004). Low salaries and unpleasant work conditions lead health providers in some low-income nations to migrate to better opportunities (Brown & Connell, 2004). Such "brain drain" compounds the negative health effects of underinvestment in health services by reducing the number of health providers, as well as the quality of available care (Brown & Connell, 2004; Chanda, 2001; World Health Organization, 2006). Some evidence exists that perceived poor quality of health services leads to underutilization of these services and increased use of alternative resources (Haddad & Fournier, 1995; Segall, 2000). Alternatives include traditional healers or self-medication, which may increase chances of inappropriate or insufficient treatment, possibly also encouraging drug resistance for certain pathogens (Evans et al., 2005).

Underinvestment in social resources at the national level is also an important predictor of population health (Davey Smith, 1996; Wagstaff, Bustreo, Bryce, & Claeson, 2004). Societies with a large proportion of uninsured or underinsured individuals who cannot afford health care costs are at risk for sustained transmission of communicable diseases as well as high burdens of disability due to untreated chronic diseases (Hadley, 2003; Institute of Medicine, 2002). A lack of support for people who are unemployed, unable to work, or underpaid increases poverty levels. Poverty is recognized as an important determinant of population health through a vast array of mechanisms, including increased susceptibility to disease due to poor nutrition (Wagstaff et al., 2004) and incomplete vaccination (Klevens & Luman, 2001), increased contact with disease-causing agents due to unhealthy environments and crowding, and prolonged duration of disease due to lack of appropriate treatment (Wagstaff et al., 2004).

Finally, underinvestment in environmental infrastructure, including roads, the built environment, water and sewage systems, and electricity, also holds great potential to reduce population health. For example, unpaved roads on a Native American reservation in New Mexico were shown to discourage timely access to health services in children with meningitis (Williams, 1987). Lack of potable water and sewage and waste disposal facilitates the spread of infectious diseases

(World Health Organization, 2004) and increases the stress and physical strain for families (especially women and children) who must transport water long distances to their homes (Cosgrove & Rijsberman, 1998; United Nations, 2005). Additionally, poor water quality and inadequate sewage infrastructure may create breeding sites for vectors that transport infectious disease agents (Keating et al., 2003).

3.2. Employment

The availability and nature of employment opportunities at the national level have been shown to affect population health, especially overall mortality (Gerdtham & Johannesson, 2005) and suicides (Dooley, Fielding, & Levi, 1996). National employment trends may be examined by several characteristics. Most commonly, unemployment rates are reported as an indication of the percentage of a nation's population that is unwillingly jobless. Another important element of employment is salary, with information coming from both minimum wages mandated by national law and the range and distribution of salaries in the country. Additionally, the permanence or reliability of employment and the type of job and associated work conditions are national employment trends that shape population health.

Unemployment, underemployment and nonstandard employment affect population health through several mechanisms. First, joblessness usually accompanies loss of income, which limits the purchase or attainment of necessary resources. Unemployment or part-time or seasonal employment may lead to loss of medical insurance to cover disease prevention and treatment (Ostry & Spiegel, 2004). Another important mechanism by which unemployment affects health is by elevating acute stress or creating situations of chronic stress. A large body of literature on the health effects of threatened job loss in factory workers reveals many negative outcomes, such as elevated blood pressure, increased depression and anxiety (Cobb & Kasl, 1977; Ostry & Spiegel, 2004), or diminished mental health and increased stress (Hamilton, Broman, Hoffman, & Renner, 1990). A Danish study conducted on bus drivers with restructured and contracted out jobs (less stability) found high levels of urinary cortisol and elevated blood pressure (Netterstrom & Hansen, 2000). Non-standard work (part-time, contingent) may also increase risk of stress and workplace injury (Quinlan, Mayhew, & Bohle, 2001). A complete review of the health effects of stress is beyond the scope of this paper, but it includes reduced immunity to infectious diseases (Cohen, Tyrrell, & Smith, 1991; Takkouche, Regueira, & Gestal-Otero, 2001), increased adoption of unhealthy behaviors (smoking, drinking, etc.) (Adler & Newman, 2002) and increased susceptibility to inflammatory diseases (Korte, Koolhaas, Wingfield, & McEwen, 2005; McEwen & Seeman, 1999).

Even reliable employment with livable wages may affect population health through the nature of the work and the work environment. Poor work environments place workers at risk for injury, respiratory disease, exposure to toxins and infectious agents (Loewenson, 2001). For example, in African countries annual injury rates for occupations such as mining, forestry and transport all exceed

30 injuries per 1000 workers (Loewenson, 1998). The risk for such negative health outcomes at the national level depends greatly on the nature of available jobs. Current global trends concentrate the risks of poor quality work environments and insecure, low paying, low quality jobs in less industrialized countries (Loewenson, 2001). Women are disproportionately affected by these trends, which compound the health affects of the social and economic marginalization that they experience. A clear example is female employment in export processing zones. These jobs provide low wages, exposure to toxic chemicals and substances, long work hours, physical brutality and psychological stress (Hippert, 2002; Loewenson, 2001). The health effects of child labor are also important. An estimated 211 million children under the age of 14 and 352 million under the age of 17 are part of the worldwide workforce, most in developing countries (Habenicht, 1994; International Program on the Elimination of Child Labor, 2002). Child labor detracts from the benefits of education and has been shown to be associated with stunting and wasting (Hawamdeh & Spencer, 2003).

3.3. Income Growth

National income growth is generally assumed to be beneficial for population health (Marmot, 2002). More income means more resources that can be used to meet the health needs of the population. In reality, the association between national income growth and health is much more complex and depends on a wide array of contextual factors. The important factors likely include fiscal and regulatory policies, level of dependence on imports and exports, level of indebtedness and loan stipulations, and baseline income level as well as the distribution of the income (Ayala-Carcedo & Gonzalez-Barros, 2005). Considerable economic literature on globalization argues that opening economies to the global market stimulates economic growth, which, in turn, reduces poverty (Dollar & Kraay, 2002; Frankel & Romer, 1999). Assuming that poverty reduction is good for health, it logically follows that opening national economies will lead to healthier nations. There are several problems with this argument. First, it is controversial whether opening economies to the global market promotes national income growth (Cornia, 2001). Support for this hypothesis is informed by Dollar and Kraay's (2002) findings. Their work relies heavily on data from India and China, presumably because those countries represent such a large percentage of the world's population; however, the experiences of Indian and Chinese economies post-trade liberalization are not necessarily representative of all nations. Second, population health indicators seem to be more sensitive to changes in national incomes with lower baselines (Marmot & Wilkinson, 2001). Globalization's effect on income inequalities at both the global and national levels has been hotly debated (Lynch et al., 2004; Subramanian & Kawachi, 2004; Wilkinson & Pickett, 2006) as has the relative importance of income inequality versus income growth on health outcomes (Lynch et al., 2000; Ross & Mirowsky, 2001). While readers can draw their own conclusions in this debate, we present several mechanisms by which national income growth may influence population health.

Income growth provides government revenues and other societal resources needed to supply goods and services (Dodgson, Lee, & Drager, 2002; Diaz-Bonilla, Babinard, & Pinstrup-Andersen, 2002). Income growth may stimulate national labor markets, thereby providing more jobs for the population. Dependable employment with livable wages provides means for people to purchase necessary resources such as food and health care (Collins, 2003). Being securely employed also encourages feelings of self-worth and increases social cohesion (Sen, 1997). However, if national income growth is based on volatile economies, employment may be insecure and layoffs unexpected (Sen, 1997). Various potential health effects of job insecurity were described in Section 3.2. Another result of volatile income growth is sudden unexpected reductions in household wealth, which may result in children leaving school to join the workforce and sometimes engaging in high risk jobs such as prostitution (Cornia, 2001). Sudden decline in wealth may also compromise health by reducing quantity and quality of nutrition (Cornia, 2001).

3.4. Population Density

Population density has long been associated with population health. Historic studies of environmental determinants of disease in urban settings during the era of industrialization in Europe comprise the backbone of modern social epidemiologic science. Conditions during that era, including rapid industrial development, the breakdown of traditional social and ideological structures, and urban blight followed by suburban flight of the wealthy, led to concentrated poverty, crowding, death and disease in many urban settings (McMichael, 2000; Szreter, 1997). Although these trends may be less relevant for societies in Western Europe and other developed nations today, they are reality for nations in the developing world. Population density is rising in many parts of the world due to rural-to-urban migration (urbanization) and population growth (McMichael, 2000). People searching for economic opportunities, employment and a better standard of living, combined with destruction of habitats in rural areas, are among the plethora of reasons for migration to cities in the developing world (see Section 4.3). By 2007 it is estimated that over half of the world's population will live in urban settings, contrasted with only 5% at the beginning of the 19th century (United Nations Department of Economic and Social Affairs, 2003). The proportion of urban dwellers is expected to grow to 60% by 2030 (United Nations Department of Economic and Social Affairs, 2003). Additionally, the size of urban populations is continuing to expand. From 1940 to the present, the number of "megacities" with more than 10 million inhabitants rose from one (New York City) to fifteen (Satterthwaite, 2000).

Among urban residents, crowding may occur due to poverty or lack of habitable physical space. Evidence suggests that population density may predict many health effects, including infectious diseases such as tuberculosis (Antunes & Waldman, 2001) and acute respiratory infection (Lee, Jordan, Sanchez, & Gaydos, 2005), chronic diseases such as stomach cancer (Barker,

Coggon, Osmond, & Wickham, 1990), and poor mental health (Lepore, Evans, & Palsane, 1991). In addition, people living in dense populations experience higher rates of violent death (Wallace & Wallace, 1998) and injury (LaScala, Gerber, & Gruenewald, 2000) than do less dense populations.

Illuminating the mechanisms through which increased population density may affect population health is more challenging than showing an association exists. Perhaps the most intuitive relationship to discuss is that between population density and risk of infectious disease. High population density means that individuals will have a greater number of contacts with others. Contact rates are an essential parameter in the risk of infectious disease transmission, particularly for those diseases with person-to-person modes of transmission (Anderson & May, 1991). A higher contact rate generally corresponds to more transmission, all other factors being equal. Therefore, areas with high population densities are more conducive to disease spread. In addition, populations living in crowded conditions are also often those with the fewest resources (Baum, Garofalo, & Yali, 1999). Crowding in situations of poor sanitation increases the spread of infectious disease through increased risk of exposure to infectious agents in the environment (Krieger & Higgins, 2002). These factors contribute to the ongoing cholera pandemic, especially, for example, in areas such as the peri-urban slums of Brazil (Nations & Monte, 1996). Similar concerns appear in other parts of the world, such as Russia, where overcrowded prisons and insufficient public health measures contribute to multi-drug resistant tuberculosis (TB) (Holden, 1999). In Saudi Arabia, Muslim pilgrims gather annually during the Hajj, increasing risks of meningococcal outbreaks, hemorrhagic fever and even SARS (Ahmed, Arabi, & Memish, 2006), and in Palestinian refugee camps in the Gaza strip, crowding and poor sanitation contribute to intestinal parasites and diarrheal diseases (Abu Morad, 2004). Where dense populations coexist in poverty and inadequate infrastructure, environments may also increase the risk of vector-borne diseases by increasing contact with vector breeding sites (Afrane et al., 2004; McMichael, 2000).

Urban settings have been linked to high rates of certain chronic diseases, including cardiovascular disease and type II diabetes (Diez Roux, 2003; McMichael, 2000). These associations might be explained in part by aspects of the built environment that allow easier access to energy-dense foods and a decline in physical activity (Handy, Boarnet, Ewing, & Killingsworth, 2002). Concentration of cars, trucks, and buses in densely populated areas elevates noxious emissions exposure. Urban traffic is therefore linked to increased risk of respiratory disease (McMichael, 2000), not to mention the risk of transportation related accidents (LaScala et al., 2000). Furthermore, dense populations tend to have higher rates of suicides, violent crimes, drug use and mental diseases due to social tension, competition for resources, lack of social cohesion or psychosocial stress (Galea & Vlahov, 2005). Stress is also a risk factor for many chronic conditions such as atherosclerosis and depression (McEwen, 2004) and is associated with lowered immune response, making it a risk factor for infectious disease as well (McEwen & Seeman, 1999).

3.5. Governance and Policies

National policies may include health policies as well as other legislation affecting the social and environmental domains of society. National health policies dictate to what extent national governments have control over and responsibility for providing health services to the population. Some countries support a nationalized system of health care whereby the government both pays for and provides health services. Other nations have privatized health care such that individuals are responsible for meeting their health care needs through the private market. Even nations with privatized health care usually subsidize the costs of such services for certain members of the population (the elderly or poor) as in the Medicare and Medicaid programs of the US.

Other aspects of health policy important for population health include economic decisions about resource allocation. Governments may decide to invest in the development of primary care and disease prevention services to maximize cost-benefit indices, or tertiary care and treatment may be prioritized for fund distribution. Judgments must also be made about investment in research and development of medications, technologies and vaccines. Resource allocation decisions about health services relative to other national services are necessary. These decisions are political and vary greatly by nation and ideologies (Coburn, 2004). They are likely to influence health by determining what kinds of services are available, how accessible and affordable they are and what sectors of the population have access (Mehrotra, 2006). National policies regarding other domains of public life, including welfare, education, social security, subsidized housing, and employment, are also likely to play an important role in determining both quality of population health, as well as distribution of health outcomes in the population (Marmot, 2002). Finally, political ideologies at the national level have been hypothesized to influence health by differential support of welfare policies and recognition of and attention to the needs of the population (Franco, Alvarez-Dardet, & Ruiz, 2004). For example, a recent study found a link among good governance measured by accountability, political stability, absence of violence, government effectiveness, regulatory quality, rule of law and the control of corruption and national HIV prevalence (Menon-Johansson, 2005; Widdus, 2005)

Economic decisions regarding resource allocation and distribution are likely to influence population health through various pathways with resounding health effects. For example, Freudenberg and colleagues (2006) describe the impact of city, state and federal budget cuts on a TB/HIV/homicide combined epidemic in New York City during the 1980s and 1990s, which they term a "syndemic". These authors argue that budget cuts undermined the ability of city health and social service infrastructures to respond to health emergencies and emerging health threats; reduced education, policing and drug treatment services; and amplified social trends. These factors then contributed to increased risk of violence and disease in the population. Other authors have posited that national policies influence health through the mechanisms of social capital, empowerment and access to information, which are differentially accorded to populations living under different political economic systems (Franco et al., 2004). Perhaps most relevant to globalization and health are arguments delineating relationships between government policies shaped by capitalist ideology and health outcomes mediated by increasing income inequalities and lowered social cohesion (Coburn, 2000; Muntaner & Lynch, 1999). National governance therefore affects population health both through national-level and community-level pathways.

4. Global-Level Processes

Epidemiologic research on the health effects of global-level factors is inadequate. We consider global-level factors to involve the processes of globalization that extend beyond national borders (outlined in Section 1.1). Understanding the differential effects of national-level factors on health in the global system will enhance opportunities for effective health interventions through a focus on global-level structural changes to achieve sustainable improvements in health.

4.1. Global Trade

One important component of globalization is increased trade in goods and services both between and within nations. Exchanges of goods and services shape nations' economies through imports and exports and levied taxes. In effect, trade serves to redistribute commodities and wealth throughout the world, and it is the patterning of this redistribution and its associations with health that interests us. Some global health researchers seek to determine whether trade and increased access to material resources leads to more equitable redistribution of wealth or to a concentration of wealth in the hands of a few.

The nature of the dynamic global exchange of resources is likely to be affected by enduring conditions such as geographical location, location of exploitable natural resources, and history of past interactions in the global market (Gallup, Sachs, & Mellinger, 1999; Moore et al., 2006). For example, Moore et al. (2006) found that tropical and landlocked countries were more likely to have higher infant mortality rates than were other countries even after adjusting for the position of the country in the world system. Increasingly, nations are becoming dependent on the global economy and on trade with others for the well being and survival of their citizens.

Increased trade provides an opportunity for the exchange of both essential, salubrious resources and those that may be deleterious for health. Commerce in essential goods, such as food, improves access to good nutrition in areas of the world with poor quality agricultural land or short growing seasons (Hawkes, 2006; Shetty, 2006). Trade in medicinal products such as vaccines and pharmaceuticals helps to protect the quality and duration of life in areas of the world without the technological or industrial capabilities to produce their own supplies (World Health Organization, 2004; Widdus, 2005). Exchanges in services such as health care and education also provide opportunities to improve population health in disadvantaged nations (Bettcher, Yach, & Guindon, 2000; Widdus, 2005). However, expanding markets have also provided a venue for the dissemination of goods that are deleterious to health such as tobacco, illegal drugs and weapons (Huynen et al., 2005; McMichael & Beaglehole, 2000; Yach & Bettcher, 2000). In addition, global trade creates an opportunity for contaminated products or infectious agents to cause widespread illness, facilitating the speed and distance of disease outbreaks. For example, the transportation of *Aedes aegypti* mosquito eggs in used tires being shipped across the oceans led to the rapid expansion of dengue virus infections worldwide (McMichael, 2000). Indeed, a multitude of food-borne pathogens are transported globally each year; for example, *Cyclospora cayetanensis* in raspberries imported to the US caused an outbreak of diarrheal disease in 1996 (Centers for Disease Control and Prevention (CDC), 1996).

The dynamics of global trade are complex and influence health at the same time that they are influenced by national-level and community-level factors. For example, increased global trade does not ensure even distribution of commerce throughout the world (Subramanian, Belli, & Kawachi, 2002). Some countries may be denied access to the world market due to national-level factors such as governance, lack of marketable products or lack of income with which to purchase commodities (Ayala-Carcedo & Gonzalez-Barros, 2005). These countries are unlikely to experience the health benefits of increased global trade. Minimal access to the global market may also affect population health by restricting the growth of national economies, which in turn limits funds available for infrastructure development and health services at the community level. Limited national funds for health workers salaries also contributes to poor population health as doctors, nurses, teachers, and other skilled workers emigrate in search of better opportunities, thereby depriving communities of quality health services (Brown & Connell, 2004; World Health Organization, 2006). Even countries experiencing positive income growth due to trade activities on the global market may experience poor population health outcomes if the money is not used to provide necessary social services or infrastructure development. Additionally, unequal distribution of resources at the community level may contribute to deterioration of the physical and social environments, which has deleterious health effects as previously discussed (see Sections 2.3 and 2.4).

4.2. Income Distribution

Unequal distribution of goods and services contributes to unbalanced global trade as well as to income inequalities among nations. Why do we care about the distribution of wealth? We know that on an individual level rising income leads to better nutrition, lower child mortality, and better maternal health (Filmer & Pritchett, 1999; Pritchett & Summers, 1996). Whether this relationship between income and health holds at the population level is less clear. Some economists argue that nations with more open trade policies experience more rapid income growth, which leads directly to better population health (Dollar, 2001; Dollar & Kraay, 2002). Others provide evidence that increased global integration leads to increasing inequality both in wealth and in health and both within and between nations

(Coburn, 2000; Lynch et al., 2004; Wilkinson & Pickett, 2006). The debate on income inequality and its potential health effects is multifaceted. Does globalization encourage increasing income inequality, and if so, is this inequality within nations, between nations or both? Is income inequality bad for population health? What are the mediating factors of the income inequality-population health relationship?

Global income distribution may shape population health through its influence on global, national, and community level factors. At the global level, rising income inequality encourages migration and fosters conflict (Wade, 2004). Coburn (2000) hypothesizes that neo-liberal economic policies affect health by encouraging intra-national income inequality and decreased social cohesion. At the national level, unequal global income distribution provides differential access to necessary goods and services (Baum, 2001). These goods and services help to determine national income which affects community-level access to resources necessary for good health through providing the means for infrastructural development, provision of social services, and provision of employment opportunities. Differential global income distribution therefore affects the local distribution of health resources. Sizeable income inequality also suppresses income growth at the national level (Cornia, 2001) and reduces the rate of poverty alleviation (Ravillion, 2001).

The health effects of global income inequality may be moderated or mediated by national-level characteristics, such as national policies and type of governance. For example, Navarro and Shi (2001) found that countries with predominantly social democratic government traditions between 1945 and 1980 experienced more economic growth, lower levels of income inequality and unemployment, and lower infant mortality rates than did countries with liberal or fascist government traditions. Community-level characteristics may act as mediators of the health effects of income distribution as well. For example, poor communities in nations with high income inequality may experience reduced social cohesion and the associated health effects due to a lack of employment opportunities and higher poverty (Wade, 2004).

4.3. Population Movement

Population movement is another important component of globalization with significant health implications. Improvements in transportation technology in the past century have drastically amplified the speed and distance of human travel (Smolinski et al., 2003). Ease of travel, both domestically and internationally, has lead to an unprecedented magnitude of travelers both for business and for tourism (World Trade Organization, 2005). Yet any economic benefits must be evaluated in the context of increased transport and transmission of infectious diseases (Wilson, 2003). Migration is another reason for international and domestic travel. Motivations for migration are diverse and include search for better economic situations, flight from violent conflict or repressive government, and pursuance of educational opportunities, to name a few. Rural to urban migration, also known as urbanization, is an increasingly important phenomenon in the consideration of determinants of population health (Galea, Freudenberg et al., 2005; McMichael, 2000). The driving factors behind trends in population movement also change population demographics. For example, in developing countries, rural villages are aging due to the rural-urban migration of youth looking for work in the cities (Stloukal, 2001). In many villages in Southern Africa, men leave to work in the mines (Quinn, 1994), altering the male to female ratio in the communities. In Mexico and Asia it is women who leave the home to work in the export processing zones (Hippert, 2002).

Mobility of human populations has the potential to affect health through a variety of mechanisms. At the global level, population movement facilitates spread of culture and technology, which can be beneficial for population health by expanding health knowledge and encouraging healthy behaviors (Frenk, 2005). However, the globalization of culture has been seen as "Westernization" or "Americanization", which threatens other ways of life and can sometimes lead to conflict (Frenk, Sepulveda, Gomez-Dantes, McGuinness, & Knaul, 1997; Holton, 2000).

The effects of global population movement on population health may be mediated by national factors. Take, for example, the enhanced spread of infectious diseases facilitated by novel patterns of human to human contact, as well as by changing eco-social environments (McMichael, 2000). The magnitude of morbidity and mortality due to increased infectious disease spread is likely to depend on national capacity to respond to disease outbreaks, which is a function of income, infrastructure and health knowledge and resources. The recent SARS pandemic provides an appropriate opportunity for comparison of population health outcomes for affected nations with different mediating characteristics. We might compare the SARS mortality rates in Canada, China and Singapore as a function of national infrastructure or of per capita income. Community-level effects of the spread of infectious diseases due to increased population movement are demonstrated by the SARS outbreak in Toronto, Canada. The social environment of the city was affected by the psychosocial effects of fear and local resources were disrupted by the economic effects of isolation and quarantine (Gupta, Moyer, & Stern, 2005; Hawryluck et al., 2002).

Another example of population health effects of human mobility involves the dynamics of population flows. At the global level, population movement is increasing, but this movement is not uniform among nations or regions of the world. The classic example is that of "brain drain", in which highly educated or skilled individuals from poor countries are recruited for employment in more wealthy nations. This differential migration exacerbates national and community-level problems of poor education, poor access to health services, and poor quality health services in the neediest regions of the world (Brown & Connell, 2004; World Health Organization, 2006). At the national level, changing demographics associated with mobile populations include rapid urbanization, especially in the developing world (Galea & Vlahov, 2005; McMichael, 2000; Moore et al., 2006). This phenomenon, coupled with high fertility rates, threatens population health by increasing pressures on limited national and community resources (McMichael, 2000).

At the community level, the physical environment is affected; poor urban infrastructure fails to provide potable water and sewage facilities to these burgeoning populations, resulting in increased disease burdens (McMichael, 2000). Local conflicts may also arise from competition over limited food or arable land. Psychosocial stress resulting from high population densities and difficult living conditions may also seriously influence community health outcomes (McEwen & Seeman, 1999).

4.4. Global Governance

All the aforementioned components of globalization are affected, to some extent, by the nature and extent of global governance. Governance is defined by Dodgson et al. (2002) as "the actions and means adopted by a society to promote collective action and deliver collective solutions in pursuit of common goals," and has typically been conceptualized at local and national levels. As trends of globalization change our delineation of societies, the concept of governance must take on a new dimension: Increasingly globalized societies need governance on a global scale.

Pursuit of global governance is challenging due to the historical precedent of national sovereignty, the right of each nation to govern its citizens. Reorganizing governmental hierarchies and establishing common goals for the entirety of the world's people is not an easy task. Some forms of governance do exist on a global scale, however. The World Trade Organization (WTO) has developed trade agreements that guide exchanges in goods and services among nations (Kinnon, 1998). Two examples include the Agreement on Trade-Related Aspects of Intellectual Property Rights (TRIPS) and the General Agreement on Trade in Services (GATS). TRIPS establishes minimum standards of protection of intellectual property, thereby safeguarding industrially applicable inventions, such as pharmaceuticals, under patent laws. GATS regulates trade in health services. The World Health Organization (WHO) also governs global health through the legally binding International Health Regulations. These regulations aim to reduce global disease spread with minimal trade interference.

Before discussing the mechanisms through which global governance affects population health, we must mention one key caveat. It is questionable to what extent governance has truly globalized despite the existence of international organizations such as the WTO and the WHO. These organizations are charged with defending the trade interests and health interests, respectively, of member states. However, not all nations are members of these organizations despite the fact that all nations share trans-border health risks. Additionally, member states do not all have equal representation in these organizations. Many poor countries cannot pay the fees needed to send representatives to meetings (Bowman, 2004).

Mechanisms by which trends in global governance affect population health are many and varied. At the global level, international policies regulate trade in goods. As this partially predicts income distribution, governance, trade, and income are closely intertwined. At the national level, income mediates the effect of global governance on population health. A classic example is the debate over generic pharmaceutical production in developing countries that arose over the need for antiretroviral (ARV) medication for HIV. Under the TRIPS agreement created by the WTO, the production of patented medications was prohibited at the global level. The result was that national access to expensive medications was determined by national income; rich countries could afford to buy life-saving medication for their populations and poor countries could not. To pursue this example to the community level, countries with enough income to purchase limited supplies of ARVs might offer better health outcomes to high income communities that could afford the high prices. Alternatively, these nations might choose other distribution criteria, offering the medications to government employees or to those seeking care at a certain health facility. It is easy to understand how, in a community with high HIV prevalence, differential access to ARVs might erode social cohesion and trust (Bennett & Chanfreau, 2005). High medication prices may also divert resources from other necessities, such as food and school fees, producing resounding population health effects.

Two other potential mechanisms are worth noting. An addition of a global dimension to governance of health issues may be counterproductive, undermining the authority and the ability of national governments to protect the health of their citizens (Collins, 2003). This argument can similarly be made for all neo-liberal trade policies in that the tenets of economic globalization, including decentralization, may lead to disempowered national governments (Coburn, 2000; Navarro & Shi, 2001). Finally, in the current era of globalization, an increasing number of non-state actors (e.g., NGOs, private corporations, religious organizations) may influence health governance, thereby eroding national resources for addressing health issues (Dodgson et al., 2002). Despite the increasing influences of these non-state actors in health decisions, the WHO focuses its efforts on working with Ministries of Health of sovereign member states. Neglecting to bring NGOs and private sector actors into negotiations results in a lost opportunity for valuable input (Dodgson et al., 2002).

4.5. Communications and Technology

Global communications include radio, telephone, television, and media in general, as well as the internet. The scope of global communications is enormous; in 2004 over 30 minutes per person were spent on international telephone calls worldwide, and 69% of the world's population was covered by mobile telephony (World Bank, 2006). In addition, the number of global internet users increased by 189% from 2000 to 2005, with more than one billion people now having access (Internet World Stats, 2006).

Enhanced global communications affects population health through the dispersion of ideas, information, knowledge and technologies. Telephone networks provide avenues for emergency communications and foster social connections between friends and families (Berkman, Glass, Brissette, & Seeman, 2000).

The internet provides opportunities for education and information sharing, which can lead to healthier behaviors and, perhaps, more informed and effective health interventions (Frenk, 2005). Nations and communities can use the internet to store and communicate health data and statistics, allowing more targeted and efficient use of resources (Frenk, 2005). Global media also may influence population health by informing individuals, communities and nations about global issues that may have local impacts and allowing an opportunity for prevention or intervention. Media coverage of global events allows collective awareness of political, social and ecologic realities across the world. Global media also presents the potential for views and ideologies of powerful people or groups to dominate and skew the objectivity of reporting of events of global importance.

Despite the rapid growth in global information technologies in recent years, some evidence exists that the gap in access to these technologies is widening, particularly between rich and poor nations as well as between rural and urban areas within nations (Arnett, 2002; United Nations Development Programme, 2001). This suggests that the relationship between global communications and population health may be mediated by various national and community level factors. We might consider the mediating effect of culture, for example. Research by Holton (2000) examines three cultural responses to the global information influx: homogenization, polarization and hybridization. Homogenization occurs when a local culture merges with global culture, a phenomenon sometimes called "Coca-Colonization" or "McDonaldization". This may result in adoption of poor health behaviors, such as smoking and drinking alcohol, as well as healthy behaviors, such as increased hand washing. Polarization consists of diametrically opposed cultural groups that create conflict and brew hatred for one another. In that such hatred ends in war or ethnic cleansing, the negative health implications are obvious. Finally, global communications may also lead to the formation of hybridized cultures, which incorporate elements from a variety of cultural sources. The health effects of hybridization of culture may be beneficial if it leads to enhanced understanding and cooperation among different local cultures. Some evidence exists to support the "politics of difference" theory, whereby group members become empowered by drawing upon identities and beliefs that are counter-hegemonic (Williams, Labonte, & O'Brien, 2003). This empowerment may provide enhanced collective actions of communities to seek healthier environments and encourage healthier behaviors. In contrast, some individuals in a culture may resist hybridization while others support it, creating inter-group conflict and a dissolution of social trust and cohesion. One example involves intergenerational differences in responses to global media in Japan (Arnett, 2002). Attempts have been made to mathematically model the dynamic between global processes, such as population density, and the maintenance of cultural identities in order to quantify the potential for homogenization, polarization or hybridization of cultures (Hochberg, 2004). However, few have investigated how these cultural adaptations affect health outcomes, suggesting that much more research is needed.

5. Example Mechanisms

Here we present three specific examples to illustrate mechanisms through which global factors exert influences on population health. Consider that these pathways are likely to be highly complex and multidirectional and aspects of national- and community-level environments may mediate or modulate the effects of global factors on health. In addition, one global factor may influence health outcomes via multiple pathways. We present simplified examples, which serve to highlight the logistical and methodological challenges, as well as the importance of including the global context in epidemiologic population health research.

5.1. Diarrheal Mortality Rates

A common theme presented in this chapter is the health importance of access to clean water. We may use community mortality rates due to diarrheal disease caused by unclean water sources to examine how population movement may influence one particular health indicator. In order to understand the causes of high rates of deaths due to diarrhea in a community we have to consider community-level factors that have been shown to be important predictors, such as the age distribution of the population, local environmental conditions (sanitation), breast-feeding practices, malnutrition, personal hygiene and access to medical supplies and services (such as oral rehydration solutions, ORS) (Feachem, 1984; Kosek, Bern, & Guerrant, 2003; VanDerslice, Popkin, & Briscoe, 1994). Limiting our study to community-level factors may be misleading, however. By including national-level variables, we might find that although community hygiene practices significantly predict diarrheal mortality rates at the community level, when we take national population densities into account, hygiene practices are no longer predictive. This might be because personal hygiene is associated with protection from infectious diarrhea-causing agents in countries with low population densities where these behaviors are mostly sufficient to protect against disease. In highly populated countries these behaviors may not be sufficient to provide protection (maybe due to high contact rates with the infectious agents). For example, high regional population densities have been found to be associated with greater child mortality rates in Zimbabwe (Root, 1997) and to be predictive of cholera outbreaks in Bangladesh (Myaux, Ali, Felsenstein, Chakraborty, & de Francisco, 1997). Global factors may be essential in understanding and predicting the pathway between national population densities, community hygiene and population diarrheal mortality rates. National population densities may be highly dependent on global migration patterns and not just on domestic fertility rates as is the case in the United States, France and Germany (Cohen, 2003). This example demonstrates how our understanding of the underlying causality of health outcomes is improved by widening the scope of study to include the global context.

5.2. Maternal Mortality Rates

Maternal mortality rates are one of the few standard measures of health used to compare health conditions across nations or regions. We argue that in order to study the factors that contribute to high maternal mortality rates it is important to investigate community-, national- and global-level conditions. For example, at the community level, past research has shown that maternal anemia, poor health care and lack of skilled birth attendants predict high maternal mortality (Rush, 2000). These factors are likely to be influenced by national-level factors such as infrastructural resources available for health services. Evidence for this surfaces from a study in which maternal mortality rates were shown to be negatively correlated with national health expenditures (Betran, Wojdyla, Posner, & Gulmezoglu, 2005). The relationship between national health spending and maternal mortality rates may in turn be determined by global level factors such as integration into the global market. According to a report by Global Health Watch (2005), "many macro-economic factors that help to keep poor countries poor, by extension, keep levels of health care expenditure low." For example, for many developing countries well integrated in the global economy the 1979–1981 global increase in oil prices led to financial crises due to reduced trade revenues and greatly inflated debt service payments (Global Health Watch, 2005). Maternal mortality rates are therefore likely to be determined not only by local or national conditions, but also by global factors.

5.3. Severe Acute Respiratory Syndrome

One final example that illustrates the importance of global-level health determinants in studies of population health is the recent severe acute respiratory syndrome (SARS) pandemic that menaced the globe in 2002–2003. In examining the causal factors related to the SARS outbreak, community-level determinants have been shown to be crucial in the emergence of the disease in human populations. Some key factors that have been identified with SARS are densely populated communities and close, repeated contact with wild animals, especially palm civets (*Paguna* larvata) and raccoon dogs (*Nyctereutes procuyoinboides*) (Breiman et al., 2003; Poon, Guan, Nicholls, Yuen, & Peiris, 2004; Webster, 2004). On a national level, China's deficiencies in health infrastructure allowed the emergence and continued spread of the disease without appropriate response measures (Liu, 2004). In contrast, Singapore rapidly introduced strict infection control measures resulting in low numbers of secondary cases (World Health Organization, 2003). This illustrates how national infrastructures and health policies can influence disease spread at the community level. At the global level, intercontinental travel facilitated disease spread (World Health Organization, 2003), whereas the existence of global health infrastructures and global communication networks allowed enhanced information exchange and rapid implementation of appropriate control and prevention measures worldwide (Fidler, 2004; Heymann, 2004). SARS provides a recent and fitting example of how global factors influence health at local levels and illustrates the importance of global perspectives in preserving population health.

As these examples illustrate, asking questions about the global context of causal pathways leading to health and disease deepens our understanding of the eco-social mechanisms responsible and allows for more opportunities to intervene.

6. Future Research

The pathways through which community-, national- and global-level factors affect population health that are presented in our conceptual model and discussed above are far from exhaustive. Nevertheless, these examples are illustrative of the importance of context in public health research. We argue that the global context, hitherto largely overlooked in epidemiologic studies, is essential for fully understanding the determination of population health. Indeed, inclusion of global-level factors in epidemiologic analyses may reveal complexity of relationships between more proximal-level factors and health indicators that were previously thought to be simple and well characterized.

Clarification of research goals is of paramount importance in developing epidemiologic investigation of population health determinants in a global context. First, there is a need for identification of gaps in currently existing knowledge. We have presented some examples as illustration, but a more systematic examination of the literature should be undertaken. Second, research needs to focus on hypothesizing and testing specific pathways through which global factors affect health. The results of such analysis will enable policy makers to prioritize areas of intervention and to restructure inefficient or ineffective policies. Furthering this research will ultimately require enhanced multidisciplinary collaboration, as changes are likely to be needed not only in health policy, but in economic, social, and ecologic domains as well.

Achieving these research goals is challenging due to methodological limitations. For example, the measurement of key global-level constructs is complicated by the scale and the lack of precedent. Unstandardized measurements draw into question the comparability of results across studies. Additionally, the data collection methods and the data themselves vary in accuracy and completeness among different countries. Data quality depends on available resources and training of data collectors, as well as on logistical obstacles to data collection. All these factors are likely to vary by country or region of the world. Finally, the individuals and the institutions funding research influence what data are collected and how they are measured, which may affect the results and policy recommendations that follow. This is an issue of concern in studies of global contexts since the number of players is small and largely limited to international organizations with political agendas, such as the World Bank and the International Monetary Fund.

Analytic limitations also hinder the pursuit of epidemiologic research on pathways in a global context. One important issue is the potential for reciprocal interactions among the various levels of health determinants presented in our framework. For example, income growth may have a positive effect on health, but alternatively, the association seen between these variables may be due to reverse causation, in which good health may stimulate income growth. Although longitudinal studies can be designed to illuminate the directionality of this association, it is possible that the reality is bidirectional. In this case, current epidemiologic methods are unable to measure the relative importance of the directions of association. Another analytic challenge lies in the examination of multiple interactions between inter-level and intra-level components. Current analytic tools are capable of investigating interactions, but sample size and power become insufficient as multiple interactions are included in regression models.

Despite these challenges, epidemiologic research must strive to include the global context in analyses. We must avoid becoming "prisoners of the proximate," to borrow McMichael's (1999) terminology, and instead focus on identifying modifiable contextual factors likely to have a large impact on population health. Studying the global context will enable development of effective interventions and improved promotion and protection of population health.

References

Abarca, J., Casiccia, C., & Zamorano, F. (2002). Increase in sunburns and photosensitivity disorders at the edge of the Antarctic ozone hole, Southern Chile, 1986–2000. *Journal of the American Academy of Dermatology (JAAD), 46*(2), 193–199.

Abu Morad, T. (2004). Palestinain refugee conditions associated with intestinal parasites and diarrhoea: Nuseirat refugee camp as a case study. *Public Health, 188*(2), 131–142.

Adler, N. E., & Newman, K. (2002). Socioeconomic disparities in health: Pathways and policies. *Health Affairs, 21*(2), 60–76.

Adler, N. E., & Ostrove, J. M. (1999). Socioeconomic status and health: What we know and what we don't. *Annals of the New York Academy of Science, 896*(1), 3–15.

Afrane, Y., Klinkenberg, E., Drechsel, P., Owusu-Daaku, K., Garms, R., & Kruppa, T. (2004). Does irrigated urban agriculture influence the transmission of malaria in the city of Kumasi, Ghana? *Acta Tropica, 89*, 125–34.

Agnew, R. (1992). Foundation for a general strain theory of crime and delinquency. *Criminology, 30*, 47–87.

Ahmed, Q. A., Arabi, Y. M., & Memish, Z. A. (2006). Health risks at the Hajj. *The Lancet, 367*(9515), 1008–1015.

Anderson, R., & May, R. (1991). *Infectious diseases of humans: Dynamics and control.* New York: Oxford University Press.

Antunes, J. L. F., & Waldman, E. A. (2001). The impact of AIDS, immigration and housing overcrowding on tuberculosis deaths in Sao Paulo, Brazil, 1994–1998. *Social Science & Medicine, 52*(7), 1071–1080.

Arnett, J. (2002). The psychology of globalization. *American Psychologist, 57*(10), 774–783.

Atherholt, T., LeChevallier, M., Norton, W., & Rosen, J. (1998). Effect of rainfall on giardia and cryptosporidium. *Journal of the American Water Works Association, 90*(9), 66–80.

Ayala-Carcedo, F. J., & Gonzalez-Barros, M. R. Y. (2005). Economic underdevelopment and sustainable development in the world: Conditioning factors, problems and opportunities. *Environment, Development and Sustainability, 7*(1), 95–115.

Barker, D., Coggon, D., Osmond, C., & Wickham, C. (1990). Poor housing in childhood and high rates of stomach cancer in England and Wales. *British Journal of Cancer, 61*(4), 575–578.

Baum, A., Garofalo, J. P., & Yali, A. M. (1999). Socioeconomic status and chronic stress: Does stress account for SES effects on health? *Annals of the New York Academy of Sciences, 896*(1), 131–144.

Baum, F. (2001). Health, equity, justice and globalisation: Some lessons from the People's Health Assembly. *Journal of Epidemiology and Community Health, 55*, 613–616.

Bennett, S., & Chanfreau, C. (2005). Approaches to rationing antiretroviral treatment: Ethical and equity implications. *Bulletin of the World Health Organization, 83*(7), 541–547.

Berkman, L. F., Glass, T., Brissette, L., & Seeman, T. E. (2000). From social integration to health: Durkheim in the new millennium. *Social Science & Medicine, 51*(6), 843–857.

Betrán, A., Wojdyla, D., Posner, S., & Gülmezoglu, M. (2005). National estimates for maternal mortality: An analysis based on the WHO systematic review of maternal mortality and morbidity. *BMC Public Health, 5*, 131.

Bettcher, D., & Lee, K. (2002). Globalisation and public health. *Journal of Epidemiology and Community Health, 56*(1), 8–17.

Bettcher, D., Yach, D., & Guindon, G. (2000). Global trade and health: Key linkages and future challenges. *Bulletin of the World Health Organization, 78*(4), 521–534.

Bobak, M., Hertzman, C., Skodova, Z., & Marmot, M. (1999). Socioeconomic status and cardiovascular risk factors in the Czech Republic. *International Journal of Epidemiology, 28*(1), 46–52.

Bouma, M., Dye, C., & Van der Kaay, H. (1996). Falciparum malaria and climate change in the northwest frontier province of Pakistan. *American Journal of Tropical Medicine and Hygiene, 55*, 131–137.

Bowman, C. (2004). The pacific island nations: Towards shared representation. Managing the challenges of WTO participation. Geneva: World Trade Organization.

Breiman, R. F., Evans, M. R., Preiser, W., Maguire, J., Schnur, A., Li, A., Bekedam, H., & Mackenzie, J.S. (2003). Role of China in the quest to define and control Severe Acute Respiratory Syndrome. *Emerging Infectious Diseases, 9*(9), 1037–041.

Brown, R. P. C., & Connell, J. (2004). The migration of doctors and nurses from south Pacific island nations. *Social Science & Medicine, 58*(11), 2193–2210.

Bruce, N., Perez-Padilla, R., & Albalak, R. (2000). Indoor air pollution in developing countries: A major environmental and public health challenge. *Bulletin of the World Health Organization, 78*(9), 1078–1092.

Carneiro, F., Cifuentes, E., Tellez-Rojo, M., & Romieu, I. (2002). The risk of ascaris lumbricoides infection in children as an environmental health indicator to guide preventive activities in Caparaó and Alto Caparaó, Brazil. *Bulletin of the World Health Organization, 80*(1), 40–46.

Centers for Disease Control and Prevention (CDC). (1996). Outbreaks of cyclospora cayetanensis infection — United States, 1996. Morbidity and Mortality Weekly Report, *14*(25), 549–551.

Chanda, R. (2001). Trade in health services. *Bulletin of the World Health Organization 80*, 158–163.

Cheadle, A., Psaty, B. M., Curry, S., Wagner, E., Diehr, P., Koepsell, T., & Krystal, A. (1991). Community-level comparisons between the grocery store environment and individual dietary practices. *Preventive Medicine, 20*(2), 250–261.

Chen, L., Evans, T., Anand, S., Boufford, J. I., Brown, H., Chowdhury, M., Caeto, M., Dare, L., Dussault, G., Elzinga, G., Fee, E., Habte, D., Hanvoravongchai, P., Jacobs, M., Kurowski, C., Mchael, S., Pablos-Mendez, A., Sewankambo, N., Solimano, G., Stilwell, B., de Waal, A., & Wilbulpolprasert, S. (2004). Human resources for health: Overcoming the crisis. *The Lancet, 364*(9449), 1984–1990.

Cobb, S., & Kasl, S. (1977). *Termination: The consequences of job loss.* Cincinnati, OH: Department of Health, Education and Welfare (NIOSH).

Coburn, D. (2000). Income inequality, social cohesion and the health status of populations: The role of neo-liberalism. *Social Science & Medicine, 51*(1), 135–146.

Coburn, D. (2004). Beyond the income inequality hypothesis: Class, neo-liberalism, and health inequalities. *Social Science & Medicine, 58*, 41–56.

Cohen, D. A., Farley, T. A., & Mason, K. (2003). Why is poverty unhealthy? Social and physical mediators. *Social Science & Medicine, 57*(9), 1631–1641.

Cohen, D. A., Mason, K., Bedimo, A., Scribner, R., Basolo, V., & Farley, T. A. (2003). Neighborhood physical conditions and health. *American Journal of Public Health, 93*(3), 467–471.

Cohen, D., Spear, S., Scribner, R., Kissinger, P., Mason, K., & Wildgen, J. (2000). "Broken windows" and the risk of gonorrhea. *American Journal of Public Health, 90*(2), 230–236.

Cohen, J. E. (2003). Human population: The next half century. *Science, 302*, 1172–1175.

Cohen, S., Tyrrell, D., & Smith, A. (1991). Psychological stress and susceptibility to the common cold. *New England Journal of Medicine, 325*(9), 606–612.

Collins, T. (2003). Globalization, global health and access to health care. *International Journal of Health Planning and Management, 18*(2), 97–104.

Cornia, G. (2001). Globalization and health: Results and options. *Bulletin of the World Health Organization, 79*(9), 834–841.

Cosgrove, W., & Rijsberman, F. (1998). Creating a vision for water, life, and the environment. *Water Policy, 1*(1), 115–122.

Cunningham-Rundles, S., McNeeley, D. F., & Moon, A. (2005). Mechanisms of nutrient modulation of the immune response. *Journal of Allergy and Clinical Immunology, 115*(6), 1119–1128.

Curriero, F., Patz, J., Rose, J., & Lele, S. (2001). The association between extreme precipitation and waterborn disease outbreaks in the United States, 1948–1994. *American Journal of Public Health, 91*(8), 1194–1200.

Davey Smith, G. (1996). Income inequality and mortality: Why are they related? *British Medical Journal, 312*(7037), 987–988.

de Onis, M., Monteiro, C., Akre, J., & Glugston, G. (1993). The worldwide magnitude of protein-energy malnutrition: An overview from the WHO Global Database on Child Growth. *Bulletin of the World Health Organization, 71*(6), 703–712.

Diaz-Bonilla, E., Babinard, J., & Pinstrup-Andersen, P. (2002). *Opportunities and risks for the poor in developing countries.* Working Paper No. 83. New Delhi: Indian Council for Research on International Economic Relations.

Diez Roux, A. (2003). Residential environments and cardiovascular risk. *The Journal of Urban Health, 80*(4), 569–589.

Dodgson, R., Lee, K., & Drager, N. (2002). *Global health governance: A conceptual review.* Discussion paper no. 1, Center on Global Change and Health. London: London School of Hygiene and Tropical Medicine.

Dollar, D. (2001). Is globalization good for your health? *Bulletin of the World Health Organization, 79*(9), 827–833.

Dollar, D., & Kray, A. (2002). Spreading the wealth. *Foreign Affairs, 81*(1), 120–133.

Dooley, D., Fielding, J., & Levi, L. (1996). Health and unemployment. *Annual Review of Public Health, 17*, 449–465.

Draper, C., Brubaker, G., Geser, A., Kilimali, A., & Wernsdorfer, W. (1985). Serial studies on the evolution of chloroquine resistance in an area of east African receiving intermittent malaria chemosuppression. *Bulletin of the World Health Organization, 63*(1), 109–118.

Elliott, M. (2000). The stress process in neighborhood context. *Health Place, 6*, 287–299.

Evans, J. A., May, J., Tominski, D., Eggelte, T., Marks, F., Abruquah, H. H., Meyer, C.G., Timmann, C., Agbenyega, T., & Horstmann, R.D. (2005). Pre-treatment with chloroquine and parasite chloroquine resistance in Ghanaian children with severe malaria. *The Quarterly Journal of Medicine, 98*(11), 789–796.

Evans, J., Hyndman, S., Stewart-Brown, S., Smith, D., & Petersen, S. (2000). An epidemiological study of the relative importance of damp housing in relation to adult health. *Journal of Epidemiology and Community Health, 54*(9), 677–686.

Feachem, R. (1984). Interventions for the control of diarrhoeal diseases among young children: Promotion of personal and domestic hygiene. *Bulletin of the World Health Organization, 62*, 467–476.

Fidler, D. P. (2004). Germs, governance, and global public health in the wake of SARS. *The Journal of Clinical Investigation, 113*(6), 799–804.

Filmer, D., & Pritchett, L. (1999). The impact of public spending on health: Does money matter? *Social Science & Medicine, 49*, 1309–1323.

Fischer, G., Shah, M., Tubiello, F., & van Velhuizen, H. (2005). Socio-economic and climate change impacts on agriculture: An integrated assessment, 1990–2080. *Philosophical Transactions of The Royal Society B: Biological Sciences, 360*(1463), 2067–2083.

Franco, A., Alvarez-Dardet, C., & Ruiz, M. T. (2004). Effect of democracy on health: Ecological study. *British Medical Journal, 329*(7480), 1421–1423.

Frankel, J., & Romer, D. (1999). Does trade cause growth? *American Economic Review, 89*, 379–398.

Frenk, J. (2005). Globalization, health, and the role of telemedicine. *Telemedicine and e-Health, 11*(3), 291–295.

Frenk, J., Sepulveda, J., Gomez-Dantes, O., McGuinness, M. J., & Knaul, F. (1997). The future of world health: The new world order and international health. *British Medical Journal, 314*(7091), 1404–1407.

Freudenberg, N., Fahs, M., Galea, S., & Greenberg, A. (2006). The impact of New York City's 1975 fiscal crisis on the tuberculosis, HIV, and homicide syndemic. *American Journal of Public Health, 96*(3), 424–434.

Frumkin, J. (2002). Urban sprawl and public health. *Public Health Reports, 117*(3), 201–217.

Galea, S., & Ahern, J. (2005). Distribution of education and population health: An ecological analysis of New York City neighborhoods. *American Journal of Public Health, 95*(12), 2198–2205.

Galea, S., Freudenberg, N., & Vlahov, D. (2005). Cities and population health. *Social Science & Medicine, 60*(5), 1017–1033.

Galea, S., Rudenstine, S., & Vlahov, D. (2005). Drug use, misuse and the urban environment. *Drug and Alcohol Review, 24*, 127–136.

Galea, S., & Vlahov, D. (2005). Urban health: Evidence, challenges and directions. *Annual Review of Public Health, 26*, 341–165.

Gallup, J., Sachs, J., & Mellinger, A. (1999). Geography and economic development. *International Regional Science Review, 22*(2), 179–232.

Gemmell, I. (2001). Indoor heating, house conditions, and health. *Annual Review of Public Health, 55*(12), 928–929.

Gerdtham, U.-G., & Johannesson, J. (2005). Business cycles and mortality: Results from Swedish microdata. *Social Science & Medicine, 60*(1), 205–218.

Global Health Watch (2005). *Global health watch 2005–2006: An alternative world health report.* London: Zed Books.

Gopalan, C. (2001). Achieving household nutrition security in societies in transition: An overview. *Asia Pacific Journal of Clinical Nutrition, 10*(Supplement), S4–S12.

Gracey, M. (2002). Child health in an urbanizing world. *Acta Paediatrica, 91*, 1–8.

Gupta, A. G., Moyer, C. A., & Stern, D. T. (2005). The economic impact of quarantine: SARS in Toronto as a case study. *Journal of Infection, 50*(5), 386–393.

Habenicht, H. (1994). The international programme on the elimination of child labour: An international response to child labour. *International Child Health, 2*, 19–25.

Haddad, S., & Fournier, P. (1995). Quality, cost and utilization of health services in developing countries. A longitudinal study in Zaire. *Social Science & Medicine, 40*(6), 743–753.

Hadley, J. (2003). Sicker and poorer—the consequences of being uninsured: A review of the research on the relationship between health insurance, medical care use, health, work, and income. *Medical Care Research and Review, 60*(supplement 2), 3S–75.

Hamilton, V., Broman, C., Hoffman, W., & Renner, D. (1990). Hard times and vulnerable people: Initial effects of plant closing on autoworkers' mental health. *Journal of Health and Social Behavior, 31*(2), 123–140.

Handy, S., Boarnet, M., Ewing, R., & Killingsworth, R. (2002). How the built environment affects physical activity: Views from urban planning. *American Journal of Preventive Medicine, 23*(2), 64–73.

Hawamdeh, H., & Spencer, N. (2003). The effects of work on the growth of Jordanian boys. *Child: Care, Health and Development, 29* (3), 167–172.

Hawkes, C. (2006). Uneven dietary development: Linking the policies and processes of globalization with the nutrition transition, obesity and diet-related chronic diseases. *Globalization and Health, 2* (1), 4.

Hawryluck, L., Gold, W. L., Robinson, S., Pogorski, S., Galea, S., & Styra, R. (2002). SARS control and psychological effects of quarantine, Toronto, Canada. *Emerging Infectious Diseases, 10*(7), 1206–1212.

Hemingway, H., Shipley, M., Macfarlane, P., & Marmot, M. (2000). Impact of socioeconomic status on coronary mortality in people with symptoms, electrocardiographic abnormalities, both or neither: The original Whitehall study 25 year follow up. *Journal of Epidemiology and Community Health, 54*(7), 510–516.

Heymann, D. (2004). The international response to the outbreak of SARS in 2003. *Philosophical Transactions of the Royal Society B: Biological Sciences, 359*(1447), 1127–1129.

Hippert, C. (2002). Multinational corporations, the politics of the world economy, and their effects on women's health in the developing world: A review. *Health Care for Women International, 23*, 861–869.

Hochberg, M. (2004). A theory of modern cultural shifts and meltdowns. *Proceedings of the Royal Society of London, Section B: Biological Sciences, 271* (Supplement), S313–S316.

Holden, C. (1999). Stalking a killer in Russia's prisons. *Science, 286*(5445), 1670.

Holton, R. (2000). Globalization's cultural consequences. *Annals of the American Academy of Political and Social Science, 570*, 140–152.

Huynen, M., Martens, P., & Hilderink, H. (2005). The health impacts of globalisation: A conceptual framework. *Globalization and Health, 1*(1), 14.

Institute of Medicine. (2002). *Care without coverage: Too little, too late.* Washington, DC: National Academy Press.

International Program on the Elimination of Child Labor. (2002). *Every child counts: New global estimates on child labour.* Geneva: International Labour Office.

Internet World Stats (2006). Internet usage statistics – The big picture. (2006); http://www.internetworldstats.com/stats.htm

Jones, M. B., & Jones, D. R. (1995). Preferred pathways of behavioral contagion. *Journal of Psychiatric Research, 29*(3), 193–209.

Jones, R. (1987). Ozone depletion and cancer risk. *The Lancet, 2,* 443–446.

Kaplan, G. (1999). What is the role of the social environment in understanding inequalities in health? *Annals of the New York Academy of Sciences, 896,* 116–119.

Kaplan, G. A., Pamuk, E. R., Lynch, J. W., Cohen, R. D., & Balfour, J. L. (1996). Inequality in income and mortality in the United States: Analysis of mortality and potential pathways. *British Medical Journal, 312*(7037), 999–1003.

Kawachi, I., & Berkman, L. (2001). Social ties and mental health. *Journal of Urban Health, 78* (3), 458–67.

Kawachi, I., Kennedy, B., Lochner, K., & Prothrow-Stith, D. (1997). Social captial, income inequality, and mortality. *American Journal of Public Health, 87,* 1491–1498.

Kawachi, I., Kennedy, B. P., & Wilkinson, R. G. (1999). Crime: Social disorganization and relative deprivation. *Social Science & Medicine, 48*(6), 719–731.

Keating, J., MacIntyre, K., Mbogo, C., Githeko, A., Regens, J. L., Swalm, C., Ndenga, B., Steinberg, L.J., Kibe, L., Githure, J.I., & Beier, J.C. (2003). A geographic sampling strategy for studying relationships between human activity and malaria vectors in urban Africa. *American Journal of Tropical Medicine and Hygiene, 68*(3), 357–365.

Kennedy, B. P., Kawachi, I., Prothrow-Stith, D., Lochner, K., & Gupta, V. (1998). Social capital, income inequality, and firearm violent crime. *Social Science & Medicine, 47*(1), 7–17.

Kinnon, C. (1998). World trade: Bringing health into the picture. *World Health Forum, 19,* 397–406.

Klevens, R. M., & Luman, E. T. (2001). U.S. children living in and near poverty: Risk of vaccine-preventable diseases. *American Journal of Preventive Medicine, 20*(4, Supplement 1), 41–46.

Konradsen, F., Amerasinghe, P., Van Der Hoek, W., Amerasinghe, F., Perera, D., & Piyaratne, M. (2003). Strong association between house characteristics and malaria vectors in Sri Lanka. *American Journal of Tropical Medicine and Hygiene, 68*(2), 177–181.

Korte, S. M., Koolhaas, J. M., Wingfield, J. C., & McEwen, B. S. (2005). The darwinian concept of stress: Benefits of allostasis and costs of allostatic load and the trade-offs in health and disease. *Neuroscience & Biobehavioral Reviews, 9*(1), 3–38.

Kosek, M., Bern, C., & Guerrant, R. (2003). The global burden of diarrhoeal disease, as estimated from studies published between 1992 and 2000. *Bulletin of the World Health Organization, 81,* 197–204.

Krieger, J., & Higgins, D. (2002). Housing and health: Time again for public health action. *American Journal of Public Health, 92*(5), 758–768.

Labonte, R., Muhajarine, N., Abonyi, S., Woodard, G., Jeffery, B., Maslany, G., Mc Cubbin, M., & Williams, S.A., (2002). An integrated exploration into the social and environmental determinants of health: The Saskatchewan Population Health and Evaluation Research Unit (SPHERU). *Chronic Diseases in Canada, 23*(2), 71–76.

LaScala, E. A., Gerber, D., & Gruenewald, P. J. (2000). Demographic and environmental correlates of pedestrian injury collisions: A spatial analysis. *Accident Analysis & Prevention, 32*(5), 651–658.

Latkin, C., & Curry, A. (2003). Stressful neighborhoods and depression: A prospective study of the impact of neighborhood disorder. *Journal of Health and Social Behavior, 44*(1), 34–44.

LaVeist, T. A., & Wallace, J. M., Jr. (2000). Health risk and inequitable distribution of liquor stores in African American neighborhood. *Social Science & Medicine, 51*(4), 613–617.

Lee, K. (2000). Globalization and health policy: A conceptual framework and research and policy agenda. In A. Bambas, J. A. Drayton, H. A. Drayton, & A. Valdez (Eds.), *Health and human development in the new global economy: The contributions and perspectives of civil society in the Americas*. Washington, DC: Pan American Health Organization.

Lee, T., Jordan, N. N., Sanchez, J. L., & Gaydos, J. C. (2005). Selected nonvaccine interventions to prevent infectious acute respiratory disease. *American Journal of Preventive Medicine, 28*(3), 305–316.

Lepore, S., Evans, G., & Palsane, M. (1991). Social hassles and psychological health in the context of chronic crowding. *Journal of Health and Social Behavior, 32*(4), 357–367.

Lindsay, S. W., Emerson, P. M., & Charlwood, J. D. (2002). Reducing malaria by mosquito-proofing houses. *Trends in Parasitology, 18*(11), 510–514.

Link, B. G., & Phelan, J. (1995). Social conditions as fundamental causes of disease. *Journal of Health and Social Behavior, 92*(5), 730–732.

Liu, Y. (2004). China's public health-care system: Facing the challenges. *Bulletin of the World Health Organization, 82*(7), 532–538.

Loevinsohn, M. E. (1994). Climatic warming and increased malaria incidence in Rwanda. *The Lancet, 343*(8899), 714–718.

Loewenson, R. (1998). Assessment of the health impact of occupational risk in Africa: Current situation and methodological issues. *Epidemiology, 10*(5), 632–639.

Loewenson, R. (2001). Globalization and occupational health: A perspective from southern Africa. *Bulletin of the World Health Organization, 79*(9), 863–868.

Lynch, J., Kaplan, G. A., Salonen, R., Cohen, R. D., & Salonen, J. T. (1995). Socioeconomic status and carotid atherosclerosis. *Circulation, 92*(7), 1786–1792.

Lynch, J., Smith, G., Harper, S., Hillemeier, M., Ross, N., Kaplan, G. A., & Wolfson, M. (2004). Is income inequality a determinant of population health? Part 1. A systematic review. *The Milbank Quarterly, 82*(1), 5–99.

Lynch, J. W., Smith, G. D., Kaplan, G. A., & House, J. S. (2000). Income inequality and mortality: Importance to health of individual income, psychosocial environment, or material conditions. *British Medical Journal, 320*(7243), 1200–1204.

Marmot, M. (2002). The influence of income on health: Views of an epidemiologist. *Health Affairs, 21* (2), 31–46.

Marmot, M., & Wilkinson, R. G. (2001). Psychosocial and material pathways in the relation between income and health: A response to Lynch et al. *British Medical Journal, 322*(7296), 1233–1236.

Mayberry, R. M., Mili, F., & Ofili, E. (2000). Racial and ethnic differences in access to medical care. *Medical Care Research and Review, 57*(supplement 1), 108–145.

McEwen, B. S. (2004). Protection and damage from acute and chronic stress: Allostasis and allostatic overload and relevance to the pathophysiology of psychiatric disorders. *Annals of the New York Academy of Sciences, 1032* (1), 1–7.

McEwen, B. S., & Seeman, T. (1999). Protective and damaging effects of mediators of stress: Elaborating and testing the concepts of allostasis and allostatic load. *Annals of the New York Academy of Sciences, 896*(1), 30–47.

McLeod, J., & Kessler, R. (1990). Socioeconomic status differences in vulnerability to undesirable life events. *Journal of Health and Social Behavior, 31*(2), 162–172.

McMihael, A.J., (1999). Prisoners of the proximate: loosening the constraints on epidermiology in an age of change. *American Journal of Epidemiology, 149*(10), 887–897.

McMichael, A. (2000). The urban environment and health in a world of increasing globalization: Issues for developing countries. *Bulletin of the World Health Organization, 78*(9), 1117–1126.

McMichael, A., & Beaglehole, R. (2000). The changing global context of public health. *The Lancet, 356*(9228), 495–499.

McMichael, A. J., Bolin, B., Costanza, R., Daily, G. C., Folke, C., Lindahl-Kiessling, K., Lingren, E., & Niklasson, B. (1999). Globalization and the sustainability of human health: An ecological perspective. *BioScience, 49*(3), 205–210.

Meerman, L., Ord, R., Bousema, J. T., van Niekerk, M., Osman, E., Hallett, R., Pinder, M., Walraven, G., & Sutherland, C.J. (2005). Carriage of chloroquine-resistant parasites and delay of effective treatment increase the risk of severe malaria in Gambian children. *Journal Infectious Diseases, 192*(9), 1651–1657.

Mehrotra, S. (2006). Governance and basic social services: Ensuring accountability in service delivery through deep democratic decentralization. *Journal of International Development, 18*, 263–283.

Menon-Johansson, A. S. (2005). Good governance and good health: The role of societal structures in the human immunodeficiency virus pandemic. *BMC International Health and Human Rights, 5*(1), 4.

Moore, M., Gould, P., & Keary, B. S. (2002). Global urbanization and impact on health. *International Journal of Hygiene and Environmental Health, 206*, 269–278.

Moore, S., Teixeira, A. C., & Shiell, A. (2006). The health of nations in a global context: Trade, global stratification, and infant mortality rates. *Social Science & Medicine, 63*(1), 165–178.

Muntaner, C., & Lynch, J. (1999). Income inequality, social cohesion, and class relations: A critique of Wilkinson's neo-Durkheimian research program. *International Journal of Health Services, 29*(1), 59–81.

Myaux, J., Ali, M., Felsenstein, A., Chakraborty, J., & de Francisco, A. (1997). Spatial distribution of watery diarrhoea in children: Identification of risk areas in a rural community in Bangladesh. *Health & Place, 3*(3), 181–186.

Nations, M. K., & Monte, C. M. J. (1996). I'm not dog, no: Cries of resistance against cholera control campaigns. *Social Science & Medicine, 43*(6), 1007–1024.

Navarro, V., & Shi, L. (2001). The political context of social inequalities and health. *Social Science & Medicine, 52*(3), 481–491.

Netterstrom, B., & Hansen, A. (2000). Outsourcing and stress: Physiological effects on bus drivers. *Stress Medicine, 16*, 149–60.

Newman, O. (1986). *Defensible space: Crime prevention through urban design.* New York: MacMillan.

Ostry, A. S., & Spiegel, J. M. (2004). Labor markets and employment insecurity: Impacts of globalization on service and healthcare-sector workforces. *International Journal of Occupational and Environmental Health, 10*(4), 368–374.

Pascual, M., Rodo, X., Ellner, S. P., Colwell, R., & Bouma, M. J. (2000). Cholera dynamics and El Nino-Southern Oscillation. *Science, 289*(5485), 1766–1769.

Phillips, D., & Carstcnsen, L. (1986). Clustering of teenage suicides after television news stories about suicide. *New England Journal of Medicine, 315*(11), 385–389.

Pick, W. M., & Obermeyer, C. M. (1996). Urbanisation, household composition and the reproductive health of women in a South African city. *Social Science & Medicine, 43*(10), 1431–1441.

Poon, L., Guan, Y., Nicholls, J., Yuen, K., & Peiris, J. (2004). The aetiology, origins, and diagnosis of Severe Acute Respiratory Syndrome. *The Lancet Infectious Diseases, 4*(11), 663–671.

Pritchett, L., & Summers, L. (1996). Wealthier is healthier. *Journal of Human Resources, 31*, 841–868.

Quinlan, M., Mayhew, C., & Bohle, P. (2001). The global expansion of precarious employment, work disorganization, and consequences for occupational health: A review of recent research. *International Journal of Health Services, 31*(2), 335–414.

Quinn, T. C. (1994). Population migration and the spread of types 1 and 2 human immunodeficiency viruses. *Proceedings of the National Academy of Sciences, 91*, 2407–2414.

Ravillion, M. (2001). Growth, inequality and poverty: Looking beyond averages. UNU/WIDER Conference on Growth and Poverty, Helsinki.

Root, G. (1997). Population density and spatial differentials in child mortality in Zimbabwe. *Social Science & Medicine, 44*(3), 413–421.

Ross, C., & Mirowsky, J. (2001). Neighborhood disadvantage, disorder, and health. *Journal of Health and Social Behavior, 42*(3), 258–276.

Ross, C., & Wu, C. (1995). The links between education and health. *American Sociological Review, 60*(5), 715–745.

Rush, D. (2000). Nutrition and maternal mortality in the developing world. *American Journal of Clinical Nutrition, 72*(1), 212S–240S.

Sampson, R., & Groves, W. (1989). Community structure and crime: Testing social-disorganization theory. *The American Journal of Sociology, 94*(4), 774–802.

Sampson, R. J., Raudenbush, S. W., & Earls, F. (1997). Neighborhoods and violent crime: A multilevel study of collective efficacy. *Science, 277*(5328), 918–924.

Satterthwaite, D. (2000). Will most people live in cities? *British Medical Journal, 321*, 1143–1145.

Schilling, J., & Linton, L. (2005). The public health roots of zoning: In search of active living's legal genealogy. *American Journal of Preventive Medicine, 28*(2 Supplement 2), 96–104.

Segall, M. (2000). From cooperation to competition in national health systems – and back? Impact on professional ethics and quality of care. *The International Journal of Health Planning and Management, 15*(1), 61–79.

Semenza, J. C., Rubin, C. H., Falter, K. H., Selanikio, J. D., Flanders, W. D., Howe, H. L., & Wilhelm, J. (1996). Heat-related deaths during the July 1995 heat wave in Chicago. *New England Journal of Medicine, 335*(2), 84–90.

Sen, A. (1997). Inequality, unemployment and contemporary Europe. *International Labor Review, 136*(2), 155–172.

Shaw, C., & McKay, H. (1942). *Juvenile delinquency and urban areas.* Chicago: University of Chicago Press.

Shetty, P. (2006). Achieving the goal of halving global hunger by 2015. The Summer Meeting of the Nutrition Society, Norwich, Proceedings of the Nutrition Society.

Skrabski, A., Kopp, M., & Kawachi, I. (2004). Social capital and collective efficacy in Hungary: Cross sectional associations with middle aged female and male mortality rates. *Journal of Epidemiology and Community Health, 58*(4), 340–345.

Smith, A., Lingas, E., & Rahman, M. (2000). Contamination of drinking-water by arsenic in Bangladesh: A public health emergency. *Bulletin of the World Health Organization, 78*(9), 1093–1103.

Smolinski, M. S., Hamburg, M. A., & Lederberg, J. (Eds.). (2003). *Microbial threats to health: Emergence, detection and response.* Washington, D.C., Institute of Medicine.

Spiegel, J. M., Labonte, R., & Ostry, A. S. (2004). Understanding globalization as a determinant of health determinants: A critical perspective. *International Journal of Occupational Medicine and Environmental Health, 10*(4), 360–367.

Stevenson, L., Latham, M., & Ottesen, E. (2000). Global malunutrition. *Parasitology, 121*(7), S5–S22.

Stloukal, L. (2001). Rural population ageing in poorer countries: Possible implications for rural development. *SDdimensions.* (2001); http://www.fao.org/sd/2001/pe0501a_en.htm

Subramanian, S., Belli, P., & Kawachi, I. (2002). The macroeconomic determinants of health. *Annual Review of Public Health, 23*, 287–302.

Subramanian, S., Kim, D., & Kawachi, I. (2002). Social trust and self-rated health in US communities: A multilevel analysis. *Journal of Urban Health, 79*(4 Supplement 1), S21–S34.

Subramanian, S. V., & Kawachi, I. (2004). Income inequality and health: What have we learned so far? *Epidemiologic Reviews, 26*(1), 78–91.

Sundquist, K., Theobald, H., Yang, M., Li, X., Johansson, S., & Sundquist, J. (2006). Neighborhood violent crime and unemployment increase the risk of coronary heart disease: A multilevel study in an urban setting. *Social Science & Medicine, 62*(8), 2061–2071.

Szreter, S. (1997). Economic growth, disruption, deprivation and death: On the importance of the politics of public health for development. *Population and Development Review, 23*, 702–703.

Takkouche, B., Regueira, C., & Gestal-Otero, J. (2001). A cohort study of stress and the common cold. *Epidemiology, 12*(3), 345–349.

The Eurowinter Group. (1997). Cold exposure and winter mortality from ischaemic heart disease, cerebrovascular disease, respiratory disease, and all causes in warm and cold regions of Europe. *Lancet, 349*(9062), 1341–1346.

United Nations. (2002). *International migration report 2002.* New York: United Nations.

United Nations. (2005). *UN Millennium Project 2005. Health, dignity, and development: What will it take?* New York: United Nations.

United Nations Department of Economic and Social Affairs. (2003). *World urbanization prospects: The 2003 Revision.* New York: United Nations.

United Nations Development Programme. (2001). Human development report. New York: Oxford University Press.

United Nations High Commissioner for Refugees. (2004). Basic facts. United Nations High Commissioner for Refugees. New York: United Nations.

VanDerslice, J., Popkin, B., & Briscoe, J. (1994). Drinking-water quality, sanitation, and breastfeeding: their interactive effects on infant health. *Bulletin of the World Health Organization, 72*, 589–601.

Vitousek, P., Mooney, H., Lubchenco, J., & Melillo, J. (1997). Human domination of the earth's ecosystems. *Science, 277*, 494–499.

Wade, R. (2004). Is globalization reducing poverty and inequality? *World Development, 32*(4), 567–589.

Wagstaff, A., Bustreo, F., Bryce, J., & Claeson, M. (2004). Child health: Reaching the poor. *American Journal of Public Health, 94*(5), 726–736.

Wakefield, S. E. L., & Poland, B. (2005). Family, friend or foe? Critical reflections on the relevance and role of social capital in health promotion and community development. *Social Science & Medicine, 60*(12), 2819–2832.

Wallace, D., & Wallace, R. (1998). Scales of geography, time, and population: The study of violence as a public health problem. *American Journal of Public Health, 88*(12), 1853–1858.

Webster, R. G. (2004). Wet markets—a continuing source of severe acute respiratory syndrome and influenza? *The Lancet, 363*(9404), 234–236.

Weich, S., Blanchard, M., Prince, M., Burton, E., Erens, B., & Sproston, K. (2002). Mental health and the built environment: Cross-sectional survey of individual and contextual risk factors for depression. *British Journal of Psychiatry, 180*(5), 428–433.

Weinreb, L., Wehler, C., Perloff, J., Scott, R., Hosmer, D., Sagor, L., & Gundersen, C. (2002). Hunger: Its impact on children's health and mental health. *Pediatrics, 110*(4), e41.

Weisbrot, M., Baker, D., Kraev, E., & Chen, J. (2002). The scorecard on globalization 1980–2000: Its consequences for economic and social well-being. *International Journal of Health Services, 32*(2), 229–253.

Wellington, M., Ndowa, F., & Mbengeranwa, L. (1997). Risk factors for sexually transmitted disease in Harare: A case-control study. *Sexually Transmitted Diseases, 24*(9), 528–532.

Widdus, R. (2005). Public-private partnerships: An overview. *Transactions of the Royal Society of Tropical Medicine and Hygiene, 99*(Supplement 1), 1–8.

Wilkinson, R. G., & Pickett, K. E. (2006). Income inequality and population health: A review and explanation of the evidence. *Social Science & Medicine, 62*(7), 1768–1784.

Williams, L., Labonte, R., & O'Brien, M. (2003). Empowering social action through narratives of identity and culture. *Health Promotion International, 18*(1), 33–40.

Williams, R. (1987). Meningitis and unpaved roads. *Social Science & Medicine, 24*(2), 109–115.

Williamson, J. B., & Boehmer, U. (1997). Female life expectancy, gender stratification, health status, and level of economic development: A cross-national study of less developed countries. *Social Science & Medicine, 45*(2), 305–317.

Wilson, M.E. (2003). The traveller and emerging infections: sentinel courier, transmitter. *Journal of Applied Microbiology, 94*(1), 1S–11S

Woodward, D., Drager, N., Beaglehole, R., & Lipson, D. (2001). Globalization and health: A framework for analysis and action. *Bulletin of the World Health Organization, 79*(9), 875–881.

World Bank. (2006). World Development Indicators 2006. Washington, DC: The World Bank.

World Health Organization. (2003). Consensus document on the epidemiology of Severe Acute Respiratory Syndrome (SARS). Geneva: World Health Organization.

World Health Organization. (2004). Water, sanitation and hygiene links to health: Facts and figures. Geneva: World Health Organization.

World Health Organization. (2006). World health report 2006: Working together for health. Geneva: World Health Organization.

World Trade Organization. (2000a). World merchandise trade by selected region and economy, 1980–99. Geneva: World Trade Organization.

World Trade Organization. (2000b). World trade in commercial services by selected region and economy, 1980–99. Geneva: World Trade Organization.

World Trade Organization. (2005). World tourism barometer. Geneva: World Trade Organization.

Yach, D., & Bettcher, D. (2000). Globalisation of tobacco industry influence and new global responses. *Tobacco Control, 9*(2), 206–216.

Yé, Y., Hoshen, M., Louis, V., Séraphin, S., Traoré, I., & Sauerborn, R. (2006). Housing conditions and Plasmodium falciparum infection: Protective effect of iron-sheet roofed houses. *Malaria Journal*, 5, 8.

Zenk, S. N., Schulz, A. J., Israel, B. A., James, S. A., Bao, S., & Wilson, M. L. (2005). Neighborhood racial composition, neighborhood poverty, and the spatial accessibility of supermarkets in metropolitan Detroit. *American Journal of Public Health, 95*(4), 660–667.

Zenk, S. N., Schulz, A. J., Israel, B. A., James, S. A., Bao, S., & Wilson, M. L. (2006). Fruit and vegetable access differs by community racial composition and socioeconomic position in Detroit, Michigan. *Ethnicity & Disease, 16*(1), 275–280.

Zhou, G., Minakawa, N., Githeko, A. K., & Yan, G. (2004). Association between climate variability and malaria epidemics in the East African highlands. *Proceedings of the National Academy of Sciences of the United States of America, 101*(8), 2375–2380.

Chapter 3
Urbanicity, Urbanization, and the Urban Environment

Danielle C. Ompad, Sandro Galea, and David Vlahov

1. Introduction

During the Second Session of the World Urban Forum in 2004, world leaders and mayors warned that " . . . rapid urbanization was one of the greatest challenges facing humanity in the new millennium" (United Nations Human Settlements Programme (UN-HABITAT), 2004). In 1950, approximately 29 percent of the world's population lived in urban areas (United Nations, 2004). By 2000, 47 percent lived in urban areas, and the United Nations projects that approximately 61 percent of the world's population will live in cities by 2030. Overall, the world's urban population is expected to grow from 2.86 billion in 2000 to 4.94 billion in 2030 (United Nations, 2004).

With population migration into cities comes the expansion of urban centers. The number of cities with populations of 500,000 or greater grew from 447 in 1975 to 804 in 2000. Table 3.1 presents world megacities (population over ten million) between 1950 and 2015. In 1950 there were two megacities; by 2000 there were 18, and 23 are projected worldwide by 2015 (United Nations, 2006). Urban centers are not evenly distributed among resource-poor and wealthy countries. Middle- to low-income countries contained 72% of the world's cities in 2000 (Figure 3.1) and most growing cities are in developing countries.

Given the massive movement of the world's population into cities, understanding the particular role of city living in shaping population health becomes central to public health planning. We provide here a summary of the key issues that pertain to our understanding of the role urbanization and urbanicity play in shaping population health. We refer the reader to other published work that discusses these issues in substantially more detail (Galea, Freudenberg, & Vlahov, 2005; Galea & Vlahov, 2005a, b).

2. Defining Urban Areas

There is little consensus among national and international entities and disciplines about the definition of urban and what constitutes a city. The US Bureau of the Census defines an urbanized area as "a place and the adjacent densely settled

TABLE 3.1. World megacities and their populations in thousands, 1950–2015 (United Nations, 2006)

1950		1975		2000		2015 (projected)	
City	Pop.	City	Pop.	City	Pop.	City	Pop.
New York-Newark	12338	Tokyo	26615	Tokyo	34450	Tokyo	35494
Tokyo	11275	New York-Newark	15880	Mexico City	18066	Mumbai	21869
		Mexico City	10690	New York-Newark	17846	Mexico City	21568
				São Paulo	17099	São Paulo	20535
				Mumbai	16086	New York-Newark	19876
				Shanghai	13243	Delhi	18604
				Kolkata	13058	Shanghai	17225
				Delhi	12441	Kolkata	16980
				Buenos Aires	11847	Dhaka	16842
				Los Angeles-Long Beach-Santa Ana	11814	Jakarta	16822
				Osaka-Kobe	11165	Lagos	16141
				Jakarta	11065	Karachi	15155
				Rio de Janeiro	10803	Buenos Aires	13396
				Cairo	10391	Cairo	13138
						Los Angeles-Long Beach-Santa Ana	13095
				Dhaka	10159	Manila	12917
				Moscow	10103	Beijing	12850
				Karachi	10020	Rio de Janeiro	12770
						Osaka-Kobe	11309
						Istanbul	11211
						Moscow	11022
						Guangzhou, Guangdong	10420

surrounding territory that together comprise a minimum population of 50,000 people," where the "densely settled surrounding territory" is defined as "one or more contiguous block having a population density of at least 1,000 people per square mile." The US Census Bureau thus provides a dichotomy whereby territory, population, and housing units within specific size and density parameters are designated urban, and those that are outside those parameters are non-urban. However, there are inherent limitations to these definitions. Urban areas exist in contrast to rural or, more simply, to non-urban areas. In the 21st century, few cities exist in extreme isolation such that what is not defined as city is rural (e.g., Las Vegas). Most cities (e.g., New York City, London, Bangkok, etc.) are actually

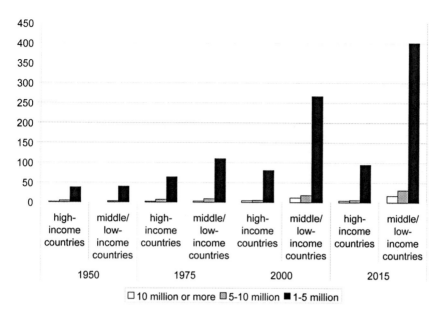

FIGURE 3.1. Number of cities with populations of 1 million or greater, 1950–2015 (United Nations, 2004)

a far-reaching densely populated area, containing peri-urban and suburban areas, which continue relatively un-interrupted for miles beyond the municipal city boundaries and the city-center.

The definition of "urban" varies widely between countries. Among 228 countries for which the United Nations had data in 2000, almost half (100) included size and density as criteria, 96 included administrative definitions of urban (e.g., living in the capital city), 33 included functional characteristics (e.g., economic activity, available services, etc.), 24 had no definition of urban, and 12 defined all (e.g., Anguilla, Bermuda, the Cayman Islands, Gibraltar, the Holy See, Hong Kong, Monaco, Nauru, Singapore) or none (e.g., Pitcairn Island, Tokelau, and Wallis and Futuna Islands) of their population as urban (United Nations, 2004). Official statistics (e.g., United Nations statistics detailed above) rely on country-specific designations and therefore vary widely. In specific instances, definitions of "urban" in adjacent countries differ tremendously. For example, Cambodia defines urban as towns, while Vietnam defines urban as cities, towns and districts with 2,000 or more inhabitants, and Thailand defines urban as municipal areas. Furthermore, definitions of urban have changed over time in different ways in different countries. Thus, global statistics are subject to country-level differences in the definition of urban that may be based on population density or specific urban features (e.g., proportion of agricultural workers, municipal services).

The variability in definitions across settings presents a challenge for those interested in examining the relationship between cities and health. Clearly, rates of disease, risk, and protective behaviors will vary between definitions. In any given study, the definition of "urban" or "city" will be a function of both the research question and the available data sources. For example, if a researcher wanted to examine the impact of restaurant smoking laws among cities, the definition of city would be defined by the municipal boundaries that are affected by city ordinances. In contrast, if a researcher wanted to use US Census data to examine the relation between socioeconomic measures and a specific health outcome in rural and urban settings, the definition of urban would be based on the US Census definitions because that is how the data on socioeconomic measures are provided. Ultimately, if the research question requires data from publicly available data sets like a census, the definition of a city or urban area will have to conform to the definitions of the data sources.

3. Conceptualizing Urban "Exposure" as a Determinant of Health

Until relatively recently, urban living and its related exposures were considered mainly in terms of their detrimental effects on health (Vlahov, Galea, & Freudenberg, 2005). This "urban health penalty" perspective has focused attention on poor health outcomes in "inner city" environments (Andrulis, 1997) and on disparities in the burden of morbidity and mortality, as well as disparities in health care access, among specific sub-groups (Vlahov, Gibble, Freudenberg, & Galea, 2004). Yet in many ways, urban living may be health promoting. Urban areas can provide access to cultural events, educational opportunities, cutting-edge medical facilities, and a plethora of health and social services (Leviton, Snell, & McGinnis, 2000; Wandersman & Nation, 1998). Moving forward, researchers must consider features that both promote and harm population health.

We can conceptualize exposure to the urban environment in the context of production of health and disease in three main ways: urbanicity, urbanization, and the urban environment, defined in Sections 3.1–3.3 below. These three urban aspects may differentially influence health in particular settings. In most developing countries urbanicity, urbanization, and the urban environment are all important determinants of health. Many of those countries are in the process of dramatic change, as their populations move from rural areas into cities. In the majority of developed countries, the pace of urbanization has slowed considerably. In both developed and developing countries, substantial differences exist between and even within cities, with respect to health outcomes and access to health and social services.

3.1. Urbanicity

Urbanicity, simply defined, is urban living. Measures of urbanicity, then, are usually in contrast to non-urban (e.g., rural and suburban) living and are subject to the definition of the urban area. Urbanicity characterizes the presence of conditions at a particular point in time (i.e., prevalence) that are particular to urban areas or present in urban areas to a much greater or lesser extent than in non-urban areas. The focus on urbanicity is important to public health assessments on prioritizing current needs and approaches.

Figure 3.2 presents the relationship between urbanicity (defined as percent urban) and the infant mortality rate for 182 countries (World Health Organization, 2005). These data suggest that the infant mortality rate is lower in countries where more people live in urban areas. One might conclude that urban living is therefore associated with improved infant mortality. However, this type of ecological analysis is limited in helping identify what it is *about* urban living that influences the health of populations. We contrast this figure with one considering the role of urbanization in the next section.

3.2. Urbanization

Urbanization refers to changes in the size, density and heterogeneity of cities over time and provides a perspective for public health planning. Urbanization is related to movement of populations and resources from rural and suburban areas to urban areas and traditionally has been linked to industrialization, although current patterns of migration toward cities in the developing world appears to be independent of industrialization (Davis, 2006). More simply stated, urbanization

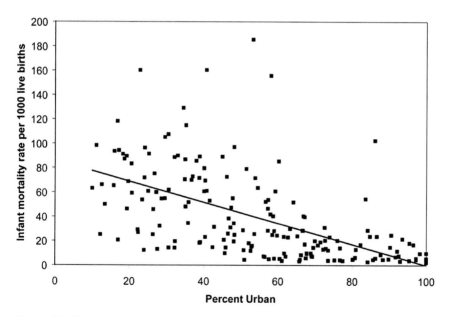

FIGURE 3.2. The relation between urbanicity and infant mortality rate for 182 countries (World Health Organization, 2005)

is the process that involves the emergence and growth of cities. Thus, urbanization is not dependent on the definition of urban per se, but rather on the dynamics of agglomeration of individuals. Although the pace of urbanization is independent of the base size of the population, the population size/density of surrounding areas may be a factor in its determination.

Characteristics of urbanization, including the intensity, rate, and duration of these changes, may influence the health of urban residents. Common mechanisms may exist through which urbanization affects health independent of the size of the city in question. Investigations of urbanization often consider "push" and "pull" factors as driving forces of urban migration (Godfrey & Julien, 2005). "Push" factors include natural disasters, civil disturbances, and economic hardship. "Pull" factors include opportunity for upward mobility, family, and desire for a "modern" lifestyle. For instance, in sub-Saharan Africa, the rapid migration into cities is related to high urban fertility rates and "push" factors such as the escape from rural poverty (McMichael, 2000). On the other hand, in South America urban growth is related to "pull" factors such as industrialization and economic opportunities (McMichael, 2000).

In addition to population changes, urbanization is associated with geographic changes, particularly changes in land use. Land use change is important not only for urban planning and resource management, but also for public health planning. Overall, a fundamental concern is the consequences on health when the pace of urbanization outstrips infrastructure development.

Urbanization is generally more of a concern for developing countries. Indeed, the growth rate of megacities in the developing world is anticipated to be higher than that of more developed countries. For example, the anticipated growth rate for Calcutta, India, between 2000 and 2015 is 1.9%, compared to an anticipated growth rate of 0.4% for New York City, USA (Hinrichsen, Blackburn, & Robey, 2001).

From a population perspective, measures of urbanization include variables such as the average annual rate of change of the urban population and the average annual rate of change of the percentage urban (Arriaga, 1970; United Nations, 2006). Figure 3.3 presents the relationship between the urbanization rate and the infant mortality rate for 182 countries (World Health Organization, 2005). These data show that the infant mortality rate is higher in countries where urbanization is occurring at a faster rate. This is in contrast to Figure 3.2, which showed lower infant mortality rates in countries that are already urbanized. These two figures simply illustrate the dramatic difference in urbanicity and urbanization as features of nations worldwide. Countries that are already substantially urbanized are typically richer countries with better health infrastructure and salutary conditions that are associated with better health. Conversely, more rapidly urbanizing countries are largely low- and middle-income countries (see Figure 3.1) where several macroeconomic and infrastrucutral factors are probably responsible for higher infant mortality rates. Therefore, simple considerations of urbanicity or urbanization cross-nationally can illuminate substantially different intra-national processes, but they do not provide information on the potential variability in the populations moving into and out of the urban areas nor about the static processes

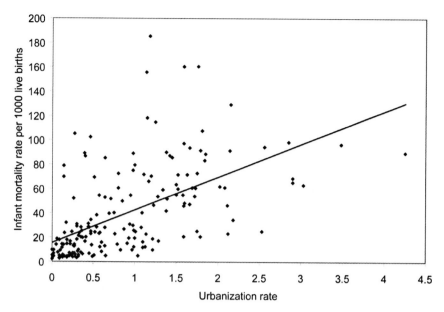

FIGURE 3.3. The relation between urbanization rate and infant mortality rate for 182 countries (World Health Organization, 2005)

that are shaping population health at one point in time. As we discuss below, understanding the elements of the urban environment, including both static elements and changing features of the urban environment, and how these constituent factors influence population health may be much more instructive in the long term.

3.3. The Urban Environment

The urban context or urban environment can be defined as the specific characteristics or features of cities that influence health. It is helpful to think about the urban environment as three distinct concepts: the social environment, the physical environment and the urban resource infrastructure. These are shaped in turn by municipal, national, and global forces and trends.

3.3.1. Social Environment

The urban social environment is the collective norms and values shared by members of social groups along with the interpersonal relationships and interactions shared among urban residents and communities (Coutts & Kawachi, 2006). Features of the social environment can both harm and promote health. Although we summarize some key pathogenic and salutogenic features of the social environment, the list provided here is by no means exhaustive. We refer the reader to other works for a more comprehensive consideration of the urban social environment (Berkman & Kawachi, 2000; Kawachi & Berkman, 2003; McCarthy, 2000).

Social disorganization theory grew out of work of the Chicago School in the early twentieth century. In 1918, Thomas and Znaniecki described social disorganization as "a decrease of the influence of existing social rules of behavior upon individual members of the group . . . " (Thomas & Znaniecki, 1999). Park and Burgess (1925) noted that social disorganization was associated with specific features of urban landscapes. These features aggregate into zones reflective of both the socioeconomic position of the zone residents and varying levels of social disorganization. From a practical standpoint, social disorganization can be measured by the prevalence of abandoned housing and neighborhood crime rates.

Several studies have demonstrated the relationship between social disorganization and health. For example, Cohen and colleagues (2000) found an association between the deteriorated physical conditions of local neighborhoods with gonorrhea rates using an index based on Wilson's "broken windows" theory (Wilson & Kelling, 1982) that measured housing quality, abandoned cars, graffiti, trash, and public school deterioration. In a study of syphilis in North Carolina, an increase in drug activity in the counties along the Interstate 95 corridor preceded a rise in syphilis cases (Cook, Royce, Thomas, & Hanusa, 1999).

Social norms are patterns of behaviors that are considered accepted and expected by a given society (Birenbaum & Sagarin, 1976) and can be conceptualized as a form of informal social control. From the perspective of urban health, societal and cultural norms are important considerations when thinking about the behavior of urban dwellers and may exist on several levels. For example, Frye, et al. (2006) considered the role of social norms in shaping behaviors among men who have sex with men (MSM) in urban communities. The authors posited that MSM may be influenced by the social norms of the gay community, with its unique physical and social structures and cultural characteristics, as well as by social norms of smaller subpopulations within the gay community. These communities may not be limited to one geographic location, however. Thus, MSM also may be influenced by the norms operating within their geographical neighborhood, which may operate in conjunction with, or in opposition to, the prevailing norms of the broader gay community.

Social capital refers to the features of social relationships or organizations that can facilitate collective action aimed at the improvement of society (Coleman, 1990). These features may include trust, reciprocity, norms, and information networks (Coleman, 1990; Putnam, 1993). However, there is no single definition or measure of the construct (Lochner, Kawachi, & Kennedy, 1999; Pilkington, 2002). Social capital is a multi-dimensional concept and is sometimes conceived of as structural and conceptual. Structural social capital refers to the quantity of relationships while cognitive social capital refers to the quality of those relationships (Bain & Hicks, 1998).

Generally, higher levels of social capital are associated with positive health outcomes. For example, in a study of children in four developing countries

(Ethiopia, India, Peru and Vietnam), cognitive social capital was positively associated with child nutritional status (De Silva & Harpham, 2006). In a cross-national study among adolescents in Chicago (United States) and Maastricht (Netherlands), higher levels of social capital (as measured by informal social control, social cohesion and trust) were associated with higher levels of perceived health (Drukker, Buka, Kaplan, McKenzie, & Van, 2005). Conversely, there is evidence to suggest that the absence of social capital is associated with negative health outcomes such as increases in mortality, poor self-rated perception of health, and higher crime rates and violence (Kawachi, Kennedy, Lochner, & Prothrow-Stith, 1997; Kennedy, Kawachi, Prothrow-Stith, Lochner, & Gupta, 1998).

3.3.2. Physical Environment

The urban physical environment refers to the built environment, pollution, and the geological and climate conditions of the area the city occupies. Similar to features of the urban social environment, features of the physical environment can be pathogenic or salutogenic. Klitzman, Matte, & Kass (2006) have proposed a useful framework for considering the physical environment when study its affect on health; the model considers underlying community factors and mediating, proximate-level factors. Community factors include population density, land use patterns, physical infrastructure systems (e.g., transportation and sanitation) and buildings. Proximate-level factors include air and water quality, dust and noise level, local climate, pestilence (e.g., insects and rodents), and physical safety and security.

The built environment refers to "housing form, roads and footpaths, transport networks, shops, markets, parks and other public amenities, and the disposition of public space" (Weich et al., 2001). Examination of the association of built environment and health overall is a relatively recent area of inquiry (see the September 2003 issues of the *Journal of Urban Health* and the *American Journal of Public Health* that examined health and the built environment), but associations between poor quality built environments and depression drug overdose, and physical activity have been found. A recent study noted that access to increased access to physical activity facilities was associated with decreased likelihood of overweight and increased likelihood of moderate to vigorous physical activity (Gordon-Larsen, Nelson, Page, & Popkin, 2006). Greenspace (e.g., parks, esplanades, community gardens, etc.) has the potential to significantly contribute to the health of urban dwellers. Living in areas with walkable greenspace has been associated with increased longevity among elderly urban residents in Japan, independent of their age, sex, marital status, baseline functional status, and socioeconomic status (Takano, Nakamura, & Watanabe, 2002). Drawing on the rapid advances in remote sensing, spatial metrics and spatial modeling and the use of satellite imagery and geographic information systems (Herold, Goldstein, & Clarke, 2003), researchers have been able to examine changes in the urban physical environment over time and to assess the role of urbanization in shaping health. For example, Ramadan, Feng, & Cheng, (2004) documented an average annual expansion of 7 km^2 in the areas surrounding Shaoxing City (China). This rapid expansion had an impact on surrounding agricultural areas and water resources, which have direct bearing on the health of urban residents.

Urban transportation systems include mass transit systems (i.e., subways, light rail and buses) as well as streets and roads. According to the Light Rail Transit Association, there are 135 subways currently operating in 67 countries worldwide. Urban transportation systems are key in the economic livelihoods of city residents as well as cities as a whole; thus, they can be considered salutogenic with respect to access to employment, health care, cultural activities and other opportunities and services. On the other hand, there are significant health considerations for mass transit and roadways, including security and violence, noise, and exposure to pollutants that may be pathogenic. These exposures are relevant not only for transit workers, but also for transit riders.

Pollution is one of the well-studied aspects of the urban physical environment. Urban dwellers are exposed to both outdoor and indoor air and water pollutants that include heavy metals, asbestos, and a variety of volatile hydrocarbons. For example, one study in Bangkok (Thailand) reported high levels of benzene and polycyclic aromatic hydrocarbons among street vendors and school children sampled from traffic-congested areas as compared to monks and nuns sampled from nearby temples (Ruchirawat et al., 2005).

3.3.3. Urban Resource Infrastructure

The urban resource infrastructure can have both positive and negative affects on health. Urban infrastructure may include both explicit health-related resources, such as health and social services, as well as municipal structures (e.g., law enforcement), which are shaped by national and international policies (e.g., legislation and cross-border agreements).

The relation between availability of health and social services and urban living is complicated and varies between and within cities and countries. In wealthy countries, cities are often characterized by a catalog of health and social services. Even the poorest urban neighborhood often has dozens of social agencies, both governmental and non-governmental, each manifesting a distinct mission and providing different services. Many of the health successes in urban areas in the last two decades, including reductions in HIV transmission, teen pregnancy rates, tuberculosis control, and new cases of childhood lead poisoning, have depended in part on the efforts of these groups. For example, social and health services are frequently more available in cities than they are in non-urban areas, which may contribute to better health and well-being among urban residents. Despite wider availability of social and health services in cities, however, many cities experience remarkable disparities in wealth between relatively proximate neighborhoods; these disparities are often associated with differences in the availability and quality of care. Low-income urban residents face significant obstacles in finding health care both in wealthy and less-wealthy countries.

Local legislation and governmental policies can have substantial influence on the health of urban dwellers. Historically, municipal regulations regarding sanitation in the 19th and 20th centuries facilitated vast improvements in population health and led to the formation of national groups dedicated to improving population health like the American Public Health Association (Brieger, 1966). A contemporary example of the power of legislation to influence health has been ongoing in New York City (USA) since 2002. The city government implemented a comprehensive tobacco control strategy that included increased taxes on cigarettes, smoke free workplaces (including bars and restaurants), and health services aimed at cessation (including a free nicotine-patch program) (Frieden, Mostashari, Kerker, Miller, Hajat, & Frankel, 2005). Health department surveys indicated that, from 2002 to 2003, smoking prevalence among adults in New York City decreased by 11%.

4. Studying the Relation Between Cities and Population Health

There is a long and rich tradition of studying how cities and city living may influence population health. It is useful to think about empiric work that has explored this issue in three categories: urban vs. rural, inter-urban, intra-urban. In the following section we consider these three categories in turn, highlighting the contributions and limitations of each of these designs.

4.1. Urban vs. Rural

Urban vs. rural studies typically contrast urban areas with rural areas in the same country or consider morbidity and mortality in urban vs. non-urban areas. Essentially, these studies seek to determine whether morbidity and mortality due to a specific health outcome is different in specific urban areas as compared to specific non-urban areas.

Urban versus rural (or non-urban) comparisons are useful in drawing attention to particular health outcomes that may be more or less prevalent in urban areas and merit further investigation to examine the specific features of the urban (or rural) environment that are associated with that outcome. It is important to consider the substantial variability within urban, suburban and rural areas. Within a city there can be wide variation with respect to housing quality, retail establishments, parks, racial/ethnic and socioeconomic characteristics of residents and many other variables between neighborhoods. Using a factor analysis approach, McDade and Adair (2001) sought to empirically evaluate different definitions of urbanicity in Cebu City (Philippines). They concluded that urban-rural comparisons are useful for only the most general studies of urbanicity and health.

More recent work has refined distinctions such as urban core, urban adjacent, urban non-adjacent and rural. Even these categories become blurred when considering newer phenomenon such as "edge cities", cities at major suburban transportation intersections (Garreau, 1991). Even with such refinements in the definition of urban, urban-rural comparisons remain limited in their ability to identify what those factors may be and the pathways through which they affect the health of urban dwellers. Features of cities change over time, and some factors may not be conserved between cities (e.g., racial/ethnic distribution). It is unsurprising, then that different urban-rural comparisons have provided conflicting evidence about the relative burden of disease in urban and non-urban areas. At best, these studies reveal gross estimates of the magnitude and scope of health measures in broad geographical areas typically defined by size and population density.

4.2. Inter-Urban

Inter-urban studies typically compare health outcomes between two or more urban areas between or within countries. Such studies can simply identify differences between cities, or they can begin to examine specific features of cities that influence health. Examples of the former are numerous. For instance, Vermeiren and colleagues (2003) have compared mental health outcomes among adolescents in New Haven (United States), Arkhangelsk (Russia) and Antwerp (Belgium), providing insights on cross-cultural and cross-urban similarities and differences in antisocial behavior, depression, substance use, and suicide. A study of Puerto Rican injection drug users in New York City (United States) and Bayamón (Puerto Rico) revealed several differences between the two ethnically similar populations; injection drug users in Puerto Rico injected more frequently (Colon et al., 2001) and had higher rates of needle sharing as compared to their New York counterparts (Deren et al., 2001). The authors pointed to similarities in drug purity (Colon et al., 2001) and differences in the onset of the crack epidemic (Deren et al., 2001) as city-level factors that influenced injector risk behaviors. When using the city as the unit of analytic interest, one implicitly assumes that city-level exposures are equally important for all residents. Studying differences in drug use risk behaviors among two cities does not permit analysis of differences in behaviors within cities due to location of residence, variability in barriers to safer behaviors, or variations in access to key services (e.g., drug treatment, needle exchange) provided to different urban residents. However, inter-urban studies such as the examples mentioned here can help guide municipal and state policy makers when making decisions on service provision throughout a city.

4.3. Intra-Urban

Intra-urban studies typically compare health outcomes within cities and are becoming widely used to investigate specific features of the urban environment. These studies often focus on neighborhoods, specific geographic areas within a city that are generally administrative groupings (e.g., census tracts in Canada, sub-areas or suburbs in South Africa). However, it is important to note that these areas may not represent residents' perceptions of their neighborhoods. The Project for Human Development in Chicago Neighborhoods (PHDCN), which identified collective efficacy as a determinant of violence in urban neighborhoods (Sampson, Raudenbush, & Earls, 1997), is an example of such studies and has demonstrated their potential to guide specific interventions to improve urban health. As a result of findings from the PHDCN, public health interventions have been developed that attempt to increase collective efficacy and social capital in particular urban neighborhoods.

Recent innovations in statistical methodology have enabled the consideration of multi-level determinants of health (see Chapters 15 and 17 in this book for a fuller description of statistical methodologies). Many of these studies have empirically shown that living in disadvantaged areas is associated with poor health and that there are substantial inequalities in health. For example, evidence has shown an association between neighborhood-level poverty and all-cause mortality (Hahn et al., 1996), AIDS incidence (Zierler et al., 2000), low birthweight (Krieger et al., 2003), sexually transmitted diseases (Luke, 2004), and tuberculosis (Luke, 2004).

Intra-urban studies may contribute important insights into the relations between specific urban features and health outcomes. However, it may be difficult to generalize from one city to another. For instance, the relation between collective efficacy and violence may be modified by differential access to illicit substances within a given city. Furthermore, it is important to consider that neighborhood residence is a function of geographical location and social ties that are facilitated or necessitated by the urban environment (Bond, Valente, & Kendall, 1999).

5. Conclusion

Urban living and urbanization can have substantial influence on health and disease among urban populations. Evaluating the cross-national role of urbanicity alone as a construct has limited utility in illuminating the pathways through which urban living can impact health. Investigating the way in which the process of urbanization together with features of the urban environment affect health can help to elucidate these pathways and thus provide potential targets for public health interventions and governmental policies. Recent empirical research has begun to evaluate the independent associations between specific characteristics of the social environment and health within specific cities. Much more work will need to be done to establish cross-national comparisons that may enable us to draw conclusions that are generalizable across cities and across countries.

It is important to consider that the specific features of the urban environment do not exist in a vacuum. In other words, the interactions between the physical environment, urban resource infrastructure, and the social environment are important. The process of urbanization then intersects with the urban environment at any one point in time through demographic change and changes in land use, availability, and the impact on agriculture and natural resources. Additionally, regional, national and international politics, events and governance can have substantial impact on the features of the urban environment. Moving forward, investigations into the nature of the interactions between these macro-level determinants of health may offer new understanding of how urban living shapes the health of populations and may suggest avenues for potential intervention.

Acknowledgements   Parts of this paper are adapted from Galea, S., & Vlahov, D. (2005a). Urban health: Evidence, challenges, and directions. *Annual Review of Public Health,* 26,341–65 and from Galea, S., Freudenberg, N., Vlahov, D. (2005). Cities and population health. *Social Science & Medicine,* 60(5),1017–1033. Fuller discussions of the role urbanization and urbanicity play in shaping population health can be found in several chapters in Galea, S., & Vlahov, D. (2005b) *Handbook of Urban Health: Populations, methods, and practice.* Springer Science and Business Media Publishers.

References

Andrulis, D. P. (1997). The urban health penalty: New dimensions and directions in inner-city health care. In American College of Physicians (Ed.), *Inner city health care.* Philadelphia: American College of Physicians.

Arriaga, E. E. (1970). A new approach to the measurements of urbanization. *Economic Development & Cultural Change, 18,* 206–219.

Bain, K., & Hicks, N. (1998). Building social capital and reaching out to excluded groups: The challenge of partnerships. Presentation at: CELAM meeting on the struggle against poverty towards the turn of the millennium, Washington, DC.

Berkman, L. F., & Kawachi, I. (2000). *Social epidemiology.* New York: Oxford University Press.

Birenbaum, A., & Sagarin, E. (1976). *Norms and human behavior.* New York: Praeger.

Bond, K. C., Valente, T. W., & Kendall, C. (1999). Social network influences on reproductive health behaviors in urban northern Thailand. *Social Science & Medicine, 49,* 1599–1614.

Brieger, G. H. (1966). Sanitary reform in New York City: Stephen Smith and the passage of the Metropolitan Health Bill. *Bulletin of the History of Medicine, 40,* 407–429.

Cohen, D., Spear, S., Scribner, R., Kissinger, P., Mason, K., & Wildgen, J. (2000). "Broken windows" and the risk of gonorrhea. *American Journal of Public Health, 90,* 230–236.

Coleman, J. S. (1990). *Foundations of social theory.* Cambridge, MA: Harvard University Press.

Colon, H. M., Robles, R. R., Deren, S., Sahai, H., Finlinson, H. A., Andia, J., et al. (2001). Between-city variation in frequency of injection among Puerto Rican injection drug users: East Harlem, New York, and Bayamon, Puerto Rico. *Journal of Acquired Immune Deficiency Syndromes, 27,* 405–413.

Cook, R. L., Royce, R. A., Thomas, J. C., & Hanusa, B. H. (1999). What's driving an epidemic? The spread of syphilis along an interstate highway in rural North Carolina. *American Journal of Public Health, 89,* 369–373.

Coutts, A., & Kawachi, I. (2006). The urban social environment and its effects on health. In N. Freudenberg, S. Galea, & D. Vlahov (Eds.), *Cities and the health of the public*. Nashville: Vanderbilt University Press.

Davis, M. (2006). *Planet of slums*. New York: Verso.

Deren, S., Robles, R., Andia, J., Colon, H. M., Kang, S. Y., & Perlis, T. (2001). Trends in HIV seroprevalence and needle sharing among Puerto Rican drug injectors in Puerto Rico and New York: 1992–1999. *Journal of Acquired Immune Deficiency Syndromes, 26*, 164–169.

De Silva, M. J., & Harpham, T. (2006). Maternal social capital and child nutritional status in four developing countries. *Health & Place*, Epub ahead of print.

Drukker, M., Buka, S. L., Kaplan, C., McKenzie, K., & Van, O. J. (2005). Social capital and young adolescents' perceived health in different sociocultural settings. *Social Science & Medicine, 61*, 185–198.

Frieden, T. R., Mostashari, F., Kerker, B. D., Miller, N., Hajat, A., & Frankel, M. (2005). Adult tobacco use levels after intensive tobacco control measures: New York City, 2002–2003. *American Journal of Public Health, 95*, 1016–1023.

Frye, V., Latka, M. H., Koblin, B., Halkitas, P. N., Putnam, S., Galea, S., et al. (2006). The urban environment and sexual risk behavior among men who have sex with men. *Journal of Urban Health, 83*, 308–324.

Galea, S., Freudenberg, N., Vlahov, D. (2005). Cities and population health. *Social Science & Medicine, 60*(5),1017–1033.

Galea, S., & Vlahov, D. (2005a). Urban health: Evidence, challenges, and directions. *Annual Review of Public Health, 26*, 341–65.

Galea, S., & Vlahov, D. (2005b) *Handbook of Urban Health: Populations, methods, and practice*. Springer Science and Business Media Publishers.

Garreau, J. (1991). *Edge city: Life on the new frontier*. New York: Doubleday.

Godfrey, R., & Julien, M. (2005). Urbanisation and health. *Clinical Medicine, 5*, 137–141.

Gordon-Larsen, P., Nelson, M. C., Page, P., & Popkin, B. M. (2006). Inequality in the built environment underlies key health disparities in physical activity and obesity. *Pediatrics, 117*, 417–424.

Hahn, R. A., Eaker, E. D., Barker, N. D., Teutsch, S. M., Sosniak, W. A., & Krieger, N. (1996). Poverty and death in the United States. *International Journal of Health Services, 26*, 673–690.

Herold, M., Goldstein, N. C., & Clarke, K. C. (2003). The spatiotemporal form of urban growth: Measurement, analysis and modeling. *Remote Sensing of Environment, 86*, 286–303.

Hinrichsen, D., Blackburn, R., & Robey, B. (2001). Cities at the forefront – population growth and urbanization. *Population Reports*, preview edition.

Kawachi, I., & Berkman, L. (2003). *Neighborhoods and health*. New York: Oxford University Press.

Kawachi, I., Kennedy, B. P., Lochner, K., & Prothrow-Stith, D. (1997). Social capital, income inequality, and mortality. *American Journal of Public Health, 87*, 1491–1498.

Kennedy, B. P., Kawachi, I., Prothrow-Stith, D., Lochner, K., & Gupta, V. (1998). Social capital, income inequality, and firearm violent crime. *Social Science & Medicine, 47*, 7–17.

Klitzman, S., Matte, T. D., & Kass, D. E. (2006). The urban physical environment and its effects on health. In N. Freudenberg, S. Galea, & D. Vlahov (Eds.), *Cities and the health of the public*. Nashville: Vanderbilt University Press.

Krieger, N., Chen, J. T., Waterman, P. D., Soobader, M. J., Subramanian, S. V., & Carson, R. (2003). Choosing area based socioeconomic measures to monitor social inequalities in low birth weight and childhood lead poisoning: The Public Health Disparities Geocoding Project (US). *Journal of Epidemiology and Community Health, 57,* 186–199.

Leviton, L. C., Snell, E., & McGinnis, M. (2000). Urban issues in health promotion strategies. *American Journal of Public Health, 90,* 863–866.

Lochner, K., Kawachi, I., & Kennedy, B. P. (1999). Social capital: A guide to its measurement. *Health & Place, 5,* 259–270.

Luke, D. A. (2004). *Multilevel modeling.* Thousand Oaks, CA: Sage.

McCarthy, M. (2000). Social determinants and inequalities in urban health. *Reviews on Environmental Health, 15,* 97–108.

McDade, T. W., & Adair, L. S. (2001). Defining the "urban" in urbanization and health: A factor analysis approach. *Social Science & Medicine, 53,* 55–70.

McMichael, A. J. (2000). The urban environment and health in a world of increasing globalization: Issues for developing countries. *Bulletin of the World Health Organization, 78,* 1117–1126.

Park, R. E., & Burgess, E. W. (1925). *The city.* Chicago: University of Chicago Press.

Pilkington, P. (2002). Social capital and health: Measuring and understanding social capital at a local level could help to tackle health inequalities more effectively. *Journal of Public Health Medicine, 24,* 156–159.

Putnam, R. D. (1993). *Making democracy work: Civic traditions in modern Italy.* Princeton, NJ: Princeton University Press.

Ramadan, E., Feng, X. Z., & Cheng, Z. (2004). Satellite remote sensing for urban growth assessment in Shaoxing City, Zhejiang Province. *Journal of Zhejiang University Science, 5,* 1095–1101.

Ruchirawat, M., Navasumrit, P., Settachan, D., Tuntaviroon, J., Buthbumrung, N., & Sharma, S. (2005). Measurement of genotoxic air pollutant exposures in street vendors and school children in and near Bangkok. *Toxicology and Applied Pharmacology, 206,* 207–214.

Sampson, R. J., Raudenbush, S. W., & Earls, F. (1997). Neighborhoods and violent crime: A multilevel study of collective efficacy. *Science, 277,* 918–924.

Takano, T., Nakamura, K., & Watanabe, M. (2002). Urban residential environments and senior citizens' longevity in megacity areas: The importance of walkable green spaces. *Journal of Epidemiology and Community Health, 56,* 913–918.

Thomas, W. I., & Znaniecki, F. (1999). The concept of social disorganization, reprinted from The Polish peasant in Europe and America, Chicago: University of Chicago Press, 1918. In S. H. Traub & C. B. Little (Eds.), *Theories of deviance.* 5th edition. Itasca, Il: F.E. Peacock.

United Nations. (2004). *World urbanization prospects: The 2003 revision, data tables and highlights.* New York: United Nations.

United Nations. (2006). *World urbanization prospects: The 2005 revision population database.* New York: United Nations.

United Nations Human Settlements Programme (UN-HABITAT). (2004). *Second session of the World Urban Forum: Executive summary.* Geneva: United Nations.

Vermeiren, R., Schwab-Stone, M., Deboutte, D., Leckman, P. E., & Ruchkin, V. (2003). Violence exposure and substance use in adolescents: Findings from three countries. *Pediatrics, 111,* 535–540.

Vlahov, D., Galea, S., & Freudenberg, N. (2005). The urban health "advantage". *Journal of Urban Health, 82,* 1–4.

Vlahov, D., Gibble, E., Freudenberg, N., & Galea, S. (2004). Cities and health: History, approaches, and key questions. *Academic Medicine, 79,* 1133–1138.

Wandersman, A., & Nation, M. (1998). Urban neighborhoods and mental health – psychological contributions to understanding toxicity, resilience, and interventions. *American Psychologist, 53,* 647–656.

Weich, S., Burton, E., Blanchard, M., Prince, M., Sproston, K., & Erens, B. (2001). Measuring the built environment: Validity of a site survey instrument for use in urban settings. *Health & Place, 7,* 283–292.

Wilson, J. Q., & Kelling, G. L. (1982). Broken windows: The police and neighborhood safety. *The Atlantic Monthly, 249,* 29–38.

World Health Organization. (2005). *Global health atlas.* New York: World Health Organization.

Zierler, S., Krieger, N., Tang, Y., Coady, W., Siegfried, E., DeMaria, A., et al. (2000). Economic deprivation and AIDS incidence in Massachusetts. *American Journal of Public Health, 90,* 1064–1073.

Chapter 4
Corporate Practices

Nicholas Freudenberg and Sandro Galea

1. Introduction

In the 21st century, corporations are the dominant global organizational form. Of the 100 largest economies in the world in 2000, 51 were corporations and the combined sales of the world's top 200 corporations were larger than the combined economies of all countries excluding the biggest 10 (Anderson & Cavanagh, 2000). Today corporations influence every aspect of human experience, from diet, air pollution, work, and health care to personal identity, life style, sexuality, and governance. As corporations have displaced prior social influences, such as religion, family, community, and government, their impact on health has also increased. Although the preponderance of evidence suggests that the overall burden of disease imposed by consumer products such as tobacco, high fat-low nutrient foods, automobiles, and firearms is large and growing (Choi, Hunter, Tsou, & Sainsbury, 2005; Richmond, Cheney, & Schwab, 2005; Yach, Hawkes, Gould, & Hofman, 2004) public health researchers have rarely studied corporations or the free markets in which they are embedded as direct social determinants of health. Instead, they have focused on the social stratification, stresses, and inequities that the market system creates, leaving relatively unexamined the pathways by which corporate decisions influence population health.

In this chapter, we summarize the various ways that corporations influence health, then describe in more detail one increasingly important pathway – the impact on health of the products corporations manufacture and sell and their practices to maximize such sales. Finally, we examine the public health response to health-damaging corporate behaviors and suggest research and practice strategies to reduce their harm.

2. Corporations as a Social Determinant of Health

The corporation first emerged in Europe in the 16th and 17th centuries as a way of pooling capital in order to invest in commercial opportunities that no single investor could realize on his own. In the 19th century, corporations helped to amass the capital necessary for building the railways, canals, and other infrastructure needed to sustain the Industrial Revolution. By the end of that century, both England and United States had passed laws that limited the personal liability of investors for the harm caused by their business activity and that loosened controls on mergers and acquisitions (Bakan, 2004; Berle & Means, 1968; Galbraith, 1952). These changes set the framework for the modern corporation, which Ambrose Bierce jocularly defined in 1911 as "an ingenious device for obtaining individual profit without individual responsibility" (Bierce, 1911).

In the past century, corporations have penetrated almost every sector of human experience. They set patterns of employment and working conditions for a significant sector of the working population (Hippert, 2002; LaDou, 2003), are a dominant voice in welfare, tax, trade, health care, and environmental policies within many nations and global organizations (Fort, Mercer, & Gish, 2004; Pollock & Price, 2003; Waitzkin, Jasso-Aguilar, Landwehr, & Mountain, 2005), and shape patterns of consumption and life style through the products they make and their advertising (Cross, 2002; De Graaf, Wann, & Naylor, 2001; Hawkes, 2006; Schor, 2004). They also increasingly operate privatized services, such as health care, education, corrections, and security, that were previously public (Sclar & Leone, 2001); control growing sectors of public space and media (Bagdikian, 2004; Mitchell, 2003); and influence individual consciousness in such diverse areas as family life, sexuality, body image, and self-worth (Schor & Holt, 2000). Through these and other pathways, corporations have become a major influence on individual and population health.

2.1. Levels of Analysis

The multiple pathways by which corporations influence health require researchers to focus their investigations on a specific level of analysis. In previous health research, these have included the free market capitalist system as a whole, a specific national economy, a particular industry, a single company, or a single product. Table 4.1 lists examples of research questions and selected studies at these different levels. Each approach has distinct advantages and disadvantages, depending on the objectives of the analyst. For example, advocates seeking to reduce gun violence might choose to look at the firearms industry as a whole to identify opportunities for policy intervention, while those seeking to remove *trans* fat from food products to prevent cardiovascular disease and diabetes may focus on this single but pervasive product.

Since a comprehensive review of the findings of each level of analysis is beyond the scope of this chapter, we seek to more generally explore the health impact of the business and political activities of corporations. These practices result from companies' decisions about production, pricing, distribution, and promotion of their products and from their political efforts to create an environment favorable for their business. Our focus is less "fundamental" than the capitalist

TABLE 4.1. Levels of analysis of health consequences of corporate system.

Level	Research questions	Selected references
Free market system as a whole	What are the overall health consequences of free market capitalism? How does global economic system explain global disparities in health?	Navarro, 2004; Engels, 1987;
National/regional economy	What is the relationship of a nation's or region's (e.g. European Union, NAFTA nations) economic and political system on health and health disparities? How do differences in market systems between two nations/regions explain differences in health?	Stillman, 2006; Navarro & Schmitt, 2005
Specific industry	What are the health benefits and costs of an industry (e.g. tobacco) on a nation, region or the globe?	Stebbins, 1990
Specific company	What are the health consequences of a specific company (e.g. McDonald's) on global, national or local health?	Spencer, Frank, & McIntosh, 2005
Specific product	What are the health consequences of a particular product (e.g., SUVs) on global, national or local health?	Cummings, 2002
Industry practices	What is the impact of specific practices (e.g., advertising, retail practices) on global, national or local population health? What is the attributable risk of a specific practice to selected outcomes or compared to other practices (e.g. impact of tobacco advertising or comparison of advertising and pricing)?	Austin, Melly, Sanchez, Patel, Buka, & Gortmaker, 2005

system as a whole but less proximate than the individual behaviors that corporate practices encourage.

Compared to analyses that study the health impact of the capitalist system (or any other system) as a whole, the focus employed here has greater potential for informing policies that can improve population health in the medium term. Given the current absence of social forces that can promise substantive transformation of the dominant global socioeconomic system, our more modest perspective appears to have more pragmatic public health value. Nevertheless, some believe that the system of social stratification, unequal distribution of resources, and market displacement of the public sector is itself the cause of current patterns of mortality and morbidity. For them, our perspective suggests more limited changes that may seem more symbolic than substantive. For example, ending advertising of harmful products to children and promoting strict regulation of products whose social costs may exceed their benefits, such as trans fats or Sport Utility Vehicles (SUVs), may seem too modest for those seeking more fundamental changes.

2.2. Corporate Practices that Influence Health

Corporations have an impact on health through their production processes, through their engagement in the political process, and through public consumption of the goods and services they produce. Production processes can influence health by exposing workers to unhealthy or unsafe working conditions. The International Labour Organization (ILO) estimates that among the world's 2.7 billion workers, at least 2 million deaths per year and many more illnesses and injuries are attributable to occupational diseases and injuries. The ILO also estimates that on average about 4 percent of the gross domestic product (GDP) of a nation is lost because of work-related diseases and injuries (Rosenstock, Cullen, & Fingerhut, 2006). In the United States, the economic costs of job-related injuries ($145 billion) and illnesses ($26 billion) are much higher than those for AIDS and Alzheimer's disease and are on par with those for cancer and circulatory diseases (Leigh, Markowitz, Fahs, Shin, & Landrigan, 1997). Studies of the proportion of deaths attributable to the practices of corporations are generally lacking; however, the recent history of occupational health shows strong corporate opposition to health and safety measures that reduce profit, challenge managerial authority, or increase government involvement in corporate oversight (Gochfeld, 2005; Rosner & Markowitz, 1989).

Production processes can also have a larger impact on health by exposing the population as a whole to the various pollutants or environmental damage that are manufacturing by-products Corporate influence on environmental health has increased dramatically in the 20th century. Corporate actions have contributed to global warming, deforestation, ozone depletion, and air pollution (McNeill, 2000), each associated with specific causes of mortality and morbidity (Guerra, Snow, & Hay, 2006; Haines & Patz, 2004; McMichael, 2001). Business decisions regarding which manufacturing products to use and which control technologies to install determine the environmental consequences of their production processes.

Corporations also influence health through their engagement in the political process. Their activities in this arena have a direct effect on health through their efforts to create favorable occupational, environmental, consumer regulatory, and other policies. Corporations shape health indirectly through lobbying on trade, taxation, defense, human services, education, and other issues. For example, free trade policies espoused by multinational food companies have increased the availability and lowered the cost of high fat, high sugar foods, contributing to obesity and diabetes (Hawkes, 2006). Corporations seek to lower taxes both by locating operations off shore and by changing tax law, thus reducing government revenues available for health and human services. In health care, global health companies advocate for privatization of health services, making these services less available to the poor and less accessible to public oversight (Waitzkin et al., 2005).

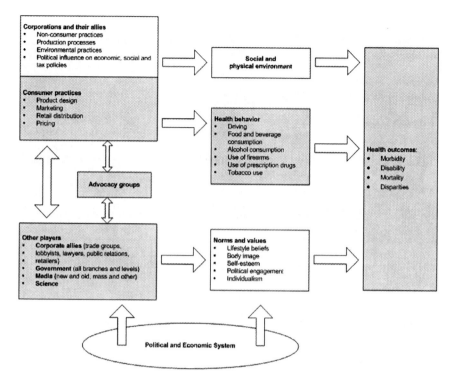

FIGURE 4.1. A conceptual model of the influence of corporate practices on health.

Figure 4.1 provides a conceptual model for the hypothesized pathways by which corporations influence health; the focus of this chapter is on the shaded portions of the figure that describe the impact of corporate practices on consumers. For the sake of brevity, we consider corporations and their allies, e.g., trade groups, lobbyists, lawyers, public relations firms, and retailers, as a single system. In fact, empirical research demonstrates complex relationships among these corporate partners (e.g., Hemenway, 2004; Kluger, 1997; Nestle, 2002), suggesting the need for further work to clarify the implications for public health intervention.

We further focus on six industries – alcohol, automobiles, firearms, food and beverages, pharmaceuticals, and tobacco. We selected these six because their products play a central role in mortality and morbidity in the developed world, their size makes them key players in the economy of the US as well as other developed and developing nations, and each has elicited public health efforts to modify harmful practices (illustrated by the box labeled "advocacy groups" in Figure 4.1). In addition, an extensive literature describes the health consequences of their products and, to a lesser extent, the role of corporate practices in shaping health risks, thus permitting a more systematic review of the findings of this body of literature. Table 4.2 summarizes the health impact of the products of these industries.

TABLE 4.2. Health impact of selected consumer products.

Industry/products	Health impact	Selected references
Alcohol	Motor vehicle accidents, cirrhosis, liver cancer, homicide, and suicide	Centers for Disease Control (CDC), 2004
Automobiles and other motor vehicles	Air pollution related respiratory diseases and cancer; driver, passenger, and pedestrian injuries and deaths	White, 2004; Environmental Protection Agency, 2004
Food and beverages	Obesity, heart disease, diabetes, some cancers	Katz, O'Connell, Yeh, Nawaz, Njike, Anderson, Cory, & Dietz, 2005
Firearms	Homicide, suicide, accidental and intentional injuries	Centers for Disease Control (CDC), 1999
Pharmaceuticals	Overuse, toxic effects	Centers for Disease Control (CDC), 2005
Tobacco	Cancers, heart disease, respiratory diseases	Stratton, Shetty, Wallace, & Bondurant, 2001

3. Summary of Evidence on Impact of Corporate Practices on Health

Four broad corporate practices have been linked to health outcomes: production and design, marketing, retail distribution, and pricing. Figure 4.2 lists the various mechanisms through which decisions in each practice can influence health. In this section, we review selected evidence to illustrate the pathways and mechanisms by which corporate practices in the target industries (alcohol, automobiles, firearms, food and beverages, pharmaceuticals, and tobacco) influence health and to illuminate future research needs and opportunities for intervention. In order to consider a wide range of relevant research, we include not only studies that have explicitly linked corporate practices to particular health indicators, but also those that examine the associations between corporate practices and health behaviors, e.g., tobacco use, diets associated with obesity, etc. We note that the availability and previous synthesis of evidence varies widely by industry. Tobacco, for example, has been studied most systematically; the literature on the food industry and health is only now expanding rapidly, while the literature on the firearms and pharmaceutical industries is sparser. Our goal is to highlight evidence that illustrates how practitioners and researchers have gone about examining the link between corporate practices and health. In the future, systematic reviews of the health impact of corporate practices by industry, practice, and health outcome are needed to advance our understanding.

3.1. Production and Design

Production and design refers to business decisions about where to invest capital and about the specific characteristics of a product. In market economies, corporate managers are expected to maximize profit for shareholders; failure to do so

---

Overview of Corporate Practices that Harm Health

Production and Design
1. Shift capital to production of more profitable but less healthy products
2. Add design features that harm health but increase profits
3. Resist addition of health enhancing features in order to avoid increasing production costs.
4. Shift investment or redesign products to reach new market where harm to health may be greater
5. Fail to test for safety prior to production or marketing

Marketing
1. Increase population exposure to harmful products
2. Misrepresent health consequences of product in order to encourage consumption
3. Target vulnerable populations for marketing of harmful products
4. By-pass legal restrictions on sale of unsafe or unhealthy products

Retail distribution
1. Increase access to and availability of unhealthy products
2. Decrease access to and availability of healthy products

Pricing
1. Lower prices of unhealthy products to attract new customers
2. Raise prices of health-enhancing products to increase profit

---

FIGURE 4.2. Overview of Corporate Practices that Harm Health

constitutes fiduciary neglect of their main responsibility (Friedman, 1982). A first step in maximizing profit is to assure that capital is invested in the most profitable ventures available, which are constrained by corporate history, technology, competitors, and law. A second step is to design a particular product so as to maximize profits. Unfortunately, as the following examples illustrate, the decisions about where to invest capital and how to design products may run counter to health.

3.1.1. Shifting Capital to Production of more Profitable but Less Healthy Products

To maximize profits, a company or industry can decide to shift its capital from the production of a less damaging to a more health damaging product in order to maximize profit. Sport Utility Vehicles (SUVs) provide a recent example. From the early 1990s to 2005, SUVs have been the best-selling and most profitable vehicles made by the US auto industry; each vehicle returns a profit 10–12 times higher than for conventional cars. During the 1990s, US auto makers invested billions of dollars in new factories to build these vehicles, meanwhile reducing their focus on producing less polluting and more fuel-efficient vehicles.

SUVs are characterized by a pick-up truck underbody, high ground clearance, enclosed rear cargo area, and available 4-wheel drive (Bradsher, 2002). SUVs, together with pickup trucks and minivans, are considered "light trucks," a category that has its own regulatory standards separate from that of passenger cars. By 2000, light trucks accounted for 40 percent of US motor vehicles, double the 1980 rate (Coate & Vanderhoff, 2001).

SUVs pose several health and environmental problems. Because of their design, compared with other vehicles they are more likely to roll over, more likely than sedans to kill pedestrians and occupants of cars they hit, harder to steer, take longer to stop, and more likely to give their drivers a false sense of security that leads to riskier driving. They also produce more pollution than passenger cars, contributing to respiratory disease, cancer, global warming, and other conditions (Bradsher, 2002; Environmental Protection Agency, 2004; Haines & Patz, 2004; National Highway Traffic Safety Administration, 2005; White, 2004). Based on a review of scientific and government reports, Bradsher (2002) estimates that through the previously described mechanisms, SUVs account for roughly 3,000 excess deaths per year.

In recent years, rising gas prices and increased public concerns about SUV safety and pollution led to sharp declines in sales. US auto manufacturers find it difficult to abandon this sector of the market, however, because of their heavy investment in SUV production, the high unit profitability of SUVs, and the stiff competition from foreign auto makers in other sectors of the business (Wald, 2006).

In the last several decades, the food and beverage industries has chosen to use corn-based fructose rather than other sweeteners in processed foods and sweetened drinks. Between 1970 and 1990, the consumption of high fructose corn syrup increased by more than 1000%, far exceeding the changes in intake of any other food or food group (Bray, Nielsen, & Popkin, 2004). A variety of evidence suggests that these products have contributed to the epidemics of obesity and diabetes (Bray et al., 2004), yet government subsidies and changes in food production make corn syrup cheap and therefore highly profitable (Pollan, 2006).

Similarly, the decision by several domestic gun manufacturers to invest in and significantly increase production of "Saturday night special" handguns in the 1980s and 1990s contributed to an increase in homicides in that period (Hemenway, 2004: 133). According to one study, 60 percent of guns traced to crimes in the early 1990s were produced by Southern California's "Ring of Fire" gun makers, who had recently expanded production of Saturday night specials (Wintemute, 1994).

In another example, pharmaceutical companies make investment decisions that adversely affect population health when they do not develop products that are life saving but unprofitable (e.g., vaccines (Andre, 2002)), often known as "orphan drugs" (Schieppati, Remuzzi, & Garattini, 2001), or to create products that are unnecessary but profitable, a practice labeled as "disease mongering" (Moynihan & Cassels, 2005).

3.1.2. Designing Features that Harm Health but Increase Profit

A second mechanism by which corporate practices can influence health is when producers modify their products in ways that harm health, often in order to increase sales or profits or reduce costs. The addition of trans fats to hundreds of US food products in the last four decades illustrates how product design intended to increase shelf life, and therefore profitability, can have dire health consequences. Trans fats are solid fats produced artificially by heating liquid vegetable oils in the presence of metal catalysts and hydrogen (Ascherio, Stampfer, & Willett, 1999). They are used to enhance the crispness, creaminess, stability, flavor, and shelf life of many processed and fast foods. By the late 1990s, roughly 40 percent of supermarket products contained trans fats, commonly identified on labels as partially-hydrogenated fats. In 1994, the Center for Science in the Public Interest (CSPI), a national advocacy organization, petitioned the Food and Drug Administration (FDA) to require that food manufacturers label the *trans* fatty acid (trans fat) content of their food products. The petition was based on new research showing that replacing trans fat with healthier oils could prevent between 30,000 and 100,000 premature cardiovascular deaths in the United States each year (Willett et al., 1993). In 1999, the FDA estimated that strengthening food labeling was likely to yield significant health and economic benefits, including saving 2,100 to 5,600 lives a year and $3 billion to $8 billion a year (Food and Drug Administration, 1999). Not until 2006, however, did new regulations go into effect requiring food companies to list the trans fat content on nutritional labels.

3.1.3. Resisting Addition of Health Enhancing Features in Order to Avoid Increasing Production Costs

In some cases, failure to change product design harms health. The auto industry has initially resisted almost every proposed safety or pollution reduction feature: e.g., mandatory seat belts, air bags, and improved fuel efficiency (Doyle, 2000). As early as 1965, Ralph Nader, in his book *Unsafe at Any Speed: The Designed-In Dangers of the American Automobile* (1965), described many examples of auto industry reluctance to spend money on improving safety.

The food industry also resists making changes. If the next 100 billion McDonald's burgers sold were vegetable-based rather than beef-based burgers, they would provide an additional 1 billion pounds of fiber and 660 million pounds of protein and would reduce saturated fats and total fat by 550 million pounds and 1.2 billion pounds, respectively (Spencer, Frank, & McIntosh, 2005). The higher profitability of meat-based products in the present economy makes such a transformation unlikely.

In another example, redesigning handguns and other firearms to include trigger locks, magazine safety devices, and owner identification systems and avoiding making guns that can be mistaken for toys could substantially reduce accidental and intentional injuries and deaths (Carbone, Clemens, & Ball, 2005; Hemenway, 2004). Despite evidence that gun locks and other safety features can mitigate the adverse consequences of guns in the home (Carbone et al., 2005), gun makers have resisted government efforts to make such features required or more routinely available (Siebel, 2000).

3.1.4. Shifting Investment or Redesigning Products to Reach New Markets where Harm to Health may be Greater

In another pathway, companies or industries make production or design decisions that result in new populations being exposed to harmful products. For example, liberalization of trade policies beginning in the 1980s and culminating in the 1994 North American Free Trade Agreement opened new opportunities for transnational food companies to invest and profit in Mexico. Between 1987 and 1999, for example, direct US investment in Mexican food processing companies increased from US$210 million to US$5.3 billion, a 25-fold increase. As a result, these companies sold more processed food in Mexico, per capita consumption of snack foods and carbonated beverages increased substantially, and obesity rates increased by more than 75 percent (Hawkes, 2006).

Similarly, when the regulatory environment and public opinion became less favorable to tobacco in the United States, the tobacco industry decided to invest in developing nations with less burdensome regulations (Mackay, 1992; Stebbins, 1990). In these nations, not only does tobacco directly impose future health problems on millions of people, expenditures on tobacco and its health consequences divert precious limited resources away from desperately needed basic human requirements (Stebbins, 1990).

Designing products to appeal to a new demographic group can expose additional people to a harmful product. If the targeted population happens to have a greater vulnerability (e.g., because of age, socioeconomic status, gender or other characteristics), these corporate decisions may contribute to the exacerbation of health disparities. For example, RJ Reynolds redesigned Camel cigarettes by including an additive to reduce throat irritation (Wayne & Connolly, 2002), and some companies have introduced cigarette brands with candy-like flavors (Carpenter, Wayne, Pauly, Koh, & Connolly, 2005); both of these changes were designed to appeal to young smokers. The tobacco industry also added menthol to attract women (O'Keefe & Pollay, 1996) and African-Americans (Sutton & Robinson, 2004), contributing to increased smoking rates among these groups (Ezzati & Lopez, 2003).

Similarly, in the last decade, the alcohol industry has developed and marketed wine coolers and "alcopops," sweetened alcoholic drinks designed to appeal to young drinkers (Mosher & Johnsson, 2005). Alcopops are frozen sweetened products that contain fruit juices and alcohol, a product that has been called "training wheels for drinkers" by public health advocates and that an industry spokesperson called "the perfect bridging beverage." The tobacco and alcohol industries invest capital in designing products that attract and retain future customers, counting on the addictive properties of their products to hold on to at least some portion of initiators.

3.1.5. Failing to Test for Safety Prior to Production or Marketing

To save money or the time needed to get a product to market, companies sometimes fail to test a product for safety adequately or ignore early warnings about possible harm. It now seems apparent that Merck failed to test Vioxx sufficiently prior to production and marketing and ignored potentially troublesome findings in its own research (Topol, 2004). Both the Bridgestone/Firestone North American Tire Company and Ford Motor Company blamed each other for failing to act earlier on information that Ford Explorer SUVs equipped with Firestone tires had higher rates of accidents than comparable vehicles with other tires (Vernick, Mair, Teret, & Sapsin, 2003).

3.2. Marketing

Marketing describes corporate strategies and activities to encourage consumption and increase demand. It includes advertising, sales promotions, sponsorship of sports and music events, product placement, viral marketing, and websites and Internet campaigns (Ewen, 1977; Hawkes, 2006).

Corporations rely heavily on advertising as a tool to encourage consumption of their products, and evidence shows that for many products advertising is associated with increased consumption (Chen, Cruz, Schuster, Unger, & Johnson, 2002; Collins, Schell, Ellickson, & McCaffrey, 2003; Grube & Wallack, 1994; Mastro & Atkin, 2002; Wakefield, Flay, Nichter, & Giovino, 2003) and positive brand identification, itself associated with subsequent increases in consumption (Donovan, Jancey, & Jones, 2002).

Between 1990 and 2005, total inflation-adjusted expenditures on advertising in the United States increased by 50 percent, a measure of its growing role in business spending. In 2005, US advertisers spent $933 per capita. The industries profiled here were among the biggest advertisers; of the nearly $100 billion the top 100 global marketers spent in 2004, 24 percent was devoted to automotive advertising; 17 percent to food, restaurants, soft drinks, and candy; and 9 percent to pharmaceuticals (Assadourian, 2006).

3.2.1. Increasing Population Exposure to Harmful Products

Most directly, advertising can increase exposure to harmful products, thus magnifying their adverse impact on population health. For example, between 1999 and 2004, Merck spent more than $500 million advertising Vioxx to consumers (Topol, 2004), and in 2003 alone the company spent another $500 million advertising Vioxx to physicians (Brown, 2004). By 2004, when Merck withdrew the drug because of safety concerns, more than 20 million people had used Vioxx, generating $10 billion in revenues for the company (Topol, 2004).

Despite the previously described health hazards associated with SUVs, the automobile industry, the nation's largest advertiser, has promoted the profitable SUVs heavily; automakers spent more than $9 billion on SUV ads between 1990 and 2001 (Coate & Vanderhoff, 2001).

3.2.2. Misrepresenting Health Consequences of Products in Order to Encourage Consumption

Advertising can also contribute to health problems by understating risks inherent in products and overstating their potential benefits, leading consumers to choose a more dangerous product than they would if they were fully informed. For example, despite evidence to the contrary, auto advertisements often suggested that SUVs were safer than passenger cars (Claybrook, 2003) and that they offered a way to escape the stresses of every day life by enabling drivers to scale mountains, ford rivers, and enter primal forests.

Merck advertisements implied that Vioxx and other COX-2 inhibitors (drugs in the same class as Vioxx) were superior painkillers compared to the much less expensive over-the-counter alternatives (Brown, 2004). Unfortunately, the evidence about the superiority of Vioxx and other COX-2 inhibitors is flimsy (Modica, Vanhems, & Tebib, 2005). This became particularly important when evidence emerged about the increased risk of stroke and myocardial infarction that attended Vioxx use (Topol, 2004).

Further, even when manufactures alert consumers to the adverse consequences of their products, they often do so in a way intended to minimize the impact. Although much public health effort has been expended on adding health warnings to tobacco products and to alcohol and tobacco advertisements, studies have suggested that these notices are developed to minimize their impact (Hammond, Fong, McNeill, Borland, & Cummings, 2006). One study found that the majority of adolescents viewing these advertisements do not even notice the public health warnings (Fischer, Richards, Berman, & Krugman, 1989).

3.2.3. Targeting Vulnerable Populations for Marketing of Harmful Products

All industries seek to target their advertising to potential customers. This practice affects public health when harmful products are more heavily advertised to populations who are already at higher risk of health problems. The tobacco industry has been particularly sophisticated in its use of targeted advertising to increase smoking in particular age, gender, racial/ethnic, and socioeconomic groups. For example, tobacco companies have conducted systematic and extensive research to design cigarette packaging in a way that it is most appealing to target customers (Wakefield, Morley, Horan, & Cummings, 2002). In addition, several studies have shown that Black and Latino groups and neighborhoods are disproportionately exposed to cigarette advertisements (Alaniz & Wilkes, 1998; Balbach, Gasior, & Barbeau, 2003; King, Siegel, & Pucci 2000; Muggli, Pollay, Lew, & Joseph, 2002; Wildey et al., 1992), as are poorer persons and neighborhoods (Luke, Esmundo, & Bloom, 2000). Similarly, tobacco advertising has targeted women, specifically appealing to their perceived needs and wants (Anderson, Glantz, & Ling, 2005; Toll & Ling, 2005). Targeted advertising of tobacco to youth occurs in venues frequented by youth, including bars and clubs (Gilpin, White, & Pierce, 2005; Sepe & Glantz, 2002) and stores where adolescents shop frequently (Celebucki & Diskin, 2002; Henriksen, Feighery, Schleicher, Haladjian, & Fortmann, 2004). Analyses of tobacco industry documents have suggested that industry marketing has explicitly aimed to target young smokers (Cummings, Morley, Horan, Steger, & Leavell, 2002), and studies have shown that nearly 90 percent of 13 year olds report exposure to cigarette marketing (Schooler, Feighery, & Flora, 1996).

The food industry similarly often targets children. Research has shown that food advertising during the television programs children watch most is dominated by advertisements for snack, convenience, and fast foods (Harrison & Marske, 2005), which may have a substantial impact on children's dietary habits and subsequent adult obesity (Henderson & Kelly, 2005). It has been estimated that American children see on average 40,000 commercials per year on television, the majority of which are for unhealthy foods (Horgen, 2005). The food industry has also targeted schools for marketing campaigns, seeking to capitalize on a captive population of future lifetime consumers (Shaul, 2000). When faced with growing evidence about the link between advertising for unhealthy foods and obesity and the looming threat of regulatory action to control such advertising, large food companies like Kraft have put a moratorium on food advertising for children (Mayer, 2005).

The alcohol industry has also targeted advertising at promising customers, including children and youth, women, minorities, and problem drinkers. These ads seek to introduce people to drinking and to encourage profitable patterns of consumption. Tobacco and alcohol billboards have been shown to be more prevalent in poor neighborhoods than adjoining better-off neighborhoods (Hackbarth, Silvestri, & Cosper, 1995; Hackbarth, Schnopp-Wyatt, Katz, Williams, Silvestri, & Pfleger, 2001), and alcohol advertising in magazines has specifically targeted gender groups (Alaniz & Wilkes, 1998; Jernigan, Ostroff, Ross, & O'Hara, 2004) and racial/ethnic groups (Jones-Webb, Baranowski, Fan, Finnegan, & Wagenaar, 1997). The alcohol industry has also used targeted advertising to shape drinking patterns among minorities (Cui, 2000), college students (DeJong, 2002), adolescents (Ellickson, Collins, Hambarsoomians, & McCaffrey, 2005; Garfield, Chung, & Rathouz, 2003; Grube & Wallack, 1994), and problem drinkers. One study found that alcohol advertisements in magazines expose young people aged 12 to 20 – and thus below legal drinking age – to 48 percent more beer advertisements, 20 percent more distilled spirits advertisements, and 92 percent more "alcopops" advertising than adults 21 and over (Center on Alcohol Marketing and Youth, 2005). National studies have demonstrated an association between increased exposure to alcohol advertising and increased adolescent consumption of alcohol (Snyder, Milici, Slater, Sun, & Strizhakova, 2006).

Another study found that in the same period that alcohol drinking among teenage girls increased dramatically, more alcohol advertising reached young women than young men (Jernigan et al., 2004). A study by the Center on Addiction and Substance Abuse (Foster, Vaughan, Foster, & Califano, 2006) estimated that 17.5 percent of US alcohol sales in 2001 came from underage drinking and 20.1 percent from adult "pathological" drinking, a category that used clinical definitions for alcohol abuse or dependence. These data illustrate the financial value of targeting these groups for advertising or other promotion.

In the late 1980s and early 1990s, gun manufacturers targeted women for advertising, using ads that highlighted fear of violence (Hemenway, 2004). Some studies claim that gun ads target children and youth (Langley, 2001) and that others demonstrate misleading claims about the safety benefits of firearms (Vernick, Teret, & Webster, 1997).

3.2.4. Bypassing Legal Restrictions on Sale of Unsafe or Unhealthy Products

Advertising also connects buyers to sellers, sometimes bypassing legal controls or safety standards. For example, one study found that 53 percent of 184 major city newspapers in the US accepted gun ads for all types of guns, regardless of whether or not the seller was a licensed gun dealer (Jacobs, 2002: 132). These advertising practices make it easier for those who cannot purchase guns legally to acquire a firearm. Similarly, tobacco and alcohol advertising and Internet sales can help underage consumers to buy these products (Ribisl, Williams, & Kim, 2003).

In another example, the drug company Parke-Davis promoted off-label use of gabapentin (brand name Neurontin, an agent to control epilepsy). A review of industry documents found that the company recruited local doctors to communicate favorable messages about gabapentin to their physician colleagues and paid medical communication companies to develop and publish articles about gabapentin in the medical literature and to suppress unfavorable study results (Steinman, Bero, Chren, & Landefeld, 2006). Ultimately, Warner-Lambert, then owner of Parke-Davis, agreed to plead guilty and pay more then $430 million to resolve criminal charges and civil liabilities in connection with its illegal and fraudulent promotion of unapproved uses for the drug ("Drug maker to pay," 2004).

3.3. Retail Distribution

Retail distribution refers to industry practices that affect product availability at the consumer level; manufacturers seek a retail distribution system that makes their products readily accessible to as many potential consumers as possible. Placement of fast food outlets, supermarkets or liquor stores; location of products within stores; adherence with legal industry restrictions on retail practices; or industry oversight of retail distribution of prescription drugs, firearms, or tobacco are examples of business decisions that affect product availability and therefore impact health.

The relationships between producers and retailers are complex and influenced by both national and local factors. At the national level, the state of the economy, profit margins in the industry, and the degree to which retailers have independent political muscle influence their ability to negotiate with producers. Locally, the competitive environment within various sectors and neighborhoods and the degree of vertical and horizontal integration with other retailers (e.g., Wal-Mart vs. the local bodegas) also influence the process and outcome of retailing decisions and thus their impact on health.

3.3.1. Increasing Access to and Availability of Unhealthy Products

Companies use retail distribution systems to make their products widely available and demonstrate ingenuity and flexibility in devising new retail strategies. For example, when laws have restricted or banned advertising, the tobacco industry has moved to its retail network to find new customers. Tobacco companies have used incentive programs to ensure placement of tobacco products in visible locations (Feighery, Ribisl, Clark, & Haladjian, 2003) and made extensive use of point-of-purchase (POP) promotions (e.g., "buy two, get one free" specials) (Feighery, Ribisl, Schleicher, Lee, & Halvorson, 2001) to enhance tobacco sales. Evidence suggests that such promotions increase when limits are imposed on more traditional advertising. One analysis has shown that POP cigarette promotions increased notably in the aftermath of the tobacco Master Settlement Agreement (MSA) that imposed price increases and tobacco control programs (Loomis, Farrely, Nonnemaker, & Mann, 2006). Studies of POP tobacco promotion have found that they increase positive images of smoking and beliefs in the availability of cigarettes (Donovan et al., 2002; Wakefield, Germain, Durkin, & Henriksen, 2006).

The food industry also uses POP promotions. Producers and distributors pay supermarkets to give prominent shelf space to higher-profit food items, often high-calorie, low-nutrient processed foods or sweetened beverages that contribute to obesity (Nestle, 2006a). In addition, supermarkets place products in such a way as to encourage young children to nag their parents to buy heavily advertised, often sweet and processed food (Nestle, 2006a).

As with tobacco, evidence suggests that retail availability of alcohol influences patterns of drinking. Point-of-purchase marketing has been shown to increase alcohol sales and consumption substantially, with one study showing that such promotions increased beer sales by as much as 17 percent (Beverage Industry, 2001). In a CDC study (2003) of nearly 4,000 alcohol outlets, 94 percent had some form of POP marketing.

Retail automobile dealers serve as the link between car manufacturers and consumers. The products they choose to promote most heavily, the discounts they offer, and their role in safety issues influence the vehicles customers purchase. Because SUVs were more profitable for dealers as well as manufacturers, dealers played an active role in promoting these vehicles, even though they were less safe and more polluting than other products (Bradsher, 2002). For example, some dealers built off-road tracks to allow adventuresome customers to test drive their SUVs, even though few owners actually go off road.

Retail availability of firearms influences who can get guns for what price. Use of largely unregulated guns shows, distribution of guns to unlicensed retailers, and willingness to accept straw purchasers are among the practices that have been associated with increased access to guns for those who would otherwise be barred from buying a weapon (Hemenway, 2004). One anecdote illustrates the practice: In 1999, a Milwaukee gun dealer posted a billboard bragging that his store had been rated first in sales of guns later used in crimes. The owner reported that the advertising and ranking helped business (McBride, 1999).

The density of retail outlets also affects product use. For example, a study in Chicago found that both minors and adults living in neighborhoods with a higher density of tobacco retail outlets were more likely to smoke than those living in lower density neighborhoods (Novak, Reardon, Raudenbush, & Buka, 2006).

Tobacco vending machines and sales of tobacco over the Internet make the products more readily available to minor and adult smokers (Centers for Disease Control, 1996; Ribisl, 2003).

Similarly, several analyses have shown spatial clustering of fast-food restaurants closer to schools, making it easier for children to find products that can contribute to overweight and obesity. Austin and colleagues (2005) showed that 78 percent of Chicago schools had at least one fast-food restaurant within 800 meters and that there was an estimated 3–4 times as many fast-food restaurants within 1.5 kilometers of schools than would be expected if fast-food restaurants were randomly distributed throughout the city. A national analysis, using data from the Behavioral Risk Factor Surveillance Survey, suggested that square miles per fast-food restaurant and residents per restaurant accounts for 6 percent of the variance in state obesity rates in multivariable hierarchical models that account for potential confounders including physical activity and fruit and vegetable intake (Maddock, 2004). These observations suggest that availability of obesogenic food may well be deleterious to health in and of itself and may be contributing to the obesity epidemic that has been extensively documented in the past 15 years.

Higher alcohol outlet density is also associated with higher consumption of alcohol and higher rates of alcohol-related health problems, including homicide and gonorrhea (Cohen et al., 2006; Gruenwald & Remer, 2006; Pollack, Cubbin, Ahn, & Winkleby, 2005).

In the alcohol, firearms and tobacco industries, laws often regulate retail distribution of these products, limiting access to certain populations. When producers or retailers oppose these laws or advocate against enforcement, they contribute to wider availability. One study found that the vigor of enforcement of retail tobacco laws influences tobacco availability to young people (Jason, Pokorny, Muldowney, & Velez, 2005). In addition, alcohol retailers seek to use the law to maximize the venues and hours in which they can sell alcohol in stores, bars, and other settings, further influencing alcohol availability. In the automobile industry, retail auto dealers play an active role in lobbying against safety and fuel efficiency regulations, providing the auto industry with a more acceptable public face (Doyle, 2000).

3.3.2. Decreasing Access to and Availability of Healthy Products

Distributors of lower cost and healthier foods, such as chain supermarkets, may be less likely to open retail facilities in low-income neighborhoods, in part because of the perception of lower profit margins, fears of crime, or neighborhood instability. As a result of such business decisions, disadvantaged communities have less access to affordable fresh fruits and vegetables and low-fat products. Several recent studies have documented the lower prevalence of supermarkets in low-income than in high-income neighborhoods (Moore & Diez-Roux, 2006; Morland, Wing, Diez-Roux, & Poole, 2002; Zenk et al., 2005).

To what extent are the locations of retail food outlets the result of decisions by major food companies as compared to more impersonal market forces or choices by local retailers? Evidence suggests that factors influencing these decisions are specific to company, product, time, and place. For example, a vertically-integrated company such as McDonald's or Wal-Mart can decide when and where to open facilities or award franchises, thus giving these corporations a powerful voice in shaping the retail landscape, the American diet, and inequities in access to healthy and unhealthy foods (Quinn, 2005; Schlosser, 2001; Spencer et al., 2005). In contrast, the observation that the small grocery stores and bodegas prevalent in low-income urban neighborhoods (Moore & Diez-Roux, 2006) are less likely to stock fresh fruits and vegetables or low-fat dairy products (Glanz & Yaroch, 2004) appears to be a result of various market forces, e.g., turnover and economies of scale, rather than a central decision by any company.

Pharmacists and retail pharmacy chains make decisions that affect pricing, drug availability, and the information consumers have about drugs. Studies have shown that pharmacists often fail to inform consumers about available discounts (Lewis et al., 2002), thus increasing the price of drugs and presumably decreasing their availability to some consumers. In addition, some pharmacies have failed to substitute less expensive generics for more expensive brand name drugs, raising costs to consumers and profits for retailers and manufacturers. In some cases, these practices have led to legal action against retail drug stores (National Legislative Association on Prescription Drug Prices, 2005).

Retailers can also influence gun safety practices. It has been shown that gun locks are only sporadically available through gun retailers (Milne & Hargarten, 1999), and retailers rarely educate customers about safe gun storage (Sanguino, Dowd, McEnaney, Knapp, & Tanz, 2002).

3.4. Pricing

Pricing practices determine who pays how much for a product; therefore these practices influence who is exposed to what level of harmful products. Companies and their retail affiliates decide how much to charge various customers, whether or not to engage in legal or illegal price fixing, whether to oppose or support excise taxes, and how to relate to illicit markets (e.g., untaxed tobacco products).

Producers price products in order to maximize sales. Among the strategies they use are pricing loss leaders to attract customers who will then become loyal consumers, offering discounts or rebates, fixing prices with other producers to reduce competition (often an illegal practice), winning public subsidies so as to lower costs to consumers, and resisting taxes that will increase prices. Pricing practices influence health when unhealthy products become more attractive because of their lower price or health-promoting products become less attractive because of higher prices. We illustrate with a few examples from each of the target industries.

3.4.1. Lowering Prices of Unhealthy Products to Attract New Customers

A variety of evidence shows that as the price of tobacco increases, demand falls. One estimate suggests that a 10 percent increase in cigarette prices would reduce overall cigarette consumption by between 2.5 and 5 percent (Chaloupka,

Wakefield, & Czart, 2001). A review of tobacco company documents showed that the industry carefully studied the impact of price on demand and developed pricing strategies, such as promoting lower-cost generic brands, absorbing the cost of increased excise taxes, and offering discounts and coupons in order to retain more price-sensitive customers (Chaloupka, Cummings, Morley, & Horan, 2002). In addition, the tobacco industry has aggressively resisted increased excise taxes at local, state, and federal levels (Morley, Cummings, Hyland, Giovino, & Horan, 2002).

The federal government has long subsidized the US food industry, providing growers and manufacturers with the financial support needed to maintain prices lower than would be dictated by market forces alone. In recent decades, these policies have made corn-based products such as corn sweeteners the foundation of a significant portion of processed food both in the United States and globally; each year the federal government provides corn growers with $4 billion in direct payments (Pollan, 2006). Some observers have linked the growing proportion of calories in the US diet derived from corn sweeteners with the parallel rise of obesity and diabetes (Gross, Li, Ford, & Liu, 2004).

Like other products, alcohol consumption is subject to price elasticity – higher prices lead to lower consumption. Studies show that beer consumption is insensitive to price while wine and distilled spirits are more sensitive (Chaloupka, Grossman, & Saffer, 2002). The alcohol industry has been relatively successful in resisting increased excise taxes, contributing to the decline in the real price of alcohol in recent decades (Chaloupka, Grossman et al., 2002). In California in 2005, the alcohol industry unsuccessfully campaigned to classify "alcopops" as a beer rather than a distilled spirit in order to benefit from the lower tax rate for beer and thus make the product more accessible to the price-sensitive youth market (Marin Institute, 2006).

As the allure of SUVs declined in recent years, the auto industry has offered a variety of price incentives, including rebates, discounts, and low-cost loans, in order to stimulate demand (Warner, 2004). While these efforts have not been able to reverse the trend, they have served to put more of these unsafe and polluting vehicles on the road, thus perpetuating their adverse health impact.

In the gun industry, the previously described increase in production of cheap Saturday night special guns (Wintemute, 1994) in the 1980s and 1990s ensured that low cost weapons would be available in the low-income communities most sensitive to price. This pricing strategy contributed to rising gun homicide rates in these areas in that period. Young people and low-level criminals seeking to purchase guns benefit most from low-cost weapons (Wintemute, 2002).

3.4.2. Raising Prices of Health-Enhancing Products to Increase Profit

Raising prices of health-enhancing products can discourage their use. For example, car manufacturers sometimes make new safety technology an option available at additional cost rather than a standard feature. Although this practice allows consumers to tailor the purchase to their own economic and safety needs, it eliminates the lower price benefits from economies of scale. Thus, the average customer chooses a lower sticker price – and a less safe vehicle.

The pharmaceutical industry seeks to maintain control of drug prices – usually advocating for higher prices in order to preserve profits. It opposes more rapid introduction of generic drugs in order to sustain the monopoly benefits from high-priced drugs that a company has patented, opposes competition from manufacturers in other countries that sell at lower prices, opposes legislation that would allow the government to negotiate bulk discounts on drugs, and supports federal programs that subsidize drug costs for populations such as senior citizens (Angell, 2004; Baker, 2004). These practices make good business sense but often make it harder for individuals to get the drugs they need.

4. Interactions with Other Sectors

In order to achieve their business objectives in investment and product design, marketing, retail distribution, pricing, and other areas not reviewed here, corporations and their business associations interact with government, scientists, and mass media. To the extent that that these interactions influence the health consequences of various corporate practices, they are of interest to public health researchers. In this section, we describe some of the ways that corporations in the six target industries seek to influence government, scientists, and mass media to support their goals.

4.1. Government

Corporations seek to influence all levels and branches of government to advance business policy objectives that contribute to profitability. In their interactions with government, corporations and their allies seek to advance their business goals in the four areas previously described, i.e., investment and product design, marketing, retail distribution, and pricing. Their broad goals are to avoid regulation or other types of public oversight of these and other practices, minimize taxes or other charges that reduce profits, maximize direct public support for their activities through subsidies or tax breaks, and retain the right to shift external costs imposed by their products or practices (e.g., pollution or health harm) to other sectors. To achieve these objectives, businesses carry out a variety of activities including lobbying, campaign contribution, litigation, public relations, and encouragement of a revolving door between government and business. In some cases, businesses resort to illegal activities such as bribery or influence peddling. Industry interactions with government are of public health interest when they prevent public officials from acting to protect health and safety or when they result in the wider availability and distribution of health-damaging products.

Lobbying and other legislative activities are a central tool for advancing corporate objectives. In 2000, the Center for Responsive Politics estimated that there were more than 20,000 registered lobbyists in Washington, D.C.

About 1,000 lobbyists work in the nation's capital for the food industry (Nestle, 2002) and 675 for the pharmaceutical industry (Brown & Doyle, 2004). More lobbyists work in state capitals. In the mid-1990s, for example, the tobacco industry had 25 lobbyists in Minnesota alone (Wolfson, 2001), working to defeat or water down that state's tobacco regulations. Between 1998 and 2005, total reported spending on lobbying increased by 160 percent to $2.28 billion (Center for Responsive Politics, 2006).

Lobbyists work both to pass beneficial legislation and to defeat harmful laws. In 2003, for example, the pharmaceutical industry poured millions of dollars into a concerted – and successful – lobbying effort to convince Congress to pass legislation that would increase coverage of senior citizens for some prescription drugs and defeat provisions that would have allowed the federal government to negotiate lower prices on behalf of Medicare patients or import lower-cost medicines from Europe or Canada. Analysts estimated the law would increase drug company profits by $13 billion a year. Pharmaceutical companies acted despite overwhelming public support for the restrictions they opposed and expert opinion that the measure would leave major gaps in coverage and fail to contain costs (Connolly, 2003). In 1994, lobbyists for the dietary supplement industry persuaded Congress and the President to label dietary supplements as foods rather than drugs, thus escaping FDA requirements for safety and effectiveness. A few years later, after aggressive advertising of the benefits of these products, deaths from supplements, such as ephedra, illustrated the public health costs of this deregulation and led to calls for renewed public oversight (Fontarosa, Drummond, & DeAngelis, 2003).

Campaign contributions and other electoral activities help to cement the friendly relationships between elected officials and industry by increasing the chances that the legislators or executive branch officials will be grateful or indebted to lobbyists. Many industry political action committees contribute to both parties, ensuring influence no matter what the outcome of an election. In 2002, for example, the drug industry contributed about $22 million to the Republicans and almost $8 million to Democrats (Brown & Doyle, 2004). The NRA and its gun industry allies offer not only financial support to sympathetic candidates, but also assistance in voter mobilization and campaigning (Diaz, 1999). This helps to explain why the gun industry and the NRA consistently win legislative victories even though public opinion polls show high levels of public support for restrictions on assault rifles and opposition to exempting gun manufacturers from liability suits.

Litigation allows industry to delay, weaken, or overturn laws and regulations it dislikes. Corporations and their allies go to court to seek action against individuals, organizations, and government agencies that they perceive as threats to their business goals. In 2000, for example, seven gun makers filed a suit against the US Secretary for Housing and Urban Development, the New York State Attorney General, and other state and local officials, claiming they were violating the gun makers' right to sell legal firearms by seeking to force them to accept a code of conduct on the sale and design of handguns. The manufacturers did not

seek monetary damages but instead asked the court to bar the officials from trying to convince local police departments to buy weapons only from companies
that had signed the agreement (Brown & Abel, 2003). The automobile industry
has regularly gone to court to challenge state and federal clean air and emission
control legislation (Doyle, 2000).

Public relations fosters a positive public image for corporate America and
blocks proposals that harm its perceived interests (Marchand, 1998). In some
cases, the use of public relations strategies also involve interactions with the
media, described in Section 4.3. When critics challenge the safety of a product,
corporations and their trade associations often respond forcefully, looking to
preclude action to limit profits, to restrict advertising, or to regulate manufacturing or distribution. For example, when the FDA proposed new regulations for
vitamins, industry groups sponsored television ads showing soldiers storming
suburban homes to seize vitamin C bottles (Kessler, 2001). To make their public
messages more credible, industries may create front groups to act as their public
voice. Philip Morris formed the National Smokers Alliance to contest tobacco
regulation (Kessler, 2001), the tobacco, food, and restaurant industries funded the
Center for Consumer Freedom to oppose smoking bans in public places and
lower legal limits on blood alcohol levels (Brownell, 2003: 269), and the auto
industry hired a Washington lobbying firm to create Nevadans for Fair Fuel
Economy Standards, a paper organization that opposed higher mileage standards
that would reduce pollution (Bradsher, 2002: 64).

Public relations seeks to frame the public dialogue on issues relevant to the
industry (Dorfman, Wallack, & Woodruff, 2005), often articulating strikingly
similar messages. These include "market mechanisms, not government action,
provide the best remedies for dangers to consumers," "it is wrong to restrict
advertising of legal products," "individuals are responsible for their own behavior," and "having choices is the American way" (Brownell, 2003; Diaz, 1999;
Menashe & Siegel, 1998). In many cases, public relations expenses are tax
deductible, creating a public subsidy for messages intended to thwart policy
changes to protect health.

The revolving door between government and business ensures that both sides
of the interaction are friendly to corporate interests. For example, presidential
adviser Karl Rove had been chief political strategist for Philip Morris before
working for Bush, and President Bush's first chief of staff, Andrew Card, had
been General Motors' top lobbyist in Washington, D.C. (Bradsher, 2002). Daniel
Glickman, secretary of agriculture in the Clinton administration, left office to join
a law firm that lobbies for agriculture and food companies (Nestle, 2002). In
1994, when Philip Morris needed someone to testify against FDA regulation of
tobacco before Congress, it hired former FDA Commissioner Charles Edwards,
paying him $120,000 for the consultancy (Kessler, 2001). In 1998, 128 former
members of Congress were listed as lobbyists, 12 percent of all senators and representatives who had left office since 1970 (Abramson, 1998; Nestle, 2002).
Compared to the handful of lobbyists who advocate for public health, these personal and professional associations between elected and appointed officials and

corporate lobbyists provide industry with a competitive advantage in influencing legislation and regulation.

Illegal activities, such as bribery, influence peddling, or price fixing, are another strategy some corporations have used to advance their objectives. In the early 1970s, Ford Motor Company fabricated auto safety test data that it submitted to the government, leading to a $7 million fine (Yates, 1983). In 1994, tobacco industry executives lied under oath to Congress about their prior knowledge of nicotine's addictiveness (Kessler, 2001), and in 1999, the US Justice Department reached a $255 million settlement with the vitamin industry for price fixing, a practice that made its products more expensive for consumers (Nestle, 2002). Given spotty enforcement of regulations on corporate behavior, data are not available to ascertain whether illegal activities constitute the renegade actions of a few bad apples or a common business practice that endangers public health.

In sum, a variety of evidence shows that corporations act to increase the likelihood that the government will support or at least not oppose their business agenda. In some cases, these actions prevent or undermine government efforts to protect public health. To date, systematic investigation of the burden of disease that can be attributed to these activities has been lacking, suggesting the need for more research.

4.2. Science

Companies seek to influence the scientific community in order to develop or redesign more profitable products, win regulatory approval (e.g., FDA approval of Vioxx), and challenge scientific research that threatens their business interests (e.g., food industry-sponsored research to challenge university research on role of trans fats in cardiovascular disease). This strategy contributes to the development of unsafe or unhealthy products. Activities to influence science include sponsorship and publication of research by their own research departments, trade associations (e.g. the now defunct Tobacco Institute), university-based researchers, or scientific and professional organizations, as well as contributions to universities and professional organizations. Examples include food industry support for nutrition researchers who emphasize exercise rather than diet as the cause of obesity and several recent cases in which pharmaceutical companies have been accused of withholding evidence from their own research on the side effects of their drug products such as Vioxx, Paxil, and others (Harris, 2004; Topol, 2004).

Krimsky (2003), who has studied corporate behavior related to scientific research, uses the term "manufactured doubt" to describe the practice of sowing confusion to avoid or delay regulatory action. In some cases, scientists have hidden the industry sponsorship of their work, limiting the ability of the scientific community, policy makers, and the public to assess bias or conflict of interest (Hardell, Walker, Walhjalt, Friedman, & Richter, 2006). More broadly, some academic leaders have warned against growing corporate influence on the scientific research enterprise, compromising universities' ability to be an independent voice (Bok, 2003).

4.3. Mass Media

Corporations seek to influence mass media in order to create a social and political climate favorable to their agenda, to frame their messages, to combat threats to profitability, and to advance their specific economic, electoral, legislative, legal, and other policy goals (Ewen, 1996; Marchand, 1998). Activities include public relations, communications, philanthropy, organization of front groups, and public service campaigns. For the most part, these activities are seen as standard business practices and are therefore tax deductible. Corporations and their allies interact with the media in order to communicate their messages to the general public and government and more broadly to influence the public discourse on corporations and their role in society. Activities such as public relations (described above in Section 4.1), corporate philanthropy, and corporate (as opposed to product) advertising are of interest to public health to the extent they enable industry to better distribute products that harm health. Industry can also use its advertising power to discourage coverage of certain topics. For example, in a stark display of the power of the tobacco industry, in the 1980s no women's magazine that accepted tobacco advertising published a single article, editorial, or column on the harmful effects of tobacco, despite the fact that it was then that lung cancer surpassed breast cancer as the leading cause of cancer deaths among women (Anderson, 1995; Hertz, 2001).

As US and global media ownership becomes more concentrated among a handful of large multinational corporations (Bagdikian, 2004), often with links to industries that produce harmful products, the willingness of major media outlets to investigate corporate malfeasance or disease promotion may further diminish.

5. Societal Responses to Health-Damaging Corporate Practices

In the 19th century, reformers and public health and social science researchers called attention to the health impact of the emerging capitalist system. Engels' *The Condition of the Working Class in England* described how the English factory system contributed to the "wretched conditions" of the working class in England. Nine years later, John Snow, a physician-epidemiologist, convinced a local London parish to remove the handle from the Broad Street pump that a private company used to bring drinking water from a polluted river, contributing to the epidemic of cholera. Removing the pump handle was an early form of direct public oversight of corporate practices.

Later, health researchers called attention to the health consequences of working conditions, documenting higher rates of cancer, injuries, and other conditions among workers in particular industries. These occupational illnesses were often exacerbated by corporate unwillingness to sacrifice profits for improved working conditions. Recent research, for example, has demonstrated that from the

1920s on, the lead industry hid its knowledge of the toxic results of lead exposure (Markowitz & Rosner, 2002).

In the 20th century, reformers as well as public health professionals publicized the risks associated with the practices of various industries. In 1906, Upton Sinclair published *The Jungle*, an exposé of dangerous working conditions and the unsanitary products of the meat industry. In 1964, the US Surgeon General published the first report on smoking and health, beginning a continuing campaign to reduce the harm from the products of the tobacco industry. A year later, Ralph Nader published *Unsafe at Any Speed*, an investigation of the automobile industry's failure to protect car owners from known safety hazards. By the 1970s, consumer advocates were pressing for a federal agency to protect consumers against industries intent on profiting at the expense of public health.

Today, health professionals; consumer, health and environmental advocates; local officials; and others are modifying old strategies and developing new ones to contest corporations' power to shape health. Like the corporations they challenge, they have used a variety of strategies and tactics to achieve their goals of reducing the harm from corporate practices. These include electoral, legislative and legal strategies, media advocacy, community organizing, and others (Freudenberg, 2005).

While a review of this emerging domain of public health practice is beyond the scope of this chapter, several questions warrant further investigation. These include:

1. To what extent do the disparate activities designed to change corporate practices in several industries that have been launched by consumer, health and environmental activists constitute an emerging social movement (Wiist, 2006)? What are the relative advantages and disadvantages of a more comprehensive approach to changing corporate behavior as compared to the more common piece-meal approach?
2. What is the potential for establishing collaborative partnerships with industry to modify health-damaging practices? Under what political and economic circumstances will corporations engage in genuine joint ventures, and when are some efforts more cosmetic than substantive? Some recent evidence suggests that even when companies agree to cooperate, their practice does not necessarily match their commitment to achieving public health goals (Nestle, 2006b).
3. What are the characteristics of effective public health campaigns to change corporate practices? Are local or regional campaigns more effective than national ones? What "frames" serve to best mobilize constituencies in support of public health goals (Dorfman et al., 2005)?
4. What role can state and local health departments play in modifying corporate practices? Recent efforts to change the practices or density of food, tobacco, gun and alcohol retailers (Bragg, Galloway, Spohn, & Trotter, 2003; Schneider, Reid, Peterson, Lowe, & Hughey, 2005; Webster, Vernick, Bulzacchelli, 2006) or to institute local bans of trans fats in restaurant foods provide examples of potential roles.

5. Conclusion

We suggest that in the early part of the 21st century, corporate practices play a growing role in shaping daily behavior and well-being. In this chapter we have considered how corporate practices influence the health of populations through multiple mechanisms. Clearly, the link between corporate practices and any particular health indicator is complex, and a full understanding of each of the pathways linking corporate practices to population health can suggest multiple opportunities for intervention. Future research in the area can fruitfully both elucidate the precise links between corporate practices and population health and suggest avenues for intervention.

Acknowledgements.   Parts of this paper are adapted from Freudenberg, N. (2005). Public health advocacy to change corporate practices: implications for health education practice and research. *Health Education and Behavior. 32*(3), 298–319. The work in this chapter was supported in part by an American Legacy Foundation Innovative Project Award to Freudenberg. The authors would like to thank Emily Goldmann for editorial assistance.

References

Abramson, J. (1998, September 29). Ring of law and lobbying concerns circling White House have banner year. *New York Times*, p. A1.

Alaniz, M. L., & Wilkes, C. (1998). Pro-drinking messages and message environments for young adults: The case of alcohol industry advertising in African American, Latino, and Native American communities. *Journal of Public Health Policy, 19*(4), 447–472.

Anderson, R. (1995). *Consumer culture and TV programming*. Boulder, CO: Westview.

Anderson, S., & Cavanagh, J. (2000). The rise of corporate global power. Washington, DC (December 4, 2000); http://www.ips-dc.org/downloads/Top_200.pdf.

Anderson, S., Glantz, S., & Ling, P. (2005). Emotions for sale: Cigarette advertising and women's psychosocial needs. *Tobacco Control, 14*(2), 127–135.

Andre, F. E. (2002). How the research-based industry approaches vaccine development and establishes priorities. *Developments in Biologicals, 110*, 25–29.

Angell, M. (2004). *The truth about the drug companies: How they deceive us and what to do about it*. New York: Random House.

Ascherio, A., Stampfer, M. J., & Willett, W.C. (1999). *Background and scientific review trans fatty acids and coronary heart disease*. Boston, MA: Departments of Nutrition and Epidemiology, Harvard school of Public Health, The Channing Laboratory, Department of Medicine, Brigham and Women's Hospital.

Assadourian, E. (2006). Advertising spending sets another record. In The Worldwatch Institute (ed.), V*ital signs 2006–2007*. Washington, DC: World Watch Institute.

Austin, S., Melly, S., Sanchez, B., Patel, A., Buka, S., & Gortmaker, S. L. (2005). Clustering of fast-food restaurants around schools: A novel application of spatial statistics to the study of food environments. *American Journal of Public Health, 95*(9), 1575–1581.

Bagdikian, B. (2004). *The new media monopoly*. Boston: Beacon Press.

Bakan, J. (2004). *The corporation: The pathological pursuit of profit and power*. New York: Free Press.

Baker, D. (2004). A free market solution for prescription drug crises. *International Journal of Health Services, 34*(3), 517–526.

Balbach, E. D., Gasior, R .J., & Barbeau, E. M. (2003). RJ Reynolds' Targeting of African Americans: 1988–2000. *American Journal of Public Health, 93*(5), 822–827.

Berle, A. A., & Means, G. C. (1968). *The modern corporation and private property*. New York: Harcourt Brace & World.

Beverage Industry. (2001). POP proves its worth. *Beverage Industry, 92,* 44–47.

Bierce, A. (1911). The devil's dictionary. Berkeley, CA (July 8, 1998); http://sunsite.berkeley.edu/Literature/Bierce/DevilsDictionary/

Bok, D. (2003). *Universities in the marketplace: The commercialization of higher education*. Princeton and Oxford: Princeton University Press.

Bradsher, K. (2002) *High and mighty SUVs: The world's most dangerous vehicles and how they got that way*. New York: Public Affairs.

Bragg, B., Galloway, T., Spohn, D. B., & Trotter, D. E. (2003). Land use and zoning for the public's health. *The Journal of Law, Medicine & Ethics , 31*(4 Supplement), 78–80.

Bray, G. A., Nielsen, S. J., & Popkin, B. M. (2004). Consumption of high-fructose corn syrup in beverages may play a role in the epidemic of obesity. *American Journal of Clinical Nutrition, 79*(4), 537–543.

Brown, D. (2004, October 3). Promise and peril of Vioxx casts harsher light on new drugs. *Washington Post*, p. A14.

Brown, P. H., & Abel, D. G. (2003). *Outgunned: Up against the NRA*. New York: Free Press.

Brown, S., & Doyle, S. (2004, January 28). The Medicare index. *The New York Times*, p. A25.

Brownell, K. D. (2003). *Food fight: The inside story of the food industry, America's obesity crisis and what we can do about it*. New York: McGraw-Hill.

Carbone, P. S., Clemens, C. J., & Ball, T. M. (2005). Effectiveness of gun-safety counseling and a gun lock giveaway in a Hispanic community. *Archives of Pediatrics and Adolescent Medicine, 159*(11), 1049–1054.

Carpenter, C. M., Wayne, G. F., Pauly, J. L., Koh, H. K., & Connolly, G. N. (2005). New cigarette brands with flavors that appeal to youth: Tobacco marketing strategies. *Health Affairs, 24*(6), 1601–1610.

Celebucki, C. C., & Diskin, K. (2002). A longitudinal study of externally visible cigarette advertising on retail storefronts in Massachusetts before and after the Master Settlement Agreement. *Tobacco Control, 11*(Supplement 2), ii47–ii53.

Center for Responsive Politics. (2006). Lobbying Database. Washington, DC (2006); http://www.opensecrets.org/lobbyists/index.asp.

Center on Alcohol Marketing and Youth. (2005). Youth overexposed: Alcohol advertising in magazines, 2001–2003. Washington, DC (2006); http://camy.org/research/mag0405/ mag0405.pdf.

Centers for Disease Control and Prevention (CDC). (1996). Accessibility to minors of cigarettes from vending machines—Broward County, Florida, 1996. *MMWR Morbidity and Mortality Weekly Reports, 45*(47), 1036–1038.

Centers for Disease Control and Prevention (CDC). (1999). Nonfatal and fatal firearm-related injuries – United States, 1993–1997. *MMWR Morbidity and Mortality Weekly Reports, 48*(45), 1029–1034.

Centers for Disease Control and Prevention (CDC). (2003). Point-of-purchase alcohol marketing and promotion by store type—United States,2000–2001. *MMWR Morbidity and Mortality Weekly Reports*, *52*(14), 310–313.

Centers for Disease Control and Prevention (CDC). (2004). Alcohol use among adolescents and adults – New Hampshire, 1991–2003. *MMWR Morbidity and Mortality Weekly Reports*, *53*(8), 174–175.

Centers for Disease Control and Prevention (CDC). (2005). Increase in poisoning deaths caused by non-illicit drugs – Utah, 1991–2003. *MMWR Morbidity and Mortality Weekly Reports*, *54*(2), 33–36.

Chaloupka, F. J., Cummings, K. M., Morley, C. P., & Horan, J. K. (2002). Tax, price and cigarette smoking: Evidence from the tobacco documents and implications for tobacco company marketing strategies. *Tobacco Control*, *11*(Supplement 1), I62–172.

Chaloupka, F. J., Grossman, M., & Saffer, H. (2002). The effects of price on alcohol consumption and alcohol-related problems. *Alcohol Research and Health*, *26*(1), 22–34.

Chaloupka, F. J., Wakefield, M., & Czart, C. (2001). Taxing tobacco: The impact of tobacco taxes on cigarette smoking and other tobacco use. In R. L. Rabin & S. D. Sugarman (Eds.), *Regulating tobacco*. New York: Oxford University Press.

Chen, X., Cruz, T. B., Schuster, D. V., Unger, J. B., & Johnson, C. A. (2002). Receptivity to protobacco media and its impact on cigarette smoking among ethnic minority youth in California. *Journal of Health Communication*, *7*(2), 95–111.

Choi, B. C., Hunter, D. J., Tsou, W., & Sainsbury, P. (2005). Diseases of comfort: Primary cause of death in the 22nd century. *Journal of Epidemiology and Community Health*. *59*(12), 1030–1034.

Claybrook, J. (2003). Profit-driven myths and severe public damage: The terrible truth about SUVs. Washington, DC (2006); www.citizen.org/documents/JC_SUV_testimony.pdf

Coate, D., & Vanderhoff, J. (2001). The truth about light trucks. *Regulation, 24*(1), 22–27.

Cohen, D. A., Ghosh-Dastidar, B., Scribner, R., Miu, A., Scott, M., Robinson, P., et al. (2006). Alcohol outlets, gonorrhea, and the Los Angeles civil unrest: A longitudinal analysis. *Social Science & Medicine*, *62*(12), 3062–3071.

Collins, R. L., Schell, T., Ellickson, P. L., & McCaffrey, D. (2003). Predictors of beer advertising awareness among eighth graders. *Addiction*, *98*, 1297–1306.

Connolly, C. (2003, November 21). Drugmakers protect their turf: Medicare bill represents success for pharmaceutical lobby. *The Washington Post*, p. A4.

Cross, G. (2002). *An all-consuming century: Why commercialism won in modern America*. New York: Columbia University Press.

Cui, G. (2000). Advertising of alcoholic beverages in African-American and women's magazines: Implications for health communication. *Howard Journal of Communications*, *11*(4), 279–293.

Cummings, K. M. (2002). Programs and policies to discourage the use of tobacco products. *Oncogene, 21*(48), 7349–7364.

Cummings, K., Morley, C., Horan, J., Steger, C., & Leavell, N. R. (2002). Marketing to America's youth: Evidence from corporate documents. *Tobacco Control, 11*(supplement 1), i1–i17.

De Graaf, J., Wann, D., & Naylor, T. H. (2001). *Affluenza: The all-consuming epidemic*. San Francisco: Berrett-Kohler.

DeJong, W. (2002). The role of mass media campaigns in reducing high-risk drinking among college students. *Journal of Studies on Alcohol, 2002*(14), 182–192.

Diaz, T. (1999). *Making a killing: The business of guns in America*. New York: New Press.

Donovan, R., Jancey, J., & Jones, S. (2002). Tobacco point of sale advertising increases positive brand user imagery. *Tobacco Control, 11*(3), 191–194.

Dorfman, L., Wallack, L., & Woodruff, K. (2005). More than a message: Framing public health advocacy to change corporate practices. *Health Education & Behavior, 32*, 320–336.

Doyle, J. (2000). *Taken for a ride: Detroit's big three and the politics of pollution.* New York: Four Walls Eight Windows.

Drug maker to pay $430 million in fines, civil damages. (2004). *FDA Consumer, 38*(4), 36–37.

Ellickson, P., Collins, R., Hambarsoomians, K., & McCaffrey, D. F. (2005). Does alcohol advertising promote adolescent drinking? Results from a longitudinal assessment. *Addiction, 100*(2), 235–246.

Engels, F. (1987). *The condition of the working class in England.* (reprint). New York: Penguin Classics.

Environmental Protection Agency (EPA). (2004). *Control of emissions from new and in-use highway vehicles and engines,* 40 CFR 86.

Ewen, S. (1977). *Captains of consciousness: Advertising and the social roots of the consumer culture.* New York: Basic Books.

Ewen, S. (1996). *PR!.* New York: Basic Books.

Ezzati, M., & Lopez, A. D. (2003). Estimates of global mortality attributable to smoking in 2000. *Lancet, 362*(9387), 847–852.

Feighery, E. C., Ribisl, K. M., Clark, P. I., & Haladjian, H. H. (2003). How tobacco companies ensure prime placement of their advertising and products in stores: Interviews with retailers about tobacco company incentive programmes. *Tobacco Control, 12*(2), 184–188.

Feighery, E. C., Ribisl, K. M., Schleicher, N., Lee, R. E., & Halvorson, S. (2001). Cigarette advertising and promotional strategies in retail outlets: Results of a statewide survey in California. *Tobacco Control, 10*(2), 184–188.

Fischer, P. M., Richards, J. W., Berman, E. J., & Krugman, D. M. (1989). Recall and eye tracking study of adolescents viewing tobacco advertisements. *Journal of the American Medical Association, 261*(1), 84–89.

Fontarosa, P., Drummond, R., & DeAngelis, C. D. (2003). The need for regulation of dietary supplements: Lessons learned from Ephedra. *Journal of the American Medical Association, 289*, 1568–1570.

Food and Drug Administration (FDA). (1999). Food labeling: Trans fatty acids in nutrition labeling, nutrient content claims and health claims. *Federal Register, 64*, 62746.

Fort, M., Mercer, M. A., & Gish, O. (Eds.). (2004). *Sickness and wealth: The corporate assault on global health.* Cambridge, MA: South End Press.

Foster, S. E., Vaughan, R. D., Foster, W. H., & Califano, J. A., Jr. (2006). Estimate of the commercial value of underage drinking and adult abusive and dependent drinking to the alcohol industry. *Archives of Pediatrics and Adolescent Medicine, 160*(5), 473–478.

Freudenberg, N. (2005). Public health advocacy to change corporate practices: Implications for health education practice and research. *Health Education and Behavior, 32*(3), 298–319.

Friedman, M. (1982). *Capitalism and freedom.* Chicago: University of Chicago Press.

Galbraith, J. K. (1952). *American capitalism: The concept of countervailing power.* Boston: Houghton Mifflin.

Garfield, C., Chung, P., & Rathouz, P. (2003). Alcohol advertising in magazines and adolescent readership. *Journal of the American Medical Association, 289*, 2424–2429.

Gilpin, E. A., White, V. M., & Pierce, J. P. (2005). How effective are tobacco industry bar and club marketing efforts in reaching young adults? *Tobacco Control, 14*(3), 186–192.

Glanz, K., & Yaroch, A. L. (2004). Strategies for increasing fruit and vegetable intake in grocery stores and communities: Policy, pricing, and environmental change. *Preventive Medicine, 39*(Supplement 2), S75–S80.

Gochfeld, M. (2005). Occupational medicine practice in the United States since the industrial revolution. *Journal of Occupational and Environmental Medicine, 47*(2), 115–131.

Gross, L. S., Li, L., Ford, E. S., & Liu, S. (2004). Increased consumption of refined carbohydrates and the epidemic of type 2 diabetes in the United States: An ecologic assessment. *American Journal of Clinical Nutrition, 79*(5), 774–779.

Grube, J. W., & Wallack, L. (1994). Television beer advertising and drinking knowledge, beliefs, and intentions among schoolchildren. *American Journal of Public Health, 84*(2), 254–259.

Gruenewald, P. J., & Remer, L. (2006). Changes in outlet densities affect violence rates. *Alcoholism, Clinical and Experimental Research, 30*(7), 1184–1193.

Guerra, C. A., Snow, R. W., & Hay, S. I. (2006). A global assessment of closed forests, deforestation and malaria risk. *Annals of Tropical Medicine and Parasitology, 100*(3), 189–204.

Hackbarth, D. P., Schnopp-Wyatt, D., Katz, D., Williams, J., Silvestri, B., & Pfleger, M. (2001). Collaborative research and action to control the geographic placement of outdoor advertising of alcohol and tobacco products in Chicago. *Public Health Reports, 116*(6), 558–567.

Hackbarth, D. P., Silvestri, B., & Cosper, W. (1995). Tobacco and alcohol billboards in 50 Chicago neighborhoods: Market segmentation to sell dangerous products to the poor. *Journal of Public Health Policy, 16*(2), 213–230.

Haines, A., & Patz, J. A. (2004). Health effects of climate change. *Journal of the American Medical Association, 291*(1), 99–103.

Hammond, D., Fong, G. T., McNeill, A., Borland, R., & Cummings, K. M. (2006). Effectiveness of cigarette warning labels in informing smokers about the risks of smoking: Findings from the International Tobacco Control (ITC) Four Country Survey. *Tobacco Control, 15*(Supplement 3), iii19–iii25.

Hardell, L., Walker, M. J., Walhjalt, B., Friedman, L. S., & Richter, E. D. (2006). Secret ties to industry and conflicting interests in cancer research. *American Journal of Industrial Medicine.* Epub ahead of print.

Harris, G. (2004, June 3). Spitzer sues a drug maker, saying it hid negative data. *The New York Times*, p. A1.

Harrison, K., & Marske, A. L. (2005). Nutritional content of foods advertised during the television programs children watch most. *American Journal of Public Health, 95*(9), 1568–1574.

Hawkes, C. (2006). Uneven dietary development: Linking the policies and processes of globalization with the nutrition transition, obesity and diet-related chronic diseases. *Global Health, 2*, 4.

Hemenway, D. (2004). *Private guns public health.* Ann Arbor, MI: University of Michigan Press.

Henderson, V. R., & Kelly, B. (2005). Food advertising in the age of obesity: Content analysis of food advertising on general market and African American television. *Journal of Nutrition Education and Behavior, 37*(4), 191–196.

Henriksen, L., Feighery, E. C., Schleicher, N. C., Haladjian, H. H., & Fortmann, S. P. (2004). Reaching youth at the point of sale: Cigarette marketing is more prevalent in stores where adolescents shop frequently. *Tobacco Control, 13*(3), 315–318.

Hertz, N. (2001). *The silent takeover: Global capitalism and the death of democracy.* New York: Free Press.

Hippert, C. (2002). Multinational corporations, the politics of the world economy, and their effects on women's health in the developing world: A review. *Health Care for Women International, 23*(8), 861–869.

Horgen, K. B. (Ed.). (2005). *Big food, big money, big children.* Westport, CT: Praeger Publishers/Greenwood Publishing Group, Inc.

Jacobs, J. B. (2002). *Can gun control work?* New York: Oxford University Press.

Jason, L. A., Pokorny, S. B., Muldowney, K., & Velez, M. (2005). Youth tobacco sales-to-minors and possession-use-purchase laws: A public health controversy. *Journal of Drug Education, 35*(4), 275–290.

Jernigan, D. H., Ostroff, J., Ross, C., & O'Hara 3rd, J. A. (2004). Sex differences in adolescent exposure to alcohol advertising in magazines. *Archives of Pediatrics & Adolescent Medicine, 158*(7), 629–634.

Jones-Webb, R., Baranowski, S., Fan, D., Finnegan, J., & Wagenaar, A. C. (1997). Content analysis of coverage of alcohol control policy issues in black-oriented and mainstream newspapers in the U.S. *Journal of Public Health Policy, 18*(1), 49–66.

Katz, D. L., O'Connell, M., Yeh, M., Nawaz, H., Njike, V., Anderson, L. M., et al. (2005). Public health strategies for preventing and controlling overweight and obesity in school and worksite settings: A report on recommendations of the Task Force on Community Preventive Services. *MMWR. Recommendations and Reports: Morbidity and Mortal Weekly Reports, 54*(RR–10), 1–12.

Kessler, D. (2001). *A question of intent: A great American battle with a deadly industry.* New York: Public Affairs.

King 3rd, C., Siegel, M., & Pucci, L. G. (2000). Exposure of black youths to cigarette advertising in magazines. *Tobacco Control, 9*(1), 64–70.

Kluger, R. (1997). *Ashes to ashes: America's hundred year cigarette war, the pubic health, and the unabashed triumph of Philip Morris.* New York: Vintage.

Krimsky, S. (2003). *Science in the private interest: Has the lure of profits corrupted biomedical research?* Lanham, MD: Rowman and Littlefield.

LaDou, J. (2003). International occupational health. *International Journal of Hygeine and Environmental Health, 206*(4–5), 303–313.

Langley, M. (2001). *A .22 for Christmas: How the gun industry designs and markets firearms for children and youth.* Washington, DC : Violence Policy Center.

Leigh, J. P., Markowitz, S. B., Fahs, M., Shin, C., & Landrigan, P. J. (1997). Occupational injury and illness in the United States. Estimates of costs, morbidity, and mortality. *Archives of Internal Medicine, 157*(14), 1557–1568.

Lewis, J. H., Schonlau, M., Munoz, J. A., Asch, S. M., Rosen, M. R., Yang, H., et al. (2002). Compliance among pharmacies in California with a prescription-drug discount program for Medicare beneficiaries. *New England Journal of Medicine, 346*(11), 830–835.

Loomis, B. R., Farrelly, M. C., Nonnemaker, J. M., & Mann, N. H. (2006). Point of purchase cigarette promotions before and after the Master Settlement Agreement: Exploring retail scanner data. *Tobacco Control, 15*(2), 140–142.

Luke, D., Esmundo, E., & Bloom, Y. (2000). Smoke signs: Patterns of tobacco billboard advertising in a metropolitan region. *Tobacco Control, 9*(1), 16–23.

Mackay, J. (1992). US tobacco export to Third World: Third World War. *Journal of the National Cancer Institute. Monographs, 12*, 25–28.

Maddock, J. (2004). The relationship between obesity and the prevalence of fast food restaurants: State-level analysis. *American Journal of Health Promotion, 19*(2), 137–143.

Marchand, R. (1998). *Creating the corporate soul. The rise of public relations and corporate imagery in American big business*. Berkeley, CA: University of California Press.

Marin Institute. (2006). Alcohol industry loses alcopop tax battle in California. San Rafael, CA (2006); http://www.marininstitute.org/alcohol_policy/hot.htm.

Markowitz, G., & Rosner, D. (2002). *Deceit and denial: The deadly politics of industrial pollution*. Berkeley, CA: University of California Press.

Mastro, D. E., & Atkin, C. (2002). Exposure to alcohol billboards and beliefs and attitudes toward drinking among Mexican American high school students. *Howard Journal of Communications, 13*(2), 129–151.

Mayer, C. E. (2005, January 12). Kraft to curb snack-food advertising. Move phases out ads aimed at kids under 12. *Washington Post* p. E01.

McBride, J. (1999, November 29). Store's sign brags of top rank for selling guns tied to crime. *Milwaukee Journal Sentinel*.

McMichael, A. J. (2001). Impact of climatic and other environmental changes on food production and population health in the coming decades. *The Proceedings of the Nutrition Society, 60*(2), 195–201.

McNeill, J. R. (2000). *Something new under the sun: An environmental history of the twentieth century*. New York: Norton.

Menashe, C. L., & Siegel, M. (1998). The power of a frame: An analysis of newspaper coverage of tobacco issues-United States, 1985–1996. *Journal of Health Communication, 3*, 307–325.

Milne, J. S., & Hargarten, S. W. (1999). The availability of extrinsic handgun locking devices in a defined metro area. *Western Medical Journal, 98*(7), 25–28

Mitchell, D. (2003). *The right to the city: Social justice and the fight for public space*. New York: Guildford Press.

Modica, M., Vanhems, P., & Tebib, J. (2005). Comparison of conventional NSAIDs and cyclooxygenase-2 inhibitors in outpatients. *Joint Bone Spine, 72*(5), 397–402.

Moore, L. V., & Diez-Roux, A. V. (2006). Associations of neighborhood characteristics with the location and type of food stores. *American Journal of Public Health, 96*(2), 325–331.

Morland, K., Wing, S., Diez-Roux, A., & Poole, C. (2002). Neighborhood characteristics associated with the location of food stores and food service places. *American Journal of Preventive Medicine, 22*(1), 23–29.

Morley, C. P., Cummings, K. M., Hyland, A., Giovino, G. A., & Horan, J. K. (2002). Tobacco Institute lobbying at the state and local levels of government in the 1990s. *Tobacco Control, 11*(Supplement 1), I102–I109.

Mosher, J. F., & Johnsson, D. (2005). Flavored alcoholic beverages: An international marketing campaign that targets youth. *Journal of Public Health Policy, 26*(3), 326–342.

Moynihan, R., & Cassels, A. (2005). *Selling sickness: How the world's biggest pharmaceutical companies are turning us all into patients*. New York: Nations Books.

Muggli, M. E., Pollay, R. W., Lew, R., & Joseph, A. M. (2002). Targeting of Asian Americans and Pacific Islanders by the tobacco industry: Results from the Minnesota Tobacco Document Depository. *Tobacco Control, 11*(3), 201–209.

Nader, R. (1965). *Unsafe at any speed: The designed-in dangers of the American automobile*. New York: Grossman.

National Highway Traffic Safety Administration, U.S. Department of Transportation. (2005). *Federal motor vehicle safety standards: Roof crush resistance*. 49 CFR Part 571.

National Legislative Association on Prescription Drug Prices. (2005). New York settles with pharmacies for 6.7 million In Medicaid overbilling. *National Legislative Association on Prescription Drug Prices Newsletter, May 25*(2005), 11–12.

Navarro, V. (2004). The world health situation. *International Journal of Health Services, 34*(1), 1–10.

Navarro, V., & Schmitt, J. (2005). Economic efficiency versus social equality? The U.S. liberal model versus the European social model. *International Journal of Health Services, 35*(4), 613–630.

Nestle, M. (2002). *Food politics: How the food industry influences nutrition and health.* Berkeley: University of California Press.

Nestle M. (2006a). *What to eat.* New York: North Point Press.

Nestle, M. (2006b). Food industry and health: Mostly promises, little action. *Lancet, 368*(9535), 564–565.

Novak, S. P., Reardon, S. F., Raudenbush, S. W., & Buka, S. L. (2006). Retail tobacco outlet density and youth cigarette smoking: A propensity-modeling approach. *American Journal of Public Health, 96*(4), 670–676.

O'Keefe, A. M., & Pollay, R. W. (1996). Deadly targeting of women in promoting cigarettes. *Journal of the American Medical Women's Association, 51*(1–2), 67–69.

Pollan, M. (2006). *The omnivore's dilemma.* New York: Penguin Press.

Pollock, A. M., & Price, D. (2003). The public health implications of world trade negotiations on the general agreement on trade in services and public services. *Lancet, 362*(9389), 1072–1075.

Pollack, C. E., Cubbin, C., Ahn, D., & Winkleby, M. (2005). Neighbourhood deprivation and alcohol consumption: Does the availability of alcohol play a role? *International Journal of Epidemiology, 34*(4), 772–780.

Quinn, B. (2005). *How Walmart is destroying America and the world: And what you can do about it.* 3rd Edition. Berkeley, CA: Ten Speed Press.

Ribisl, K. (2003). The potential of the internet as a medium to encourage and discourage youth tobacco use. *Tobacco Control, 12*(90001), i48–i59.

Ribisl, K., Williams, R., & Kim, A. (2003). Internet sales of cigarettes to minors. *Journal of the American Medical Association, 290*(10), 1356–1359.

Richmond, T. S., Cheney, R., & Schwab, C. W. (2005). The global burden of non-conflict related firearm mortality. *Injury Prevention, 11*(6), 348–352.

Rosenstock, L., Cullen, M., & Fingerhut, M. (2006). Occupational health. In D. T. Jamison, J. G. Breman, A. R. Measham, G. Alleyne, M. Claeson, D. B. Evans, P. Jha, A. Mills, & P. Musgrove (Eds.), *Disease control priorities in developing countries.* 2nd edition. Washington, DC: World Bank.

Rosner, D., & Markowitz, G., (Eds.). (1989). *Dying for work: Worker's safety and health in twentieth-century America.* Bloomington, IN: Indiana University Press.

Sanguino, S. M., Dowd, M. D., McEnaney, S. A., Knapp, J., & Tanz R. R. (2002). Handgun safety: What do consumers learn from gun dealers? *Archives of Pediatrics and Adolescent Medicine, 156*(8), 777–780.

Schieppati, A., Remuzzi, G., & Garattini, S. (2001). Modulating the profit motive to meet needs of the less-developed world. *Lancet, 358*(9293), 1638–1641.

Schlosser, E. (2001). *Fast food nation. The dark side of the all American meal.* Boston: Houghton-Mifflin.

Schneider, J. E., Reid, R. J., Peterson, N. A., Lowe, J. B., & Hughey, J. (2005). Tobacco outlet density and demographics at the tract level of analysis in Iowa: Implications for environmentally based prevention initiatives. *Prevention Science, 6*(4), 319–325.

Schooler, C., Feighery, E., & Flora, J. A. (1996). Seventh graders' self-reported exposure to cigarette marketing and its relationship to their smoking behavior. *American Journal of Public Health, 86*(9), 1216–1221.

Schor, J. B. (2004). *Born to buy: The commercialized child and the new consumer culture.* New York: Scribner.

Schor, J. B., & Holt, D. B., (Eds.). (2000). *The consumer society reader.* New York: New Press.

Sclar, E. D., & Leone, R. C. (2001). *You don't always get what you pay for: The economics of privatization.* Ithaca, NY: Cornell University Press.

Sepe, E., & Glantz, S. A. (2002). Bar and club tobacco promotions in the alternative press: Targeting young adults. *American Journal of Public Health, 92*(1), 75–78.

Shaul, M. S. (2000). Public education: Commercial activities in schools. United States General Accounting Office report to congressional requesters. GAO/HEHS 00–156. 2000. Washington, DC (September, 2000); http://eric.ed.gov/ERICDocs/data/eric-docs2/content_storage_01/0000000b/80/22/93/f1.pdf

Siebel, B. J. (2000). The case against the gun industry. *Public Health Reports, 115*(5), 410–418.

Snyder, L. B., Milici, F. F., Slater, M., Sun, H., & Strizhakova, Y. (2006). Effects of alcohol advertising exposure on drinking among youth. *Archives of Pediatrics and Adolescent Medicine, 160*(1), 18–24.

Spencer, E. H., Frank, E., & McIntosh, N. F. (2005). Potential effects of the next 100 billion hamburgers sold by McDonald's. *American Journal of Preventive Medicine, 28*(4), 379–381.

Stebbins, K. R. (1990). Transnational tobacco companies and health in underdeveloped countries: Recommendations for avoiding a smoking epidemic. *Social Science & Medicine, 30*(2), 227–235.

Steinman, M. A., Bero, L. A., Chren, M. M., & Landefeld, C. S. (2006). Narrative review: The promotion of gabapentin: An analysis of internal industry documents. *Annals of Internal Medicine, 145*(4), 284–293.

Stillman, S. (2006). Health and nutrition in Eastern Europe and the former Soviet Union during the decade of transition: A review of the literature. *Economics and Human Biology, 4*(1), 104–146.

Stratton, K., Shetty, P., Wallace, R., & Bondurant, S. (Eds.). (2001). *Clearing the smoke: Assessing the science base for tobacco harm reduction.* Washington, DC: National Academy Press.

Sutton, C. D., & Robinson, R. G. (2004). The marketing of menthol cigarettes in the United States: Populations, messages, and channels. *Nicotine & Tobacco Research, 6*(Supplement 1), S83–S91.

Toll, B. A., & Ling, P. M. (2005). The Virginia Slims identity crisis: An inside look at tobacco industry marketing to women. *Tobacco Control, 14*(3), 172–180.

Topol, E. J. (2004). Failing the public health—rofecoxib, Merck, and the FDA. *The New England Journal of Medicine, 351*(17), 1707–1709.

Vernick, J. S., Mair, J. S., Teret, S. P., & Sapsin, J. W. (2003). Role of litigation in preventing product-related injuries. *Epidemiologic Reviews, 25*, 90–98.

Vernick, J. S., Teret, S. P., & Webster, D. W. (1997). Regulating firearm advertisements that promise home protection. A public health intervention. *Journal of the American Medical Association, 277*(17), 1391–1397.

Waitzkin, H., Jasso-Aguilar, R., Landwehr, A., & Mountain, C. (2005). Global trade, public health, and health services: Stakeholders' constructions of the key issues. *Social Science & Medicine, 61*(5), 893–906.

Wakefield, M., Flay, B., Nichter, M., & Giovino, G. (2003). *Role of the media in influencing trajectories of youth smoking. Addiction, 98*, 79–103.

Wakefield, M., Germain, D., Durkin, S., & Henriksen, L. (2006). An experimental study of effects on schoolchildren of exposure to point-of-sale cigarette advertising and pack displays. *Health Education Research, 21*(3), 338–347.

Wakefield, M., Morley, C., Horan, J. K., & Cummings, K. M. (2002). The cigarette pack as image: New evidence from tobacco industry documents. *Tobacco Control, 11*(supplement 1), i73–i80.

Wald, M. L. (2006, March 30) Automakers use new technology to beef up muscle, not mileage. *New York Times*, p. C1.

Warner, F. (2004, September 26). Climbing down from the S.U.V., and liking the view. *New York Times*.

Wayne, G. F., & Connolly, G. N. (2002). How cigarette design can affect youth initiation into smoking: Camel cigarettes 1983–93. *Tobacco Control, 11*(supplement 1), i32–i39.

Webster, D. W., Vernick, J. S., & Bulzacchelli, M. T. (2006). Effects of a gun dealer's change in sales practices on the supply of guns to criminals. *Journal of Urban Health, 83*(5), 778–787.

White, M. J. (2004). The "arms race" on American roads: The effect of sports utility vehicles and pickup trucks on traffic safety. *Journal of Law and Economics, 47*, 333–353.

Wiist, W. H. (2006). Public health and the anticorporate movement: Rationale and recommendations. *American Journal of Public Health, 96*(8), 1370–1375.

Wildey, M. B., Young, R. L., Elder, J. P., de Moor, C., Wolf, K. R., Fiske, K. E., et al. (1992). Cigarette point-of-sale advertising in ethnic neighborhoods in San Diego, California. *Health Values, 16*(1), 23–28.

Willett, W. C., Stampfer, M. J., Manson, J. E., Colditz, G. A., Speizer, F. E., Rosner, B. A., et al. (1993). Intake of trans fatty acids and risk of coronary heart disease among women. *Lancet, 341*(8845), 581–585

Wintemute, G. J. (1994). *Ring of fire: The handgun makers of southern California.* Sacramento, CA: Violence Prevention Research Program.

Wintemute, G. J. (2002). Where the guns come from: The gun industry and gun commerce. *Future Child, 12*(2), 54–71.

Wolfson, M. (2001). *The fight against big tobacco: The movement, the state and the public's health.* New York: Aldine.

Yach, D., Hawkes, C., Gould, C. L., & Hofman, K. J. (2004). The global burden of chronic diseases: Overcoming impediments to prevention and control. *Journal of the American Medical Association, 291*(21), 2616–2622.

Yates, B. (1983). *The decline and fall of the American automobile industry.* New York: Empire Books.

Zenk, S. N., Schulz, A. J., Israel, B. A., James, S. A., Bao, S., & Wilson, M. L. (2005). Neighborhood racial composition, neighborhood poverty, and the spatial accessibility of supermarkets in metropolitan Detroit. *American Journal of Public Health, 95*(4), 660–667.

Chapter 5
Political Economic Systems and the Health of Populations: Historical Thought and Current Directions

Howard Waitzkin

1. Introduction

Today, when disease-producing features of the workplace and environment threaten the survival of humanity and other life forms, it is not surprising that conditions of society that generate illness and mortality, as well as the impact of a society's political economic system on these conditions, would receive attention. However, there is a long history of research and analysis about the relationships among political economic systems, the social determinants of health, and the health of populations that has been neglected. As such this work tends to be forgotten and rediscovered with each succeeding generation. In this chapter, I trace some historical roots of work on political economic[i] systems and their relationship to health and illness. I describe critically some of the main recent findings in this area and implications for research and potential intervention efforts that focus on the impact of political economic system on health.

2. Historical Perspectives on Political Economic Systems and Health

Three people – Friedrich Engels, Rudolf Virchow, and Salvador Allende – made major early contributions to the understanding of social origins of illness.[ii] Although other writers also have examined this topic, these three writers emphasized the importance of political economic systems as causes of illness-generating social conditions. Engels and Virchow provided analyses of the impact of political economic conditions on health that essentially created the perspective of social medicine. Both men were writing about these issues during the tumultuous years of the 1840s; both took decisive – though quite divergent – personal actions, which they saw as corrective of the conditions they described through political economic change. Allende's key work appeared later, during the 1930s, and in a different geopolitical context. While Engels and Virchow documented the impact of early capitalism, Allende focused on capitalist imperialism and underdevelopment. Although little known in North America and Western Europe, Allende's studies in social medicine have greatly influenced efforts at political economic change in order to facilitate health planning and strategy in Latin America and elsewhere in the developing world.

While Engels, Virchow, and Allende conveyed certain unifying themes, they also diverged in major ways, especially regarding the political economic structures of oppression that cause disease, the social contradictions that inhibit change, and directions of reform in political economic systems that would foster health rather than illness. The next section looks to these prior works to give an historical perspective to issues that today gain even more urgency. The works of Engels, Virchow, and Allende also have influenced a new generation of researchers and activists in Latin America, who also focus in large part on political economic systems as social determinants of health and illness; I also summarize these important directions.

2.1. Friedrich Engels

Engels wrote his first major book, *The Condition of the Working Class in England*, under circumstances whose ironies now are well known (Engels, 1952). Between 1842 and 1844, Engels was working in Manchester as a middle-level manager in a textile mill of which his father was co-owner. Engels carried out his managerial duties in a perfunctory manner while immersing himself in English working-class life. The richness of Engels' treatment of working-class existence has attracted much critical attention, both sympathetic and belligerent.[iii] In contrast, Engels' analysis of the political economic origins of illness, though central to his account of working-class conditions, has received relatively little notice.

Engels' theoretical position was unambiguous: for working-class people the roots of illness and early death lay in the organization of economic production and in the social environment (Engels, 1952). British capitalism, Engels argued, forced working-class people to live and work under circumstances that inevitably caused sickness; this situation was well known to the capitalist class. The contradiction between profit and safety worsened health problems and stood in the way of necessary improvements.

In addition to his own personal observations, Engels' work made use of public reports to the Poor Law Commission in Britain. These reports appeared in the early 1840s and culminated in 1842 with the appearance of Chadwick's *Inquiry into the Sanitary Condition of the Labouring Population of Great Britain*. In this report, Chadwick documented the connections among economic deprivation, environmental pollution, disease, and mortality (Chadwick, 1965). Engels analyzed problems similar to those Chadwick discussed. Engels' theoretical perspective, however, focused on the profound impact of political economic system and class structure, as well as the difficulties of change while the effects of social class under early industrial capitalism persisted.

Considering the effects of environmental toxins, he claimed that the poorly planned housing in working-class districts did not permit adequate ventilation of toxic substances. Workers' apartments surrounded a central courtyard without direct spatial communication to the street. Carbon-containing gases from combustion and human respiration remained within living quarters. Because disposal systems did not exist for human and animal wastes, these materials decomposed in courtyards, apartments, or the street; severe air and water pollution resulted. Next, Engels discussed infectious diseases caused in large part by poor housing conditions; tuberculosis, an airborne infection, was his major focus. He noted that overcrowding and insufficient ventilation contributed to high mortality from tuberculosis in London and other industrial cities. Typhus, carried by lice, also spread because of bad sanitation and ventilation.

Engels drew connections among social conditions, nutrition, and disease. He emphasized the expense and chronic shortages of food supplies for urban workers. Lack of proper storage facilities at markets led to contamination and spoilage. Problems of malnutrition were especially acute for children. Engels related scrofula to poor nutrition; this view antedated the discovery of bovine tuberculosis as the major cause of scrofula and pasteurization of milk as a preventive measure. He also described the skeletal deformities of rickets as a nutritional problem, long before the medical finding that dietary deficiency of vitamin D caused rickets.

Engels' analyzed the social forces that fostered excessive drinking. In Engels' view, alcoholism was a response to the miseries of working-class life. Lacking other sources of emotional gratification, workers turned to alcohol. Individual workers could not be held responsible for alcohol abuse, and instead alcoholism ultimately was the responsibility of the capitalist class:

"Liquor is their [the workers'] only source of pleasure. . . . The working man . . . must have something to make work worth his trouble, to make the prospect of the next day endurable. . . . Drunkenness has here ceased to be a vice, for which the vicious can be held responsible. . . . They who have degraded the working man to a mere object have the responsibility to bear" (Engels, 1952)

For Engels, alcoholism was rooted firmly in social structure. If the experience of deprived social conditions caused alcoholism, the solution involved basic political economic change rather than treatment programs focusing on the individual.

In this context Engels analyzed structures of oppression within the social organization of medicine. He emphasized the maldistribution of medical personnel. According to Engels, working-class people contended with the "impossibility of employing skilled physicians in cases of illness" (Engels, 1952). Infirmaries that offered charitable services met only a small portion of people's needs for professional attention. Engels criticized the patent remedies containing opiates that apothecaries provided for childhood illnesses. High rates of infant mortality in working-class districts, Engels hypothesized, were explainable partly by lack of medical care and partly by the promotion of inappropriate medications.

Engels undertook an epidemiologic investigation of mortality rates and social class, using demographic statistics compiled by public health officials. He showed that mortality rates were inversely related to social class, not only for entire cities but also within specific geographic districts of cities. He noted that in Manchester, childhood mortality was much greater among working-class children than among children of the higher classes. In addition, Engels commented on the cumulative effects of class and urbanicity on childhood mortality. He cited data that demonstrated higher death rates from epidemics of infectious diseases like smallpox, measles, scarlet fever, and whooping cough among working-class children. For Engels, features of urban life, such as crowding, poor housing, inadequate sanitation, and pollution, combined with social class position in the etiology of disease and early mortality.

The social causes of accidents drew Engels' indignation. He linked accidents to the exploitation of workers, lack of suitable childcare, and the consequent neglect of children. Because both husband and wife needed to work outside the home in most working-class families and no facilities for childcare were available, children were subject to such accidents as falls, drowning, or burns. Engels noted that deaths from children's burns were especially frequent during the winter because of unsupervised heating facilities. Industrial accidents were another source of concern, especially the risks that industrial workers faced because of machinery. The most common accidents involved loss of fingers, hands, or arms by contact with unguarded machines. Infection resulting from accidents often led to tetanus.

In other sections of his book, Engels provided early accounts of occupational diseases that did not receive intensive study until well into the twentieth century. Many orthopedic disorders, in Engels' view, derived from the physical demands of industrialism. He discussed curvature of the spine, deformities of the lower extremities, flat feet, varicose veins, and leg ulcers as manifestations of work demanding long periods of time in an upright posture. Engels commented on the health effects of posture, standing, and repetitive movements:

"All these affections are easily explained by the nature of factory work. . . . The operatives . . . must stand the whole time. And one who sits down, say upon a window-ledge or a basket, is fined, and this perpetual upright position, this constant mechanical pressure of the upper portions of the body upon spinal column, hips, and legs, inevitably produces the results mentioned. This standing is not required by the work itself." . . . (Engels, 1952)

The insight that chronic musculoskeletal disorders could result from unchanging posture or small, repetitive motions seems simple; however, this source of illness, which is quite different from a specific accident or exposure to a toxic substance, has entered occupational medicine as a serious topic of concern only within the last two decades.

Engels also singled out the eye disorders suffered by workers in textile and lace manufacturing. This work required constant fine visual concentration, often in poorly lighted conditions. Engels discussed such eye diseases as corneal inflammation, myopia, cataracts, and temporary or permanent blindness. After an exposition of ocular abnormalities, Engels returned to the passion of his political economic analysis:

"This is the price at which society purchases for the fine ladies of the bourgeoisie the pleasure of wearing lace; a reasonable price truly! Only a few thousand blind working-men, some consumptive labourers' daughters, a sickly generation of the vile multitude bequeathing its debility to its equally "vile" children and children's children. . . . Our English bourgeoisie will lay the report of the Government Commission aside indifferently, and wives and daughters will deck themselves in lace as before." (Engels, 1952)

For Engels the contradictions of class in capitalist society made themselves felt most keenly in symbolic paraphernalia like lace, which the capitalist class enjoyed at the expense of workers' eyesight.

Engels' exposition of pottery workers' "poisoning" was a clinical description of intoxication from lead and other heavy metals. His observations again are startling because this disease has evoked wide concern in modern industrial hygiene. He noted that workers absorbed lead largely from the finishing fluid that came into contact with their hands and clothing. The consequences Engels described included severe abdominal pain, constipation, and neurological complications like epilepsy and partial or complete paralysis. These signs of lead intoxication occurred not only in workers themselves, according to Engels, but also in children who lived near pottery factories. Epidemiologic evidence concerning the community hazards of industrial lead has gained appreciation in environmental health mainly since 1970, largely without recognition of Engels' observations.

Engels' discussions of lung disease were detailed and far-reaching. His presentation of textile workers' pulmonary pathology antedated by many years the medical characterization of byssinosis, or brown lung:

"In many rooms of the cotton and flax-spinning mills, the air is filled with fibrous dust, which produces chest affections, especially among workers in the carding and combing-rooms. . . . The most common effects of this breathing of dust are bloodspitting, hard, noisy breathing, pains in the chest, coughs, sleeplessness, in short, all the symptoms of asthma.'. . . (Engels, 1952)

Engels offered a parallel description of "grinders' asthma," a respiratory disease caused by inhalation of metal dust particles in the manufacture of knife blades and forks.

Engels devoted even more attention to the ravages of pulmonary disorder among coal miners. He reported that unventilated coal dust caused both acute and chronic pulmonary inflammation that frequently progressed to death. Engels observed that "black spittle" – the syndrome now called coal miners' pneumoconiosis, or black lung – was associated with other gastrointestinal, cardiac, and reproductive complications. By pointing out that this lung disease was preventable, Engels illustrated the contradiction between profit and safety as a political economic determinant of disease in capitalist industry:

"Every case of this disease ends fatally. . . . In all the coal-mines which are properly ventilated this disease is unknown, while it frequently happens that miners who go from well to ill-ventilated mines are seized by it. The profit-greed of mine owners which prevents the use of ventilators is therefore responsible for the fact that this working-men's disease exists at all." (Engels, 1952)

After more than a century, the same structural contradiction impedes the prevention of black lung.

The Condition of the Working Class in England resembled other Marxist classics in its scholarship, which the author intended mainly for the purpose of sociopolitical action. For Engels, the analysis of the political economic sources of illness was part of a much larger agenda, and he quickly focused on other theoretical and practical concerns. Despite later writings on natural and physical sciences (Engels, 1966), Engels never returned to the social origins of illness as a major issue in its own right, though in a book aimed at a broad description of working-class life, he did provide a profound analysis of the causal relationships between political economic system and physical illness. Engels' argument implied that the solution to many health problems required basic political economic change, and limited medical interventions would never yield the most needed improvements. It is unfortunate that Engels' early work on medical issues has eluded later students and activists. However, Engels' analysis exerted a major influence, both intellectual and political, on one of the founders of social medicine, Rudolf Virchow.

2.2. Rudolf Virchow

Virchow's life spanned 80 years of nineteenth-century history, more than 2,000 publications, numerous contributions in medical science and anthropology, and activity as an elected member of the German parliament. His best known work is *Cellular pathology as based upon physiological and pathological histology* (Virchow, 1971), which presented the first comprehensive exposition of the cell as the basic unit of pathologic processes. Throughout his career, however, he tried to develop a unified explanation of the physical and political economic forces that cause disease and human suffering.

After a lengthy critique of detached science pursued "for its own sake," Virchow concluded, "It certainly does not detract from the dignity of science to come down off its pedestal – and from the people science gains new strength" (Virchow, 1958). From this perspective emerged Virchow's frequent assertion that the most successful science drew its problems largely from concrete social concerns. Science and scientific medicine, according to Virchow, should not be detached from political economic reality. On the contrary, he argued, the scientist must seek to link the findings of research to political work suggested by that research.

Hegel was the main source of Virchow's dialectic approach to both biologic and political economic problems. On the biologic level, Virchow perceived natural processes as a series of antitheses, such as the humoral-solidistic or vitalistic-mechanistic dualities, that were resolved by syntheses such as cellular pathology. On the political economic level, in 1847 Virchow anticipated the revolutions of 1848 by claiming that the apparent social tranquility would be "negated" through social conflict in order to reach a higher synthesis" (Ackerknecht, 1953). Virchow used a similar dialectic analysis in tracing the process of scientific knowledge (Virchow, 1958).

While influenced by Hegel, Virchow rejected Hegelian idealism. Virchow argued for a new "materialism" in medicine that would replace dogma and spiritualism (Virchow, 1957). In attempting to construct a dialectic materialist approach in biology, Virchow cited Engels' approach in *The Condition of the Working Class in England* and used some of Engels' data to demonstrate the relationships between poverty and illness (Virchow, 1879). During his early years, Virchow was influenced most by Arnold Ruge, who with Marx edited *Die Deutsch-Französischen Jahrbücher*. Virchow referred frequently to Ruge's writings and speeches, especially those on the ambiguities of political authority and on the need to discover "natural laws" of human society (Virchow, 1957).

Virchow manifested these orientations – of applied science, dialectics, and materialism – in his analyses of specific illnesses. He emphasized the concrete historical and material circumstances in which disease appeared, the contradictory political economic forces that impeded prevention, and researchers' role in advocating reform. In the analysis of multifactorial etiology, Virchow claimed that the most important causative factors of disease were material conditions of people's everyday lives. This view implied that an effective health care system could not limit itself to treating the pathophysiological disturbances of individual patients.

Based on study of a typhus epidemic in Upper Silesia, a cholera epidemic in Berlin, and an outbreak of tuberculosis in Berlin during 1848 and 1849, Virchow developed a theory of epidemics that emphasized the political economic structures that fostered the spread of illness. He argued that defects of society were a necessary condition for the emergence of epidemics. Virchow classified certain disease entities as "crowd diseases" or "artificial diseases"; these included typhus, scurvy, tuberculosis, leprosy, cholera, relapsing fever, and some mental disorders. According to this analysis, inadequate social conditions increased the population's susceptibility to climate, infectious agents, and other specific causal factors – none of which alone was sufficient to produce an epidemic. For the prevention and eradication of epidemics, political economic change was as important as medical intervention, if not more so: "The improvement of medicine would eventually prolong human life, but improvement of social conditions could achieve this result even more rapidly and successfully" (Virchow, 1879).

The political economic contradictions that Virchow emphasized most strongly were those of class structure. For example, he noted that morbidity and mortality rates, especially infant mortality rates, were much higher in working-class districts of cities than in wealthier areas. As documentation he used the statistics that Engels cited, as well as data he gathered for German cities. Describing inadequate housing, nutrition, and clothing, Virchow criticized government officials for ignoring these root causes of illness. Virchow expressed his outrage about class conditions most forcefully in his discussion of epidemics like the cholera outbreak in Berlin:

"Is it not clear that our struggle is a social one, that our job is not to write instructions to upset the consumers of melons and salmon, of cakes and ice cream, in short, the comfortable bourgeoisie, but is to create institutions to protect the poor, who have no soft bread, no good meat, no warm clothing, and no bed, and who through their work cannot subsist on rice soup and camomile tea . . .? May the rich remember during the winter, when they sit in front of their hot stoves and give Christmas apples to their little ones, that the shiphands who brought the coal and the apples died from cholera. It is so sad that thousands always must die in misery, so that a few hundred may live well" (Virchow, 1957)

For Virchow, the deprivations of working-class life created a susceptibility to disease, so; when infectious organisms, climatic changes, famine, or other causal factors were present, disease occurred and spread rapidly through the community.

Virchow's understanding of the political economic origins of illness was the source of the broad role that he envisioned for public health and the medical scientist. He attacked structures of oppression within medicine, particularly the policies of hospitals that required payment by the poor rather than assuming their care as a matter of social responsibility. He envisioned the creation of a "public health service," an integrated system of publicly owned and operated health care facilities, staffed by health workers who were employed by the state. In this system, health care and the enjoyment of political economic conditions of life that contributed to health rather than to illness would be defined as a constitutional right of citizenship (Virchow, 1957).

The activities of public health workers, to whom Virchow referred as "doctors of the poor" (*Armendärzten*), would involve advocacy as well as direct medical care; in this sense, health workers would become the "natural attorneys of the poor." Even with the best of motivations, he argued, doctors working among the poor faced continuous overwork and impotence in changing the social conditions that foster illness. For these reasons, it was naive to argue for a public health service without also struggling for more basic political economic change.

Two other principles were central to Virchow's conception of the public health service: prevention and the state's responsibility to assure material security for citizens. Virchow's emphasis on prevention again derived mostly from his observation of epidemics, which he believed could be averted by fairly simple measures. He identified several poor potato harvests preceding the Berlin epidemic as a major cause. Government officials could have prevented malnutrition by distributing foodstuffs from other parts of the country. Therefore, prevention was largely a political economic problem: "Our politics were those of prophylaxis; our opponents preferred those of palliation" (Virchow, 1957). It was foolish to think that health workers could accomplish prevention solely by activities within the medical sphere; material security also was essential. The state's responsibilities, Virchow argued, included providing work for "able-bodied" citizens. Only by conditions of economic production that guaranteed employment could workers obtain the economic security necessary for good health. Likewise, the physically disabled should enjoy the right of public compensation (Virchow, 1957).

Virchow's vision of the political economic origins of illness pointed to a wide scope of medicine. To the extent that illness derived from political economic conditions, the medical scientist must study those conditions as a part of clinical research, and the health worker must engage in political action. Virchow frequently drew connections among medicine, social science, and politics: "Medicine is a social science, and politics is nothing more than medicine in larger scale" (Virchow, 1957). Virchow's analysis of these issues fell from sight largely because of conservative political forces that shaped the course of scientific medicine during the late nineteenth and early twentieth centuries. However, his contributions set a standard for current attempts to understand, and to change, the political economic conditions that generate illness and suffering.

2.3. Salvador Allende

Although Allende's political endeavors remain better known than his medical career, his writings and efforts to reform medicine and public health became one of several important influences on the course of social medicine in Latin America. Acknowledging intellectual debts to Chadwick, Engels, Virchow, and other analysts of the social roots of illness in nineteenth-century Europe, Allende set forth a political economic model of medical problems in the context of economic underdevelopment. This model emphasized political economic characteristics that were amenable to social policy reform.

Writing in 1939 as minister of health for a Popular Front government, Allende presented his analysis of the relationships among political economy, disease, and suffering in his book, *La Realidad Médico-Social Chilena* (Allende, 1939). *La Realidad* conceptualized illness as a disturbance of the individual that was fostered by deprived social conditions. This view implied that political economic change was the only potentially effective therapeutic approach to many health problems. After an introduction on the connections between political economic system and illness, Allende presented some geographic and demographic "antecedents" necessary to place specific health problems in context. He devoted the next part of the book, similar to Engels and Virchow, to the "living conditions of the working classes." The last sections of the book presented an exhaustive review of health care facilities and services and a plan for change.

The introduction of *La Realidad* explored the dilemmas of reformism and argued that incremental reforms within the health care system would remain ineffective unless accompanied by broad political economic changes in the society. Allende criticized capitalist imperialism, particularly the multinational corporations that extracted profit from Chilean natural resources and inexpensive labor. He claimed that to improve the health care system, a popular government must end capitalist exploitation:

"For the capitalist enterprise it is of no concern that there is a population of workers who live in deplorable conditions, who risk being consumed by diseases or who vegetate in obscurity.... [Without] economic advancement . . . it is impossible to accomplish anything serious from the viewpoints of hygiene or medicine . . . because it is impossible to give health and knowledge to a people who are malnourished, who wear rags, and who work at a level of unmerciful exploitation." (Allende, 1939)

In his account of working-class life, Allende focused first on wages, which he viewed as a primary determinant of workers' material condition in the structure of economic production. Many of his political economic observations anticipated later concerns, including wage differentials for men and women, the impact of inflation, and the inadequacy of laws purporting to assure subsistence-level income. He linked his exposition of wages directly to the problem of nutrition and presented comparative data on food availability, earning power, and economic development. Not only was the production of milk and other needed foodstuffs less efficient than in more developed countries, but Chilean workers' inferior earning power also made food less accessible. Reviewing the minimum requirement to assure adequate nutrition, he found that the majority of Chilean workers could not obtain the elements of this diet on a regular basis. He argued that high infant mortality, skeletal deformities, tuberculosis, and other infectious diseases all had roots in bad nutrition; improvements depended on changed political economic conditions.

Allende then turned to clothing, housing, and sanitation facilities. He found that working class people in Chile were inadequately clothed, largely because wages were low and the greatest proportion of income went for food and housing. The effects of insufficient clothing, Allende observed, were apparent in rates of upper respiratory infections, pneumonia, and tuberculosis, which were higher than in any economically developed country.

In his analysis of housing problems, Allende focused on population density, which largely reflected the geography of economic production. He noted that Chile had one of the highest rates of inhabitants per residential structure in the world; overcrowding fostered the spread of infectious diseases and poor hygiene. Again he cited comparative data that showed a correlation between population density and overall mortality. In a style reminiscent of both Engels and Virchow, Allende presented a concrete description of housing conditions, including details about insufficient beds, inadequate construction materials, and deficiencies in apartment buildings. He reviewed the provisions for private initiative in construction, found them unsatisfactory, and outlined the need for major public sector investment in new housing. Allende gave data on drinking water and sewerage systems for all provinces of Chile. He noted that vast areas of the country lacked these rudimentary facilities, in association with lower levels of economic production.

Allende observed that maternal and infant mortality rates generally were much lower in developed than in underdeveloped countries. After reviewing the major causes of death he concluded that malnutrition and poor sanitation, both rooted in the political economy of underdevelopment, were major explanations for this excess mortality. In the same section, Allende gave one of the first analyses of illegal abortion. He noted that a large proportion of deaths in gynecologic hospitals, about 30 percent, derived from abortions and their complications. Pointing out the high incidence of abortion complications among working-class women, he attributed this problem to economic deprivations of class structure. Again, after a statistical account of complications, Allende allowed his outrage to surface:

"There are hundreds of working mothers who, because of anxiety about the inadequacy of their wages, induce abortion in order to prevent a new child from shrinking their already insignificant resources. Hundreds of working mothers lose their lives, impelled by the anxieties of economic reality." (Allende, 1939)

Allende designated tuberculosis as a "social disease" because its incidence differed so greatly among social classes. Writing before the antibiotic era, Allende reached conclusions similar to those of modern epidemiology – the major decline in tuberculosis followed economic advances rather than therapeutic medical interventions. From statistics of the first three decades of the twentieth century, he noted that tuberculosis had decreased consistently in the economically developed countries of Western Europe and the United States. Conversely, in economically underdeveloped countries like Chile, little progress against the disease had occurred. Within the context of underdevelopment, tuberculosis exerted its most severe impact on the working class.

Allende emphasized political economic conditions that favored the spread of syphilis and gonorrhea. For example, he discussed deprivations of working-class life that encouraged prostitution. Citing the prevalence of prostitution in Santiago and other cities, as well as the early recruitment of women from poor families, he argued that social programs to eliminate prostitution through expansion of employment opportunities must precede significant improvements in venereal diseases.

Regarding other communicable diseases, Allende turned first to typhus, the same disease that had shaped Virchow's views about the relations between illness and political economic system. Allende began his analysis with a straightforward statement: "Some [communicable diseases], like typhus, are an index of the state of pauperization of the masses" (Allende, 1939). Like Virchow in Upper Silesia, Allende found a disproportionate incidence of typhus in the working class of Chile. He showed that bacillary and amebic dysentery and typhoid fever occurred because of inadequate drinking water and sanitation facilities in residential areas densely populated by working-class families. Similar problems fostered other infections, such as diphtheria, whooping cough, scarlet fever, measles, and trachoma.

Addiction troubled Allende deeply throughout his career. One of his health policies priorities as President of Chile was a large-scale alcoholism program. In *La Realidad,* Allende analyzed the social and psychological problems that motivated people to use addictive drugs. Allende's political economic analysis of the causes of alcohol intoxication was similar to Engels':

"We see that one's wages, appreciably less than subsistence, are not enough to supply needed clothing, that one must inhabit inadequate housing . . . [and that] one's food is not sufficient to produce the minimum of necessary caloric energy. . . . The worker reaches the conclusion that going to the tavern and intoxicating oneself is the apparent solution to all these problems. In the tavern one finds a lighted and heated place, and friends for distraction, making one forget the misery at home. In short, for the Chilean worker . . .alcohol is not a stimulant but an anesthetic." (Allende, 1939)

Rooted in social misery generated by the conditions of capitalist production, alcoholism exerted a profound effect on health, an impact that Allende documented for a variety of illnesses, including gastrointestinal diseases, cirrhosis, delirium tremens, sexual dysfunction, birth defects, and tuberculosis. He also traced some of the more subtle societal outcomes of alcoholism; for example, he offered an early analysis of the role of alcohol in deaths from accidents.

Allende recognized that the occupational causes of death and disability were among the most important that the country faced. The diseases of work revealed direct links between illness and the conditions of economic production. Allende noted, however, that knowledge about occupational diseases remained at a rudimentary level. (Allende, 1939)

Allende also analyzed monopoly capital and multinational expansion by the pharmaceutical industry. In perhaps the earliest discussion of its type, Allende compared the prices of brand-name drugs with their generic equivalents:

"Thus, for example, we find for a drug with important action on infectious diseases, sulfanilamide, these different names and prices: Prontosil $26.95, Gombardol $20.80, Septazina $21.60, Aseptil $18.00, Intersil $13.00, Acetilina $6.65. All these products, which in the eyes of the public appear with different names, correspond, in reality, to the same medication which is sold in a similar container and which contains 20 tablets of 0.50 grams of sulfanilamide." (Allende, 1939)

Beyond the issue of drug names, Allende also anticipated a later theme by criticizing pharmaceutical advertising: "Another problem in relation to the pharmaceutical specialties is . . . the excessive and charlatan propaganda attributing qualities and curative powers which are far from their real ones" (Allende, 1939).

Allende concluded *La Realidad* by setting forth the policy positions and plan for political economic action of the Ministry of Health within the Popular Front government. In considering reform and its dilemmas, he reviewed the political economic origins of illness and the social structural remedies that were necessary. Allende refused to discuss specific health problems apart from macro-level political economic issues. He introduced his policy proposals with a chapter entitled, "Considerations Regarding Human Capital." Analyzing the detrimental political economic impact of ill health among workers, he argued that a healthy population was a worthy goal both in its own right and also for the sake of national development. The country's productivity suffered because of workers' illness and early death, yet improving the health of workers was impossible without fundamental political economic changes in the society. These changes would include "an equitable distribution of the product of labor," state regulation of "production, distribution, and price of articles of food and clothing," a national housing program, and special attention to occupational health problems. The links between medicine and the broader political economy were inescapable: "All this means that the solution of the medico-social problems of the country would require precisely the solution of the economic problems that affect the proletarian classes" (Allende, 1939).

He proposed specific reforms that he viewed as preconditions for an effective health system. These reforms called for profound changes in existing structures of power, finance, and economic production. First, he suggested modifications of wages, which, if enacted, would have led to a major redistribution of wealth. Regarding nutrition, he developed a plan to improve milk supplies, fishing, and refrigeration and suggested land reform provisions to enhance agricultural productivity. Recognizing the need for better housing, Allende proposed a concerted national effort in publicly supported construction as well as rent control in the private sector.

According to Allende, since the major origins of illness included low wages, which were closely linked to malnutrition and poor housing, the first responsibility of the public health system, was to improve these political economic conditions. Allende did not emphasize programs of research or treatment for specific diseases; instead, he assumed that the greatest advances toward lowering morbidity and mortality would follow fundamental political economic changes. This orientation also pervaded his proposed "medico-social program." In this program he suggested innovations including the reorganization of the ministry of health, planning activities, control of pharmaceutical production and prices, occupational safety and health policies, measures supporting preventive medicine, and sanitation programs. Like Engels and Virchow before him, Allende saw major origins of illness in the structure of capitalist production. This vision implied that medical intervention without political activism would remain ineffectual and, in a deep sense, misguided.

2.4. Convergences and Divergences

Engels, Virchow, and Allende held divergent, though complementary, views about the social etiology of illness. The divergences reflect general differences in theoretical orientation. For Engels, economic production was primary; even in his early work, Engels emphasized the organization and process of production. Disease and premature death, in his view, developed directly from exposure to dusts, chemicals, time pressures, bodily posture, visual demands, and related difficulties that workers faced in their jobs. Environmental pollution, bad housing, alcoholism, and malnutrition also contributed to the poor health of the working class, but on balance these factors mainly reflected or exacerbated the structural contradictions of production itself.

Virchow shared Engels' view that the working class suffered disproportionately. Virchow's analysis, however, focused on inequalities in the distribution and consumption of social resources. Important sources of illness and early death included poverty, unemployment, malnutrition, cultural and educational deficits, political disenfranchisement, linguistic difficulties, inadequate medical facilities and personnel, and similar deficiencies that affected the working class. He believed, for example, that public officials could prevent epidemics by distributing food more efficiently. Disease and mortality, he argued, would improve if a "public health service" made medical care more available. Though Virchow did criticize profiteering by businessmen and the high fees of the private medical profession, he did not emphasize the illness-generating conditions of production itself. Instead, he viewed unequal access to society's products as the principal problem of social medicine.

Allende also concerned himself with the impact of class structure, but chiefly in the context of underdevelopment and imperialism. The deprivations that the working-class experienced in countries like Chile reflected the exploitation of the developing world by advanced capitalist nations. Allende attributed low wages, malnutrition, poor housing and related problems directly to the extraction of wealth by international imperialism. He recognized that production itself could produce illness but, unlike Engels, devoted less attention to occupational illness per se. He did document distributional inequalities of goods and services that, as in Virchow's analysis, ravaged the working class. However, for Allende, the most crucial political economic determinant of illness and death was the contradiction of development and underdevelopment. Economic advancement of the society as a whole, although impeded by imperialism, was the major precondition for meaningful improvements in medical care and individual health.

The contributions of Engels, Virchow, and Allende shared the framework of multifactorial causation, a vision of multiple social structures and processes impinging on the individual. Disease was not the straightforward outcome of an infectious agent or pathophysiological disturbance. Instead, a variety of problems – including malnutrition, economic insecurity, occupational risks, bad housing, and lack of political power – created an underlying predisposition to disease and death. Although these writers differed in the specific factors they emphasized, they each saw illness as deeply embedded in the complexities of social reality. To the extent that social contradictions affected individual disease, therapeutic intervention that limited itself to the individual level was both naive and futile. Multifactorial etiology implied social change as therapy, linking medical practice to political practice. Despite this common belief, Engels, Virchow, and Allende differed in their views of the strategies needed to achieve the policies they sought and visions of the society in which these policies would take effect. Although their explanations of the social origins of illness complemented one another, the question of how to change illness-generating conditions evoked quite different strategic analyses.

Engels' strategy involved revolution, not reform. He intended his data to serve, at least in part, as propaganda. The purpose was to provide a focus of political organizing among the working-class. Notably, Engels did not advocate specific changes in the conditions he described. While he detailed, for instance, the defects of housing, sanitation, occupational safety, maldistribution of medical personnel, and promotion of drugs, he did not explicitly seek reforms in any of these areas. The alternatives that he occasionally suggested, such as the cursory outlines of a public health service, were always speculations about how a more effective system might appear in a post-revolutionary society. The many deprivations of working-class life required fundamental change in the entire social order rather than limited improvements in each separate sphere. Though Engels' later writings sometimes adopted a more flexible stance about reform in the context of capitalism, the companion piece to *The Condition of the Working Class in England* was clearly *The Communist Manifesto*. The strategic implications of Engels' analysis of health problems were congruent with his role as a primary organizer of the First Internationale. From this perspective, reformism in health care made as little sense as any other piecemeal tinkering with capitalist society.

Virchow's strategic approach was quite different. Although he participated in the agitation of the late 1840s and doubted that the ruling circles would permit needed changes in response to peaceful challenges alone, he ultimately opted for reform rather than for revolution. While the conditions he witnessed in the Upper Silesian typhus epidemic were horrifying, for instance, he believed that a series of reforms could correct the problem. He proposed rationalized food distribution, modifications in the educational system, political enfranchisement, and other changes at the level of social structure. He also adopted a broad view of the systematic reforms that were necessary in health care. An adequate health system, for example, demanded a public health service. In this service, health care professionals would work as employees of the state and would act to correct maldistribution across class, geographical, and ethnic lines. As an overall political goal, Virchow favored a constitutional democracy that would reduce the power of the monarchy and nobility. He supported principles of socialism, particularly those that involved public ownership and rational organization of health and welfare facilities. However, Virchow argued against communism, mainly because of its view that a just society was feasible without a strong state apparatus. Virchow clearly believed that limited reforms within capitalist society were both appropriate and desirable, and he was optimistic that they would be effective. During his later life, the reformist slant of his strategic thinking became even clearer.

Allende's conceptualization of political strategy was more complex and differentiated than Engels' or Virchow's. In *La Realidad Médico-Social Chilena,* he stated unambiguously that the health problems of the working class were inherent in the contradictions of class structure and underdevelopment and in the oppressive international relations of capitalist imperialism. Without basic modification of these structural problems, he argued, limited medical reform would prove futile (Allende, 1939).

In Allende's view, revolutionary social change was necessary, but could be achieved through peaceful means . Throughout his life, Allende believed that progressive forces could achieve a socialist transformation of society through a sequence of peaceful actions within the framework of constitutional democracy. He and his co-workers based this position on a reading of prior socialist strategists, examples of other revolutions and, most of all, a detailed analysis of Chile's concrete historical and material reality. From this viewpoint, the most important health-related reforms transcended medicine or public health. Allende called for improvements in housing, nutrition, employment, and other concrete manifestations of class oppression. Such reforms were preconditions for reduced morbidity and mortality; without them, changes in health care services could not succeed. On the other hand, structural reforms in the social organization of medicine, including a public health service and a nationalized pharmaceutical and equipment industry, were desirable goals en route to a socialist society. Allende did not accurately anticipate the violence of national and international groups about to be dispossessed on the peaceful road to socialism. The balance between reform and revolutionary alternatives remains a crucial and incompletely resolved problem in strategic planning.

3. Latin American Social Medicine

Partly stimulated by Allende's work, linking health outcomes to political economic conditions has become a key emphasis in the field of Latin American social medicine. Although social medicine is a widely respected field of research, teaching, and clinical practice in Latin America, its accomplishments remain little known in the English speaking and reading world. This gap in knowledge derives partly from the fact that important publications remain untranslated from Spanish into English. In addition, the lack of impact reflects a frequently erroneous assumption in richer countries that the intellectual and scientific productivity of poorer countries manifests a less rigorous and relevant approach to the important questions of our age.

3.1. European Influences

Most Latin American accounts of social medicine's history emphasize its European origins. In general, Latin American reports allude to the same history of social medicine published in English-language studies. Some of these historical accounts have appeared in widely distributed Spanish translations (Foucault, 1977; Rosen, 1985) and usually cite the work of Rudolf Virchow in Germany as an important intellectual source for the development of Latin American social medicine (Nunes, 1991).

In the United States, where (as noted earlier) Virchow remains best known for his work in cellular pathology, social medicine oriented to the vision of Virchow and his followers became one of many conceptual approaches advanced at the turn of the twentieth century. These competing approaches included allopathic medicine emphasizing unifactorial etiology, homeopathy, chiropractic practice, midwifery and related practices in women's health care, and various traditions of folk healing. By the early 1900s, these competing orientations had created a wide spectrum of explanatory frameworks for education and clinical practice. At that time, however, powerful forces within the United States began to exert pressure to legitimate a unifactorial model, rooted in laboratory-based "science," as the only suitable framework for modern medicine. The Flexner Report (Flexner, 1972) advocated for laboratory-based medicine and unifactorial causation. Soon after its publication, the American Medical Association and the Rockefeller Foundation coordinated legislative and regulatory efforts to reduce or eliminate the vast majority of medical schools not oriented to these principles. With this change, Virchow's vision of social medicine and political economic determinants of illness and death declined rapidly in influence (Brown, 1979).

The historical processes affecting medical education and practice in Latin America were very different. Adherents to Virchow's vision of social medicine immigrated to both North America and to Latin America near the turn of the twentieth century. In Chile, Argentina, Mexico, and several other countries, Virchow's followers helped establish major medical schools and initiated courses in social medicine. Often these European immigrants worked in academic departments of pathology. As one of several examples, an influential German pathologist, Max Westenhofer, for many years directed the department of pathology at the medical school of the University of Chile (Illanes, 1993). Westenhofer was to become the teacher of another great pathologist, innovator in social medicine, and resident of Chile: Salvador Allende.

Such academic leaders, inspired by Virchow's efforts to link pathology and political economic conditions, advanced social medicine as a focus of medical education and research. No analogy to the Flexner Report became influential in Latin America, and by the beginning of the 1930s, social medicine had become firmly rooted in several Latin American countries.

3.2. The "Golden Age" of Latin American Social Medicine

Although similar tendencies occurred in several countries, Chile's history, leading to what has been termed the "golden age of social medicine," illustrated several typical and conflicting orientations. We already have considered Allende's contributions. However, Ricardo Cruz-Coke, a prominent academic physiologist, became minister of health during the mid-1930s. In this role, Cruz-Coke wrote a monograph, which remains a well-known classic of Chilean social medicine (Cruz-Coke, 1938). Cruz-Coke argued that infectious and cardiovascular diseases reduced the productivity of the labor force. From this political economic perspective, preventive and curative health services aiming to reduce these disorders promised to boost the economy. Cruz-Coke claimed that economic reforms would prove inadequate to enhance the productivity of labor but that improved health care services would achieve this goal more efficiently. The book concludes with the legislation on preventive medicine that Cruz-Coke presented to the national legislature in 1938, which, in large part, went into effect.

The efforts of Cruz-Coke led in a very different direction from those of Allende. While Allende placed a value on health in its own right and economic development as route to improve health for Chile's population, Cruz-Coke emphasized the contribution of health to economic productivity. In that sense, Cruz-Coke's orientation reflected that of the Rockefeller Foundation, which during the same time period initiated efforts in less developed countries to improve the productivity of labor (Birn & Solórzano, 1999; Brown, 1979; Cueto, 1994). Cruz-Coke also anticipated more recent efforts to enhance labor productivity and economic development by "investing in health" (Waitzkin, 2003; World Bank, 1993).

3.3. Danger and Productivity in Contemporary Latin American Social Medicine

During the last half century, Latin American social medicine has advanced in many countries. For some people active in this field, their intellectual work has proven very dangerous indeed, in several instances leading to torture, imprisonment, or exile. The main reason for this threat derives from the intellectual point of view that political economic conditions determine patterns of illness and death.

To the extent that improvement of these conditions warrants fundamental social change, the perspective can prove challenging to those groups that currently hold power in society.

Several centers and investigators – based in Argentina, Brazil, Chile, Colombia, Cuba, Mexico, Venezuela – now carry out research and programs in this tradition (Waitzkin, 1998; Waitzkin, Iriart, Estrada, & Lamadrid, 2001a, b) (Table 5.1 summarizes the participants and foci of these groups). While these investigators and activists have achieved varying influence on medical practice, public health programs, and medical education in their respective countries, they have built an important network of groups working in the tradition of social medicine. For the most part, their work has not been published in English and is little known outside Latin America. Yet their contributions have much to offer in the United States and other developing world countries, where the connections between political economic conditions and health outcomes have received much less emphasis. Such efforts also deserve attention because of the courage demonstrated by these individuals and groups to continue under dangerous working conditions.

A theoretical distinction that Latin American practitioners of social medicine draw between their field and traditional public health concerns the static versus dynamic nature of health versus illness, as well as impact of the social context. Social medicine conceptualizes "health-illness" as a dialectic process rather than a dichotomy between two static conditions. Influenced by Engels' earlier and Levins and Lewontin's more recent interpretations of dialectic processes in biology (Engels, 1940; Levins & Lewontin, 1985), critical epidemiologists in social medicine have studied disease processes in a contextualized model that considers the changing effects of political economic conditions over time. From this standpoint, the epidemiologic profile of a society or a group within a society consists of a multi-level analysis of how social conditions such as economic production, reproduction, marginalization, and political participation affect the dynamic process of health-illness. From this theoretical vision, multivariate models in public health – such as logistic regression models with disease as a dichotomized dependent variable, either present or absent – obscure health-illness as a dialectic process.

This dialectic approach to health-illness has led to criticisms about traditional explanations of causality in medicine and public health (Franco, 1989; Laurell, 1982). At a basic level, social medicine practitioners have criticized monocausal explanations of disease. Taking a perspective similar to Virchow's, they argue that simplistic explanations that a specific agent causes a specific disease do not adequately consider the political economic conditions that either increase or decrease the likelihood of disease in the presence of a specific agent. However, even multicausal models, such as those that consider the interactions among agent, host, and environment, still define disease in a relatively static fashion. Critiques from the standpoint of social medicine have argued that by dichotomizing the presence or absence of a disease, traditional multicausal models do not adequately consider the dynamic linkages by which social conditions affect the health-disease dialectic process. These analyses have suggested a more

TABLE 5.1. Groups in Latin American social medicine that conduct research on the political economic determinants of health

Country	Group	Leaders	Foci	Comments
Argentina	Buenos Aires	Mario Testa, Celia Iriart Laura Nervi, Francisco Leone, Silvia Faraone	Strategic planning, history of public health, health policy, environmental health, mental health	Courses at University of Buenos Aires; collaborations with labor unions
	Buenos Aires	José Carlos Escudero, Enrique Kreplak, Matilde Ruderman, Alicia Stolkiner, Marco Buchbinder, Deborah Tajer, Liliana Mayoral	Environmental health, mental health, health policy, research methods	Journal: *Salud, Problema y Debate*; help coordinate Latin American Association of Social Medicine
	Rosario	Carlos Bloch, Susana Belmartino, Irene Luppi, Zulema uinteros, maria del Carmen Troncoso	Medical profession, social epidemiology, health policy	Research center: *Centro de Estudios Santiarios y Sociales*; journal: *Cuadernos Médico Sociales*
	Córdoba	Horacio Barri, Norma Fernández, Sylvia Bermann, Héctor Seia	Medical education, occupational health, community-based epidemiology, health communication	Maintains values of Movement for an Integral Health System; journal: *Salud y Sociedad*; collaborates with labor unions
	Brazil		"Collective health", influence of theology of liberation and empowerment education, nacional organization: *Asociación Brasiliera de Pós-Graduação em Saúde Colectiva*	
	São Paulo	Maria Cecilia Donnangelo, Ricardo Bruno Mendes Gonçalves, Amelia Cohn, Paulo Elías, Lilia Shraiber, José Ricardo Ayres, Paulette Goldemberg, Rita Baradas Barrata	Work process in health, economic policies, medical education, philosophy of epidemiology	Collaborates with Workers Party
	Campinas	Emerson Merhy, Gastão Wagner de Sousa Campos, Everardo Duarte Nunes	Health policy and planning, history of public health, health administration, micro-level processes	Laboratory of Administration and Planning; collaborations with municipal and state

TABLE 5.1. (*Continued*)

Country	Group	Leaders	Foci	Comments
	Rio de Janeiro	Sergio Arouca, Paulo Buss, Hesio Cordeiro, Madel Luz, Sonia Fleury, Cristina Possas	Health policy, critical epidemiology, institutional analysis	governments, labor unions, Workers Party; journal:*Saúde em Debate*
	Bahía	Naomar de Almedia Filho, Sebastián Loureiro Carmen Fontes Teixeira, Jairnilson Paim, Mauricio Lima Barreto	Multi-method epidemiology, public health planning, conferences	Importance of Oswaldo Cruz Founcation; National School of Public Health; journal: *Cadernos de Saúde Pública*; Epidemiologic teaching
Chile	Santiago	Alfredo Estrada, Adriana Vega, Jaime Sepúlveda, Carlos Montoya, Mariano Requena, Marilú Soto, Enrique Barilari, Silvia Riquelme, Felipe Cabello, Hugo Behm	Mental health, gender and health, occupational and environmental health, social epidemiology, health policy	Medicina Social; journal: *Salud y Cambio*
Columbia	Bogotá, Medellín, Cali	Saúl Franco, Alberto Vasco	Urban poverty and marginalization, infectious diseases, occupational health, gender, violence, social class	Affected by recurrent violence
Cuba	Havana	Francisco Rojas Ochoa, Cosmé Ordóñez, Silvia Martínez Calvo	History of social medicine, community-oriented medical education, geriatric medicine,interface with primary care	Debate about need for social medicine; journal: *Boletín de Ateneo Juan César García*
Ecuador	Quito	Jaime Breilh, Arturo Campaña, Oscar Betancourt, Edmundo Granda, Francisco Hidalgo *Estudios y Asesoría en Salud*; work with nacional coalition	Critical epidemiology, multi-method research, work process, gender, mental health, health policy	Research and consulting center: Centro de
Mexico	Mexico City, Guadalajara	Asa Cristina Luarell, Catalina Eibenschutz, Carolina Tetelboin, Mariano Noriega, José BlancoGil, Olivia López, Eduardo Menéndez, Francisco Mercado	Occupational health, community health, multi-method and participatory research, health policy	Graduation program, Autonomous Metropolitan University; journal: *Salud Problema*; collaborations with labor unions, Revolutionary Democratic Party, Zapatista Army for National Liberation

complex approach to causality, in which political economic conditions receive more explicit emphasis.

4. Political Economic Determinants of Illness and Health in Western Countries Today

With the coming of a new millennium, research on the political economic determinants of illness and health has burgeoned. This work rarely acknowledges its roots in the classical studies of Engels and Virchow or its similarities to the efforts of Allende and current researchers in Latin America. Nevertheless, the recent investigations on political economic determinants, conducted in both Europe and North America, have advanced knowledge about the social conditions that underlie morbidity and early death. The findings of these studies again lead to humility about the impact of improved access to medical services. Instead, the conclusions from this field (a brief summary of which follows) suggest that, in addition to improved access, basic change in social conditions will be needed if the goal is to improve the health outcomes of populations.

In the United States, class and race remain the most important determinants of the population's health outcomes. Research continues to accumulate showing that the poor suffer much worse overall mortality than the wealthy. In addition, poverty predicts life expectancy, infant mortality, and outcomes from medical conditions such as cardiovascular disease, cancer, and diabetes mellitus (Marmot & Feeney, 1997; Marmot et al., 1998; Martikainen, Stansfeld, Hemingway, & Marmot, 1999). Although the impact of poverty on health continues as the object of research, the findings have changed very little from those that Engels, Virchow, and Allende described many years ago.

Income inequality has emerged as one of the most important class-based predictors of health outcomes, perhaps as important as poverty itself. For instance, research comparing states, counties, and metropolitan areas throughout the United States has found that geographical units with the highest measures of income inequality manifest the most unfavorable mortality, life expectancy, and outcomes from problems such as cardiovascular disease (Kaplan, Pamuk, Lynch, Cohen, & Balfour, 1996; Kennedy, Kawachi, & Prothrow-Stith, 1996; Lynch et al., 1998; Lynch, Smith, Kaplan, & House, 2000; Schalick, Hadden, Pamuk, Navarro, & Pappas, 2000). Other studies have determined that among economically developed countries, those with higher levels of income inequality manifest worse disease outcomes. Researchers have argued that the perception of one's economic position as unfavorable becomes a major psychosocial stressor that mediates the effects of social inequality at the individual level (Kawachi, Kennedy, & Wilkinson, 1999; Wilkinson, 1996). Epidemiologists have developed more sophisticated methods that attempt to trace the "multi-level," psychosocial processes by which social conditions like income inequality exert their impacts on individuals' health (Diez Roux, 2000; Diez Roux, Link, & Northridge, 2000; Kennedy, Kawachi, Glass, & Prothrow-Stith, 1998).

Race also remains a major predictor of adverse outcomes. As of 1999, average life expectancy at birth for African American men in the United States was about seven years shorter than for white men and about five years shorter for African American women than for white women. In Harlem, rates of survival until 65 years of age for African American males has been worse than for males living in Bangladesh, one of the poorest countries in the world (Fang, Madhavan, & Alderman, 1996; Geronimus, Bound, Waidman, & Hillemeier, 1996; Kramarow, Lentzner, Rooks, Weeks, & Saydah, 1999; Mackay, Fingerhut, & Duran, 2000; McCord & Freeman, 1990). African American infant mortality is more than twice that for whites. Similarly, outcomes for cardiovascular disease, cancer, and AIDS remain much worse among African Americans (Carmichael & Iyasu, 1998; Carmichael, Iyasu, & Hatfield-Timajchy, 1998). Physicians exert more extensive diagnostic and therapeutic efforts for white patients than for African American patients with similar medical conditions. These differences in practice patterns appear to derive from racially based bias in evaluating symptoms experienced by white versus African American patients (Schulman et al., 1999). Racial differences in disease outcomes appear to be mediated by psychosocial processes such as the reaction to the disrespect inherent in racism (Kennedy, Kawachi, Lochner, Jones, & Prothrow-Stith, 1997). As Williams and others have shown, the impact of race and racial discrimination on outcomes is often difficult to separate from the impact of social class (Ren, Amick, & Williams, 1999; Williams, 1997, 1999a, b).

Gender-based differences in health outcomes also are linked to social conditions, although the associations often interact with class and race. While women continue to show overall mortality advantages compared to men in economically developed countries, age-adjusted outcomes in some conditions become unfavorable for women. For instance, cardiovascular outcomes for older women past the age of menopause are similar or worse than those for men. Although the reasons for women's deteriorating outcomes with age remain unclear, one possibility supported by evidence from research is that gender bias in diagnostic procedures and treatments may reduce their use when indicated.[iv] Gender clearly interacts with class and race in affecting health outcomes. For instance, in cancers affecting women, such as cancer of the breast and cervix, indicators such as rates of diagnosis, screening procedures like mammography and pap testing, and survival rates all are worse for poor than for non-poor women and for African-American women than for white women (Mandelblatt et al., 1999; Mandelblatt et al., 2000; Mandelblatt, Yabroff, & Kerner, 1999; McDonough, Williams, House, & Duncan, 1999; Rathore et al., 2000; Sheifer, Escarce, & Schulman, 2000). Under conditions of greater income inequality, gender differences in mortality increase, as men tend to die earlier from deaths related to violence, accidents and alcohol; a "culture of inequality" also leads to more violence against women (Kawachi, Kennedy, Gupta, & Prothrow-Stith, 1999; Wilkinson, 1999).

In particular, epidemiological research has documented the impact of income inequality on health outcomes so clearly that mammoth social policy initiatives designed to redistribute income appear completely warranted. To the extent that they would reduce income inequality, such measures as new tax policies, welfare payments, family allowances, and food subsidies probably would exert very favorable effects on the adverse mortality patterns and health outcomes that many studies have reported. However, because income inequality is so firmly rooted in the political structure of the United States and some (but not all) other advanced capitalist countries, such drastic policy changes remain a daunting task.

The improbability of basic change in income inequality has led some researchers, as well as agencies of the US government, to emphasize policies that aim to improve the "social capital" of low-income communities, rather than policies to achieve income redistribution (Baron, Field, & Schuller, 2001; Coleman, 1988; Kawachi, Kennedy, Lochner, & Prothrow-Stith, 1997; Kennedy, Kawachi, Prothrow-Stith, Lochner, & Gupta, 1998; Putnam, 2000). Social capital in communities involves higher levels of social support, cohesiveness, networking, and friendships. Such characteristics do appear associated with improved health outcomes, although less so than reduced income inequality. While interventions to increase social capital predictably will not improve outcomes to the same extent as policies to reduce inequality, such interventions have attracted support since they appear easier to achieve in the political context of the United States. It will be unfortunate if the worthwhile concern with social relationships within communities diverts attention in policy away from the importance of income inequality itself.

Access to health care services remains an important goal in the United States, yet it is very unlikely that improved access alone will lead to substantial improvements in outcomes linked to social class, race, and gender. Evidence for this claim also has arisen from countries with national health programs that provide universal access to health care services. For instance, in the United Kingdom, social class differentials in mortality and health outcomes have persisted despite the improvements in access achieved by the British National Health Service. As an example of research in this area, the Whitehall study of British civil servants assessed mortality, overall health status, and outcomes from cardiovascular and other specific diseases during the 1960s and again during the early 1990s. In this research, the all subjects held jobs in the British civil service but ranged from highly paid administrators to lowly paid clerical and manual workers. For overall mortality and outcomes in nearly all diseases studied, workers from the lower income levels did much worse than workers at the higher income levels. In fact, for most conditions a gradient appeared that indicated a direct correlation between outcomes and social class, as measured by income and position in the hierarchy of civil service jobs (Marmot et al., 1991; van Rossum, Shipley, van de Mheen, Grobbee, & Marmot, 2000).

Class and race differentials have appeared in Canada, whose national health program has won wide international admiration (Bell, Crystal, Detsky, & Redelmeier, 1998; Katz, Charles, Lomas & Welch, 1997; Katz, Hofer, & Manning, 1996; Williamson & Fast, 1998; World Health Organization, 1999). Again, studies of overall mortality and outcomes for specific diseases show worse results for lower-income subjects. Further, Canada manifests regional variations, with adverse outcomes in rural, economically undeveloped areas, especially in the northern part of the country. These regional variations also are linked with the proportion of Native American residents in the population. In regions with higher proportions of Native Americans, mortality and disease-specific outcomes are worse than in regions with fewer racial minorities. In short, despite Canada's overall prosperity and a national health program that has improved access for people throughout the country, evidence of social class and racial disparities in health outcomes persists. The important differences in outcomes that persist despite universal access again leads to the conclusion that in addition to national policies that assure access, much more fundamental change in the structure of society is required.

The maladies that workers in social medicine have described for more than a century remain with us. Even in rich nations that have achieved high levels of economic development, wide disparities in mortality and key indicators of health outcomes reflect the social class and racial distribution of the societies. In the United States, national health policies cannot afford to overlook the problems that have remained when similar countries have enacted successful programs to improve access. The persistence of these problems implies that broader changes in society are required for meaningful improvements in health outcomes.

5. Political Economic Systems, Socioeconomic Development, and Population Health

Is a population's health related to a country's political economic system? Despite much speculation and rhetoric, there has been remarkably little research that has compared the achievements of capitalist and socialist systems at similar levels of economic development in both health care and health outcomes. Whether a country adopts one system or another exerts a profound influence on social policy in general and on development strategies in particular.

Large cross-national studies, such as those conducted by the World Health Organization, have assessed the relationship of economic development to health outcomes, without taking political economic system into account.[v] In the mid-1980s, Shirley Cereseto and I did a research project using data from the World Bank, which focused on measures of the "physical quality of life" (PQL) (Cereseto & Waitzkin, 1986). In this analysis, we compared PQL in capitalist and socialist countries, grouped by level of economic development. The PQL measures included indicators of health, health services, and nutrition (infant mortality rate, child death rate, life expectancy, population per physician, population per nursing person, and daily per capita calorie supply); measures of education (adult literacy rate, enrollment in secondary education, and enrollment in high education); and a composite PQL index (PQLI). We analyzed data for 123 countries, which comprised 97 percent of the world's population. In the data analysis, we compared countries with capitalist versus socialist political economic systems, within each level of economic development. We also performed multivariate analyses that assessed the relative impact of economic development versus political economic system on PQLI outcomes (Table 5.2)

Our data showed that all PQLI measures improved as economic development increased; however, at the same level of economic development, the socialist countries showed more favorable outcomes than the capitalist countries in all these measures. In 28 of 30 comparisons between countries at similar levels of economic development, socialist countries showed more favorable PQL outcomes. Differences between capitalist and socialist countries in PQL were greatest at lower levels of economic development and tended to narrow at the higher levels of development.

TABLE 5.2. Physical quality of life variables, economic development, and political-economic system: Mean values

Variables	Capitalist countries	Socialist countries
Infant-mortality rate (per 1,000)		
Low income	131	71
Lower-middle income	81	38
Upper-middle income	42	22
Child death rate (per 1,000)		
Low income	26	7
Lower-middle income	11	2
Upper-middle income	4	1
Life expectancy (years)		
Low income	48	67
Lower-middle income	60	68
Upper-middle income	69	72
Population per physician		
Low income	19,100	1,920
Lower-middle income	5,832	638
Upper-middle income	1,154	488
Daily per-capita calorie supply (% requirement)		
Low income	94	107
Lower-middle income	106	117
Upper-middle income	122	137
Adult literacy rate (%)		
Low income	34	69
Lower-middle income	63	87
Upper-middle income	81	97
Secondary education (%)		
Low income	15	34
Lower-middle income	38	74
Upper-middle income	59	74
Higher education (%)		
Low income	2	1
Lower-middle income	12	12
Upper-middle income	16	19
PQL index		
Low income	35	76
Lower-middle income	62	83
Upper-middle income	81	92

Within each level of economic development, the socialist countries showed infant mortality and child death rates approximately two to three times lower than the capitalist countries. Though less striking, similar relationships emerged for life expectancy. Differences were again largest for the low-income and lower-middle-income countries and narrowed for the upper-middle-income countries.

Countries at higher levels of economic development provided more favorable ratios of medical and nursing personnel for their populations. Socialist countries consistently showed higher numbers of health professionals per population than capitalist countries at equivalent levels of economic development. These differences were again sharpest at the low-income and lower-middle-income levels. The ratio of upper-middle-income socialist societies was comparable to that of high-income capitalist societies.

Socialist countries also provided a higher daily per capita calorie supply as a percentage of requirement than did the capitalist countries at a similar level of development. The difference between capitalist and socialist countries averaged 12 to 15 percent. Nutritional supply of all socialist countries exceeded the 100 percent requirement.

With the exception of one tie, all measures of education improved with the level of economic development. Within each level of economic development, socialist countries showed more favorable adult literacy rates and numbers enrolled in secondary schools as a percentage of age group. Socialist countries at the upper-middle-income level showed a greater degree of participation in higher education, although the difference was not large. Low-income and lower-middle-income capitalist countries showed a fraction of a percent greater participation in higher education than the socialist countries.

As a composite and derived measure, the PQLI closely paralleled the other findings, increasing with level of economic development. In all three comparisons within given levels of development, socialist countries achieved markedly higher PQLIs. Our analysis of the World Bank's data supported a conclusion that, in the aggregate, the socialist countries achieved more favorable PQL outcomes than capitalist countries at equivalent levels of economic development.

Statistical information published by the World Bank represented the most comprehensive and accurate body of data on PQL that was available from Western sources. The primary tabulations were readily available in published form for reanalysis. Data collection and reporting from the socialist countries were likely to be at least as accurate as in the capitalist countries. All the socialist countries maintained statistical bureaus that gathered and published these data as one phase of planning and policy formulation. These efforts periodically led to findings that were not necessarily favorable. For example, infant mortality, crude death rate, and cardiovascular mortality in the Soviet Union worsened during the 1970s. In Cuba, reported mortality rates rose during the early 1960s and later improved rapidly; the temporary increase in mortality reflected improved data gathering, as the Ministry of Public Health expanded its efforts after the Cuban Revolution. Underreporting morbidity and mortality statistics frequently occurred in the low-income and lower-middle-income capitalist countries. However, better reporting would have tended to increase morbidity and mortality rates and would strengthen the finding of more favorable outcomes in the socialist countries.

Historically, there was some evidence that the discrepancies between capitalist and socialist nations reflected varying social policies. All the socialist countries initiated major public health efforts. These initiatives aimed at improved sanitation, immunization, maternal and child care, nutrition, and housing. In every case, the socialist countries also created national health services based on the principle of universal entitlement to care. These policies led to greater accessibility of preventive and curative services for previously deprived groups. Expanded educational opportunity also was a major priority of the socialist nations, as publicly subsidized education became more widely available. Literacy campaigns in these countries brought educational benefits to sectors of the population who earlier had not gone to school.

Nevertheless, national health policies, including national health insurance and/or a national health service, were not initiated solely by socialist countries. In fact, all the high-income capitalist countries except the United States enacted such national health policies. While capitalist countries at higher levels of economic development enjoyed the fruits of public health and educational improvements, poorer capitalist countries seldom succeeded in implementing such drastic changes in policy.

Cross-national differences in income inequality and the distribution of wealth may have contributed to the socialist countries' favorable PQLI outcomes. The socialist countries manifested a higher proportion of income received by the lowest 20 percent of the population, a lower proportion of income received by the highest 5 percent of the population, and a markedly lower index of inequality. Inequality continued to exist in all the socialist societies, but the range of inequality tended to be much narrower than in the capitalist countries.

In the less developed countries, the differences in PQLI between the capitalist and socialist systems were profound. There, the options in public health and education that a socialist political-economic system provided seemed to overcome some of the grueling deprivations of poverty. Our findings indicated that countries with socialist political economic systems could make great strides toward meeting basic human needs and population health, even without extensive economic resources.

Obviously, these PQLI advantages, demonstrated through the World Bank's conservative and relatively reliable data, did not prevent the collapse of several socialist governments. Clearly, other factors, including repressive governmental structures and the attractions of a consumerist ideology, motivated citizens in these countries to seek public policies compatible with capitalist values. Several socialist regimes in Eastern Europe manifested very antidemocratic and authoritarian policies. Despite some apparent advantages for health outcomes, the prior political economic systems in Eastern Europe (compared, for instance, with a more favorable situation in Cuba[vi]) should not be used as a model for a just society.

The political repression that fostered the collapse of socialism during the late 1980s and early 1990s leads to a question of the impact of political economic change on population health. Recent reports from Eastern Europe have documented the dismantling of public-sector national health programs, as well as fundamental changes in social policies concerning education, housing, and nutrition. Analyses of data from the 1990s have revealed a marked deterioration in the advantages in PQLI that were observed in the previously socialist countries. For instance, in Russia, life expectancy for men declined from 63.8 years in 1990 to 59.0 years in 1993 and for women from 74.3 years in 1990 to 71.5 years in 1993 – one of the most remarkable reported deteriorations in population health during all world history (Barr & Field, 1996; Bobak & Marmot, 1999; Bobak, Pikhart, Hertzman, Rose, & Marmot, 1998; Cockerham, 1997; Marmot, 1999a, b; Murphy, Bobak, Nicholson, Rose, & Marmot, 2006; Notzon et al., 1998; Tulchinsky & Varavikova, 1996; Walberg, McKee, Shkolnikov, Chenet, & Leon, 1998; Wilkinson, 1996; Wyon, 1996). Life expectancy and other indicators of population health probably started to decline during the 1980s before the collapse of socialism in the Soviet Union and the "triumph of capitalism," but the most drastic deteriorations have occurred after the collapse.

The precise causes of this massive worsening in indicators of population health, in association with a change of political economic system, remain unexplained. Some evidence points to the importance of increasing alcoholism and violence, associated with the end of guaranteed employment in economic production, as sources of early death. Replicating the cross-national research done during the 1980s, again controlling for level of economic development, will clarify the extent to which the previous advantages in PQL persisted or (more likely) disappeared with the transition to capitalism.

6. Political Economic Origins and Political Economic Reconstruction

The political economic origins of illness are not mysterious. Yet more than a century and a half after Engels' analysis first appeared, these problems remain. Public health generally has adopted the medical model of etiology. In this model, though social conditions may increase susceptibility or exacerbate disease, but primary causes are microbial agents or disturbances of normal physiology. Partly because research rarely has clarified the causes of illness within political economic systems, political strategy – both within and outside medicine – seldom has addressed the political economic roots of disease.

We need more empirical investigation that explores the short-term and long-term effects of political economic change on population health. For instance, such research will examine more carefully the apparently deleterious impact of capitalism's "triumph" on population health, initially in the Soviet Union and Eastern Europe, and, more recently, in Asia. Cross-national research on political economic determinants of health outcomes also may take advantage of the conceptual and methodological advances in Latin American social medicine in extending these perspectives to other regions of the world. In political economic research, the changing impacts of economic neo-imperialism and militarism on health outcomes also deserve greater attention.

Political economic pathologies – those that distressed Engels, Virchow, Allende – continue to create suffering and early death. Inequalities of class, exploitation of workers, and conditions of capitalist production cause disease now as previously. Likewise, the constraints of profit and lack of societal responsibility for individual economic security still inhibit even incremental reforms. The links between political economic conditions and disease become ever more urgent, as economic instability, unreliable food supplies, petroleum depletion, nuclear and toxic chemical wastes, global warming, and related problems threaten the survival of human beings and other life forms. Understanding political economic roots of illness also reveals the scope of reconstruction that is necessary for meaningful solutions. Given the inexorable relation between political economic systems and population health, public health professionals ignore such an important upstream determinant of health at our peril.

Endnotes

i. Due to the varying usages of the term *political economy*, a brief definition may prove helpful. In this chapter, political economy refers to the conditions under which economic production is organized. This definition follows the usage of the term in Marxian and neo-Marxian studies, as well as their prior antecedents in the works of Adam Smith and David Ricardo. In this sense, *political economic systems* refer to the different organizational frameworks for organizing economic production, such as capitalism and socialism. From this viewpoint, class structure, particularly the distinction between those who do own or control the means of production (capitalists) and those who do not (workers), comprises a crucial focus of political economy.

ii. Early works that considered the social origins of illness, but with a different analytic perspective, include:

Rosen, G. (1947). What is social medicine? *Bulletin of the History of Medicine*, 21, 674–733.

Rosen, G. (1958). *A history of public health*. New York: MD Publications. [especially pp. 192–293]

Sand, R. (1952). *The advance to social medicine*. London: Staples Press. [especially pp. 295–343, 507–589]

Sigerist, H. E. (1944). *Civilization and disease*. Ithaca, NY: Cornell University Press. [especially pp. 6–64]

For more extensive discussions of this history, see:

Waitzkin, H. (2000). *The second sickness: Contradictions of capitalist health care*. Lanham, MD: Rowman & Littlefield. [pp. 55–73]

Waitzkin, H. (2001). At the front lines of medicine: How the health care system alienates doctors and mistreats patients . . . and what we can do about it. Lanham, MD: Rowman and Littlefield. [pp. 41–75]

iii. For a sympathetic critique, see S. Marcus, *Engels, Manchester, and the Working Class* (New York: Vintage, 1974).

iv. For an overview of this literature on gender bias in diagnosis and treatment, see V. Elderkin-Thompson and H. Waitzkin, Difficulties in clinical communication with female patients: Are there diagnostic and treatment implications? *Journal of General Internal Medicine* 14 (1999): 112–121.

v. For instance: J.D. Wark, Osteoporosis: a global perspective, *Bulletin of the World Health Organization* 77 (1999): 424–426; Cervical cancer in developing countries: memorandum from a WHO meeting, *Bulletin of the World Health Organization* 74 (1996): 345–351; J.T. Boerma, K.I. Weinstein, S.O. Rustein, and A.E. Sommerfelt, Data on birth weight in developing countries: can surveys help? *Bulletin of the World Health Organization* 74 (1996): 209–216.

vi. For example, see: H. Waitzkin, Health policy and social change: a comparative history of Chile and Cuba, *Social Problems* 31 (1983): 235–248; H. Waitzkin, *The Politics of Medical Encounters: How Patients and Doctors Deal with Social Problems* (New Haven, CT: Yale University Press, 1991), pp. 265–272; H. Waitzkin, K. Wald, R. Kee, R. Danielson and L. Robinson, Primary care in Cuba: low- and high-technology developments pertinent to family medicine *Journal of Family Practice* 45 (1997). 250–258.

Aknowledgements.   This chapter was adapted from: Howard Waitzkin. (2001). *At the front lines of medicine: How the health care system alienates doctors and mistreats patients . . . and what we can do about it.* Lanham, MD: Rowman and Littlefield. and Howard Waitzkin. (2000). *The second sickness: Contradictions of capitalist health care.* 2nd edition. Lanham, MD: Rowman and Littlefield.

References

Ackerknecht, E. H. (1953). *Rudolf Virchow: Doctor, statesman, anthropologist.* Madison, WI: University of Wisconsin Press.

Allende, S. (1939). *La realidad médico-social Chilena.* Santiago, Chile: Ministerio de Salubridad, Prevision y Asistencia Social.

Baron, S., Field, J., & Schuller, T. (2001). *Social capital: Critical perspectives.* New York: Oxford University Press.

Barr, D., & Field, M. (1996). The current state of health care in the former Soviet Union: implications for health care policy and reform. *American Journal of Public Health, 86*(3), 307–12.

Bell, C., Crystal, M., Detsky, A., & Redelmeier, D. A. (1998). Shopping Around for hospital services: A comparison of the United States and Canada. *Journal of the American Medical Association, 279*(13), 1015–1017.

Birn, A., & Solorzano, A. (1999). Public health policy paradoxes: Science and politics in the Rockefeller Foundation's hookworm campaign in Mexico in the 1920s. *Social Science & Medicine, 49*(9), 1197–1213.

Bobak, M., & Marmot, M. (1999). Alcohol and mortality in Russia: Is it different than elsewhere? *Annals of Epidemiology, 9*(6), 339–340.

Bobak, M., Pikhart, H., Hertzman, C., Rose, R., & Marmot, M. (1998). Socioeconomic factors, perceived control and self-reported health in Russia. A cross-sectional survey. *Social Science & Medicine, 47*(2), 269–279.

Brown, E. R. (1979). *Rockefeller medicine men: Medicine and capitalism in America.* Berkeley, CA: University of California Press.

Carmichael, S., & Iyasu, S. (1998). Changes in the black-white infant mortality gap from 1983 to 1991 in the United States. *American Journal of Preventive Medicine, 15*(3), 220–227.

Carmichael, S., Iyasu, S., & Hatfield-Timajchy, K. (1998). Cause-specific trends in neonatal mortality among black and white infants, United States, 1980–1995. *Maternal and Child Health Journal, 2*(2), 67–76.

Cereseto, S., & Waitzkin, H. (1986). Capitalism, socialism, and the physical quality of life. *International Journal of Health Services, 16*(4), 643–58.

Chadwick, E. (1965). *Inquiry into the sanitary condition of the labouring population of Great Britain.* Edinburgh: Edinburgh University Press.

Cockerham, W. (1997). The social determinants of the decline of life expectancy in Russia and Eastern Europe: A lifestyle explanation. *Journal of Health and Social Behavior, 38*(2), 117–130.

Coleman, J. (1988). Social capital in the creation of human capital. *American Journal of Sociology, 94*, 95.

Cruz-Coke, E. (1938). *Medicina preventiva y medicina dirigida.* Santiago, Chile: Editorial Nascimento.

Cueto, M. (Ed.). (1994). *Missionaries of science: The Rockefeller Foundation and Latin America.* Bloomington, IN: Indiana University Press.

Diez Roux, A. V. (2000). Multilevel analysis in public health research. *Annual Review of Public Health, 21*, 171–192.

Diez Roux, A., Link, B., & Northridge, M. (2000). A multilevel analysis of income inequality and cardiovascular disease risk factors. *Social Science & Medicine, 50*(5), 673–687.

Engels, F. (1940). *Dialectics of nature.* New York: International publishers.

Engels, F. (1952). *The condition of the working class in England.* London: Allen and Unwin.

Engels, F. (1966). *Herr Eugen Dühring's revolution in science (anti-Dühring).* New York: International Publishers.

Fang, J., Madhavan, S., & Alderman, M. (1996). The association between birthplace and mortality from cardiovascular causes among black and white residents of New York City. *New England Journal of Medicine, 335*(21), 1545–1551.

Flexner, A. (1972). *Medical education in the United States and Canada: A report to the Carnegie Foundation for the Advancement of Teaching.* New York: Arno Press.

Foucault, M. (1977). El nacimento de la medicina social. *Revista Centroamericana de Ciencieas de la Salud, 3*(6), 89–108.

Franco, S. (1989). *La cuestión de la causalidad en medicina. Desarrollo de la medicina social en America Latina, OPS-ALAMES.* Mexico City: Organización Panamericana de la Salud.

Geronimus, A., Bound, J., Waidmann, T., Hillemeier, M. M., & Burns, P. B. (1996). Excess mortality among blacks and whites in the United States. *New England Journal of Medicine, 355*(21), 1552–1558.

Illanes, M. A. (1993). *"En el nombre del pueblo, del estado y de la ciencia, . . .": Historia social de la salud pública, Chile 1880–1973.* Santiago, Chile: Colectivo de Atención Primaria.

Kaplan, G. A., Pamuk, E. R., Lynch, J. W., Cohen, R. D., & Balfour, J. L. (1996). Inequality in income and mortality in the United States: Analysis of mortality and potential pathways. *British Medical Journal, 312*, 999–1003.

Katz, S., Charles, C., Lomas, J., & Welch, H. G. (1997). Physician relations in Canada: Shooting inward as the circle closes. *Journal of Health Politics, Policy, & Law, 22*(6), 1413–1431.

Katz, S., Hofer, T., & Manning, W. (1996). Hospital utilization in Ontario and the United States: The impact of socioeconomic status and health status. *Canadian Journal of Public Health, 87*(4), 253–256.

Kawachi, I., Kennedy, B., Gupta, V., & Prothrow-Stith, D. (1999). Women's status and the health of women and men: A view from the States. *Social Science & Medicine, 48*(1), 21–32.

Kawachi, I., Kennedy, B. P., Lochner, K., & Prothrow-Stith, D. (1997). Social capital, income inequality, and mortality. *American Journal of Public Health, 87*(9), 1491–1498.

Kawachi, I., Kennedy, B., & Wilkinson, R. (1999). *The society and population health reader. Income inequality and health.* New York: New Press.

Kennedy, B., Kawachi, I., Glass, R., & Prothrow-Stith, D. (1998). Income distribution, socioeconomic status, and self rated health in the United States: Multilevel analysis. *British Medical Journal, 317*(7163), 917–921.

Kennedy, B., Kawachi, I., Lochner, K., Jones, C., & Prothrow-Stith, D. (1997). (Dis) respect and black mortality. *Ethnicity & Disease, 7*(3), 207–214.

Kennedy, B., Kawachi, I., & Prothrow-Stith, D. (1996). Income distribution and mortality: Cross sectional ecological study of the Robin Hood index in the United States. *British Medical Journal, 312*(7037), 1004–1007.

Kennedy, B., Kawachi, I., Prothrow-Stith, D., Lochner, K., & Gupta, V. (1998). Social capital, income inequality, and firearm violent crime. *Social Science & Medicine, 47*(1), 7–17.

Kramarow, E., Lentzner, H., Rooks, R., Weeks, J., & Saydah, S. (1999). *Health and aging chartbook. Health, United States, 1999.* Hyattsville, MD: National Center for Health Statistics.

Laurell, A. C. (1982). La salud-enfermedad como proceso social. *Revista Latinoamericana De Salud, 2,* 7–25.

Levins, R., & Lewontin, (1985). *The dialectical biologist.* Cambridge, MA: Harvard University Press.

Lynch, J. W., Kaplan, G. A., Pamuk, E. R., Cohen, R. D., Heck, K. E., Balfour, J. L., et al. (1998). Income inequality and mortality in metropolitan areas of the United States. *American Journal of Public Health, 88*(7), 1074–1081.

Lynch, J. W., Smith, G. D., Kaplan, G. A., & House, J. S. (2000). Income inequality and mortality: Importance to health of individual income, psychosocial environment, or material conditions. *British Medical Journal, 320,* 1200–1204.

MacKay, A., Fingerhut, L., & Duran, C. (2000). *Adolescent health chartbook. Health, United States, 2000.* Hyattsville, MD: National Center for Health Statistics.

Mandelblatt, J., Gold, K., O'Malley, A. S., Taylor, K., Cagney, K., Hopkins, J. S., et al. (1999). Breast and cervix cancer screening among multiethnic women: Role of age, health, and source of care. *Preventive Medicine, 28*(4), 418–425.

Mandelblatt, J., Hadley, J., Kerner, J., Schulman, K. A., Gold, K., Dunmore-Griffith, J., et al. (2000). Patterns of breast carcinoma treatment in older women. *Cancer, 89*(3), 561–573.

Mandelblatt, J., Yabroff, K., & Kerner, J. (1999). Equitable access to cancer services. *Cancer, 86*(11), 2378–2390.

Marmot, M. (1999a). Epidemiology of socioeconomic status and health: Are determinants within countries the same as between countries? *Annals of the New York Academy of Sciences, 896*(1), 16–29.

Marmot, M. (1999b). Introduction. In M. Marmot & R. G. Wilkinson (Eds.), *Social determinants of health.* Oxford: Oxford University Press.

Marmot, M., & Feeney, A. (1997). General explanations for social inequalities in health. *IARC Scientific Publications, 138*, 207–28.

Marmot, M., Fuhrer, R., Ettner, S., Marks, N. F., Bumpass, L. L., & Ryff, C. D. (1998). Contribution of psychosocial factors to socioeconomic differences in health. *The Milbank Quarterly, 76*(3), 403–448.

Marmot, M., Smith, G., Stansfeld, S., Patel, C., North, F., Head, J., et al. (1991). Health inequalities among British civil servants: The Whitehall II study. *Lancet, 337*(8754), 1387–1393.

Martikainen, P., Stansfeld, S., Hemingway, H., & Marmot, M. (1999). Determinants of socioeconomic differences in change in physical and mental functioning. *Social Science & Medicine, 49*(4), 499–507.

McCord, C., & Freeman, H. (1990). Excess mortality in Harlem. *New England Journal of Medicine, 322*(3), 173–177.

McDonough, P., Williams, D., House, J., & Duncan, G. J. (1999). Gender and the socioeconomic gradient in mortality. *Journal of Health and Social Behavior, 40*(1), 17–31.

Murphy, M., Bobak, M., Nicholson, A., Rose, R., & Marmot, M. (2006). The widening gap in mortality by educational level in the Russian Federation, 1980–2001. *American Journal of Public Health, 96*(7), 1293–1299.

Notzon, F., Komarov, Y., Ermakov, S., Sempos, C. T., Marks, J. S., & Sempos, E. V. (1998). Causes of declining life expectancy in Russia. *Journal of the American Medical Association, 279*, 793–800.

Nunes, E. D. (1991). Trayectoría de la medicina social en América Latina: Elementos para su configuración. In S. Franco, E. D. Nunes, J. Breilh, & C. Laurell (Eds.), *Debates en medicina social*. Quito, Ecuador: Organización Panamericana de la Salud/ ALAMES.

Putnam, R. (2000). *Bowling alone: The collapse and revival of American community*. New York: Simon & Schuster.

Rathore, S., Berger, A., Weinfurt, K., Feinleib, M., Oetgen, W. J., Gersh, B. J., et al. (2000). Race, sex, poverty, and the medical treatment of acute myocardial infarction in the elderly. *Circulation, 102*, 642–648.

Ren, X., Amick, B., & Williams, D. (1999). Racial/ethnic disparities in health: The interplay between discrimination and socioeconomic status. *Ethnicity & Disease, 9*(2), 151–165.

Rosen, G. (1985). *De la politica médica a la medicina social*. Mexico City: Siglo XXI.

Schalick, L. M., Hadden, W. C., Pamuk, E., Navarro, V., & Pappas, G. (2000). The widening gap in death rates among income groups in the United States from 1967–1986. *International Journal of Health Services, 30*(1), 13–26.

Schulman, K. A., Berlin, J.A., Harless, W., Kerner, J. G., Sistrunk, S., Gersh, B. J., et al. (1999). The effect of race and sex on physicians' recommendations for cardiac catheterization. *New England Journal of Medicine, 340*(8), 618–627.

Sheifer, S., Escarce, J., & Schulman, K. (2000). Race and sex differences in the management of coronary artery disease. *American Heart Journal, 139*(5), 848–857.

Tulchinsky, T., & Varavikova, E.A. (1996). Addressing the epidemiologic transition in the former Soviet Union: Strategies for health system and public health reform in Russia. *American Journal of Public Health, 86*, 313–320.

van Rossum, C., Shipley, M., van de Mheen, H., Grobbee, D. E., & Marmot, M. G. (2000). Employment grade differences in cause specific mortality. A 25 year follow up of civil servants from the first Whitehall study. *British Medical Journal, 54*(3), 178–184.

Virchow, R. L. K. (1879). *Gesammelte abhandlungen aus dem gebiet der offentlichen medicin und der seuchenlehre*. Berlin: Hirschwald.

Virchow, R. L. K. (1957). *Werk und wirkung*. Berlin: Rütten & Loenig.

Virchow, R. L. K. (1958). *Disease, life, and man, selected essays.* Stanford, CA: Stanford University Press.

Virchow, R. L. K. (1971). *Cellular pathology as based upon physiological and pathological histology.* New York: Dover Publications.

Waitzkin, H. (1998). Is our work dangerous? Should it be? *Journal of Health and Social Behavior, 39*(1), 7–17.

Waitzkin, H. (2003). Report of the WHO Commission on Macroeconomics and Health: A summary and critique. *Lancet, 361*(9356), 523–526.

Waitzkin, H., Iriart, C., Estrada, A., & Lamadrid, S. (2001a). Social medicine in Latin America: Productivity and dangers facing the major national groups. *Lancet, 358*(9278), 315–323.

Waitzkin, H., Iriart, C., Estrada, A., & Lamadrid, S. (2001b). Social medicine then and now: Lessons from Latin America. *American Journal of Public Health, 91*(10), 1592–1601.

Walberg, P., McKee, M., Shkolnikov, V., Chenet, L., & Leon, D. A. (1998). Economic change, crime, and mortality crisis in Russia: Regional analysis. *British Medical Journal, 317*(7154), 312–318.

Wilkinson, R. (1996). *Unhealthy societies: The afflictions of inequality.* New York: Routledge.

Wilkinson, R. G. (1999). Putting the picture together: Prosperity, redistribution, health, and welfare. In M. Marmot & R. G. Wilkinson (Eds.), *Social determinants of health.* Oxford: Oxford University Press.

Williams, D. (1997). Race and health: Basic questions, emerging directions. *Annals of Epidemiology, 7*(5), 322–333.

Williams, D. (1999a). The monitoring of racial/ethnic status in the USA: Data quality issues. *Ethnicity & Health, 4*(3), 121–137.

Williams, D. R. (1999b). Race, socioeconomic status, and health: The added effects of racism and discrimination. *Annals of the New York Academy of Sciences, 896*(1), 173–188.

Williamson, D., & Fast, J. (1998). Poverty and medical treatment: When public policy compromises accessibility. *Canadian Journal of Public Health, 8* (2), 120–124.

World Bank. (1993). *World development report 1993: Investing in health.* Oxford: Oxford University Press for the World Bank.

World Health Organization. (1999). *Basic health statistics.* Geneva: World Health Organization.

Wyon, J. (1996). Comment: Deteriorating health in Russia—a place for community-based approaches. *American Journal of Public Health, 86*(3), 321–323.

Chapter 6
Climate Change

Marie S. O'Neill and Kristie L. Ebi

1. Introduction

For centuries, climate and weather have been recognized as important influences on human health (Haines, Kovats, Campbell-Lendrum, & Corvalan, 2006; McMichael, Campbell-Lendrum, Corvalan, Ebi, Githeko, Scheraga, Woodward, 2003). Climate, defined as the average weather over decades, is always changing. However, recent human activities, primarily fossil fuel combustion and deforestation have contributed to historically unprecedented concentrations of heat-trapping gases in the lower atmosphere. The elevated levels of these gases have begun to alter the global climate, with consequences that include increased surface temperatures, changes in the hydrological cycle, increased climate variability, and sea level rise (Albritton & Meira-Filho, 2001; Karl & Trenberth, 2003; Schiermeier, 2005; Ebi, Lewis, & Corvalan, 2006; Haines, McMichael, Kovats, & Saunders, 1998; Karl & Trenberth, 2003; McMichael et al., 2003; Schiermeier, 2005)

The health and social implications of this phenomenon transcend generations (McMichael, 2003) and geographic boundaries. There are major challenges in researching this macrosocial determinant of population health. These include the scale and complexity of the problem and the uncertainties inherent in projecting future consequences that depend on complicated system dynamics across multiple geographic, temporal, and operational scales that range from ecologic systems to actions taken by individuals and governments. Nonetheless, there is a growing imperative to produce and communicate scientific knowledge that will effectively inform and garner public support for sustainable, health-enhancing and equitable policies (Ebi & Gamble, 2005; McMichael, 2001a; Patz & Khaliq, 2002; Patz et al., 2000; Staropoli, 2002).

The goal of this chapter is to introduce the reader to the links between climate change and population health in research and practice. The chapter is divided into five sections. The first (Section 2) describes the science and evidence of anthropogenic (human-influenced) climate change. However, as health impacts due to climate variability and change do not depend on the drivers of climate change (i.e. deaths during a heat wave do not depend on whether the heat wave was due to natural influences or anthropogenic emissions of heat-trapping gases), the remaining sections examine aspects of climate change due to both natural and anthropogenic causes. Section 3 discusses climate change influences on the health of human populations. Section 4 describes how specific populations are affected by climate change, highlighting the relevant health outcomes from Section 3. Section 5 addresses societal actions to modify the course of human-influenced climate change, and Section 6 considers the specific role for public health action.

2. Climate Change Science

The earth's physical climate is principally determined by the sun's interactions with the atmosphere, oceans, land surface, and biosphere. Direct solar radiation is one source of warming of the earth; another key source is atmospheric levels of greenhouse gases (GHG), such as water vapor, carbon dioxide, methane, nitrous ozide, ozone, and others. The GHG absorb and re-radiate solar radiation that has been reflected by the earth's surface, thus increasing surface temperature. Both naturally occurring phenomena (volcanoes, forest fires) and human activities are sources of GHG. Human activities that emit carbon dioxide and other GHG include fossil fuel combustion for transportation, industrial processes, cooking, and heating and cooling, as well as methane emissions from landfills and agricultural activities.

Human influence on the earth's vegetative cover can also affect the climate. For example, land use and urbanization have contributed to the observed decrease in diurnal temperature range over the past 50 years (Kalnay & Cai, 2003), although other factors also play an important role (Vose, Karl, Easterling, Williams, & Menne, 2004). Land use also can influence the localized urban heat island effect, in which air temperatures in cities during hot weather are 2–10° F higher than in rural and suburban areas due to lack of vegetation and trees; heat emitted from vehicles, air conditioners and buildings; and reduced air flow around buildings (Environmental Protection Agency, 2005; Vose et al., 2004; Xu & Chen, 2004).

Temperature records over thousands of years can be approximated from gases trapped in polar ice cores, coral reefs, and other sources. These estimates provide compelling evidence that the climate has been warming at an unprecedented rate in the last 100 years and that these changes are strongly correlated with atmospheric carbon dioxide levels. Based on observations made at globally distributed land and sea surface monitors since 1880, Figure 6.1 depicts temperature departures from an average reference period (1951–1980), clearly demonstrating the strong upward trend in recent decades. Global surface temperature has increased about 0.2°C per decade in the past 30 years, and global mean surface temperature may be within about 1°C of the maximum temperature in the past million years (Hansen, Sato, Ruedy, Lo, Lea, & Medina-Elizade, 2006).

In addition to changing global average surface temperature, climate change will alter the hydrologic cycle, raise sea levels (due to both thermal expansion of warmer water and to melting of ice caps and glaciers), and increase the frequency

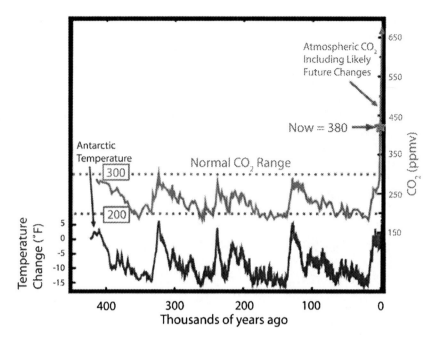

FIGURE 6.1. Temperature departures from an average reference period (1951–1980) based on observations made at globally distributed land and sea surface monitors since 1880.

Reprinted from Alley, R. B. (2004). Climate changes: Oceans, ice and us. *Oceanography*, 17 (4) 194–206.

of extreme weather events, such as droughts and floods (Easterling, Meehl, Parmesan, Changnon, Karl, & Mearns, 2000; Gaffen & Ross, 1998; Houghton, Ding, Griggs, Noguer, van der Linden, & Xiaosu, 2001; Karl, Knight, & Plummer, 1995; Karl & Trenberth, 2003; McGeehin & Mirabelli, 2001; National Research Council, 2001a). These projected changes take into account the counterbalancing effects of the reflective properties of aerosols (airborne particles) that result from both anthropogenic and natural sources. The inherent inertia in the climate system means that the world is committed to decades of climate change, even if drastic reductions in GHG emissions were accomplished immediately.

Already there is extensive evidence of ecological effects in response to recent climate change. Scientists have noted shifts in geographical distributions of animals and plants (Parmesan & Galbraith, 2004; Root, MacMynowski, Mastrandrea, & Schneider, 2005); multi-decade studies in Europe and North America found that birds, butterflies and foxes are shifting their habitual ranges northward, and many species of birds are laying their eggs earlier (Parmesan & Galbraith, 2004). Changes have been documented in plant growing seasons, from earlier springs to later fall colors, with an average lengthening of the European growing season of 11 days since 1960 (Menzel, 2000). These changes have important implications for agriculture. Recently, vintners and olive farmers in southern England had successful harvests, demonstrating the possible regional benefits to climatic changes. A survey of climate change-related impacts on life and livelihood in Nepal found both positive and negative changes (Dahal, 2005). For example, apples grow larger and more flavorful at high altitudes where it used to be too cold for apple farming. Older adults are finding their homes and villages more comfortable due to the warmer winters. However, other areas, including small island states and many mountain regions, are projected to experience significant adverse effects (Ebi, Lewis et al., 2006).

Although climate change is not the only factor affecting observed alterations in ecosystems, it can be an important driver that may impact biodiversity, habitat conservation, and endangered species. These ecosystem changes ultimately affect human health as well, as described in the next section.

3. Climate Change Influences on Population Health

3.1. Specific Health Outcomes

The cause-and-effect chain from climate change to changing patterns of health determinants and outcomes is often extremely complex and includes factors such as wealth, distribution of income, status of the public health infrastructure, provision of medical care, access to adequate nutrition, safe water, and sanitation, and population density (Woodward, Hales, Litidamu, Phillips, & Martin, 2000). Table 6.1 shows major health outcomes that can result from climate-related stressors, both direct and indirect. Information on each of these outcomes is provided in several recent reviews (McMichael, Woodruff, & Hales, 2006; Patz, Epstein, Burke, & Balbus, 1996; Patz, Graczyk, Geller, & Vittor, 2000; Woodward & Hales, 2003).

Three broad categories of health impacts are associated with climatic conditions: impacts relatively directly related to weather and climate variability; impacts resulting from environmental changes that occur in response to climate variability and change; and impacts resulting from consequences of climate-induced economic dislocation and environmental decline (Ebi, Mills, Smith, & Grambsch, 2006; McMichael et al., 2006; Patz, Campbell-Lendrum, Holloway, & Foley, 2005). The first two categories of climate-sensitive health determinants and outcomes include (1) changes in the frequency and intensity of thermal extremes and extreme weather events (i.e. floods and droughts) that directly affect population health and (2) indirect impacts that occur through changes in the geographic range and incidence of infectious diseases and food- and waterborne diseases, and changes in the prevalence of diseases associated with air pollutants and aeroallergens. Ecosystem changes can facilitate the emergence and re-emergence of disease, even under current climatic conditions (National Research Council, 2001b). For example, infectious agents (viruses, protozoa, etc) and their vectors e.g., mosquitoes, ticks) have evolved under particular ranges of temperature and precipitation; changes in weather patterns can affect their geographic distribution (Patz et al., 2005; Patz et al., 1996). Another example is foodborne illnesses, such

TABLE 6.1. Summary of the known effects of weather and climate

Health outcome	Known effects of weather and climate
Cardiovascular respiratory mortality and heat stroke mortality	• Short-term increases in mortality during heat waves • V- and J-shaped relationship between temperature and mortality in populations in temperate climates • Deaths from heat stroke increase during heat waves
Allergic rhinitis	• Weather affects the distribution, seasonality and production of aeroallergens
Respiratory and cardiovascular diseases and mortality	• Weather affects concentrations of harmful air pollutants
Deaths and injuries Infectious diseases and mental disorders	• Floods, landslides and windstorms cause death and injuries • Flooding disrupts water supply and sanitation systems and may damage transport systems and health care infrastructure • Floods may provide breeding sites for mosquito vectors and lead to outbreaks of disease • Floods may increase post-traumatic stress disorders
Starvation, malnutrition and diarrhoeal and respiratory diseases	• Drought reduces water availability for hygiene • Drought increases the risk of forest fires • Drought reduces food availability in populations that are highly dependent on household agriculture productivity and/or economically weak
Mosquito, tick-borne diseases and rodent-borne diseases (such as malaria, dengue, tick-borne encephalitis and Lyme disease)	• Higher temperatures shorten the development time of pathogens in vectors and increase the potential transmission to humans • Each vector species has specific climate conditions (temperature and humidity) necessary to be sufficiently abundant to maintain transmission
Malnutrition and undernutrition Waterborne and foodborne diseases	• Climate change may decrease food supplies (crop yields and fish stocks) or access to food supplies • Survival of disease-causing organisms is related to temperature • Climate conditions affect water availability and quality • Extreme rainfall can affect the transport of disease-causing organisms into the water supply

Modified from Kovats, R. S., Ebi, K. L., & Menne, B. (2003). *Methods for assessing human health vulnerability and public health adaptation to climate change.* World Health Organization / Health Canada / United Nations Environment Programme.

as salmonellosis, that are associated with ambient temperature in many regions (Patz et al., 2005). Climate change can further alter natural systems, making it possible for diseases to spread or emerge in areas where they had been limited or had not existed, or for diseases to disappear by making areas less hospitable to the vector or the pathogen.

Short-term weather patterns, climate variability, and climate change can affect the incidence of climate-sensitive health determinants and outcomes. An important mode of climate variability is the El Niño/Southern Oscillation (ENSO), a periodic change in sea pressure and circulation in the Indian and Pacific Oceans that results in changes in temperature, precipitation, and other weather variables patterns in the Pacific and worldwide. El Niño events are correlated with the distribution and incidence of malaria, hantavirus vectors, and other infectious diseases (Glass et al., 2002; Hales, Edwards, & Kovats, 2003). El Niño events also are of concern because they result in droughts and floods, which are of particular relevance to low-lying countries, island states, and coastal settlements (Ebi, Lewis et al., 2006). Various aspects of the ecology also can be influenced by ENSO, including growing seasons and precipitation patterns relevant to health (Walther et al., 2002). Although the impact of anthropogenic climate change on the ENSO is uncertain (Hales et al., 2003), it can be a useful indicator of future vulnerability to climate change for some regions and health outcomes.

Temperature-related mortality is directly quantifiable. Although cold can affect health, heat-related mortality has been emphasized given the expected upward shift in the temperature distribution and the trend for increasing minimum temperatures (Basu & Samet, 2003; Braga, Zanobetti, & Schwartz, 2002; Curriero et al., 2002; Hajat, Kovats, Atkinson, & Haines, 2002; Keatinge et al., 2000; O'Neill, Zanobetti, & Schwartz, 2003; Semenza et al., 1996; Whitman et al., 1997). Excess deaths occur during heat waves (Robinson, 2001), on days with higher-than-average temperatures, and in places where summer temperatures vary more (Braga, Zanobetti, & Schwartz, 2001). Other studies have evaluated hospitalizations during hot weather (Kovats, Hajat, & Wilkinson, 2004; Schwartz, Samet, & Patz, 2004; Semenza, McCullough, Flanders, McGeehin, & Lumpkin, 1999), finding less consistent associations than for mortality. Particular medical conditions, including diabetes, emphysema, and nervous system disorders, may affect risk (Semenza et al., 1999). Factors related to housing also affect vulnerability; for example, heat stroke risk is higher among individuals with no access to air conditioning or with few trees and shrubs shading their dwellings (Kilbourne, Choi, Jones, & Thacker, 1982). Identifying sources of vulnerability is important for designing public health interventions related to hot weather and heatwaves, an issue receiving increased attention after the recent devasting consequences of hot summer weather in Europe and elsewhere.

In addition to the health outcomes identified in Table 6.1, climate change has the potentially to "fundamentally alter" the conditions of life in a way that transforms population health risks (Schwartz, Parker, Glass, & Hu, 2006). Potential implications of water scarcity, for example, might be increases in violent conflict and social disruption, with far-reaching consequences for population and individual health.

3.2 Aggregate Estimates of the Health Impacts of Climate Change

An important challenge in identifying how climate change influences population health is that the causes of ill-health are multi-factorial, making attribution of health consequences to climate change difficult (Githeko & Woodward, 2003). Complexities in projecting how climate change might alter future disease patterns include uncertainties about the magnitude and timing of climate change, the extent of demographic change, how exposure-response relationships could change (i.e. the shape of the heat-mortality relationship under higher temperatures), how socioeconomic and technical development will alter public health, and other factors (Hitz & Smith, 2004). Although the extent and rate of projected climate change is uncertain (Stainforth et al., 2005), the scientific consensus is that, on balance, the health impacts will be largely negative, particularly in low-income countries (McMichael, 2001b). The World Health Organization conducted a regional and global comparative risk assessment to quantify the amount of premature morbidity and mortality due to a range of risk factors and to predict the benefit of interventions to remove or reduce these risk factors. Climate change was estimated using modeled climate exposure scenarios. According to the model, in the year 2000, climate change caused the loss of over 150,000 lives, with most of those deaths due to undernutrition and diarrheal diseases (Campbell-Lendrum, Pruss-Ustun, & Corvalan, 2003; Ezzati, Lopez, Rodgers, Vander Hoorn, & Murray, 2002; McMichael, 2004). The assessment also addressed how much of the future health burden of climate change could be avoided by stabilizing GHG emissions (Campbell-Lendrum et al., 2003). The health outcomes included were chosen based on known sensitivity to climate variation, predicted future importance, and availability of quantitative global models (or feasibility of constructing them); they included episodes of diarrheal disease, cases of *Falciparum* malaria, fatal unintentional injuries in coastal floods and inland floods/landslides, and non-availability of recommended daily calorie intake (as an indicator for the prevalence of malnutrition). Adjustments for adaptation were included in the estimates. The projected relative risks attributable to climate change in 2030 vary by health outcome and region and are largely negative; the majority of the projected disease burden is due to increases in diarrheal disease and malnutrition, primarily in low-income populations already experiencing a large burden of disease (Campbell-Lendrum et al., 2003; McMichael, 2004).

The projected risks of the WHO study highlight the need for a better understanding of the potential health impacts of climate change, particularly the distributional impacts on populations, both geographically and demographically. The next section describes four specific populations, discusses the health impacts of most relevance to them, and concludes by discussing vulnerable populations and equity.

4. Specific Populations Affected by Climate Change

4.1. Urban Populations

The proportion of the world's population living in urban centers is substantial and growing (Vlahov, Galea, Gibble, & Freudenberg, 2005), with 65% of the world's population projected to live in cities by 2025 (World Health Organization, 2000). One important climate-related concern for urban populations is exposure to extreme temperatures. Because of data availability and population concentration, much of the research on temperature and health has been conducted in urban areas in developed countries. The Intergovernmental Panel on Climate Change (IPCC) has expressed "high confidence" that heat-related morbidity and mortality will affect urban populations (partly due to urban heat-island effects) more than rural populations (Intergovernmental Panel on Climate Change, 2001a).

Aspects of urban infrastructure and personal and underlying health characteristics determine who is most affected by hot weather. Heat-related deaths occur more in areas where extreme heat is rare because those populations may be less acclimated to high temperatures (Kalkstein, 2000). Acclimatization to hot and cold temperature over the last decades is evident in studies in London (Carson, Hajat, Armstrong, & Wilkinson, 2006) and the US (Davis, Knappenberger, Michaels, & Novicoff, 2003). Projecting the future impacts of climate change on these populations is therefore complicated because of social, economic, and demographic shifts that result in differing levels of vulnerability. One important caveat to adaptive responses like increased air conditioning is that such a response could increase emissions of greenhouse gases and exacerbate climate change, depending on the energy source (O'Neill, 2003). At the same time, as poor urban air quality has been associated with health impacts in many cities worldwide (Brunekreef & Holgate, 2002; Stieb, Judek, & Burnett, 2002), reductions in air pollution as a result of GHG mitigation are projected to provide substantial health benefits in cities (Cifuentes, Borja-Aburto, Gouveia, Thurston, & Davis, 2001a, 2001b).

Urban centers may be affected strongly by floods and extreme weather events because of high population density, informal housing, and other factors. Refugees from surrounding regions are likely to congregate in cities, placing burdens on urban services and infrastructure. Certain climate-sensitive infectious diseases, such as dengue, a mosquito-borne viral disease common in urban areas of tropical countries, as well as rodent-borne diseases, are of growing concern in urban areas with increasing climate variability and climate change (Hales et al., 2003).

4.2. Small Island States

Populations in many small island states (including small islands and low lying coastal countries) are especially vulnerable to climate change-related sea level rise, flooding, and storm surges (Ahern, Kovats, Wilkinson, Few, & Matthies, 2005), and changes in temperature, rainfall patterns, and soil moisture budgets (Ebi et al., 2006). The potential for increasing frequency and severity of tropical storms is of special concern for residents of coastal and low-lying environments (Emanuel, 2005; Webster, Holland, Curry, & Chang, 2005). A common feature of many small island states is their limited ability to adapt to impacts of climate change due to small land area, limited economic and natural resources, and weaknesses in public health infrastructure. Representatives of small island states and coastal populations have appealed to international bodies for concerted preventive action given the potential catastrophic consequences of climate change.

4.3. Rural Populations

Particularly in tropical regions, climate change could adversely affect some rural populations and areas by increasing food insecurity through reducing crop yields and water resources and increasing droughts, floods, and rates of climate-sensitive diseases. Malnutrition is currently a major cause of ill health, particularly in rural areas, and there are indications that it will take approximately 35 additional years to reach the World Food Summit 2002 target of reducing world hunger by half by 2015 (Rosegrant & Cline, 2003; United Nations Millennium Project, 2005). In some regions, available food supplies are not projected to keep pace with population growth, increasing the absolute number of people malnourished. Child malnutrition is likely to persist in many low-income countries, although the overall global burden is expected to decline.

The determinants of malnutrition are complex. Due to the very large number of people that may be affected, malnutrition linked to drought and flooding may be one of the most important consequences of climate change, but limited information is available. One study estimated that climate change could increase the percentage of the Malian population at risk of hunger from 34% to 72% by the 2050s, although this could be substantially reduced by effective implementation of a range of adaptive strategies (Butt, McCarl, Angerer, Dyke, & Stuth, 2005). Projections suggest that those likely to be adversely affected are the regions already most vulnerable.

4.4. Low-Income Nations

The capacity of low-income nations to adapt to climate change is limited because the economic, transportation, and public health infrastructures are, by definition, in a state of development. Low-income countries carry 90% of the worldwide disease burden but have only 10% of resources to promote health (World Health Organization, 1992). Depending on their geographic location, the range of climate-related health risks, from thermal stress, to infectious diseases, to population displacement, can be of concern. All 191 United Nations member countries have pledged to meet the eight Millennium Development Goals by 2015 (United Nations, 2006), including goals related to improving environmental sustainability and various aspects of health, as well as eradicating extreme poverty and hunger. These goals will become more challenging as the direct and indirect consequences of climate change affect these nations.

4.5. Vulnerable Populations and Equity

Climate change does not affect the health of all members of the population or all members of the international community equally. Differential impacts by socioeconomic status, race/ethnicity, and age have been observed, and as the IPCC stated, "The impacts of climate change will fall disproportionately upon developing countries and the poor persons within all countries . . ." (Intergovernmental

Panel on Climate Change, 2001b) The global population of elderly people is increasing; physiologically and socially these groups are especially vulnerable (Khosla & Guntupalli, 1999; Klinenberg, 2002) to heat waves and hot weather. This differential vulnerability at the individual biomedical level is important, but factors beyond individuals also influence the risk of experiencing climate-related health effects and the development and deployment of adaptation strategies, policies, and measures (Diez Roux, 2004). Community attributes relevant to climate vulnerability include physical features, such as housing quality and green space; social programs, such as government programs and access to health care; population composition, such as level of education, racial/ethnic composition; and social and cultural factors, such as whether individuals believe they have responsibility for vector control.

The environmental justice movement in the United States has begun to turn its attention to the differential impacts of climate change on poor and minority populations (Environmental Justice and Climate Change, 2006), and the connection between climate change and health inequalities has been made in recent commentary (Sunyer & Grimalt, 2006).

5. Societal Actions that can Modify Climate Change

Societal actions to reduce the human influence on climate change and to adapt to the impending changes range in scope from international research activity and political treaties, to policies and activities of relevant industries and sectors, to implementation of national, state, and local strategies, policies, and measures. In 1988, the United Nations Environment Programme and the World Meteorological Organization established the Intergovernmental Panel on Climate Change (IPCC) to periodically assess the scientific evidence about the influence of human activities on climate change; to examine how these changes will affect various aspects of society, including health; and to evaluate response options (Githeko & Woodward, 2003). The IPCC reports represent international scientific consensus on these issues.

From the 1970s onward, international organizations and United Nations member states have called for preventive and adaptive action in response to growing evidence of human impact on the climate (Corvalan, Gopalan, & Llanso, 2003). The 1992 United Nations Framework Convention on Climate Change (UNFCCC) established a goal of stabilizing atmospheric concentrations of greenhouse gases in a timeframe to allow natural adaptation of ecosystems to climate change (Corvalan et al., 2003). The precautionary principle, which holds that scientific uncertainty should not be taken as a rationale for lack of action to prevent potentially severe consequences, such as environmental degradation, is embodied in the UNFCCC. Another key principle is equity; the signatories to the UNFCCC recognized a common but differentiated responsibility in which developed countries are to take the lead in combating the adverse effects of climate change.

The Kyoto Protocol is an international agreement setting specific, legally-binding commitments toward reducing concentrations of six greenhouse gases, including carbon dioxide (Corvalan et al., 2003). The Kyoto Protocol was adopted in 1997 and has been ratified by 164 countries – the United States and Australia are notable exceptions. In addition to these international frameworks and opportunities for action, local and national governments are engaged in assessing impacts of climate change and making specific commitments towards mitigation of GHG emissions (Cities for Climate Protection, 2005; Patz et al., 2000).

In spite of these activities, preventive action has not been commensurate with the magnitude of the possible consequences. This is especially true for the United States, which has 5% of the world's population and produces 25% of global carbon dioxide emissions (Schwartz et al., 2006). There are many barriers to action, including uncertainty about the magnitude and rate of climate change, the fact that the highest burden of impacts will occur in countries that contributed the least to the problem, the complexities of international negotiations, the influence of entrenched interest (both national and industrial), and the limited public awareness of the immediacy of the problem. To the last point, the US media's belief that balanced reporting requires presenting both sides equally has resulted in biased coverage that has worked against the public and policymakers' understanding of the importance and urgency of the issue (Boykoff & Boykoff, 2004). Further, there is evidence that the language commonly used to reflect the uncertainty of climate change projections is interpreted differently by scientists and the lay public (Patt & Schrag, 2003). Whatever the barriers, it is evident that human activities have and continue to influence the climate in ways that cannot be reversed.

Because of the inevitability of climate change, there is increasing focus on the importance of adaptation, which refers to actions taken to reduce the impact of actual or expected climate change (Smit et al., 2001). Population vulnerability to climate change-related health effects depends on exposure to the "climate-related hazard", how health outcomes respond to changes in climate, and the population's adaptive capacity (Bernard & Ebi, 2001; Intergovernmental Panel on Climate Change, 2001a). Therefore, the severity of future impacts will be determined by changes in climate as well as by concurrent changes in non-climatic factors and by the adaptation measures implemented to reduce negative impacts. Research is needed to understand to what degree projected impacts can be avoided by adaptation and how to achieve the appropriate balance between adaptation and mitigation to minimize the large health impacts to current and future populations. Adaptive actions might include the implementation of strategies, policies, and measures by international, national, regional, and local agencies and institutions to decrease vulnerability to current and projected impacts. Private individuals may also engage in activities that have less impact on the climate. Actions to reduce poverty and inequality, to improve environmental quality and resilience (e.g., wetland integrity), and to maintain the public health infrastructure are adaptive activities likely to reduce the health impacts of climate change.

6. Public Health Practice and Climate Change

Public health practitioners and researchers need to actively engage in understanding and planning for climate change-related health impacts. The results of the WHO comparative risk assessment suggest that health consequences of climate change are already occurring. Still, relatively little climate change has occurred compared with what is projected; therefore, unless effective actions are taken soon, it is likely that the extent of impacts will increase. Public health agencies and institutions are beginning to identify and implement specific actions to address climate change-related health impacts. However, more research is needed on the projected health effects, including quantification of the associated economic burden and the most effective and efficient policies, strategies, and measures to reduce those risks.

In the research realm, evaluating a range of health outcomes and exposures in various locations (including multi-city or multi-country studies) and on various timescales is required to understand how weather, climate variability, and climate change can negatively affect human health. The main tasks for public health in addressing the health impacts of climate change include establishing baseline relationships, finding evidence for early effects, developing scenarios, evaluating adaptation options, and estimating costs and benefits of mitigating climate change and adapting to its effects (Woodward & Scheraga, 2003). Scenarios and complex modeling processes that incorporate nonlinear associations between exposures and diseases are two useful approaches for evaluating how different futures might affect projected climate change impacts (Ebi & Gamble, 2005; Woodward & Scheraga, 2003).

The engagement of public health scientists in national and international planning processes related to climate change mitigation (e.g., GHG emissions reductions) and adaptation (e.g., urban heat island reductions, measures to increase resiliency to climate related-health effects) can help ensure that these activities promote population health. Researchers studying climate change and health take a perspective that evaluates and acknowledges the interdependence of human health and the health of ecological and physical systems of the planet (McMichael, 2003). Similarly, public health practitioners and clinicians have been encouraged to promote population health by engaging in advocacy and community participation efforts that extend beyond the traditional domain of clinical practice (Gruen, Pearson, & Brennan, 2004). Clinicians also can play a role in encouraging individual behavior changes (such as using less energy) that will reduce climate change impacts in the longer term (Schwartz et al., 2006).

Public health programs, including surveillance and response, may need to be revised, supplemented, or reoriented to measure, recognize, evaluate, anticipate, and respond to the effects of climate on health. Surveillance is a core activity of public health that provides early intelligence on whether a health outcome is increasing in incidence or geographic range (Wilson & Anker, 2005). Surveillance not only involves the systematic collection of information on health determinants and outcomes necessary to determine the occurrence and spread of these outcomes, but also the analysis, interpretation, and distribution of this information to relevant actors for timely and effective control activities.

For some diseases, surveillance programs may be coupled with an early warning system intended to prompt timely interventions to reduce the magnitude or extent of a disease outbreak. Whereas surveillance systems are designed to detect and investigate outbreaks as they occur, early warning systems are intended to alert the population and relevant authorities when an outbreak is expected. Early warning systems can be very effective in preventing deaths, diseases, and injuries (Ebi & Schmier, 2005). One example is heatwave early warning systems being implemented in the US, Canada, and Europe (Assessment and Prevention of acute Health Effects of Weather conditions in Europe (PHEWE), 2005; Grynszpan, 2003; Mattern, Garrigan, & Kennedy, 2000; Smoyer-Tomic & Rainham, 2001). System designs potentially could incorporate projected increases in climate variability and change. Early warning systems need to be flexible to adjust to changing conditions; this includes monitoring of system performance to determine when adjustments are required.

All activities mentioned above can play an integral role in efforts to prevent the health effects of climate change through societal change (Bransford & Lai, 2002; Burns, 2002; Ebi & Gamble, 2005; Haines & Patz, 2004; Patz & Khaliq, 2002; Staropoli, 2002; Sunyer & Grimalt, 2006). Like many macrosocial determinants of health, climate change is a complex phenomenon but amenable to mitigative and adaptive action if leadership and commitment is exercised at individual, local, national and international levels.

References

Ahern, M., Kovats, R. S., Wilkinson, P., Few, R., & Matthies, F. (2005). Global health impacts of floods: Epidemiologic evidence. *Epidemiologic Reviews, 27*, 36–46.

Albritton, D. L., & Meira-Filho, L. G. (Eds.). (2001). *Technical summary. Working group 1, intergovernmental panel on climate change.* Cambridge: Cambridge University Press.

Assessment and Prevention of acute Health Effects of Weather conditions in Europe. (2005). Assessment and Prevention of acute Health Effects of Weather conditions in Europe. Roma, Italy (2006); http://www.epiroma.it/phewe/.

Basu, R., & Samet, J. (2003). The relationship between elevated ambient temperature and mortality: A review of the epidemiologic evidence. *Epidemiologic Reviews, 24*(2), 190–202.

Bernard, S. M., & Ebi, K. L. (2001). Comments on the process and product of the health impacts assessment component of the national assessment of the potential consequences of climate variability and change for the United States. *Environmental Health Perspectives, 109*(Supplement 2), 177–184.

Boykoff, M., & Boykoff, J. (2004). Balance as bias: Global warming and the U.S. prestige press. *Global Environmental Change, 14*, 125–136.

Braga, A. L., Zanobetti, A., & Schwartz, J. (2001). The time course of weather related deaths. *Epidemiology, 12*, 662–667.

Braga, A. L. F., Zanobetti, A., & Schwartz, J. (2002). The effect of weather on respiratory and cardiovascular deaths in 12 U.S. cities. *Environmental Health Perspectives, 110*(9), 859–863.

Bransford, K. J., & Lai, J. A. (2002). Global climate change and air pollution: Common origins with common solutions. *Journal of the American Medical Association, 287*(17), 2285.

Brunekreef, B., & Holgate, S. T. (2002). Air pollution and health. *Lancet, 360*(9341), 1233–1242.

Burns, W. C. (2002). Climate change and human health: The critical policy agenda. *Journal of the American Medical Association, 287*(17), 2287.

Butt, T., McCarl, B., Angerer, J., Dyke, P., & Stuth, J. (2005). The economic and flood security implications of climate change in Mali. *Climatic Change, 68*, 355–378.

Campbell-Lendrum, D., Pruss-Ustun, A., & Corvalan, C. (2003). How much disease could climate change cause? In A. McMichael, D. Campbell-Lendrum, C. Corvalan, K. Ebi, A. Githeko, J. Scheraga, & A. Woodward (Eds.), *Climate change and human health: Risks and responses*. Geneva: World Health Organization.

Carson, C., Hajat, S., Armstrong, B., & Wilkinson, P. (2006). Declining vulnerability to temperature-related mortality in London over the 20th century. *American Journal of Epidemiology, 164*(1), 77–84.

Cifuentes, L., Borja-Aburto, V. H., Gouveia, N., Thurston, G., & Davis, D. L. (2001a). Assessing the health benefits of urban air pollution reductions associated with climate change mitigation (2000–2020): Santiago, Sao Paulo, Mexico City, and New York City. *Environmental Health Perspectives, 109*(Supplement 3), 419–425.

Cifuentes, L., Borja-Aburto, V. H., Gouveia, N., Thurston, G., & Davis, D. L. (2001b). Climate change. Hidden health benefits of greenhouse gas mitigation. *Science, 293*(5533), 1257–1259.

Cities for Climate Protection. (2005). Cities for Climate Protection. Toronto (2006); http://www.iclei.org/co2/

Corvalan, C. F., Gopalan, H. N. B., & Llanso, P. (2003). Conclusions and recommendations for action. In A. J. McMichael, D. H. Campbell-Lendrum, C. F. Corvalan, K. L. Ebi, A. Githeko, J. D. Scheraga, & A. Woodward (Eds.), *Climate change and human health: Risks and responses*. Geneva: World Health Organization.

Curriero, F. C., Heiner, K. S., Samet, J. M., Zeger, S. L., Strug, L., & Patz, J. A. (2002). Temperature and mortality in 11 cities of the eastern United States. *American Journal of Epidemiology, 155*(1), 80–87.

Dahal, N. (2005). Perceptions of climate change in the Himalayas. *(2005)*; http://www.tiempocyberclimate.org/newswatch/feature050910.htm

Davis, R. E., Knappenberger, P. C., Michaels, P. J., & Novicoff, W. M. (2003). Changing heat-related mortality in the United States. *Environmental Health Perspectives, 111*(14), 1712–1718.

Diez Roux, A. V. (2004). The study of group-level factors in epidemiology: Rethinking variables, study designs, and analytical approaches. *Epidemiologic Reviews, 26*, 104–111.

Easterling, D. R., Meehl, G. A., Parmesan, C., Changnon, S. A., Karl, T. R., & Mearns, L. O. (2000). Climate extremes: Observations, modeling, and impacts. *Science, 289*(5487), 2068–2074.

Ebi, K. L., & Gamble, J. L. (2005). Summary of a workshop on the development of health models and scenarios: Strategies for the future. *Environmental Health Perspectives, 113*(3), 335–338.

Ebi, K. L., Lewis, N. D., & Corvalan, C. F. (2006). Climate variability and change and their potential health effects in small island states: Information for adaptation planning in the health sector. *Environmental Health Perspectives, 114*(12), 1957–1963.

Ebi, K., Mills, D., Smith, J., & Grambsch, A. (2006). Climate change and human health impacts in the United States: An update on the results of the U.S. National Assessment. *Environmental Health Perspectives, 114*(9), 1318–1324.

Ebi, K. L., & Schmier, J. K. (2005). A stitch in time: Improving public health early warning systems for extreme weather events. *Epidemiologic Reviews, 27,* 115–121.

Emanuel, K. (2005). Increasing destructiveness of tropical cyclones over the past 30 years. *Nature, 436*(7051), 686–688.

Environmental Justice and Climate Change. (2005). Economic justice: The time is now. Oakland, CA (2005); http://www.ejcc.org/index.html

Environmental Protection Agency. (2005). Heat island effect. (October 16, 2006); http://www.epa.gov/heatisland/about/index.html

Ezzati, M., Lopez, A. D., Rodgers, A., Vander Hoorn, S., Murray, C. J. L., & Comparative Risk Assessment Collaborating Group. (2002). Selected major risk factors and global and regional burden of disease. *Lancet, 360,* 1347–1360.

Gaffen, D. J., & Ross, R. J. (1998). Increased summertime heat stress in the U.S. *Nature, 396*(6711), 529–530.

Githeko, A. K., & Woodward, A. (2003). International consensus on the science of climate and health: The IPCC third assessment report. In A. J. McMichael, D. H. Campbell-Lendrum, C. F. Corvalan, K. L. Ebi, A. Githeko, J. D. Scheraga, & A. Woodward (Eds.), *Climate change and human health: Risks and responses.* Geneva: World Health Organization.

Glass, G. E., Yates, T. L., Fine, J. B., Shields, T. M., Kendall, J. B., Hope, A. G., et al. (2002). Satellite imagery characterizes local animal reservoir populations of Sin Nombre virus in the southwestern United States. *Proceedings of the National Academy of Sciences of the United States of America, 99*(26), 16817–16822.

Gruen, R. L., Pearson, S. D., & Brennan, T. A. (2004). Physician-citizens—public roles and professional obligations. *Journal of the American Medical Association, 291*(1), 94–98.

Grynszpan, D. (2003). Lessons from the French heatwave. *Lancet, 362*(9391), 1169–1170.

Haines, A., Kovats, R. S., Campbell-Lendrum, D. H., & Corvalan, C. (2006). Climate change and human health: Impacts, vulnerability and public health. *Public Health, 120*(7), 585–596.

Haines, A., McMichael, A. J., Kovats, S., & Saunders, M. (1998). Majority view of climate scientists is that global warming is indeed happening. *British Medical Journal, 316*(7143), 1530.

Haines, A., & Patz, J. A. (2004). Health effects of climate change. *Journal of the American Medical Association, 291*(1), 99–103.

Hajat, S., Kovats, R. S., Atkinson, R. W., & Haines, A. (2002). Impact of hot temperatures on death in London: A time series approach. *Journal of Epidemiology & Community Health, 56*(5), 367–372.

Hales, S., Edwards, S. J., & Kovats, R. S. (2003). Impacts on health of climate extremes. In A. J. McMichael, D. H. Campbell-Lendrum, C. F. Corvalan, K. L. Ebi, A. Githeko, J. D. Scheraga, & A. Woodward (Eds.), *Climate change and human health: Risks and responses.* Geneva: World Health Organization.

Hansen, J., Sato, M., Ruedy, R., Lo, K., Lea, D. W., & Medina-Elizade, M. (2006). Global temperature change. *Proceedings of the National Academy of Sciences of the United States of America, 103*(39), 14288–14293.

Hitz, S., & Smith, J. (2004). Estimating impacts from global environmental change. *Global Environmental Change. 14*(3), 201–218.

Houghton, J. T., Ding, Y., Griggs, D. J., Noguer, M., van der Linden, P. J., & Xiaosu, D. (Eds.). (2001). *Climate change 2001: The scientific basis. Contribution of Working Group 1 to the Third Assessment Report of the Intergovernmental Panel on Climate Change (IPCC)*: Cambridge, UK: Cambridge University Press.

Intergovernmental Panel on Climate Change. (2001a). Climate change 2001: Impacts, adaptation, and vulnerability: Summary for policymakers. Geneva (2001); http://www.grida.no/climate/ipcc_tar/wg2/005.htm.

Intergovernmental Panel on Climate Change. (2001b). Climate change 2001: Synthesis report. http://www.ipcc.ch/pub/un/syreng/spm.pdf.

Kalkstein, L. S. (2000). Saving lives during extreme weather in summer. *British Medical Journal, 321*(7262), 650–651.

Kalnay, E., & Cai, M. (2003). Impact of urbanization and land-use change on climate. *Nature, 423*(6939), 528–531.

Karl, T. R., Knight, R. W., & Plummer, N. (1995). Trends in high-frequency climate variability in the twentieth century. *Nature, 377*(6546), 217–220.

Karl, T. R., & Trenberth, K. E. (2003). Modern global climate change. *Science, 302*(5651), 1719–1723.

Keatinge, W. R., Donaldson, G. C., Cordioli, E., Martinelli, M., Kunst, A. E., Mackenbach, J. P., et al. (2000). Heat related mortality in warm and cold regions of Europe: Observational study. *British Medical Journal, 321*(7262), 670–673.

Khosla, R., & Guntupalli, K. K. (1999). Heat-related illnesses. *Critical Care Clinics, 15*(2), 251–263.

Kilbourne, E. M., Choi, K., Jones, T. S., & Thacker, S. B. (1982). Risk factors for heatstroke. A case-control study. *Journal of the American Medical Association, 247*(24), 3332–3336.

Klinenberg, E. (2002). *Heat wave: A social autopsy of disaster in Chicago*. Chicago: The University of Chicago Press.

Kovats, R. S., Hajat, S., & Wilkinson, P. (2004). Contrasting patterns of mortality and hospital admissions during hot weather and heat waves in greater London, UK. *Occupational & Environmental Medicine, 61*(11), 893–898.

Mattern, J., Garrigan, S., & Kennedy IV, S. B. (2000). A community-based assessment of heat-related morbidity in North Philadelphia. *Environmental Research, 83*(3), 338–342.

McGeehin, M. A., & Mirabelli, M. (2001). The potential impacts of climate variability and change on temperature-related morbidity and mortality in the United States. *Environmental Health Perspectives, 109*(Supplement 2), 185–189.

McMichael, A. J. (2001a). Global environmental change as "risk factor": Can epidemiology cope? *American Journal of Public Health, 91*(8), 1172–1174.

McMichael, A. J. (2001b). Health consequences of global climate change. *Journal of the Royal Society of Medicine, 94*(3), 111–114.

McMichael, A. J. (2003). Global climate change and health: An old story writ large. In A. J. McMichael, D. H. Campbell-Lendrum, C. F. Corvalan, K. L. Ebi, A. Githeko, J. D. Scheraga, & A. Woodward (Eds.), *Climate change and human health: Risks and responses*. Geneva: World Health Organization.

McMichael, A. (2004). Climate Change. In M. Ezzati, A. Lopez, A. Rodgers, & C. Murray (Eds.), *Comparative quantification of health risks: Global and regional burden of disease due to selected major risk factors. Volume 2*. Geneva: World Health Organization.

McMichael, A. J., Campbell-Lendrum, D. H., Corvalan, C. F., Ebi, K. L., Githeko, A., Scheraga, J. D., et al. (Eds.). (2003). *Climate change and human health: Risks and responses*. Geneva: World Health Organization.

McMichael, A. J., Woodruff, R. E., & Hales, S. (2006). Climate change and human health: Present and future risks. *Lancet, 367*(9513), 859–869.

Menzel, A. (2000). Trends in phenological phases in Europe between 1951 and 1996. *International Journal of Biometeorology, 44*(2), 76–81.

National Research Council. (2001a). *Climate change science: An analysis of some key questions.* Washington, DC: National Research Council.

National Research Council. (2001b). *Under the weather: Climate, ecosystems, and infectious disease.* Washington, DC: National Academy Press.

O'Neill, M. S. (2003). Air conditioning and heat-related health effects. *Applied Environmental Science and Public Health, 1*(1), 9–12.

O'Neill, M. S., Zanobetti, A., & Schwartz, J. (2003). Modifiers of the temperature and mortality association in seven US cities. *American Journal of Epidemiology, 157*(12), 1074–1082.

Parmesan, C., & Galbraith, H. (2004). *Observed impacts of global climate change in the U.S.* Arlington, VA (November, 2004); http://www.pewclimate.org/global-warming-in-depth/all_reports/observedimpacts/index.cfm

Patt, A. G., & Schrag, D. P. (2003). Using specific language to describe risk and probability. *Climatic Change, 61*(1– 2), 17–30.

Patz, J. A., Campbell-Lendrum, D. H., Holloway, T., & Foley, J. A. (2005). Impact of regional climate change on human health. *Nature, 438*, 310–317.

Patz, J. A., Epstein, P. R., Burke, T. A., & Balbus, J. M. (1996). Global climate change and emerging infectious diseases. *Journal of the American Medical Association, 275*(3), 217–223.

Patz, J. A., Graczyk, T. K., Geller, N., & Vittor, A. Y. (2000). Effects of environmental change on emerging parasitic diseases. *International Journal for Parasitology, 30*(12–13), 1395–1405.

Patz, J. A., & Khaliq, M. (2002). Global climate change and health: Challenges for future practitioners. *Journal of the American Medical Association, 287*(17), 2283–2284.

Patz, J. A., McGeehin, M. A., Bernard, S. M., Ebi, K. L., Epstein, P. R., Grambsch, A., et al. (2000). The potential health impacts of climate variability and change for the United States: Executive summary of the report of the health sector of the U.S. National Assessment. *Environmental Health Perspectives, 108*(4), 367–376.

Robinson, P. J. (2001). On the definition of a heat wave. *Journal of Applied Meteorology, 40*(4), 762–775.

Root, T. L., MacMynowski, D. P., Mastrandrea, M. D., & Schneider, S. H. (2005). From the Cover: Human-modified temperatures induce species changes: Joint attribution. *Proceedings of the National Academy of Sciences of the United States of America, 102*(21), 7465–7469.

Rosegrant, M. W., & Cline, S. A. (2003). Global food security: Challenges and policies. *Science, 302*(5652), 1917–1919.

Schiermeier, Q. (2005). Past climate comes into focus but warm forecast stays put. *Nature, 433*(7026), 562–563.

Schwartz, B. S., Parker, C., Glass, T. A., & Hu, H. (2006). Global environmental change: What can clinicians and the environmental health community do about it now? *Environmental Health Perspectives, 114*(12), 1807–1812.

Schwartz, J., Samet, J. M., & Patz, J. A. (2004). Hospital admissions for heart disease: The effects of temperature and humidity. *Epidemiology, 15*(6), 755–761.

Semenza, J. C., McCullough, J. E., Flanders, W. D., McGeehin, M. A., & Lumpkin, J. R. (1999). Excess hospital admissions during the July 1995 heat wave in Chicago. *American Journal of Preventive Medicine, 16*(4), 269–277.

Semenza, J. C., Rubin, C. H., Falter, K. H., Selanikio, J. D., Flanders, W. D., Howe, H. L., et al. (1996). Heat-related deaths during the July 1995 heat wave in Chicago. *New England Journal of Medicine, 335*(2), 84–90.

Smit, B., Pilifosova, O., Burton, I., Challenger, B., Huq, S., Klein, R., et al. (2001). Adaptation to climate change in the context of sustainable development and equity. In J. McCarthy, O. Canziana, N. Leary, D. Dokken, & K. White (Eds.), *Climate change 2001: Impacts, adaptation, and vulnerability.* New York: Cambridge University Press.

Smoyer-Tomic, K. E., & Rainham, D. G. C. (2001). Beating the heat: Development and evaluation of a Canadian hot weather health-response plan. *Environmental Health Perspectives, 109*(12), 1241–1248.

Stainforth, D. A., Aina, T., Christensen, C., Collins, M., Faull, N., Frame, D. J., et al. (2005). Uncertainty in predictions of the climate response to rising levels of greenhouse gases. *Nature, 433*(7024), 403–406.

Staropoli, J. F. (2002). The public health implications of global warming. *Journal of the American Medical Association, 287*(17), 2282.

Stieb, D. M., Judek, S., & Burnett, R. T. (2002). Meta-analysis of time-series studies of air pollution and mortality: Effects of gases and particles and the influence of cause of death, age, and season. *Journal of the Air & Waste Management Association, 52*(4), 470–484.

Sunyer, J., & Grimalt, J. (2006). Global climate change, widening health inequalities, and epidemiology. *International Journal of Epidemiology, 35*(2), 213–216.

United Nations. (2006). UN millennium development goals. (2006); http://www.un.org/millenniumgoals/

United Nations Millennium Project. (2005). *Investing in development. A practical plan to achieve the Millennium Development Goals.* London: Earthscan.

Vlahov, D., Galea, S., Gibble, E., & Freudenberg, N. (2005). Perspectives on urban conditions and population health. *Cadernos de Saude Publica, 21*(3), 949–957.

Vose, R., Karl, T., Easterling, D., Williams, C., & Menne, M. (2004). Climate (communication arising): Impact of land-use change on climate. *Nature, 427*(6971), 213–214.

Walther, G. R., Post, E., Convey, P., Menzel, A., Parmesan, C., Beebee, T. J., et al. (2002). Ecological responses to recent climate change. *Nature, 416*(6879), 389–395.

Webster, P. J., Holland, G. J., Curry, J. A., & Chang, H. R. (2005). Changes in tropical cyclone number, duration, and intensity in a warming environment. *Science, 309*(5742), 1844–1846.

Whitman, S., Good, G., Donoghue, E. R., Benbow, N., Shou, W., & Mou, S. (1997). Mortality in Chicago attributed to the July 1995 heat wave. *American Journal of Public Health, 87*(9), 1515–1518.

Wilson, M., & Anker, M. (2005). Disease surveillance in the context of climate stressors: Needs and opportunities. In K. Ebi & J. Smith (Eds.), *Integration of public health with adaptation to climate change: Lessons learned and new directions.* London: Frances & Taylor.

World Health Organization. (1992). *World health report 1996: Fighting disease, fostering development.* Geneva: World Health Organization.

World Health Organization. (2000). *Guidelines for air quality.* Geneva: World Health Organization.

Woodward, A., & Hales, S. (2003). Weather, climate, climate change and human health. *Applied Environmental Science and Public Health, 1*(1), 3–7.

Woodward, A. Hales, S., Litidamu, N., Phillips, D., & Martin, J. (2000). Protecting human health in a changing world: The role of economic and social development. *Bulletin of the World Health Organization, 78*(1), 1148–1155.

Woodward, A., & Scheraga, J. D. (2003). Looking to the future: Challenges for scientists studying climate change and health. In A. J. McMichael, D. H. Campbell-Lendrum, C. F. Corvalan, K. L. Ebi, A. Githeko, J. D. Scheraga, & A. Woodward (Eds.), *Climate change and human health: Risks and responses.* Geneva: World Health Organization.

Xu, H. Q., & Chen, B. Q. (2004). Remote sensing of the urban heat island and its changes in Xiamen City of SE China. *Journal of Environmental Sciences (China), 16*(2), 276–281.

Chapter 7
Global Governance

Obijiofor Aginam

1. Introduction to the Concept of Global Governance

We live in an interdependent world. The dynamics of the global interdependence of nations and peoples have led to the emergence of global challenges, such as global warming, transnational spread of infectious diseases, pollution and climate change, illicit drug trade and obesity. These new challenges defy the classic Westphalian inter-state system[i] by disrespecting the geo-political boundaries of nation-states. As a result of the globalization of the world's political economy, policies at the "domestic-foreign frontier" (Rosenau, 1997) now converge and intermesh in a seamless web of global governance. The idea of global governance was popularized in the 1990s through the work of the Commission on Global Governance (1995), and the emerging discourse in international relations (Rosenau Czempiel, 1992). Governance is defined as:

" . . . the sum of the many ways individuals and institutions, public and private, manage their common affairs. It is a continuing process through which conflicting or diverse interests may be accommodated and co-operative action may be taken. It includes formal institutions and regimes empowered to enforce compliance, as well as informal arrangements that people and institutions either have agreed to or perceive to be of interest" (Commission on Global Governance, 1995).

The concept of global governance does not imply that nation-states have become irrelevant, nor does it denote a centralized enforcing authority as a global government. Instead, global governance postulates the emergence of multiple actors – states, regional and international organizations, charitable foundations, non-governmental organizations, civil society, and private sector interests like multinational corporations and international business associations – that now share power, influence, and authority in the cross-national dealings (Aginam, 2005; Bettcher & Lee, 2002; Mathews, 1997). Because of the absence of a centralized enforcing authority at the global level, global governance is not synonymous with government (Rosenau, 1997). The effectiveness of governance rule systems (Rosenau, 2002) derives from traditional norms and habits, informal agreements, shared premises, and "as the demand for governance increases with the proliferation of complex interdependencies, rule systems can be found in non-governmental organizations, corporations, professional societies, business associations, advocacy groups, and many other types of collectivities that are not considered to be governments" (Rosenau, 2002)

In an age of globalization, global issues can only be effectively regulated through a combination of a state-centric system driven by governments and a "multi-centric system" driven by a collection of non-state actors. State and non-state actors compete, cooperate, and interact (Rosenau, 2002) and the proliferating centers of authority on the global stage are now composed of actors, large and small, formal and informal, economic and social, political and cultural, liberal and authoritarian, who collectively form a highly complex system of global governance. Examples of governance frameworks based on the state-centric system include multilateral conventions, treaties, regulations, standards, and soft law declarations. These are negotiated and adopted by states either among themselves as the dominant actors in international relations, or by states under the auspices of Westphalian international organizations like the United Nations, World Trade Organization, World Health Organization, and the Food and Agriculture Organization, which admit only states as members.[ii] Multi-centric system frameworks cover regulatory approaches to global issues that either are driven by non-state actors or involve their active participation along with states in the form of public-private partnerships.

This chapter assesses the relevance of global governance to population health by focusing on the new International Health Regulations adopted by the World Health Assembly of the World Health Organization (WHO) in 2005 and by exploring the dynamics of public-private partnership, including discussion of the specific example of the Global Fund to Fight AIDS, Tuberculosis and Malaria.

2. Global Governance and Population Health

The World Health Organization's ambitious definition of health as "a state of complete physical, mental and social well-being, and not merely the absence of disease or infirmity" (WHO, 2001b) links public health to a range of other public goods in the global context (Grad 2002; Kaul, Conceicao, Le Goulven, & Mendoza, 2003; Smith, Beaglehole, Woodward, & Drager, 2003). The link between global governance and population health is driven by the phenomenon of globalization, a process that intensifies transcontinental risks and networks and adds cognitive, temporal, and spatial dimensions to global interdependence of markets, peoples and nations (Lee & Dodgson, 2000). In the health context, globalization underscores a complex web of interrelated risks and opportunities that affect the well-being of populations in rich and poor countries (Arhin-Tenkorang & Conceicao, 2003; Taylor, Bettcher, & Peck, 2003). In an interconnected world "bacteria and viruses travel almost as fast as e-mail and financial flows" (Brundtland, 2003). Globalization of public health concerns includes the challenges of infectious and non-communicable diseases in an interdependent world (Lee & Dodgson, 2000; Woodward, Drager, Beaglehole, & Lipson, 2001; Yach & Bettcher 1998a,b).

Beyond infectious diseases, tobacco marketing, environmental degradation, alcohol and illicit drug use, anti-microbial resistance, hunger and food insecurity, diet and obesity now constitute worldwide health threats.

Globalization has altered the governance architecture of global health through transformation of the spatial organization of social relations (Held, McGrew, Golblatt, & Perraton 1999; Scholte, 2000). The regulatory approaches to transnational spread of disease and other health threats pose enormous challenges that are beyond the governance capabilities of individual nation-states. Erosion of the traditional distinction between national and international health threats means states are no longer the sole actors or stakeholders in negotiating effective solutions to transnational health threats. The traditional use of treaties, regulations and formal regimes, mostly by states within international organizations like WHO, still plays an important role in global governance because countries have always used international law to solve problems that are transnational in nature (Aginam, 2005; Fidler, 1999; Kaul et al., 2003; Taylor et al., 2003). However, the globalization of public health has catalyzed emerging global health governance involving states, international organizations and non-state actors (Kickbusch, 2003). Gomez-Dantes (2001) observes, "the actors who traditionally dominated the global health arena – national governments, the World Health Organization (WHO), and various NGOs – have been joined by development banks, aid agencies, and other private sector groups who wish to shape the response to the threat of disease."

Because of the multiplicity of actors in global health governance, the implementation and coordination of global health policy have become exceedingly complex (Gomez-Dantes, 2001). One recent governance framework that links global governance and population health is the World Health Organization's new International Health Regulations (IHR).

2.1. International Health Regulations

In May 2005, the World Health Assembly of the WHO adopted the new IHR to provide the regulatory framework for WHO's global public health surveillance (Baker & Fidler, 2006). The fundamental principle of the IHR is to ensure "maximum security against the international spread of diseases with a minimum interference with world traffic." The new IHR replace the old IHR adopted in 1951. The 1951 Regulations were narrow in scope as they applied only to three diseases: cholera, plague and yellow fever. The old IHR, a legally-binding set of regulations adopted under the auspices of WHO, represent one of the earliest multilateral regulatory approaches to global surveillance for infectious diseases.

Under the old IHR, WHO member states that accepted the Regulations undertook to notify the organization of an outbreak of any of the three diseases in their territories. Notifications sent by a Member State to WHO were transmitted to all the other member states with acceptable public health measures to respond to such outbreaks. The old IHR listed maximum public health measures applicable during outbreaks, and provided for rules for international traffic and travel. These measures covered the requirements of health and vaccination certificates for travellers from areas infected by these three diseases to non-infected areas; deratting, disinfecting and disinsecting of ships and aircraft; and detailed health measures at airports and seaports in the territories of WHO member states. The old IHR were ineffective as a global health regulatory tool mainly because they were based on a classic inter-state framework. WHO had no powers to operate pro-actively and could only use information given by Member States.

The new IHR codified ambitious proposals that mark a radical shift from the traditional inter-state governance framework to global governance that would involve non-state actors. This move stemmed from the complex ways in which globalization is propelling the emergence and re-emergence of epidemics (Aginam, 2004; Baker, & Fidler, 2006; Fidler, 2005). The new IHR formalized a duty of each state to notify WHO of "all events which may constitute a public health emergency of international concern within its territory." On the basis of information received, particularly from the state party within whose territory an event was occurring, Article 12 authorizes the Director-General of WHO to determine whether an event constitutes a public health emergency of international concern. The determination shall rely on scientific principles as well as available scientific evidence and other relevant information, including consultation with the state party in whose territory the event is occurring and information from non-state actors.

The most difficult task facing the WHO is identifying optimal methods to manage the IHR in the unfolding post-Westphalian public health architecture. Practically, WHO must respond to the realities of the present international system, in which nation-states are still the dominant, but no longer the sole actors in international relations. As codified in the new IHR, WHO's global public health surveillance must transform from traditional state-centered approaches to a "post-Westphalian" global health governance (Fidler, 2004) – a combination of formal and informal governance tools that directly involves states as well as international organizations, civil society, and non-governmental organizations.

The new IHR enables the WHO to develop global governance strategies by making use of information derived not exclusively from WHO member states, as is the case with the old IHR, but from relevant non-state actors. These global governance strategies were effectively deployed by WHO during the 2004 Severe Acute Respiratory Syndrome (SARS) outbreak when WHO collaborated with the global community of epidemiologists and with civil society to contain the crisis (Aginam, 2004; Fidler, 2004). Besides SARS, the IHR's application to "all events which may constitute a public health emergency of international concern" links WHO's Global Outbreak Alert and Response Network (GOARN) to emerging epidemics and pandemics such as avian and pandemic influenza. The WHO has recently set up an advisory Task Force linked to the IHR on potential public health issues of international concern related to avian and pandemic influenza, including issues such as the appropriate phase of pandemic alert, the declaration of an influenza pandemic, and appropriate international response measures to a pandemic. The IHR are a key element in strengthening global health security and a platform for sharing knowledge and the ability to respond to rapidly-evolving emergencies globally. The IHR complement existing technical partnerships and networks of global disease surveillance (WHO, 2006). The Regulations also offer a framework to enable WHO to collaborate more effectively with other non-state actors during health emergencies.

2.2. Public-Private Partnerships

Another way to explore global governance in the context of population health is the gradual but steady proliferation of public-private partnerships (PPPs) involving international organizations, states, and non-state actors. These partnerships operate on a range of health issues: malaria, vaccines and immunization, tuberculosis, polio eradication, HIV/AIDS, and trachoma (Buse & Walt, 2000a,b, Buse & Waxman, 2001; Pinet, 2003). Global PPPs for health are "those collaborative relationships which transcend national boundaries and bring together at least three parties, among them a corporation (and/or industry association) and an intergovernmental organization, so as to achieve a shared health-creating goal on the basis of a mutually agreed and explicitly defined division of labour" (Buse & Walt, 2002). Examples of global PPPs that involve the private sector, corporate entities, civil society organizations, inter-governmental organizations, and states include the Global Alliance for Vaccines and Immunization (GAVI), Stop TB Initiative, Roll-Back Malaria Campaign, Medicines for Malaria Venture, and International Partnership for AIDS in Africa.

The extent to which PPPs affect population health outcomes directly has been debated primarily because some PPPs are "product-based partnerships" that consist mainly of drug donation programs in developing countries while the others are "systems/issue-based partnerships" that assist governments in strategizing and harmonizing approaches and raising profiles of single diseases in global health policy (Buse & Walt, 2002). Global health PPPs have been the subject of critical and analytical discourses that assess their fairness, legitimacy, accountability and transparency (Aginam, 2002; Buse & Walt, 2002; Yamey, 2002). As Buse & Walt (2002) observed, the widespread adoption of PPPs in global health policy raises challenges, including the need for "more empirical research on the institutional features that make such partnerships effective. Such empirical work should also aim to identify more generally applicable, good practice guidelines, including principles for 'good partnership governance' (transparency, accountability, etc.)." In the absence of good practice guidelines, PPPs are accountable to no one. This has largely been the case with the Roll-Back Malaria Campaign and the Medicines for Malaria Venture (Aginam, 2002; Yamey, 2002). The proliferation of PPPs, although valuable, should not be confused with optimal effectiveness for global health governance.

2.3. Global Governance of AIDS and the Global Fund to Fight AIDS, Tuberculosis and Malaria

As the WHO Commission on Macroeconomics and Health (World Health Organization, 2001a) observed, health is inexorably linked to poverty reduction as well as to long-term economic growth. Evidence in support of these linkages is powerful and much stronger than is generally understood. The mortality and morbidity burdens of disease in some low-income regions, especially Africa, impede economic growth and therefore must be addressed centrally in any comprehensive development strategy. The HIV/AIDS epidemic, for instance, represents an unprecedented urgency that can undermine Africa's development over the next generation.

With over 40 million living with HIV globally and new infections accelerating, especially in developing countries, the epidemic of HIV/AIDS has challenged the traditional international health governance framework. In a single decade, the governance of HIV/AIDS has shifted from a program within the World Health Organization (Global Program on AIDS) to a joint venture program of nine United Nations system organizations (the UNAIDS), and is presently the subject of a global PPP financing facility – the Global Fund to Fight HIV/AIDS, Tuberculosis and Malaria (Poku, 2002). The Global Fund was conceived mainly by the G8 summit as a PPP to promote an integrated approach emphasizing prevention in a continuum of treatment and care for HIV/AIDS, tuberculosis and malaria. These three diseases are poverty-related, with the heaviest burdens in developing regions of the world where the public health systems are weak and vulnerable populations cannot afford effective therapies. Therefore, the Global Fund was intended as a funding facility to compliment existing multilateral organizations, especially WHO, World Bank, and UNAIDS.

Based in Geneva, Switzerland, the Fund is a public-private collaborative financial instrument, and not an implementing agency. It is an alliance of partners from the United Nations agencies, developing countries, donor governments, foundations, corporations and non-governmental organizations, and people living with HIV/AIDS (Bartsch, 2005; Brugha & Walt, 2001). The Fund is built on basic principles that include the creation, development, and expansion of government, private and civil society partnerships and the promotion of consistency with international law and agreements and respect for intellectual property rights. At the time of its inception, it was estimated that the Global Fund would need about $7–10 billion annually to combat HIV/AIDS alone, and would obviously need more resources for tuberculosis and malaria. The Global Fund, as a PPP, has emerged as an important player in global health governance by bringing together states and non-state actors in decision-making processes nationally and globally (Bartsch, 2005).

Since its establishment in 2002, the Fund has become a leading financing mechanism for tuberculosis and malaria treatment and prevention, distributing 66% and 45% of all international funding for the two diseases respectively, and 20% of all international funding for HIV/AIDS (Bartsch, 2005). Still, the Fund is not without serious problems. One challenge for the Fund is donor fatigue; donors must be mobilized to redeem their past pledges and sustain future financial commitment to the Fund. As well, Barstch (2005) has rightly observed that the Fund "must try to handle one problem typical for public-private partnerships: the existing tensions between a vertical approach in fighting specific diseases and broader horizontal approaches in health system development and the promotion of public health." Nonetheless, the Global Fund has since its inception attracted US\$ 4.7 billion in financing through 2008. It has committed US \$ 1.5 billion in funding to support 154 programs in 93 countries worldwide. This has enabled many countries to scale up existing programs (Global Fund, 2006).

3. The Future of Global Governance for Public Health

This chapter discussed the relevance of global governance strategies to the transnational spread of diseases and health threats and argued that the traditional Westphalian governance model, while still relevant, is limited by the globalized challenges of disease-control initiatives in an interdependent world. Communicable and non-communicable diseases have both become global health issues that require new global governance strategies. The complex transcontinental networks created by the phenomenon of globalization, when applied to the global health context, are compelling enough to catalyze fresh insights on the best ways to regulate transnational spread of diseases. The codification and implementation of global health accords is becoming increasingly important as global health interdependence accelerates and nations increasingly recognize the need to cooperate to solve essential problems. Governance of global health requires collaboration between international organizations with "overlapping" mandates, such as WHO, UNAIDS, Food and Agriculture Organization of the United Nations, World Bank, World Trade Organization and many others, along with both state and non-state actors. It also requires cross-disciplinary work among scholars and researchers in public health and epidemiology, clinical medicine, international relations and international law, demography and economics, anthropology, social work, and development.

Endnotes

i. The Westphalian international system emerged from the Treaty of Westphalia, 1648, that ended thirty years of war and conflict in Europe and led to the emergence of nation-states as the primary actors in international relations. Applied to public health diplomacy, membership of multilateral health organizations like the World Health Organization is open only to states, and only states can become parties to multilateral health treaties, conventions, and regulations negotiated under the auspices of those organizations.

ii. There are numerous treaties, conventions, agreements, regulations, declarations and soft-law adopted by states under the auspices of these international organizations. While some are health-specific, others affect health in different ways. Examples include the long list of human rights and environmental treaties and conventions negotiated and adopted by states within the United Nations system; the World Health Organization's

Framework Convention on Tobacco Control (FCTC); The World Health Organization and Food and Agriculture Organization's jointly administered Codex Alimentarius Commission standards on food safety;and the trade agreements enforced by the World Trade Organization, especially the Agreements on Trade-Related Aspects of Intellectual Property Rights (TRIPS), Sanitary and Phyto-Sanitary Measures (SPS), Technical Barriers to Trade (TBT), and the General Agreement on Trade in Services (GATS).

References

Aginam, O. (2002). From the core to the peripheries: Multilateral governance of malaria in a multi-cultural world. *Chicago Journal of International Law, 3*(1), 87–103.

Aginam, O. (2004). Globalization of infectious diseases, international law and the World Health Organization: Opportunities for synergy in global governance of epidemics. *New England Journal of International and Comparative Law, 11*(1), 5 –74.

Aginam, O. (2005). *Global health governance: International law and public health in a divided world.* Toronto: University of Toronto Press.

Arhin-Tenkorang, D., & Conceicao, P. (2003). Beyond communicable disease control: Health in the age of globalization. In I. Kaul, P. Conceicao, K. Le Goulven, & R. U. Mendoza (Eds.), *Providing global public goods: Managing globalization.* New York: Oxford University Press.

Baker, M. G., & Fidler, D. P. (2006). Global public health surveillance under the new international health regulations. *Emerging Infectious Diseases, 12*(7), 1058–1065.

Bartsch, S. (2005). *The Global Fund to Fight Aids, Tuberculosis and Malaria: Establishment, current issues and future challenges.* Paper prepared for the Salzburg Seminar on the Governance of Health, Schloss Arenberg, Salzburg, Austria.

Bettcher, D., & Lee, K. (2002). Glossary: Globalisation and health. *Journal of Epidemiology and Community Health, 56*, 8–17.

Brugha, R., & Walt, G. (2001). A global health fund: A leap of faith. *British Medical Journal, 323*, 152–154.

Brundtland, G. H. (2003). Global health and international security. *Global Governance, 9*, 417–423.

Buse, K., & Walt, G. (2000a). Global public-private partnerships: Part I – a new development in health? *Bulletin of the World Health Organization, 78*(5), 549–561.

Buse, K., & Walt, G. (2000b). Global public-private partnerships: Part II – what are the issues for global governance? *Bulletin of the World Health Organization, 78*(4), 699–709.

Buse, K., & Walt, G (2002). Globalisation and multilateral public-private partnerships: Issues for health policy. In K. Lee, K. Buse, & S. Fustukian (Eds.), *Health policy in a globalising world.* Cambridge, UK: Cambridge University Press.

Buse, K., & Waxman, A. (2001). Public-private partnerships: A strategy for the WHO. *Bulletin of the World Health Organization, 79*(8), 748–754.

Commission on Global Governance. (1995). *Our global neighbourhood: The report of the Commission on Global Governance.* New York: Oxford University Press.

Fidler, D. (1999). *International law and infectious diseases.* Oxford: Clarendon Press.

Fidler, D. (2004). *SARS, governance and the globalization of disease.* Basingstoke, UK: Palgrave Macmillan.

Fidler, D. (2005). From international sanitary conventions to global health security: The new international health regulations. *Chinese Journal of International Law, 4*, 325–392.

Global Fund. (2006). The Global Fund to Fight AIDS, Tuberculosis, and Malaria. Geneva (2006); http://www.theglobalfund.org/EN/.

Gomez-Dantes, O. (2001). Health. In P. J. Simmons & C. D. J.Oudraat (Eds.), *Managing global issues: Lessons learned.* Washington, DC: Carnegie.

Grad, F. (2002). The preamble of the constitution of the World Health Organization. *Bulletin of the World Health Organization, 80*, 981–982.

Held, D., McGrew, A., Goldblatt, D., & Perraton, J. (Eds.). (1999). *Global transformations: Politics, economics and culture.* Cambridge: Polity Press.

Kaul, I., Conceicao, P., Le Goulven, K., & Mendoza, R. U. (2003). *Providing global public goods: Managing globalization.* New York: Oxford University Press.

Kickbusch, I. (2003). Global health governance: Some theoretical on the new political space. In K. Lee (Ed.), *Health impacts of globalization: Towards global governance.* London: Palgrave.

Lee, K., & Dodgson, R. (2000). Globalization and cholera: Implications for global governance. *Global Governance, 6*, 213–236.

Matthews, J. (1997). Power shift. *Foreign Affairs, 76*(1), 50–66.

Pinet, G. (2003). Global partnerships: A key challenge and opportunity for implementation of international health law. *Medicine and Law, 22*, 561–577.

Poku, N. K. (2002). The Global AIDS Fund: Context and opportunity. *Third World Quarterly, 23*, 283–298.

Rosenau, J. N. (1997). *Along the domestic-foreign frontier: Exploring governance in a turbulent world.* Cambridge: Cambridge University Press.

Rosenau, J. N. (2002). Governance in a new global order. In D. Held & A. McGrew (Eds.), *Governing globalization: Power, authority and global governance.* Cambridge: Polity Press.

Rosenau, J. N., & Czempiel, E. O. (Eds.). (1992). *Governance without government: Order and change in world politics.* Cambridge: Cambridge University Press.

Scholte, J. A. (2000). *Globalization: A critical introduction.* New York: St. Martin's Press.

Smith, R., Beaglehole, R., Woodward, D., & Drager, N. (Eds.). (2003). *Global public goods for health: Health, economic and public health perspectives.* Oxford: Oxford University Press.

Taylor, A., Bettcher, D., & Peck, R. (2003). International law and international legislative process: The WHO framework convention on tobacco control. In R. Smith, R. Beaglehole, D. Woodward, & N. Drager (Eds.), *Global public goods for health: Health, economic and public health perspectives.* Oxford: Oxford University Press.

Woodward, D., Drager, N., Beaglehole, R., & Lipson, D. (2001). Globalization and health: A framework for analysis and action. *Bulletin of the World Health Organization, 79*(9), 875–881.

World Health Organization. (2001a). *Macroeconomics and health: Investing in health for economic development – report of the commission on macroeconomics and health.* Geneva: World Health Organization.

World Health Organization. (2001b). Constitution of the World Health Organization. In World Health Organization (Ed.), *Basic documents*, 43rd edition. Geneva: World Health Organization.

World Health Organization. (2006). WHO influenza pandemic holds first meeting: WHO press release. Geneva (September 26, 2006); http://www.who.int/mediacentre/news/notes/2006/np28/en/print.html

Yach, D., & Bettcher, D. (1998a). The globalization of public health, I: Threats and opportunities. *American Journal of Public Health, 88*, 735–738.

Yach, D., & Bettcher, D. (1998b). The globalization of public health, II: The convergence of self-interest and altruism. *American Journal of Public Health, 88*, 738–741.

Yamey, G. (2002). WHO in 2002: Faltering steps towards partnerships. *British Medical Journal, 325*, 1236–1240.

Chapter 8
Macroeconomics

David M. Bishai and Yung-Ting Kung

1. Introduction

Health and survival of all organisms depends on the availability of nutrients, water, and a hospitable environment. Social animals like humans rely on social institutions to help provide these material foundations of health. Our foremost institutions are economies which govern the production, distribution and consumption of goods and services. Microeconomics describes how individuals and households make decisions to produce and consume services. Macroeconomics describes the aggregate outcomes of these individual household behaviors. Because macroeconomic phenomena emerge at the population level, a thorough understanding of individual human behavior, while necessary, will not guarantee insight into the functioning of the macroeconomy. An analogy to the world of health is instructive: Clinical medicine concerns the restoration and preservation of health at the individual level while public health describes measures to restore and preserve the health of populations. Physiological processes that are important for individual health become mere background for the predominant demographic, social, and epidemiological forces that determine the health of populations.

The most remarkable event in recent human history is the dramatic improvement in the macroeconomic well-being of the majority of the world's population during the last two centuries. It is widely agreed that macroeconomic improvements have contributed to lifting most indicators of population health in nearly all countries of the world. A rudimentary understanding of why and how economies grow and develop should thus be considered fundamental to understanding population health. As Figure 8.1 shows, macro and microeconomics affect and are affected by both individual and population health. The relationship between macro and microeconomics, and between individual and population health, is compositional, as reflected by the brackets. The health and material well-being of individuals compose the health and wealth of populations. This chapter specifically looks at arrows 1–4 in Figure 8.1 to describe how macroeconomic factors are linked to both individual health and the health of populations.

Because a macroeconomy is one of the most complex systems known to science, we can only offer a cursory explanation of economic development and

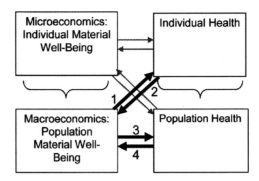

FIGURE 8.1. Conceptual framework for the relationship between the economy and health. Macroeconomics affect and are affected by both the health of the individuals and the health of the population.

hope to stimulate readers to further inquiry. A much more achievable goal for this chapter is to present the basic terminology of macroeconomics, describing "indicators" that are relevant to health. With the terminology in hand, we will review the relationship between macroeconomic indicators and health.

This chapter will strive to correct the common reductionist belief that economic progress can be examined in isolation from social, political, and cultural changes. Ascribing health gains that occur in countries with growing economies solely to improvements in the national income has been an unjustifiable error in inference and a wellspring of harmful policy decisions.

2. Indicators of Material Well-Being

Conventional macroeconomic indicators relevant to health include measures of national income, income distribution, and employment. Understanding these measures can reveal how much they capture and what they omit.

2.1. National Income Measures

The aspects of the macroeconomy most relevant to health are aggregate measures of how much "stuff" there is. To be more precise, both goods (nutrients, clean water, shelter) and services (sanitation, health information, medical care) affect population health. Goods and services are being constantly produced or provided by workers and firms and are thus said to "flow." The principal indicator of the monetized flow of goods and services in a population in a given year is the Gross Domestic Product (GDP).[i] For example, the GDP per capita of the US in 2004 was $41,400 whereas that of Bangladesh was $140. Almost every government in the world produces national income estimates like GDP, with historical series for some countries dating back to the 1700s. The availability of national income data explains their extensive use in elucidating the relationship between the macro-economy of a nation and health.

Summarizing a country's economic performance with a single indicator requires awareness of some of the limitations of the indicator. One important limitation of GDP is that the flow of goods and services includes medical goods and services as well as environmental clean up; these components of GDP increase when problems arise rather than when growth is occurring. For example, an epidemic, toxic spill, or chronic endemic disease may lead a population to use these types of remedial goods and services, which are then counted in GDP. The result is that the true relationship between good health and high GDP becomes muddled.

Another limitation in using GDP to explain population health has to do with timing. Items that last for more than a year are called "durable." Those durable items that are used to produce other goods and services (like hospital-buildings) are called "capital," while durable items that are used over time to serve consumers (like pacemakers) are called "consumer durables." Many of the items that make a population healthy today may have flowed into the population years ago. While income is the flow of resources available in a given period – goods and services moving from one person to another – wealth is an accumulated stock of resources that are controlled by a person or household. Accumulated wealth-resources can give long term benefits without having to be traded for other things. Few countries estimate their stock of wealth because it is difficult to measure. However, national wealth and its distribution may be more appropriate determinants of population health than income. Wealth need not resemble machines and buildings but can take the form of knowledge and social institutions as well, even though these are difficult to measure. One particularly important durable wealth item that is commonly owned is the discovery of biomedical knowledge and its gradual dissemination across the planet.[ii]

2.2. Income Distribution

Demographers know that the risk of death and disease is not uniformly distributed in a population, but rather is concentrated more heavily in certain subgroups with higher vulnerability, for example among the poor. As aggregate measures of the flow of goods and services, national income indicators do not reflect the distribution of income within a country. Measures of income distribution include the widely used Gini coefficient (See Figure 8.2 for definition), as well as indicators such as the Robin Hood Index, Theil's Entropy, and the Atkinson Index, all of which are closely correlated. At least one study has shown that the choice of income distribution indicator matters little in analyzing the relationship of income distribution to mortality (Kawachi & Kennedy, 1997). As would be expected, the data requirements for reliable estimation of income distribution indicators are more severe because nationally representative information on household income is required.

2.3. Unemployment

Unemployment is measured as the ratio between the number of people who are not employed and the size of the civilian labor force, i.e., those who were

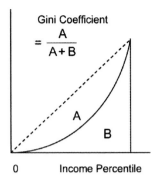

FIGURE 8.2. Income distribution and the Gini coefficient. In a plot of the contribution of each income percentile to the cumulative national income, the dashed line reflects perfect income equality and would have Gini coefficient of 0. A society where area B = 0 would have maximum inequality and a Gini coefficient of 1.

employed in or who attempted to find wage-based or self-employment jobs in the last 30 days. People who do informal jobs or housework are not considered to be in the labor force, although in many countries these categories often overlap with subsistence agriculture. The effects of unemployment on population health were once thought to be universally negative for the same reasons that individual unemployment jeopardizes individual health. However, as we shall see, there is growing evidence that increases in unemployment in some societies may be protective for a population as a whole.

2.4. Other Macroeconomic Indicators

Recognizing the limitations of current national income indicators, several groups are developing measures of natural resource wealth, human capital, and governance. These are often omitted features in standard economic statistics. To measure natural resource wealth, World Bank economists have computed the value of soil, forests, and mineral reserves. Human capital indicators include schooling and life expectancy. Governance has been measured with a broad set of indicators ranging from accountability to control of corruption (Kaufmann, Kraay, & Mastruzzi, 2003).

3. How Economic Development Relates Material Well-Being to Health

3.1. Definitions of Development

A paradigm shift is gaining among economists, most of whom would no longer identify the growth of GDP per capita – or any single other material indicator – as an adequate measure of "development." What is development? This concept is as difficult to define for populations as it is for individual human beings.[iii]

3.2. Development as the Capability to Undertake Social Tasks

The core of the modern concept is that "developed" entities have the ability to realize more of their capabilities. In achieving any goal, a more developed person or country is more likely to succeed. Having money can certainly facilitate the achievement of goals, but it is neither necessary nor sufficient for either countries or persons. One of the recurring tragedies of history is that when countries develop improved capabilities they often use their advantage to pursue goals that are ruinous for neighboring countries or for a vulnerable minority group. From a moral perspective, several have argued that the highest mark of a developed society is to extend self-determination and improved human functioning indiscriminately to each of its members (Nussbaum, 2000; Nussbaum & Sen, 1993; Sen, 1999). The United Nations' Human Development Index (HDI) is a simple average of a country's performance in improving life expectancy, education, and GDP per capita (United Nations Development Program, 2005). Although it is advanced as a more encompassing reflector of development, it cannot be used to explain health because it already encompasses life expectancy measures.

3.3. The Mechanics of Development

In bygone days when development was thought to be simply income growth, capital accumulation took on a central explanatory role. Advisors in the 1950s emphasized raising domestic savings rates and encouraged governments and individuals to invest more in machines, buildings, and infrastructure. Economies produce goods and services – the GDP – out of raw materials, labor, and capital, but raw materials, like land, increased arithmetically, while population increased geometrically. In the quotient, GDP/population, the numerator must grow faster than the denominator to achieve per capita growth. The size of the labor force can seldom grow faster than the population;[iv] thus, early theories of economic growth stressed capital accumulation to make the growth of GDP faster and fertility control to slow the growth of the denominator (Harrod, 1939). Solow was among the first to recognize that neither capital nor labor explained most of GDP growth. He emphasized the role of omitted or "residual" factors, like technology, as a significant determinant of economic growth (Solow, 1956, 1957). Modern development economics continues to focus on intangible determinants of growth but no longer characterizes these intangible determinants as exclusively technical in an engineering sense. Obsolete models predicted that any country of a given population size could achieve sustainable growth solely by acquiring sufficient capital and the right engineering formulas. Decades of investing capital and technical assistance in both small and large failed projects suggest that the process is more complicated (Bauer, 1981). Current thinking emphasizes the role of social institutions and good governance as well as technology in explaining aspects of productivity unexplained by labor and capital.

3.4. Endogenous Growth Theories

Newer theories of growth have begun to chip away at the mystery of how countries with similar amounts of labor and capital can experience different amounts of economic growth. The ability to successfully implement newer technologies, to start new businesses, and to attract new capital can vary for social, political, and cultural reasons. Different cultures and governments vary in their success at creating the right environment for growth to occur. Ultimately the societies that grow faster find a way to enter a cycle in which economic growth fosters social, political, and health improvements that then encourage the macroeconomy. A stark example would be country A and country B, similar in literacy and health. Every year each country's economy grinds out enough resources to maintain a workforce and keep all the machines in good order and have some surplus funds that can be invested in making life better. Country A invests its entire surplus in physical capital (machines), but country B invests partly in physical capital, and partly in improving schooling and health, which could be considered human capital. It is possible that the improved skill and health of the labor force in country B enable it to obtain better returns from new technology than country A. In fact, countries generally do invest some of their surplus in human capital, leading to a virtuous cycle in which health investments feed greater economic growth, which feeds greater health, and so on (Arrows 3 and 4 in Figure 8.1).

To formalize such a model consider an economy which produces its GDP or national income, Y, from capital, K, labor, L, and the health of its labor force H.

$$[1] \; Y = f(K,L,H)$$

The economy saves one portion of its income, s_K, to invest in capital, and another portion, s_H, is invested in health so that the total savings rate $s = s_k + s_H$. Then capital, despite depreciation at rate δ, will grow as described in Eq. 2.

$$[2] \; K_{t+1} = s_K Y - \delta K_t$$

Labor grows at the population's rate of natural increase, n. Health investment each year is undertaken partly by households and partly by the government. Thus, the total health budget $s_H Y = I_{HG} + I_{HH}$, where $s_H Y$ is the total health spending, I_{HG} is health investment undertaken by government, and I_{HH} is health investment undertaken by households. The final part of the model is the equation for the societal production of health and follows the work of Mokyr (Mokyr, 1993).

$$[3] \; H_{t+1} = E(H_t) + [G(B - \Phi(K))] \times s_H Y$$

Where:

E is environmental contagion, which can be thought of as the average annual risk of acquiring an infectious disease. E is a decreasing function of the health stock, H_t, in the current period because the healthier everybody is, the fewer prevalent cases of infection there are to spread disease.

G is the quality of health production technology

B is the best available health technology in area j

Φ is the gap between best and actual health technology in area j and may be a decreasing function of the capital stock

The potential for positive feedback occurs because lowering contagion in one period may make it easier to make the population healthier in the next period. Furthermore, the growth of the capital stock may make it easier to apply the latest health technology with smaller gaps in implementation. Because better health allows better economic performance, as per Eq. 1, one achieves a cycle: more health → more income → more health, etc.

4. Evidence Linking Income and Health

Having defined simple macroeconomic indicators of material well-being and discussed their limitations as being fully reflective of the development of an economy, we move on to explore the relationship of the macroeconomy to health. There are no widely available measures that can be used for this purpose, and despite its limitations, the literature we will review has used GDP per capita extensively. As shown in arrows 1–4 of Figure 8.1, the connection between macroeconomic growth and health permits bi-directional causation. Determining how much the economy is affecting health and vice versa relies on dynamic data as we shall see in Section 7.

4.1. Preston Curve

The raw relationship between the logarithm of GDP per capita and life expectancy as plotted in a cross-section of countries is an upward sloping line known as the Preston curve. Preston showed that when plotted against the log of GDP per capita, the relationship is nearly linear, and when comparing the relationship in the 1930s to the 1960s, the entire curve has shifted dramatically upwards. The upward sloping relationship between GDP and health means that one will expect improvements in GDP to move health up the curve.

The upward shift of the entire curve in the middle of the 20th century suggests that the world's population got a "free ride," in that health was being improved in the 20th century without the slow march up the curve of GDP growth. The factors shifting the Preston curve upward are interpreted to be changes in technology and social institutions, rather than income. Preston found that factors exogenous to a country's current level of income, like public health technology, accounted for 75–90% of the growth of life expectancy for the world as a whole, while income growth, per se, accounted for only 10–25% (Preston, 1975). National income matters, but it does not matter as much as a host of unmeasured exogenous factors.

Figure 8.3 shows the Preston curve as of 2004. Note that there are outliers on the curve. The ones below the curve, like Namibia and South Africa, can be termed "negative deviants." They represent places that are less healthy than their national income would suggest. Conversely, there are positive deviants who are healthier than would be expected by their national income.

A very important feature of the Preston curve is its non-linearity (the Preston curve is a straight line when the log of GDP per capita is used, but it is a curve when GDP is used without the log transform). Because the relationship shown in Figure 8.3 is drawn on a semi-log plot, the relationship implies that for high income countries national economic status has little impact on raising life expectancy (Wilkinson, 1999).

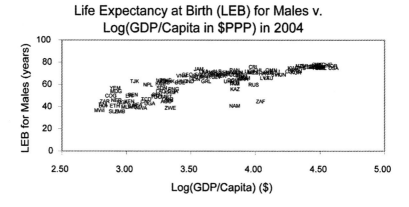

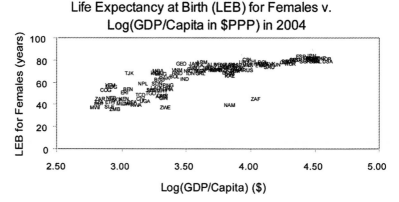

FIGURE 8.3. Plots of life expectancy v. log GDP/Capita based on 2004 data, also known as "Preston Curves." Namibia (NAM), South Africa (ZAF), and Zimbabwe (ZWE) are notable as "negative deviants" where life expectancy is lower than would be expected for their national income. Tajikistan (TJK) emerges as a "positive deviant" where life expectancy is higher than national income would predict. Data Source World Bank. World Development Report 2006.

4.2. Does National Income Level Cause Health Improvements?

The bidirectional relationship between population health and income spurs the question of to what extent economic growth causes health improvements, and vice versa. McKeown was the first to work through plausible mechanisms linking the macroeconomy to population health. In his book *The Modern Rise of the Population*, (McKeown, 1976) McKeown parsed out the role of medical and public health interventions in mortality decline, focusing on the population's ability to better fight infectious disease. He noted that airborne diseases, most of which were unaffected by public health measures, were critical in mortality reduction. Additionally, most medical therapies and immunizations were not available for infectious diseases until the 1900s, when many diseases were already declining. Therefore, as the nature of most diseases did not change, a large part of the mortality reduction must be ascribed to host factors in the population. According to McKeown, the means by which health improved was through better nutrition and hygiene. Additional money makes both better food and a better living environment possible.[v] Fogel has offered direct evidence that economic growth during the 19th and 20th century was linked to better nutritional intake (Fogel, 1997), making McKeown's claims more plausible. Fogel's evidence of gains in height for populations enjoying economic growth, however, does not constitute proof that nutrient intake was the critical factor; both a hygienic environment and a lower exposure to childhood diseases contribute significantly in determining adult height.

Szreter criticized McKeown's analysis of the mortality decline in a 1988 paper that emphasized instead the importance of "social intervention" (Szreter, 1994). He claimed that McKeown overestimated the impact of airborne diseases on mortality decline and underestimated the impact of water-borne diseases, which are more easily influenced by public health measures. Furthermore, Szreter argued that the mortality decline only occurred consistently in the late 1800s, which was precisely when many sanitation measures were implemented and public health acts established. He contended that these "social interventions" had the power to reduce both water and airborne diseases through improved housing and working conditions and offer a better explanation of the mortality decline.

The McKeown-Szreter debate epitomizes the modern policy debate between GDP-optimists, who would advise that economic growth is the main driver of improved health, and GDP-skeptics, who worry that GDP gains alone may be insufficient. The GDP-optimists would look at the Preston curve in Figure 8.3 and emphasize how dependably life expectancy seems to rise with GDP/capita throughout the curve. GDP-skeptics will point out the remarkable benefits that can be achieved when the entire Preston curve shifts upward. They would also note negative deviants like Namibia and South Africa as evidence for Szreter's point that conscientious effort is required in addition to GDP growth, or a country will fail to attain its expected place on the Preston curve. If one properly distinguishes economic development (the ability of a population to effectively pursue worthy social goals) from economic growth (simply having a higher GDP per capita), much of the dispute between GDP optimists and skeptics is resolved. Few would pursue growth to the detriment of development.

4.3. Biphasic Effects of Economic Growth on Health

As pointed out by McKeown, improvements in life expectancy over the last two centuries are tied to better income, nutrition, and public health infrastructure and help explain the upward sloping relationship between health and GDP/capita in the Preston curve. There are important exceptions where the relationship between economic growth and health is biphasic, most notably in the area of motor vehicle fatalities. As shown in Figure 8.4, the relationship takes on an inverted U-shape; motor vehicle fatalities first rise with economic growth then, at a GDP per capita around $10,000 per person, begin to fall as societies achieve the ability to salvage

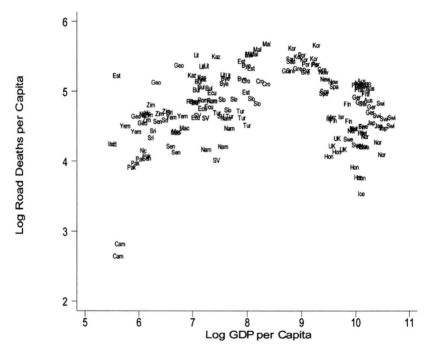

FIGURE 8.4. Scatterplot of Log Road Deaths per Capita v. Log GDP per Capita 1992–1996 KEY: Country abbreviations are initial letters from the list below with exceptions noted in ( ): Austria, Bulgaria, Belarus, Cambodia, Croatia, Ecuador, El Salvador (SV), Estonia, Finland, France, Georgia, Germany, Greece, Hong-Kong, India, Israel, Kazakhstan, Lithuania, Macedonia, Malaysia, Namibia, Netherlands, Nicaragua, Norway, Pakistan, Portugal, Republic of Korea (Kor), Romania, Saudi Arabia, Senegal, Slovakia, Sri Lanka, Sweden, Switzerland, United Kingdom (UK), United States (US), Yemen, Zimbabwe. Source author's calculations using data from (Bishai, Qureshi, James, & Ghaffar, 2005).

trauma victims and to invest in safer vehicles and roads. Other relationships that have an inverted U type relationship with economic growth include the presence of environmental pollutants and the extent of income inequality – these relationships are named Kuznets curves (Dasgupta, Laplante, Wang, & Wheeler, 2002).

4.4. Famines

Clear evidence documenting causation from the economy to health can be found when examining famines. Famines can occur during natural fluctuations in agricultural productivity due to climate or pestilence, and in rare cases famines can be attributed to health events such as plagues and epidemics. However, it is increasingly recognized that many, if not most, famines of the 20th century can be attributed to macroeconomic misadventures – sometimes intentioned, sometimes results of ineptitude[vi] (Ravallion, 1997). A macroeconomic downturn can increase the real price of food compared to real earning power to such an extent that large numbers of the population suffer starvation and death.

Sen (1981) was among the first to point out that modern famines tend to have selective effects in differentially killing certain subgroups in a process he characterized as reducing their set of entitlements.[vii] Historically, famines may have been more indiscriminate. Galloway's (1986) study of French parish register data on mortality in 16th century Rouen revealed surprisingly little variation in infant mortality rates between rich and poor arrondissements following slack grain harvests and scarcity-induced rises in the price of wheat. Analysis of more recent famines, such as the 1974 Bangladesh famine, revealed the substantial role of macroeconomic mismanagement in failing to stabilize soaring rice prices despite adequate crop yields (Ravallion, 1987). Ravallion also showed how famine mortality was concentrated more heavily among landless artisans rather than equally affecting all of the rural poor.

5. Evidence Linking Equity and Health

The concentration of famine mortality in vulnerable subgroups typifies a common finding in the study of macroeconomics and health. Whether one considers health benefits or economic benefits, there is variability in the extent to which various sub-groups benefit from economic growth. The early phases of economic growth tend to increase income inequalities as capitalists and entrepreneurs benefit disproportionately compared to laborers. According to Kuznets, income inequalities begin to diminish at advanced stages of economic development as low paid rural workers migrate towards better paying jobs in the developed economy. Sala-i-Martin (2002) has shown that income inequality in the world has declined since 1976, and the number of $1 a day poor people has decreased. However, this latter phase of reduced inequalities is contested – the evidence is mixed.

The health side of equity and macroeconomics was the subject of much research in the 1990s directed at answering the following two questions: 1) What determines the health equity of a society? and 2) Does economic inequality harm population health?

5.1. Health Equality and Equity

Conceptual clarity requires distinguishing between "health equality" and "health equity." The former refers to health outcomes in a population (e.g., age at death or healthy life expectancy) having low variance within populations and across sub-populations. The latter refers to equality of access to health services in the face of need. Economic growth can have dual effects on these processes. Kuznets-type processes that raise the Gini coefficient early in development may lead to more variation in life expectancy. If the relationship between income and health were simply linear, then a higher Gini coefficient would necessitate more health inequality. However, the non-linearity of the Preston curve denotes the gap between the health of the poorest and richest member of a rich society should be smaller than the same gap in a poor society (see Figure 8.5).

If economic development has empowered a society to address its social goals, it may use its greater capacity to address income inequality as well as health inequity and inequality. It can be costly to reduce income and health inequalities; development empowers countries to narrow the gap if their political resolve moves in that direction. For example, with the notable exception of the US,

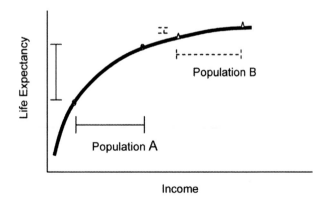

FIGURE 8.5. Effect of income growth on health equality. Population A has a lower average income and a 95% confidence interval as shown by bars. Population B has higher income but equivalent income inequality. Because of non-linearity of Preston curve, variation in life expectancy is expected to be lower in Population B than in A.

highly developed countries around the world have guaranteed access to health insurance for the entire population.

5.2. Effects of Income Inequality on Health

A large literature has documented relationships between measures of income inequality and health. The conceptual basis of these tests is that the experience of living in a population with large income inequality imposes physiological stress on individuals (known as allostatic load). However, as first pointed out by Rodgers (1979), the non-linear relationship between income and health automatically leads to a spurious, non-causal relationship between income inequality and poor health. It could be that what some call a relationship between income *inequality* and health is simply a rediscovery of the relationship between income and health and has nothing to do with income distribution. If there are two populations with the same mean income but different income variance, the population with the wider variance of income will automatically contain more poor people suffering more intensely from poor health (Rodgers, 1979). The non-linear shape of the Preston curve implies that populations with more poor people will have worse overall survival even if their average incomes are the same. This makes it difficult to test whether the stressful effects of income inequality are spilling over into the entire population without using a multilevel modeling approach that can simultaneously control for household income and population income distribution.

Studies have attempted to control for the Rodgers effect using statistical models that control for individual wealth while including area-specific measures of income inequality. These generally find that income inequalities are correlated with poorer health in certain cases but not others. Most of the multilevel studies use US states as the unit of analysis for Gini coefficients and household data and use self-rated health as the outcome (Blakely, Kennedy, Glass, & Kawachi, 2000; Blakely, Lochner, & Kawachi, 2002; Diez-Roux, Link, & Northridge, 2000; Subramanian, Belli, & Kawachi, 2002; Subramanian, Blakely, & Kawachi, 2003; Subramanian & Kawachi, 2003). Multilevel studies performed at the state level support the income inequality hypothesis, while the one (arguably more powerful) multilevel study examining 232 metropolitan areas and 216 counties did not support the hypothesis (Blakely et al., 2002).

Deaton and Lubotsky (2003) argue that the effects of income inequality in America are difficult to extricate from the effects of racial inequality. Between-group income inequality tends to be higher wherever there is a larger fraction of African Americans in the population. When city and state mortality data are re-analyzed taking account of both income inequality and racial make-up, it emerges that racial makeup, not income inequality, has dominant effects on population mortality (Deaton & Lubotsky, 2003). Deaton found, quite puzzlingly, that white mortality is higher in locations where the fraction of the black population is higher.[viii] He cautions that income inequalities are just one form of social inequality that can affect health in models that emphasize the role of stress and allostatic load.

6. Evidence Linking Employment and Health

On an individual level there is copious evidence that the experience of being unemployed is associated with significant stress, anxiety, and mental health problems (Dooley, Fielding, & Levi, 1996). Unemployed people are more likely to suffer cardiovascular disease, suicide, and total mortality (Jin, Shah, & Svoboda, 1995). Since our focus is on macroeconomic effects of unemployment, we must first ask whether intuitions about micro effects of unemployment on the unemployed carry over to macro effects of unemployment on the health of the population. With unemployment rates typically hovering between 5 and 10% of the labor force (and even smaller fractions of general population), one should not expect population health indicators to reflect the personal travails of the 1–2% of the newly unemployed individuals. Rather, one must conceptualize the social effects of a rise in unemployment on the aggregate health of the (ordinary) households that have remained employed. For example, a population experiencing unemployment has fewer cars carrying commuters on the road, hence fewer car crashes. With job scarcity, individuals need to be more careful about being the model employee; thus, there may be less alcohol use and antisocial behavior (Catalano & Bellows, 2005).

The early analyses that studied time series of unemployment and health fell victim to statistical pitfalls (Brenner, 1971, 1973, 1975, 1979). These early studies simply regressed a single country's trends in mortality rates against GDP/capita, GDP changes, unemployment and their historical values and found that unemployment and recessions increase total mortality, infant mortality, cardiac deaths, cirrhosis, suicide, and homicide. The simple statistical techniques used in the early studies were flawed because they did not fully adjust for possible secular relationships in the trends. Just because two trends are increasing does not mean they are causally connected, otherwise one could "discover" connections between global warming and the increases in the number of reality-based television shows. Although generations of economists have discredited these early findings (Bishai, 1995; Gravelle, Hutchinson, & Stern, 1981; Laporte, 2004; Wagstaff, 1985), the spurious results were long perpetuated in the medical literature (Catalano & Serxner, 1992; Jin et al., 1995). In the last few years there appears to be a wider recognition in the epidemiologic literature that mortality time series must be studied as annual fluctuations or with methods capable of handling their non-stationarity[ix] (Ruhm, 2005).

One study that used more advanced methods to control for secular trends in unemployment and mortality found higher unemployment rates associated with higher infant mortality in the US (1919–1989), mixed results in the UK (1888–1988)[x] and no relationship in Sweden (1800–1989) (Bishai, 1995). Studies of US data for 1948–1996 and 1900–1996 found a positive relationship between more unemployment and better health (Granados, 2005; Laporte, 2004). One other properly executed time series study has found that there is no impact of unemployment on rates of low birthweight (Joyce & Mocan, 1993).

On the whole, the use of time series to explore the relationship between unemployment and population health has been treacherous and unrewarding. When improper methods were originally used for time series analysis, the results were impressive but wrong. When appropriate methods are applied to time series on unemployment and health, the analysis typically must study rates of change rather than levels, so the signal is weak, wavering, and inconclusive. The weakness of the signal can be inferred from Figure 8.6, which plots the relationship between recent rates of growth of gross national income per capita and growth of life expectancy. The once robust relationship seen in the Preston curve has vanished when one studies the correlation between growth rates.

Exciting recent work on unemployment and health has turned towards shorter panel data, where the health of populations in multiple independent labor markets can be followed over time as unemployment fluctuates. The principal statistical issues become confounding of the effects of unemployment by unobservable location-specific effects and the possible endogenous migration of unhealthier people either towards or away from areas experiencing unemployment. For instance, a study of the 50 US states and District of Columbia from 1972 to 1991 that controlled for fixed effects showed that a unit increase in the state unemployment rate would lower total mortality by 0.5% (Ruhm, 2000). The study found significant effects of state unemployment on the mortality of cohorts age

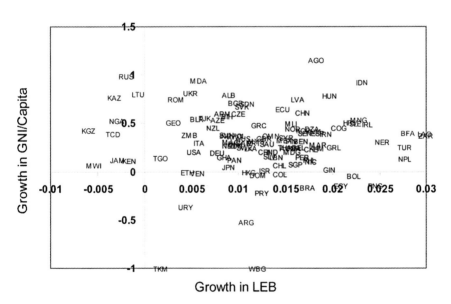

FIGURE 8.6. Scatter plot showing growth rate of Gross National Income per Capita from 2000 to 2004 vs. growth in life expectancy per capita over the same period. The plot seems to show a predominance of countries where both life expectancy and GNI/Capita grow however the raw correlation between the two variables is –0.0842. Ordinary regression yields a coefficient of –0.004 (P = 0.335).

0–30 days, 0–12 months, 20–44 years, and 65 + years. Effect sizes were highest for 20–44 year olds, where a 1 point rise in unemployment lowered mortality by 2%. Heart disease, vehicular injuries, suicide, and homicide were lowered by unemployment by 0.46%, 3%, 1.3%, and 1.9% respectively. Two studies of unemployment in 23 OECD countries between 1960–1997 found that a one point rise in country-level unemployment lowered mortality by 0.4% (Gerdtham & Ruhm, 2006; Johansson, 2004). Conditions most alleviated by higher unemployment in OECD countries were heart disease mortality (0.4%), hepatic mortality (1.8%) and vehicular injuries (2.1%). In 50 Spanish provinces for 1980–1997, Granados found that unemployment led to a 0.3% reduction in mortality, with leading effects on injuries but insignificant effects on heart disease, cancer, homicide, and suicide (Granados, 2005). Many other fixed effects panel studies with consistent findings on all cause mortality are extensively reviewed elsewhere (Ruhm, 2006).

The link between unemployment or recession and car crash mortality is intuitive. More employed people mean more commuters on the road, potentially making roads more hazardous for everybody. Alcohol use is also well known to increase when employment rates rise (Freeman, 1999; Ruhm & Black, 2002). In contrast, it is difficult to establish a plausible mechanism by which a recession will lower cardiovascular mortality within the same year. Behavioral risks for heart disease, like smoking, fat consumption, and physical inactivity, are significantly reduced during unemployment (Ruhm, 2000). However, the development of fatal atherosclerotic plaques in the coronary vessels requires 5–10 years, so it is unlikely that a phenomenon as transient as a business cycle could cause fatal coronary lesions by changing cardiac risk behaviors in this time frame. Changes in employment this year cannot create coronary lesions this year. If there is to be a link, it must be that people who already have significant coronary lesions are more likely to form blood clots at those lesions when the economy is heating up and unemployment rates are down. This scenario counters conventional wisdom that the population is under more "stress" during times of unemployment than times of employment. Similarly, suicide and homicide, mostly considered to be indicators of population stress, may be reduced when more people are unemployed (Ruhm, 2000). Note that not all panel studies agree that heart disease, suicide, and homicide are reduced during unemployment, but panel studies do reach consensus that injuries and all cause mortality are reduced.

These findings challenge the natural desire to extrapolate from the knowledge that unemployment is bad for individuals. They also challenge the intuition based on the Preston curve that being a wealthier country offers better health than being a poorer country. None of the panel studies of unemployment and health has used data from lower or middle income countries. Like any statistical finding, an association that holds on average for a large group of states or countries does not necessarily hold for each and every state and country.[xi] While being a rich country may be good for health in the long run, the process of growing the economy appears to include a rise in economic activity that can have short term adverse consequences, particularly in terms of automotive injuries as we saw in Figure 8.4. The policy impact of these findings on unemployment and health may consequently be minimal. No serious politician would recommend recession for its health benefits (Catalano & Bellows, 2005). Even an impolitic health policy maker would be ill-advised to support prolonged recession and the consequent descent down the Preston curve because the long term health losses would outweigh short term gains.

7. Health to Macroeconomic Development

In discussing Figure 8.1 we established the plausibility of a bi-directional association not only from material well being to health, but also from health to material well-being. Most of the reasoning for the health → development relationship is built on the micro-level evidence that people who become permanently disabled often become impoverished. Chronic conditions such as schistosomiasis (Fenwick & Figenschou, 1972; Ndamba, Makaza, Munjoma, Gomo, & Kaondera, 1993) and iron deficiency (Viteri & Torun, 1974) are known to lower economic productivity in workers and to affect the productivity of the farms or plantations that are tied to these workers. Several geographical determinists have conjectured that endemic diseases like malaria inhibit economic growth (Landes, 1998; Sachs, 2005). Another example would be onchocerciasis, or river blindness, an endemic disease transmitted by the black fly. Historically, the Volta river valley in Burkina Faso had areas so heavily endemic with onchocerciasis that what would otherwise be very productive land could not be farmed. Programs to control the disease by distributing ivermectin can open up productive land and generate goods and services that were previously unattainable.

The Commission on Macroeconomics and Health sponsored several studies that attempted to find evidence that investments in health were leading to economic growth (World Health Organization, 2003). Despite the inherent plausibility of the hypothesis, the commission's report itself offers little in the way of new incontrovertible evidence that health investments cause economic growth. Critics of the commission's report have noted that the relationship between health and poverty is not symmetrical and that poverty influences health much more than health influences poverty (Katz, 2004).

Finding an exogenous improvement in health that was not caused by pre-existing economic development has proven challenging. Some of the best evidence on how health interventions can improve the economy comes from a quasi-experiment conducted in Matlab by the International Centre for Diarrhoeal Disease Research, Bangladesh (ICDDR, B). This quasi-experiment took place in 141 villages in Matlab, half of which received outreach services with family planning and maternal and child health services delivered door to door during the period from 1978 to 1982. The intervention has been well known to have significantly lowered fertility by about 1 birth averted per woman in the treatment area (Fauveau, 1994). A recent analysis of data from a living standard survey conducted in a subset of treatment and comparison villages showed that the intervention appears to have improved household wealth and women's income in the macroeconomy represented by the treatment area (Joshi & Schultz, 2005). The economic benefits of the health intervention were not distributed equally among the villagers, instead being concentrated in households with greater schooling. For women in the treatment area, each additional year of schooling was worth $312 in net asset worth by 1996 (Joshi & Schultz, 2005). Unless women's schooling attainments become more evenly distributed, health interventions may widen rather than narrow socioeconomic disparities.

Another notable quasi-experimental study focused on the date when 69 low income countries adopted WHO-recommended treatment programs for the 15 leading causes of death. This adoption date was used as an exogenous instrument to predict the change in mortality between 1940 and 1980. Thus, the effect of the intervention-produced mortality reduction on the macroeconomy could be inferred. The intervention-produced mortality reduction was associated with a positive but statistically insignificant increase in GDP (numerator) and a larger statistically significant increase in population (denominator). Overall, the mortality reductions attributable to earlier introduction of WHO's disease control technologies had no significant effect on GDP per capita growth (Acemoglu & Johnson, 2006). The relationship of better health to transient rises in population may defeat attempts to find the individual level health to wealth relationship at the population level. This is an active area of research and there is much more to be learned.

8. Conclusion

We have reviewed the three primary macroeconomic indicators relevant to health: 1) national income, 2) income distribution, and 3) unemployment. The three measures differ in how one conceptualizes their effects on health. In each case, the measures may proxy multiple unmeasured properties of the population, particularly the quality of institutions that govern how the country's economy functions and the social goals to which national resources are applied. One may be tempted to view the effects of national income on health as the population aggregate of the effects of individual income on health, but income distribution and unemployment do not lend themselves to this approach. Income distribution's effects on health need to be considered independently of the income of the individual – measuring the effects of greater income equality on both rich and poor. Unemployment's effects on health reflect primarily the effects of the tempo of economic activity on the health of people in households unaffected by unemployment. These properties of the macroeconomy emerge from the whole economy and are not inherent in the individual households. This is a powerful argument for studying socioeconomic determinants of health at the level of nations, states, counties, and communities.

The other important result of this review emphasizes the shifting nature of the relationship between macroeconomics and health. The effects of the macroeconomy on health vary in magnitude depending on the stage of a country's economic development. As depicted in the Preston curve, the health of poorer populations is more responsive to the level of national income. In wealthy countries, the overall level of national income has weak effects on health, and economic upturns appear to have deleterious effects on many health conditions. One needs to be prepared for qualitative differences between the effects of the level of economic development and the effects of changes in that level on health. Being rich can have salutary effects on health while being engaged in the process of becoming rich can be detrimental. Health planners have long been cognizant of socioeconomic influences on health, but economic planners have seldom shown a reciprocal concern. Treasury secretaries do not consult the nation's health experts before changing interest rates and endorsing fiscal policy. This chapter has discussed at least one reason why this might need to be reconsidered. As economies heat up and unemployment goes down, there are increases in mortality and a broad spectrum of disease. Increasingly affluent societies find it harder and harder to derive additional enjoyment from additional income. However, death and suffering do not become any less abhorrent with affluence. At some point in the richest countries of the world, the welfare benefits from economic growth may not be worth the harms to health. Meanwhile, in poor countries the dual effects of better economic conditions and appropriately chosen public health strategies that accompany macroeconomic development will be the most powerful influences on public health.

Endnotes

i. This definition requires that the goods and services have to be flowing or exchanging ownership from seller to buyer; it also requires that the transactions be "monetized", meaning there is a market value associated with each deal. GDP is only slightly different from Gross National Product (GNP), in that GDP defines "population" geographically so that both citizens and resident aliens residing in a place contribute to GDP. In contrast, the population of interest for GNP consists of the legal citizens of that country no matter where they reside. For countries with no resident aliens and no citizens overseas, the two measures are identical.

ii. Louis Pasteur's salary from the École Normale Supérieure may have been a small flow to the GDP of France in 1862, but the global benefits from his discovery of germ theory that year are still accruing.

iii. There was a time when some (typically residing in wealthy countries) might confuse a country's higher economic wealth as the sine qua non of development. There was also a time when some (typically among the privileged) might have confused an individual's wealth with superior human development. The presence of numerous examples of depravity and baseness among the wealthy has given lie to these presumptions.

iv. An increase in women's labor force participation could produce temporary, but not sustained, increases in labor force availability.

v. Strictly speaking, additional money is not enough to ensure that better nutrition and hygiene will ensue. It is necessary that nutrition and hygiene have a positive "income elasticity of demand", meaning that human tastes are such that demand for these items will grow as income grows. It is theoretically possible that a given individual may have tastes such that additional income is used to finance debauchery and dissipation. Darwinian theory suggests that such individuals would make less competitive ancestors, and on average the population should have inherited tendencies to spend surplus income on better housing and better food inasmuch as these choices affect health and survival through child-bearing age. Exceptions occur as can be seen in evidence that salt, spices, and condiments had a superior income elasticity compared to protein and calories in a population with borderline nutrition in India (Behrman & Deolalikar, 1987).

vi. Examples where dictators have been able to geographically and socially direct famines towards politically expedient targets include Ethiopia under Mengistu (Harris, 1986) and China under Mao (Becker, 1996).

vii. The set of entitlements for an individual is his or her set freedoms and opportunities to pursue life and personal development. Given the definition of economic development as population level ability to expand entitlements for its citizens, famine is its antithesis writ large in which large sub-groups of the population lose entitlements to such a large extent that their survival is imperiled.

viii. It is worth noting that an analysis at the state level of self-rated health (SRH) found that the effects of the Gini-coefficient in worsening SRH were robust to the inclusion of state-level racial makeup indicators (Subramanian & Kawachi, 2003).

ix. Non-stationary time series are also known as random walks in which $y_t = y_{t-1} + \epsilon_t$, where ϵ_t is a random shock. As time goes on, the random shocks simply build on each other so that after T periods $y_T = y_0 + \sum_{t=0}^{T} \epsilon_t$. The variance of this time series goes to infinity as T increases so that conventional significance tests based upon an assumption that y_t is normally distributed are far too lenient and lead to the "discovery" of spurious correlations (Granger & Newbold, 1974).

x. The method used in the Bishai paper was called "cointegration" and can uncover multiple long-run relationships between time trends. In the UK, there were two cointegrating vectors, one showed a negative correlation between unemployment, and the other showed a positive correlation, suggesting that the system is capable of two contrasting long term equilibria.

xi. Similarly, the proverbial 90 year old life long smoker testifies that although smoking harms health, it does not harm health in every single case.

References

Acemoglu, D., & Johnson, S. (2006). *Disease and development: The effect of life expectancy on economic growth*. Cambridge, MA: MIT.

Bauer, P. (1981). *Equality, the Third World, and economic delusion*. Cambridge, MA: Harvard University Press.

Becker, J. (1996). *Hungry ghosts: Mao's secret famine*. New York: Free Press.

Behrman, J. R., & Deolalikar, A. B. (1987). Will developing country nutrition improve with income? A case study of rural south India. *Journal of Political Economy, 95*(108–38), 492.

Bishai, D., Qureshi, A., James, P., & Ghaffar, A. (2005). National road fatalities and economic development. *Health Economics, 15*(1), 65–81.

Bishai, D. M. (1995). Infant mortality time series are random walks with drift: Are they cointegrated with socioeconomic variables? *Health Economics, 4*(3), 157–167.

Blakely, T. A., Kennedy, B. P., Glass, R., & Kawachi, I. (2000). What is the lag time between income inequality and health status? *Journal of Epidemiology and Community Health, 54*(4), 318–319.

Blakely, T. A., Lochner, K., & Kawachi, I. (2002). Metropolitan area income inequality and self-rated health–a multi-level study. *Social Science & Medicine, 54*(1), 65–77.

Brenner, M. H. (1971). Economic changes and heart disease mortality. *American Journal of Public Health, 61*(3), 606–611.

Brenner, M. H. (1973). *Mental illness and the economy*. Cambridge, MA: Harvard University Press.

Brenner, M. H. (1975). Trends in alcohol consumption and associated illnesses. Some effects of economic changes. *American Journal of Public Health, 65*(12), 1279–1292.

Brenner, M. H. (1979). Mortality and the national economy. A review, and the experience of England and Wales, 1936–76. *Lancet, 2*(8142), 568–573.

Catalano, R., & Bellows, B. (2005). Commentary: If economic expansion threatens public health, should epidemiologists recommend recession? *International Journal of Epidemiology, 34*(6), 1212–1213.

Catalano, R., & Serxner, S. (1992). Neonatal mortality and the economy revisited. *International Journal of Health Services, 22*(2), 275–286.

Dasgupta, S., Laplante, B., Wang, H., & Wheeler, D. (2002). Confronting the environmental Kuznets Curve. *The Journal of Economic Perspectives, 16*, 147–168.

Deaton, A., & Lubotsky, D. (2003). Mortality, inequality and race in American cities and states. *Social Science & Medicine, 56*(6), 1139–1153.

Diez-Roux, A. V., Link, B. G., & Northridge, M. E. (2000). A multilevel analysis of income inequality and cardiovascular disease risk factors. *Social Science & Medicine, 50*(5), 673–687.

Dooley, D., Fielding, J., & Levi, L. (1996). Health and unemployment. *Annual Review of Public Health, 17*, 449–465.

Fauveau, V. (1994). *Matlab: Women, children, and health*. Dhaka: International Centre for Diarrhoeal Disease Research, Bangladesh.

Fenwick, A., & Figenschou, B. H. (1972). The effect of schistosoma mansoni infection of the productivity of cane cutters on a sugar estate in Tanzania. *Bulletin of the World Health Organization, 47*(5), 567–572.

Fogel, R. (1997). New findings on secular trends in nutrition and mortality: Some implications for population theory. In M. Rosenzweig & O. Stark (Eds.), *Handbook of population and family economics*. New York: Elsevier.

Freeman, D. G. (1999). A note on "Economic conditions and alcohol problems". *Journal of Health Economics, 18*(5), 661–670.

Galloway, P. R. (1986). Differentials in demographic responses to annual price variations in pre-revolutionary France: A comparison of rich and poor areas in Rouen, 1681–1787. *European Journal of Population, 2*, 269–305.

Gerdtham, U. G., & Ruhm, C. J. (2006). Deaths rise in good economic times: Evidence from the OECD. *Economics and Human Biology, 4*(3), 298–316.

Granados, J. (2005). Increasing mortality during expansions of the U.S. economy. *International Journal of Epidemiology, 34*, 1194–1202.

Granados, J. T. (2005). Recessions and mortality in Spain, 1980–1997. *European Journal of Population, 21*(4), 393–422.

Granger, C. W. J., & Newbold, P. (1974). Spurious regressions in econometrics. *Journal of Econometrics, 2*(2), 111–120.

Gravelle, H. S., Hutchinson, G., & Stern, J. (1981). Mortality and unemployment: A critique of Brenner's time-series analysis. *Lancet, 2*(8248), 675–679.

Harris, M. (1986). *Breakfast in hell: A doctor's experience of the Ethiopian famine.* London: MacMillan.

Harrod, R. F. (1939). An essay in dynamic theory. *Economic Journal, 49,* 14–33.

Jin, R. L., Shah, C. P., & Svoboda, T. J. (1995). The impact of unemployment on health: A review of the evidence. *Canadian Medical Association Journal, 153*(5), 529–540.

Johansson, E. (2004). A note on the impact of hours worked on mortality in OECD countries. *European Journal of Health Economics, 5*(4), 335–340.

Joshi, S., & Schultz, T. P. (2005). Family planning as an investment in development and female human capital: Evaluating the long term consequences in Matlab, Bangladesh. (June 10, 2005); http://team.univ-paris1.fr/espe2005/papers/schultz_paper.pdf

Joyce, T., & Mocan, N. (1993). Unemployment and infant Health: Time-Series Evidence from the State of Tennessee. *Journal of Human Resources, 28*(1), 185–203.

Katz, A. (2004). The Sachs report: Investing in health for economic development–or increasing the size of the crumbs from the rich man's table? Part I. *International Journal of Health Services, 34*(4), 751–773.

Kaufmann, D., Kraay, A., & Mastruzzi, M. (2003). *Governance matters III: Governance indicators for 1996–2002.* Washington, DC: World Bank.

Kawachi, I., & Kennedy, B. P. (1997). The relationship of income inequality to mortality: Does the choice of indicator matter? *Social Science & Medicine, 45*(7), 1121–1127.

Landes, D. S. (1998). *The wealth and poverty of nations: Why some are so rich and some so poor.* New York: W.W. Norton.

Laporte, A. (2004). Do economic cycles have a permanent effect on population health? Revisiting the Brenner hypothesis. *Health Economics, 13*(8), 767–779.

McKeown, T. (1976). *The modern rise of population.* New York: Academic Press.

Mokyr, J. (1993). Technological progress and the decline of European mortality. *American Economic Review, 83*(2), 324–330.

Ndamba, J., Makaza, N., Munjoma, M., Gomo, E., & Kaondera, K. C. (1993). The physical fitness and work performance of agricultural workers infected with schistosoma mansoni in Zimbabwe. *Annals of Tropical Medicine and Parasitology, 87*(6), 553–561.

Nussbaum, M. (2000). *Women and human development : The capabilities approach.* Cambridge: Cambridge University Press.

Nussbaum, M. C., & Sen, A. (1993). *The quality of life.* New York: Oxford Clarendon Press.

Preston, S. H. (1975). The changing relation between mortality and level of economic development. *Population Studies, 29*(2), 231–248.

Ravallion, M. (1987). *Markets and famines.* Oxford: Oxford University Press.

Ravallion, M. (1997). Famines and economics. *Journal of Economic Literature, 35,* 1205–1242.

Rodgers, G. (1979). Income and inequality as determinants of mortality: An international cross-section analysis. *Population Studies, 33,* 343–351.

Ruhm, C. J. (2000). Are recessions good for your health? *Quarterly Journal of Economics, 115*(2), 617–650.

Ruhm, C. J. (2005). Commentary: Mortality increases during economic upturns. *International Journal of Epidemiology, 34*(6), 1206–1211.

Ruhm, C. J. (2006). Macroeconomic conditions, health and mortality. In A. Jones (Ed.), *Elgar companion to health economics.* Northampton, MA: Edward Elgar Press.

Ruhm, C. J., & Black, W. E. (2002). Does drinking really decrease in bad times? *Journal of Health Economics, 21*(4), 659–678.

Sachs, J. (2005). *The end of poverty.* New York: Penguin Press.

Sala-i-Martin, X. (2002). *The world distribution of income.* New York: National Bureau of Economic Research, Working Paper 8933.

Sen, A. (1981). Ingredients of famine analysis: Availability and entitlements. *Quarterly Journal of Economics, 96*, 433–464.

Sen, A. (1999). *Development as freedom.* New York: Random House.

Solow, R. M. (1956). A contribution to the theory of economic growth. *Quarterly Journal of Economics, 70,* 65–94.

Solow, R. M. (1957). Technical change and the aggregate production function. *Review of Economics and Statistics, 39*(August), 312–320.

Subramanian, S. V., Belli, P., & Kawachi, I. (2002). The macroeconomic determinants of health. *Annual Review of Public Health, 23*, 287–302.

Subramanian, S. V., Blakely, T., & Kawachi, I. (2003). Income inequality as a public health concern: Where do we stand? Commentary on "Is exposure to income inequality a public health concern?" *Health Services Research, 38*(1), 153–167.

Subramanian, S. V., & Kawachi, I. (2003). The association between state income inequality and worse health is not confounded by race. *International Journal Epidemiology, 32*(6), 1022–1028.

Szreter, S. (1994). Mortality in England in the eighteenth and the nineteenth centuries: A reply to Sumit Guha. *Social History of Medicine, 7*(2), 269–282.

United Nations Development Program. (2005). *Human development report, 2005.* New York: United Nations Development Program.

Viteri, F. E., & Torun, B. (1974). Anemia and work capacity. *Clinics in Haematology, 3.*

Wagstaff, A. (1985). Time series analysis of the relationship between unemployment and mortality: A survey of econometric critiques and replications of Brenner's studies. *Social Science & Medicine, 21*(9), 985–996.

Wilkinson, R. G. (1999). Income distribution and life expectancy. In I. Kawachi, B. P. Kennedy, & R. G. Wilkinson (Eds.), *The society and population health reader: Income inequality and health.* New York: The New Press.

World Health Organization. (2003). *Investing in health: A summary of the findings of the commission on macroeconomics and health.* Geneva: World Health Organization.

Chapter 9
Culture

Richard M. Eckersley

1. Introduction

The 14th century English philosopher (and heretic), William of Occam, stated in his famous razor that "entities must not be unnecessarily multiplied." Roughly translated, this means "the simplest theory that fits the facts corresponds most closely to reality." Occam's razor has a wide application in science. However, when dealing with complex systems, like human societies, that comprise many entities often interacting in multiple, weak, diffuse and non-linear ways, we may have to "multiply entities" beyond what first seems to be necessary. This is certainly true in exploring the macrosocial determinants of health.

Consider the rise in youth suicide in many Western nations in the second half of the 20th century, one of the most striking adverse health trends in the developed world. Suicide rates have more than tripled among among young males in the United States, Canada, Australia and New Zealand. A recent study found that rates of youth suicide were strongly and positively correlated with several different measures of individualism, including personal freedom and control (Eckersley & Dear, 2002). The simplest explanation for the association is that the greater people's sense of freedom in life the more likely they are to choose death. Indeed, suicide might well be regarded as an ultimate expression of individual freedom of choice and control over one's life.

However, the study included a wide array of cultural and social variables which indicated that higher youth suicide is associated with not just freer youth, but happier, healthier, and more optimistic youth. Other researchers have proposed such results imply that suicide rises as social conditions and personal prospects improve and provide several plausible explanations for this possibility. However, when we cast the net of evidence wider, the facts show that rising suicide represents one end of a spectrum or gradient of distress and suffering. The less severe forms affect a much larger proportion of young people and have also become more prevalent over time. Put another way, suicidal youth are not an island of misery in an ocean of happiness but are, instead, the tip of an iceberg of suffering. Thus, to understand the social determinants of youth suicide, we have to go a fair distance from suicide and its social correlates.

The chapter includes: an account of how epidemiology and other disciplines have conceptualized and investigated culture, the case for a greator use of transdisciplinary synthesis to understand better the role of culture in health, a model of how culture affects health, drawing on psychosocial theories of health, some examples to illustrate the very different types of cultural impacts, and a description of the many streams of evidence that implicate culture in health. The basic premise is that culture, especially the dominant culture of a society, deserves more attention as a macrosocial determinant of population health.

2. Disciplinary Perspectives on Culture

This chapter employs a common definition of culture, that is, the language and accumulated knowledge, beliefs, practices, assumptions and values that are passed between individuals, groups and generations (Boyden, 2004). However, one of the issues that make the study of culture so fraught with contention and debate is that the word is used differently between, and even within, disciplines. Indeed, a review undertaken over fifty years ago identified 164 different definitions of culture (Kroeber & Kluckhohn, 1952, cited in Boyden, 2004).

2.1. Epidemiology: Culture as Difference

The mainstream or defining culture of a society has been given relatively little attention in the recent epidemiologic literature. Social epidemiology mainly focuses on "subcultures" or "difference", especially ethnic and racial, as one dimension of socio-economic status and inequality, (Corin, 1994, 1995; DiGiacomo, 1999; Eckersley, 2001a, 2006a). Generally speaking, however, the influence of the broader concept of culture on health has been seen as distal and diffuse, pervasive but unspecified.

The reasons for epidemiology's apparent neglect of culture are both epistemological and methodological. With its origins in medicine and reliance on statistical methods, epidemiology tends to treat individuals as units of disease and disability, which are the consequence of various social and personal exposures. As Corin (1994, 1995) has observed, epidemiology's "categorical" approach to sociocultural factors, which fits comfortably within prevailing scientific paradigms, strips human realities of much of their social context and disregards and dismisses other approaches to social and cultural realities. Objects and events do not possess an inherent and objective significance; instead, these are imbued with meanings that vary with individuals, times and societies and emerge from a network of associations. For Corin, there is a complex interaction between the objective and subjective worlds, between reality, expectations and values, and "every aspect of reality is seen embedded within webs of meaning that define a certain world view and that cannot be studied or understood apart from this collective frame."

Glass (2006) compares modern epidemiology with Newtonian physics, attesting that "epidemiology is the search for individual trajectories through fixed and invariant space, in which discrete, isolatable, linear forces (exposures) are necessary and sufficient causes of those trajectories." Culture, however, is profoundly counter-paradigmatic; it has no place in a Newtonian vision of cause and effect. Glass argues, "With few exceptions . . . epidemiology has great difficulty incorporating aggregate-level phenomena that exist in larger dimensional space beyond what touches or invades the individual."

Societies have developed rich, complex cultures to explain the world and to give meaning to life, raising the question of why culture has remained absent from epidemiologic investigations on health determinants. It is not that the evidence of the impact of qualities such as materialism, individualism, and religiosity on health and well-being is missing. Rather, the omission reveals a professional orthodoxy, a mindset that filters out concepts and issues that fall outside the dominant paradigms that frame thinking on the social determinants of health.

2.2. Other Disciplinary Views

Anthropology, which claims intellectual dominion over the construct of culture, eschews the broad definition of the term. Indeed, anthropologists even debate whether the term has any value, a discussion that, to the outsider, illustrates just how dauntingly arcane scholarly argument can become. Writing in the journal, *Cultural Anthropology*, Brightman (1995) notes that culture, the discipline's "longstanding darling," is increasingly embattled; he notes, "The utility, not to mention the integrity, of the construct of culture – as expounded by Tylor, relativized by Boas, and thereafter refracted through diverse functionalist, ecological, cognitive, transactionalist, structuralist, Marxian, and hermeneutic perspectives – is increasingly being challenged." Some anthropologists want to reject "culture" altogether in favor of "discourse", "hegemony" or "habitus".

If they have not yet abandoned the word, medical anthropologists have moved well away from a broad definition of culture in favor of a more restricted use of the term.. Their usage acknowledges just how fuzzy, complex and multifaceted culture is – variably distributed, locally influenced and intimately connected to history, politics and economics (Dressler, 2006; Janes, 2006). They dismiss notions that whole societies (let alone groups of societies) can be characterized by a few dominant themes (such as individualism). Instead, they focus on the details of population patterning and distribution, individual and group differences, and culture as local knowledge and daily life.

These arguments may well be valid, but not to the extent of disallowing broad cultural influences on population health and well-being (Eckersley, 2006a,b). We cannot afford to limit our study to only the small, local scale but must also investigate the societal and even global level. We can draw parallels between cultural changes and environmental or economic changes. For instance, the actual and projected impacts of global warming vary dramatically from place to place in terms of changes in temperature, rainfall, and extreme weather events. This does not mean it can only be studied at a local level; indeed, we would never under-stand the processes if this were done. The same is true of economic globalization: Its effects vary from country to country, between urban and rural areas, and among industries, but it involves global forces and must be studied at this level, as well as in more specific, focused ways.

The broader approach to culture is a part of psychology, where differences between individualism and collectivism remain a major research theme. Nevertheless, the validity and value of this distinction as a dominant way of categorizing societies are being debated in the psychological literature (e.g., Oyserman, Coon, & Kemmelmeier, 2002). Psychologists also use other ways of characterizing cultures and societies, including whether they are simple or complex, loose (tolerant) or tight (strict), vertical (hierarchical) or horizontal (egalitarian); these qualities interact with collectivism and individualism in shaping social qualities (Triandis & Suh, 2002). In sociology, individualization is a dominant theme, a defining feature of modernity and, even more so, post-modernity (e.g., Beck & Beck-Gernsheim, 2002). Sociologists sometimes distin-guish between "individualization" (self-determination, emancipation from traditional restrictions) and "individualism" (self-centeredness, selfishness). However, it is arguable that the first has led to the second, so the distinction is not essential for the purposes of this chapter. Here, individualization is the process of increasing individualism.

These different disciplinary perspectives on culture point to the potential for a rich cross-fertilization between disciplines in studying culture's effects on health. For example, anthropology does provide important insights into culture. Its view of culture as a system of meanings, a web or matrix of collective influences that shape people's lives, contrasts with epidemiology's more materialist approach. Also useful is the concept that individuals possess cultural models that derive both from their own biographies and from the collective or shared understandings that form the traditions of their society (Dressler, 2004). These models reflect a "cultural consensus" about the way the world works, but this consensus is not complete and can be contested, even bitterly. "Cultural consonance" is the extent to which individuals reveal in their own beliefs and behavior the cultural consen-sus (with one focus of research, often conducted on ethnic minorities, being the association between cultural consonance and disease risk).

It follows that, just as other social determinants, such as inequality, can be stud-ied at both population and individual levels, so too can culture. It can be measured as differences between societies (reflecting differences in cultural consensus) or as differences between individuals and groups within a society (reflecting degrees of cultural consonance). For example, some societies are more materialistic or individualistic than others (even among Western nations), and some individuals and groups within any one society will reveal these qualities more than others. Thus, the evidence for cultural impacts on health can be drawn from both individ-ual-level and population-level studies.

Different disciplines can also contribute to the range of measures and indicators of cultural difference and health, and so to empirical studies of the relationships between culture and health. Cultural variables can often be drawn from surveys of attitudes, beliefs and values (e.g., Eckersley & Dear, 2002) but can also be based on objective data like social fragmentation (renting, mobility, unmarried people, single-person households) (e.g., Whitley, Gunnell, Dorling, & Davey Smith, 1999) or social integration (divorce rates, education, labour-force participation, family relationships, social interaction, religious participation, community involvement) (e.g., Duberstein, Conwell, Conner, Eberly, Evinger, & Caine, 2004; Fernquist & Cutright, 1998). Both social fragmentation and integration reflect cultural changes, notably increasing individualism (and, like individualism, have been associated with suicide).

To summarize, the study of culture as a determinant of health would benefit from a more systematic examination of the potential of mixing disciplines in research.

2.3. Transdisciplinary Synthesis

There is growing scientific recognition of the importance of multidisciplinary, interdisciplinary and transdisciplinary research (with each term representing an increasing level of disciplinary fusion) (Bammer, 2005; Rosenfield, 1992). Transdisciplinary research is fundamentally about synthesis. While empirical research seeks to improve understanding of the world through the creation of new knowledge, synthesis creates new understanding by combining and integrating existing knowledge from across a range of fields, disciplines and sciences (Eckersley, 2005). The value of synthesis goes beyond reviewing, summarizing and multidisciplinary research, per se. Transdisciplinary investigation aims to develop new common conceptual frameworks, creating a new level of coherence (Higginbotham, Albrecht, & Connor, 2001, cited in Bammer, 2005). There are two general ways for doing this: having an individual synthesize findings from many disciplines to provide a comprehensive explanation of a complex issue or creating a team whose members work together on this task.

In reconciling perspectives and frameworks of various disciplines, synthesis yields several intellectual and policy benefits: It adds value to existing specialized knowledge; reduces disciplinary biases; transcends (at least potentially) interdisciplinary tensions; improves researchers' knowledge outside their specialization; generates new research questions; is especially useful in examining complex systems; and enhances the application of knowledge. Concerning application, synthesis improves the fit between research and policy; strengthens the links between research and advocacy; is particularly appropriate for addressing the increasing scale, magnitude, complexity and interconnectedness of human problems; and suits the complex, diffuse processes of social change. At the same time, synthesis raises several important conceptual issues (Bammer, 2005; Eckersley, 2005), it strives for coherence in the overall picture rather than precision in the detail, dispenses with expectations of scientific certainty and exactness, including with respect to cause and effect, and challenges Occam's Razor, as noted at the beginning of the chapter.

As already discussed, disciplines draw on different conceptul frameworks and approaches, which yield different evidence and interpretations. Much remains to be done to integrate and reconcile these prespectives. In doing this, synthesis yields several intellectual and policy benefits: it adds value to existing specialized knowledge, reduces disciplinary biases, transcends (at least potentially) interdisciplinary tensions, improves researchers' knowledge outside their specialization, generates new research questions, is especially useful in examining complex system, enhances the application of knowledge. Concerning application, synthesis improves the fit between research and policy, strengthens the links between research and advocacy; is particularly appropriate for addressing the increasing scale, magnitude, complexity and interconnectedness of human problems; and suits the complex, diffuse processes of social change.

In dissloving disciplinary boundaries, synthesis exposes the 'false consensus' that can develope within disciplinary, which then defines, and limits, the research question asked. Examples include, as already noted, epidemiology's focus on socio-economic inequality, and anthropology's on 'small-scale' culture effects. But such gains are not easily won. The cultures of scientific disciplines are like the cultures of societies: so ingrained that they appear to be the natural and right way to look at the world. For example, in a recent transdisciplinary project on young people's potentional and wellbeing (Eckersley, Wierenga, & Wyn, 2006), the author could not agree on key issues, and even had trouble agreeing on how to disagree. Rather than disguishing or blunting these difference with careful wording. they have highlighted them as a significant outcome of the project. Transdisciplinary approaches are especially relevant to the study of culture and health, given interest in culture spans several disciplines.

3.0. Culture and Health

3.1. A Model of Cultural Influences on Health

In the past two decades, the development of psychosocial theories of socio-economic inequalities in health has furthered the acceptance and understanding of the effects of culture on health. Researchers may still disagree on whether the sources of health inequalities are primarily, or fundamentally, material – resulting from differences in material exposures and experiences – or psychosocial – stemming from people's position in the social hierarchy and their perceptions of relative disadvantage (Eckersley, 2001a, 2005, 2006a). However, it is now commonly held that psychosocial factors are a significant pathway by which inequality and other social determinants affect health and that perceptions and emotions are important to health outcomes. Drawing on this work, this chapter argues that cultural factors are linked, via psychosocial pathways, to psychological well-being, and well-being is linked, through behavioral and physiological pathways, to physical health.

Psychosocial processes involve interactions between social conditions and individual psychology and behavior; they are associated (in their negative effects) with stress, depression, anxiety, isolation, insecurity, hostility and lack of control over one's life. Psychosocial factors affect health through health-related behaviors and also act via direct effects on the neuroendocrine and immune systems. Once we allow a role in health for psychosocial factors, culture has to be considered because it has psychosocial consequences.

Psychosocial perspectives on health acknowledge cultural influences but tend to frame these in terms of inequality, that the cultural factors that matter are consequences of inequality, a part of the psychosocial pathway. Marmot and Wilkinson (2001), for example, in noting the relationship between income inequality and social affiliation, suggest there is a "culture of inequality" that is more aggressive, less connected, more violent and less trusting. However, we can also think of such processes as going well beyond inequality. A culture of individualism and materialism could also produce these attributes. In other words, developments in thinking about inequality in essentially cultural terms invite a broader consideration of cultural factors as determinants of health. Cultural qualities are a cause of inequality as well as a consequence, and they also act on health independently of their effects on social structures.

Culture may help to explain health inequalities within societies in several ways. Culture may have direct impact through cultural differences among individuals and groups. It may influence levels of socio-economic inequality – for example, through the part individualism plays in market-oriented, or neo-liberal, political doctrines that are associated with greater inequality. Culture may also interact with socio-economic status to moderate or amplify its health effects; for example, materialism and individualism might accentuate the costs of being poor or of low social status by making money more important to social position and weakening social bonds and group identity. However, this chapter focuses on culture's role in explaining health differences among societies or changes in a population's health (or, more accurately, health potential) over time. Psychosocial theories of health have drawn of the work of Durkheim, amongst others. Durkheim's notion of social integration provides a tradition within sociological theory for understanding the link between social conditions, including culture, and ill health (Mestrovic, 1985; Mestrovic & Glassner, 1983). Social integration (of which social support is a by-product) involves the interplay between two antagonistic aspects of human existence, the individual and the social. Durkheim believed integration was optimal when the two sides were in balance, and part of this balance required constraining human needs. He saw anomie as a "malady of infiniteness"; it was a general law of all living things that needs and appetites are normal only on condition of being controlled.

In his seminal sociological study of suicide, Durkheim (1970) emphasized the role of social institutions, such as the family and religion, in binding individuals to society, in keeping "a firmer grip" on them and in drawing them out of their "state of moral isolation." He argued that "man cannot become attached to higher aims and submit to a rule if he sees nothing above him to which he belongs," and "to free him from all social pressure is to abandon him to himself and demoralise him." Durkheim saw clearly the distinction between material and moral causes of despair. In a comment particularly relevant to modern times, he says, "If more suicides occur today than formerly, this is not because, to maintain ourselves, we have to make more painful efforts, nor that our legitimate needs are less satisfied, but because we no longer know the limits of legitimate needs nor perceive the direction of our efforts."

The sociological literature on modernization and individualization elaborates on these consequences of freedom from social regulation and constraint. It is, however, characterized by ambivalence about the gains and losses and by the notion that the freedom people now have is both exhilarating and disturbing and that with freedom come both new opportunities for personal experience and growth and the anxiety of social dislocation (e.g., Bauman, 1995; Elliott, 1996).This literature can be very complex and subtle, challengingly so to the disciplinary outsider. In comparison, the focus of the social determinants of health literature on structural differences and changes in the economy, family, education and labor market seems crude. Conversely, the sociological literature would benefit from a more precise mapping of the health consequences of individualization.

3.2. Direct Cultural Impacts on Health, an Example: Female Genital Mutilation

Health research has emphasized the negative consequences of psychosocial processes, and this chapter is also primarily concerned with cultural sources of psychosocial stress, placing culture alongside inequality as a macrosocial determinant of health. However, culture can also affect health more directly by promoting or discouraging healthy and unhealthy practices (in fact, this is their more widely understood and accepted role). Behaviors such as smoking, alcohol and other drug use, sexual promiscuity, and violence (or, in the case of healthy practices, exercise and a healthy diet) vary in prevalence as social norms and values change, as well as in response to psychosocial stresses. In other words, the psychosocial pathways linking culture and health can be both specific and diffuse, direct and indirect.

Cultures tend to be "transparent" or "invisible" to those living within them because they comprise deeply internalized assumptions and beliefs, making their effects hard to discern. According to Corin (1994), cultural influences are always easier to identify in unfamiliar societies. Our own cultures appear to constitute a natural order that is not itself an object of study. This impression, she believes, is an "unsupported ethnocentric illusion." Consequently, it is worth illustrating cultural impacts on health with an example that comes from "unfamiliar" cultures (at least to those from European and Asian societies). The practice is female genital mutilation (FGM).

FGM involves partial or total removal of the external female genitalia or other injury to the female genitals for cultural or other non-therapeutic reasons. An estimated 100 million women worldwide have had FGM (World Health Organization Study Group on FGM and Obstetric Outcome, 2006). The practice aims to attenuate women's sexual desire to maintain chastity and virginity prior to marriage and to encourage fidelity; some societies also appear to consider it more "aesthetically pleasing" and more "hygienic." It is well known that FGM directly can affect the health of the women who experience it, causing, for example, genital and urinary tract infections. Its obstetric impacts, however, have only recently come under study. A WHO study of almost 30,000 women in six African countries where the practice is common found that women with FGM were significantly more likely to have adverse obstetric outcomes, with risks increasing with the extent of the mutilation. Births to women who have undergone FGM were significantly more likely to be complicated by caesarean section, postpartum bleeding, longer hospital stays, infant resuscitation, and still births or early neonatal deaths (the study estimates that FGM leads to an extra one to two perinatal deaths per 100 deliveries). A commentary on the study (Eke & Nkanginieme, 2006) argued that genital mutilation status should be included "among critical health indices for less developed countries," expressing the hope that FGM will face the fate of past cultural rituals, such as the rejection of twins, the African slave trade, Chinese foot-binding and Victorian chastity belts."

3.3. Diffuse Cultural Impacts on Health, an Example: Individualism

In marked contrast to FGM, the health impacts of a cultural quality such as individualism are much more complex and, correspondingly, more difficult to study. Individualism places the personal at the centre of a framework of values, norms and goals, notably personal freedom and choice. Fundamentally, individualism is about believing people are independent of one another.

Psychosocial theories of health emphasize the importance of social support and personal control to health. The psychological and sociological literatures suggest a variety of ways in which individualism reduces not only social support but also, paradoxically, personal control. These effects can be quite specific but, importantly, not necessarily reflected in changes in objective or external structures. However, the specific effects of individualism are not the only ways it affects health and well-being. Cultural influences are also very broad, pervasive and diffuse –profound forces that shape (and is shaped by) many facets of being human, even personality.

For example, the study of youth suicide (Eckersley & Dear, 2002) cited at the beginning of the chapter found that suicide rates were not correlated with divorce rates, but both suicide and individualism were significantly and negatively correlated with a sense of parental duty (measured as agreement that it is the parents' duty to do the best for their children even at the expense of their own well-being). Furthermore, the correlation of suicide with parental duty was much weaker than that with broader measures of individualism (for example, agreement that people have a great deal of freedom of choice and control over their lives), suggesting parental duty is not a major pathway by which individualism impacts on youth suicide. Supporting this more diffuse role of individualism in health, suicide has also been linked, as noted earlier, to a lack of social integration and social fragmentation.

These findings are consistent with the conclusions of a major international review (Rutter & Smith, 1995) of the evidence of rising trends in psychosocial problems such as depression, drug abuse, suicidal behavior and crime among young people in Western nations in the second half of the 20th century. It concluded that social disadvantage and inequality were unlikely explanations for the increases and called for further investigation of the theory that shifts in moral concepts and values were among the causes – in particular, "the shift towards individualistic values, the increasing emphasis on self-realization and fulfillment, and the consequent rise in expectations."

Historically, individualization has been a mainly progressive force, loosening the chains of religious dogma, class oppression and gender and ethnic discrimination. Thus it has been associated with the liberation of human potential and intended to free people to lead the lives they wanted. However, just as the reality of commitment differs from the ideal, so the reality of freedom differs from its ideal, especially when it is taken too far or is misinterpreted.

The costs of individualism have been described in many ways (Eckersley, 2006a): a heightened sense of risk, uncertainty and insecurity; a lack of clear frames of reference; a rise in personal expectations, coupled with a perception that the onus of success lies with the individual (despite the continuing importance of social disadvantage and privilege); a surfeit or excess of freedom and choice, which is experienced as a threat or tyranny; increased self-esteem (but of a contingent or narcissistic form that requires constant external validation and affirmation); and the confusion of autonomy with independence. As Bauman (2002) notes, there is "a nasty fly of impotence in the ointment of freedom," an impotence that is all the more upsetting in view of the empowerment that freedom was expected to deliver.

The result is a perception by individuals that they are separate from others and the environment in which they live – and so from the very things that affect their lives. The more narrowly and separately the self is defined, the greater the likelihood that the personal influences and social forces acting on it are experienced as external and alien. The creation of a "separate self" could be a major dynamic in modern life, impacting on everything from citizenship and social trust, cohesion, and engagement, to the intimacy of friendships and the quality of family life. The more culture focuses on the individual, the more impotent and insecure people seem to feel; the more diminished they feel as individuals, the more precious they become in the face of slights and insults and the more stridently they defend their personal "rights."

Therefore, the issue here is not just a matter of the changed interactions between the individual (as a physical entity) and social structures and institutions, as in the Newtonian model discussed earlier, but of the way in which the individual self is construed, especially in terms of its relationships to others. In other words, the result is not only increased objective isolation, but also more subjective loneliness. Broadly speaking, it would seem that individualism has produced a self that is socially and historically disconnected, discontented, and insecure; in pursuit of constant gratification and external affirmation; and prone to addiction, obsession and excess.

Thus there is a strong case for believing that increasing individualism is affecting psychosocial factors such as social support and personal control and is therefore harming psychological well-being and physical health. These negative impacts of individualism help to explain why societies do not appear to have reaped the full psychosocial benefits that should have flowed from other cultural changes of recent decades, also linked to individualization, such as increased social tolerance, diversity and pluralism (including greater gender, religious, ethnic and racial equality).

3.4. Evidence of Cultural Determinants of Health

Apart from the two specific examples discussed above, there are several streams of evidence, some admittedly indirect and circumstantial, that support the view that culture is an important social determinant of health. As well as illustrating the general concept, this evidence also serves as a summary of a wide-ranging critique of modern Western culture and its defining qualities of materialism (or consumerism) and individualism. Some of these qualities are becoming increasingly global in their influence.

3.4.1. The Direct Effects of Cultural Factors on Health

Individualism's health impacts, notably suicide, have already been discussed. Another quality of Western culture is materialism (attaching importance or priority to money and possessions). Many studies have shown materialism is associated with lesser satisfaction of human psychological needs and thus diminished well-being; materialism seems to breed unhappiness, depression, anxiety, anger, isolation and alienation (Eckersley, 2005; Kasser, 2002). People for whom "extrinsic goals" such as fame, fortune and glamour are a priority in life tend to experience more anxiety and depression and lower overall well-being – and to be less trusting and caring in their relationships – than people oriented towards "intrinsic goals" of close relationships, personal growth and self-understanding, and contributing to the community. In short, the more materialistic people are, the poorer their quality of life

3.4.2. Adverse Health Trends that are Better Explained by Cultural Rather Than by Structural Changes

A UK study (Collishaw, Maughan, Goodman, & Pickles, 2004) of comparable surveys conducted in 1974, 1986 and 1999 found the expected gradients in adolescent mental health problems according to socio-economic status and family-structure, but also that the prevalence increased across all social classes and family types. The authors hold that these uniform effects suggest that specific sociodemographic trends cannot fully explain time trends in adolescent adjustment and that "relatively broad societal changes (for example, in the media, youth culture or social cohesion) are affecting adolescent mental health." US researchers (Luthar, 2003; Luther & Latendresse, 2005) argue that comparative studies of rich and poor youth reveal "more similarities than differences in their adjustment patterns and socialisation processes." Their studies indicate that children in rich families, a little researched group, may be more likely than other children to suffer substance use problems, anxiety and depression. Two possible explanations are given: excessive pressures to achieve and isolation from parents, both physical and emotional.

3.4.3. Trends in Personality and Other Psychological Qualities that Affect Well-Being and Which Have Been Associated with Cultural Changes

US researchers have analyzed psychological tests of children and youth conducted over decades and have found marked increases in trait anxiety (or neuroticism), self-esteem and extraversion, while sense of control over life declined (Twenge, 2006). The findings denote broad social trends – not just genes and the family environment, as psychologists have assumed – are important influences on personality development. The changes are linked to increasing individualism and declining social connectedness. Anxiety and lack of control are associated with diminished well-being; even high self-esteem, once regarded as a source of well-being, is now seen as problematic by many psychologists.

3.4.4. Media Influences

The media are one of the most distinctive features of modern times; they are powerful and ubiquitous, employ stunning technologies and dominate people's leisure time (Eckersley, 2005; Myers, 2001). Increasingly, the media are defining a cultural frame of reference that extends well beyond the local, immediate and the personal. The images of the familiar and unfamiliar world that people see reflected in the media shape who they are and what they become. Attention has focused mainly on the links between media violence and real violence, evidence for which is now about as strong as that between smoking and lung cancer. However, negative media impacts extend far beyond encouraging aggression; their cultural effects are much more complex and pervasive. These include the promotion of: apocalyptic images of the future; a superficial, materialistic and self-indulgent lifestyle; invidious comparisons with the lives of people who are more powerful, beautiful, successful and exciting; unrealistic expectation of what life should offer; and diminished social cohesion and civic engagement.

3.4.5. The Changing Nature and Role of Religion

Religious belief and practice enhance health and well-being (Eckersley, 2007). The benefits flow from the social support, existential or spiritual meaning, sense of purpose, coherent belief system and moral code that religion provides. All these things can be found in other ways, although perhaps less easily. However, religion is no panacea. Americans stand out from the people of other developed nations in the strength of their religious belief and observance, an island of religiosity in a sea of secularism. Yet the United States compares poorly on many social indicators, including life expectancy, crime, poverty and inequality. Other cultural factors appear to be countering religion's protective role, perhaps by changing the quality of religious and spiritual experience.

3.4.6. Public Perceptions of Quality of Life

Studies in the United States, Australia and elsewhere over the past decade reveal levels of public anger and anxiety about changes in society that were not apparent thirty years ago. They show cultural factors, including declining moral standards and excessive materialism, consumerism, and individualism, are among the dominant reasons many people feel quality of life is declining (Eckersley, 2005, 2006b). People are concerned about the greed and selfishness they believe drive today's society, underlie social ills, and threaten their children's future. They yearn for a better balance in their lives, believing that when it comes to individual freedom and material abundance, people don't seem "to know where to stop" or now have "too much of a good thing."

3.4.7. People's Views of the Future of Society and the World

Futures studies across many countries consistently reveal, in people's expected futures, concerns about the pace and pressure of modern life, loss of community, too much consumerism, and destruction of the natural environment (Eckersley, 2005; Hicks, 2006). Their preferred futures (perhaps reflecting humanity's evolutionary and historical origins) emphasize close-knit communities, more conviviality and intimacy, human-scale settlements and technologies, and a clean, healthy environment.

While people's perceptions of quality of life and the future confirm concerns about the health effect of cultural patterns and trends, these visions of the world are themselves cultural constructs with implications for health (acting via the psychosocial, behavioral and physiological pathways already discussed). Psychological research suggests that being adaptable, being able to set goals and progress towards them, having goals that do not conflict, and viewing the world as essentially benevolent and controllable are all associated with well-being (Eckersley, 2005). Biomedical research has shown that people become more stressed and more vulnerable to stress-related illness if they feel they have little control over the causes of stress, don't know how long the source of stress will last or how intense it will be, interpret the stress as evidence that circumstances are worsening, and lack social support for the duress the stress causes (Sapolsky, 2005). Negative views of quality of life and the future of the world and humanity are likely to impact on several of these subjective states, most obviously by encouraging perceptions of the world as hostile and dangerous and of conditions as deteriorating.

As the streams of evidence indicate, culture's impacts are most obvious with psychological well-being. Cultural influences on physical health are likely to be hard to disentangle from the many other social and personal factors involved, as we have already learned with other distal determinants such as income inequality. These factors include health care; in attempting to measure the health effects of social and cultural determinants, we must take into account the growing role of biomedical advances. Though they are extending life, in doing so, they may be masking the health effects of the changes in the social conditions in which people live.

Nevertheless, the evidence linking culture to physical health is persuasive. Health authorities now accept that that there is strong and consistent evidence for a causal association between depression, social isolation and lack of social support, and heart disease (Eckersley, 2006a). Mortality among people who are socially isolated is two to five times higher than for those with strong ties to family, friends and community (Berkman & Glass, 2000). Cultural factors, notably consumerism, are also implicated in adverse social trends, such as growing obesity, which, in turn, is linked to physical health problems, including heart disease, diabetes and cancer (Eckersley, 2001b).

4. Conclusion

This chapter has argued that the cultures of societies are underestimated determinants of population health, and cultural factors can act on health through both specific effects and through more diffuse influences on ways of thinking and living. The chapter has also discussed different disciplinary perspectives on culture and proposed that transdisciplinary synthesis provides one powerful means to improve our understanding of how culture affects health. Drawing on psychosocial theories of health, the chapter suggested that cultural factors are linked, via psychosocial pathways, to psychological well-being, and well-being, through behavioral and physiological pathways, to physical health. Finally, it described a range of different types of evidence relating to culture and health.

The complex and subjective nature of the role of mainstream cultural factors in health makes them hard to study. There may be limits to what we can learn about these impacts, especially concerning clear proof of causation. However, the research is still useful and worth undertaking in order to further understanding of the fundamental drivers of population health.

The application of this research to improving population health is correspondingly diverse and likely cannot be accomplished primarily through specific public health policies, programs and practices. As with the more tangible matters such as smoking (or female genital mutilation, as we saw), there is probably a role for public education campaigns to inform people about the health effects of various cultural attitudes, values and practices. However, the most important application of research into culture as a determinant of health may be in the contribution it can make to a much broader political and public debate about the lives people want to lead, the societies they want to live in, and the futures they want to create. It is a forum in which science cannot claim supreme authority in the search for answers, but one in which it will jostle and mingle with other ways of knowing as people seek to improve their lives.

Science often struggles with those aspects of life that are subtle, intangible, tenuous, abstract, and subjective. Yet, these aspects make up a big part of the human condition. There is an enormous gap between what science describes and what people experience, between the mechanisms of life and what it is to be alive (Birch, 1999). Understanding population health will only be possible through a proper connection between the objective and subjective, between the outer world and the inner experience.

It may well be that science will never give us clear-cut and objective recipes for making life better. Nevertheless, it is contributing to a growing willingness to question and discuss what makes a good life. This may be a radical view in science, but it is preferable that we obtain imperfect knowledge about the important issues of the times than precise answers to what are, in the overall scheme of things, trivial questions.

References

Bammer, G. (2005). Integration and implementation sciences: Building a new specialization. *Ecology and Society, 10*(2), 6–36.

Bauman, Z. (1995). *Life in fragments: Essays in postmodern morality.* Oxford: Blackwell.

Bauman, Z. (2002). Individually, together. In U. Beck & E. Beck-Gernsheim (Eds.), *Individualization: Institutionalized individualism and its social and political consequences.* London: Sage.

Beck, U., & Beck-Gernsheim, E. (2002). *Individualization: Institutionalized individualism and its social and political consequences.* London: Sage.

Berkman, L. F., & Glass, T. (2000). Social integration, social network, social support, and health. In L. F. Berkman & I. Kawachi (Eds.), *Social epidemiology.* New York: Oxford University Press.

Birch, C. (1999). *Biology and the riddle of life.* Sydney: UNSW Press.

Boyden, S. (2004). *The Biology of civilisation: Understanding human culture as a force in nature.* Sydney: UNSW Press.

Brightman, R. (1995). Forget culture: Replacement, transcendence, relexification. *Cultural Anthropology, 10,* 509–546.

Collishaw, S., Maughan, B., Goodman, R., & Pickles, A. (2004). Time trends in adolescent mental health. *Journal of Child Psychology and Psychiatry, 45,* 1350–1362.

Corin, E. (1994). The social and cultural matrix of health and disease. In R. G. Evans, M. Barer, & T. R. Marmor (Eds.), *Why are some people healthy and others not? The determinants of health of populations.* New York: Aldine de Gruyter.

Corin, E. (1995). The cultural frame: Context and meaning in the construction of health. In B. C. Amick, S. Levine, A. R. Tarlov, & D. Chapman Walsh (Eds.), *Society and health.* New York: Oxford University Press.

Costanza, R. (2003). A vision of the future of science: Reintegrating the study of humans and the rest of nature. *Futures, 35,* 651–671.

DiGiacomo, S. M. (1999). Can there be a "cultural epidemiology"? *Medical Anthropology Quarterly, 13,* 436–457.

Dressler, W. W. (2004). Culture and the risk of disease. *British Medical Bulletin, 69,* 21–31.

Dressler, W. W. (2006). Commentary: Taking culture seriously in health research. *International Journal of Epidemiology, 35,* 258–259.

Duberstein, P. R., Conwell, Y., Conner, K. R., Eberly, S., Evinger, J. S., & Caine, E. D. (2004). Poor social integration and suicide: Fact or artifact? A case-control study. *Psychological Medicine, 34,* 1331–1337.

Durkheim, E. (1970). *Suicide: A study in sociology.* London: Routledge and Kegan Paul.

Eckersley, R. (2001a). Culture, health and well-being. In R. Eckersley, J. Dixon, & B. Douglas (Eds.), *The social origins of health and well-being.* Cambridge: Cambridge University Press.

Eckersley, R. (2001b). Losing the battle of the bulge: Causes and consequences of increasing obesity. *Medical Journal of Australia, 174,* 590–592.

Eckersley, R. (2005). *Well & good: Morality, meaning and happiness.* 2nd edition. Melbourne: Text Publishing.

Eckersley, R. (2006a). Is modern Western culture a health hazard? *International Journal of Epidemiology, 35,* 252–258.

Eckersley, R. (2006b). Author's response: Culture can be studied at both large and small scales. *International Journal of Epidemiology, 35,* 263–265.

Eckersley, R. (in press, 2007). Culture, spirituality, religion and health: Looking at the big picture. *Medical Journal of Australia.*

Eckersley, R., & Dear, K. (2002). Cultural correlates of youth suicide. *Social Science & Medicine, 55,* 1891–1904.

Eckersley, R., Wierenga, A., & Wyn, J. (2006). Flashpoints and signposts: Pathways to success and wellbeing for Australia's young people. Canberra and Melbourne: Australia 21 Ltd, Australian Youth Research Centre, and VicHealth.

Eke, N., & Nkanginieme, K. E. O. (2006). Female genital mutilation and obstetric outcome. *Lancet, 367,* 1799–1800.

Elliott, A. (1996). *Subject to ourselves: Social theory, psychoanalysis and postmodernity.* Cambridge: Polity Press.

Fernquist, R. M., & Cutright, P. (1998). Societal integration and age-standardized suicide rates in 21 developed countries, 1955–1989. *Social Science Research, 27,* 109–127.

Glass, T. A. (2006). Commentary: Culture in epidemiology – The 800 pound gorilla? *International Journal of Epidemiology, 35,* 259–261.

Hicks, D. W. (2006). *Lessons for the future: The missing dimension in education.* Victoria, BC: Trafford Publishing.

Higginbotham, N., Albrecht, G., & Conner, L. (2001). Health social science: a transdisciplinary perspective. Melbourne: Oxford University Press.

Janes, C. R. (2006). Commentary: "Culture", cultural explanations and causality. *International Journal of Epidemiology, 35,* 261–263.

Kasser, T. (2002). *The high price of materialism.* Cambridge, MA: MIT Press.

Kroeber, A.L., & Kluckhohn, C. (1952). Culture: a critical review of concepts and definition. Peabody Museum Papers 47, Cambridge, MA: Harvard University Press.

Luthar, S. S. (2003). The culture of affluence: Psychological costs of material wealth. *Child Development, 74,* 1581–1593.

Luther, S. S., & Latendresse, S. J. (2005). Children of the affluent: Challenges to wellbeing. *Current Directions in Psychological Science, 14,* 49–53.

Marmot, M., & Wilkinson, R. G. (2001). Psychosocial and material pathways in the relation between income and health: A response to Lynch et al. *British Medical Journal, 322,* 1233–1236.

Mestrovic, S. (1985). A sociological conceptualisation of trauma. *Social Science & Medicine, 21,* 835–848.

Mestrovic, S., & Glassner, B. A. (1983). A Durkheimian hypothesis on stress. *Social Science & Medicine, 17,* 1315–1327.

Myers, D. G. (2001). *The American paradox: Spiritual hunger in an age of plenty.* New Haven: Yale University Press.

Oyserman, D., Coon, H. M., & Kemmelmeier, M. (2002). Rethinking individualism and collectivism: Evaluation of theoretical assumptions and meta-analyses. *Psychological Bulletin, 128,* 3–72.

Rosenfield, P. (1992). The potential of transdisciplinary research for sustaining and extending linkages between the health and social sciences. *Social Science & Medicine, 35,* 1343–1357.

Rutter, M., & Smith, D. J. (Eds.) (1995). *Psychosocial disorders in young people: Time trends and their causes.* Chichester: John Wiley and Sons for Academia Europaea.

Sapolsky, R. (2005). Sick of poverty. *Scientific American, 293*(6), 92–99.

Triandis, H. C., & Suh, E. M. (2002). Cultural influences on personality. *Annual Review of Psychology, 53,* 133–160.

Twenge, J. M. (2006). *Generation me: Why today's young Americans are more confident, assertive, entitled – and more miserable than ever before.* New York: Free Press.

Whitely, E., Gunnell, D., Dorling, D., & Davey Smith, G. (1999). Ecological study of social fragmentation, poverty, and suicide. *British Medical Journal, 319,* 1034–1037.

World Health Organization Study Group on Female Genital Mutilation and Obstetric Outcome, Banks, E., Meirik, O., Farley, T., Akande, O., Bathija, H., et al. (2006). Female genital mutilation and obstetric outcome: WHO collaborative prospective study in six African countries. *Lancet, 367,* 1835–1841.

Chapter 10
Taxation and Population Health: "Sin Taxes" or Structured Approaches

Martin Caraher and Roy Carr-Hill

1. Introduction

Taxes traditionally fulfill three functions. Taxes raise revenues for public services and welfare programs, they redistribute income from the rich to the poor, and they can be used to modify people's behavior. Some economists would argue that any goods or activities that impose externalities or costs on others should be taxed for the public good. There is also no such thing as zero taxation; there is always some transfer of resources. Even in societies where there is a little or no infrastructure, there are taxes for the good of the community; these can often be in the form of tithes to the chief of the village or the setting aside of a proportion of goods or food for the "hungry season." Economists would classify these as public goods, meaning the goods or services offered have benefits beyond the individual level.

On the one hand, even when it has been used for the public good or to develop public services, taxation has often proved to be unpopular. For instance, Galbraith (1958) quoted the unpopularity of salt tax in France, and E.P. Thompson (1993), in his review of the "moral economy" of the English crowd in the 18th century, noted that food taxes often resulted in riots and were a flash point for the anger of the populace. On the other hand, taxation can be a means of developing community cohesion by providing a community safety net and by acting as a form of social coherence or control. The introduction of national insurance by the Prussian Chancellor Bismarck was seen as a means of knitting together otherwise disparate Prussian principalities. Post Second World War governments in Europe adopted taxation policies to help rebuild damaged economies and create welfare systems that offered a safety net for those less well off; the French system of "solidarité sociale" for social insurance was conceived as a way of healing the ruptures caused by the Second World War (Chamberlayne, 1992). Still, the recent emphasis on economic globalization has resulted in objections to taxation being voiced by the proponents of neo-liberal economic policies and those who represent the interests of trans-national corporations (TNCs). The basis for these objections is that taxation is an unnecessary barrier to trade and to the creation of wealth that would "trickle down" from rich to poor absent taxation.

Currently a large percentage of taxation revenue is spent on armaments and security (risk security) as compared to public health services or welfare programs (risk prevention). According to Oxfam (2006) and the United Nations Development Program (2005), thirty-six countries spend more on military hardware than on health and education.

However, realigning tax revenues to risk prevention and education would benefit population health status both nationally and globally. In public health terms, spending taxation revenues on risk security takes a limited perspective on national security because it ignores the benefits that come from a stable and cohesive society. This chapter explores the current trends in taxation for public health practice; it is not an exposition of tax laws and structures. We come from backgrounds in exploring taxes as influences on food choice and wider public health issues and using weighted formulas to address inequalities in health care funding and working in the poorer developing countries. We see in policy terms the issues being split between up-stream (macrosocial) and downstream (microsocial) discourses. We set out a case for the use of taxation for public health practice and explore its impact on macrosocial determinants in both direct and indirect ways. We are not suggesting that taxation can solve all the problems in modern societies but that it can be part of the public health approach. Combined with other approaches, such as primary care services, education, and legislation, taxation can contribute to health enhancement in a population alongside a host of other measures, such as promoting fairer trade, tackling corruption, cutting debt, and implementing health promotion and social marketing. We also note that taxation in low-income countries can best be used to fund developmental programs and public health services but, with existing international distributions and expectations of income and wealth, cannot be used to adequately address disparities in income levels, due to the large numbers of poor and overall low-income levels, quite simply there is not enough wealth to distribute (Beblavy & Mizsei, 2006; Oxfam, 2006).

The chapter is set out under four main headings. We start by examining taxation as a public health tool in terms of income redistribution and behavior change. The next Section (3) looks at how taxation revenues have been used to fund welfare systems. Global taxation and its importance in a globalizing world are set out in Section 4, and Section 5 focuses on current developments in taxation. Finally, we conclude with some recommendations on how public health might usefully conceive of and lobby for taxation as a major influence on macrosocial determinants of health.

2. Taxation as A Public Health Tool

Taxation policy can have an important influence on health status and behavior. In the long run, upstream taxation policy interventions are nearly always more effective than downstream ones. Downstream approaches tend to be short-term in focus and based on microsocial influences, but upstream interventions can be built into macrosocial structures and have a population effect. As noted above, there are three possible uses of tax: to raise revenues for public services and welfare programs, to redistribute income from the rich to the poor, and to modify people's behavior. The latter two are explored in this section, while the case for taxation to fund public services is considered in Section 3.

2.1. Direct and Indirect Taxes

Taxes can be direct or indirect. Direct taxes, such as income tax, tend to be progressive in that they take a larger proportion of income from the richest. Indirect taxes on items such as food and services are generally regressive in that they affect the poor to a greater degree. Indirect taxes, if used appropriately (i.e., targeted, sufficient taxes on goods to en/discourage behaviors), can be important in shifting behaviors at a group or population level. However, taxes on some goods and services may further disadvantage the poor and force them further into poverty. For instance, taxes on foods may impose barriers to healthy eating ; food is an elastic item in the household budget, so people may attempt to save money by buying cheaper and possibly unhealthy foods and divert spending to other necessities (Caraher & Cowburn, 2005; Dowler, Turner, & Dobson, 2001).

2.2. Redistributing Income

In *The Affluent Society*, Galbraith (1958) identified tensions between production and higher taxes as barriers to influencing income (re)distribution and reducing inequality. Galbraith's emphasis is on systems of regulation that focus on lowering rules for employment, privatization of previously public services and regulation as a barrier to economic growth (Deacon, Ollila, Koivusalo, & Stubbs, 2003; Lee, 2003; Lee, Buse, & Fustukian, 2002). Such developments run the risk of revenues (which might previously have been collected in the form of taxes) moving out of low and middle-income countries to middle and high-income ones and increasing the growth of inequalities both within and between countries.

This has become more problematic with the spread and pace of globalization and its application to national governments if they wish to join the global market (we deal with this in more detail in a later section on the global economy). At a global governance level, through agencies such as the International Monetary Fund and TNCs, the neo-liberal economic approach dominates. This approach is driven by the principle that wealth is created through trade and that taxes are an unnecessary barrier to trade and, therefore, wealth (Sachs, 2005). Developments such as Trade Related Intellectual Property Rights (TRIPS) and the General Agreement on Trade and Tariffs (GATT) argue for the removal of barriers to trade, including traditional access to welfare and contributions by employers to such schemes (Caraher & Coveney, 2004; Deacon et al., 2003; Lee, 2003; Lee et al., 2002; Ollila, 2003).

In contrast, the current consensus among developing countries and aid agencies (including many officials of the World Bank) holds that equity and influences on marcosocial factors are more likely to be achieved through state action, including spending from the public purse (Pieterse, 1998; Oxfam, 2006). More specifically, economists such as Hertz (2001) and de Soto (2000) argue that the neo-liberal economic model does not fit all countries as it assumes a trickle down of wealth in the free market economy as opposed to state determined and controlled redistribution of income or wealth.

2.2.1. The Evidence for Distributive Effects of Tax

In the UK, the Black Report and the Health Divide (Townsend, Davidson & Whitehead, 1988) argued that lifestyle factors such as unhealthy diets, smoking, and exercise levels are in fact symptoms of relative poverty/socio-economic position. This raises questions, especially in the long-term, as to the extent to tax/subside these "symptoms" or to focus upstream on poverty. The UK Independent Inquiry into Health Inequalities (Acheson, 1998) had a major recommendation on relative poverty, income tax and benefits, with specific sub-recommendations for women of childbearing age and pensioners.

The fact that income inequalities vary from one society to another suggests they can be influenced by interventions. Stewart-Brown (2000) proposes that the solution lies in making the rich less rich in order to reduce the inequality gap between the rich and the poor and thus make an impact at a population level (see also Carr-Hill, 1987). Stewart-Brown's argument is based on the principle that raising the income levels of the poor does not address the inequality gap as the rich become richer and the gap continues to grow. Such an approach locates the differences in inequality at a macrosocial level and considers inequity as the responsibility of all. Though such action may improve public health, it is not a policy that many governments would adopt.

The issue of child poverty has been tackled in different ways in developed countries. For example, Sweden compared to the UK has higher child poverty rates before redistribution of resources raised through taxation but less than half the rate after redistribution (Hirsch, 2006). Though raising children out of poverty has become a key plank of UK government policy, the focus has been on using tax receipts to fund welfare reforms, which focus on back-to-work for families with children.

This welfare to work approach is purportedly geared towards long-term sustainability of addressing persistent poverty. However, it is fundamentally flawed as full (meaningful) employment is neither environmentally sustainable nor welfare enhancing (Carr-Hill & Lintott, 2003). There is, of course, little dispute that economic growth has substantially increased pollution environmental degredation, but there is an increasing literature showing consistent decline in welfare in so-called developed countries since the mid 1960s linked to full employment (Carr-Hill & Lintott, 2003). The Index of Sustainable Economic Welfare (ISEW) is intended to "correct" GNP for social and environmental costs (Daly & Cobb, 1990). A relatively recent attempt to estimate ISEW for the UK showed a steady decline since 1970 (Jackson & Marks, 1994, 1999). Estimates of the ISEW for other countries have yielded similar results (Cobb & Cobb, 1994). History suggests that without improvements in welfare, populations will eventually object and use either conflict or the ballot box to remove governments with unpopular policies.

Moreover, many welfare to work approaches are based on a model of working parents and do not address the work and contributions of those parents who might choose not to return to work but to look after their children. A report from the Rowntree Foundation (Hirsch, 2006) puts the cost of halving childhood poverty in the UK by 2010 at UK£4 billion and a further UK£28 billion over the ensuing decade to reduce it to 5 percent. This is based on minimum incomes (usually defined as 60 percent of median income) and ignores the growing divide between the rich and the poor, whereby as the rich become richer the poor become poorer, although this only becomes important when comparing between countries and regions. According to work by Wilkinson and Marmot, this relative gap becomes important and an issue for health status, in high-income or developed economies (Marmot, 1999, 2001, 2005; Marmot & Wilkinson 2006; Wilkinson, 2005). However, as Carr-Hill (1987, 1990) has shown, this could simply be because for the same average income but a wider range of incomes, there are more people who are *really* poor (see also Scanlan, 2006). More formally, Gravelle (1998) demonstrates that the supposed link between inequalities in income and population mortality could easily be an artifact of the curvilinear relationship between income and health. Approaches to taxation need to be structured and progressive in order to redistribute income in a way that narrows the inequality gap and therefore reduces the numbers of very poor.

2.2.2. Progressive Taxation

Progressive taxation is being pursued as a more efficient way of redistributing income through taxation via tax benefits or credits (as in Canada, Australia and the UK), where the taxation system itself is the focus for the redistribution of benefits as opposed to redistributing taxes through benefits and grants (Howard, 2004; Whiteford, Mendelson, & Millar, 2003). Such approaches may break the link between specific benefits and spending, for example, food benefits now become part of the general package so that money need not be spent on food as other priorities squeeze. The basis behind such moves rests on the assumption that benefits tied to specific goods or services are restrictive and limit personal choice. Nevertheless the impact of tax benefits or credits may be marginal in terms of tackling inequity. For example, in Canada, as specific welfare food benefits disappear in favor of tax credits, income inequality has increased, and the use of food banks supported by the philanthropy of the private sector have begun to replace the state as major distributors of food welfare (Canadian Association of Food Banks, 2003; Riches, 2002).

Another approach used in some welfare systems is to combine progressive taxation with a universal entitlement to benefits in order to effect change at a macrosocial level. The application of a universal benefit may make it popular among all income groups and thus ensure popular support and prevent stigma. If it can ensure that the poor gain most, then it is progressive in having an impact where it matters most. Progressive benefits work in the opposite way to taxation in that they redistribute more of the collected revenues to the poor.

2.3. Indirect Taxes – Taxing Behavior or "The Price of Sin"

"Sin taxes" are indirect taxes usually applied to goods considered to be unhealthy, such as tobacco or foods high in fat ("fat taxes"), salt or sugar, and are under discussion in a number of countries (Caraher & Cowburn, 2005). Public health practitioners and economists use methodologies based on linear mathematical models to predict the outcomes of such taxes but often fail to consider the importance of the attitudes of individuals and populations to the specific behavior or item. For example, we know that consumers have embraced messages such as eating five or more fruit and vegetable portions a day while at the same time applying a different logic to "treat" foods, such as chocolate, which may balance out or even contradict to attitudes to eating fruit. It becomes apparent that taxes on goods and services do not influence health behavior in a linear fashion and that we need to balance a tax or negative association approach with one that uses taxes to subsidize healthy options (Caraher & Cowburn, 2005).

Marshall (2000) claimed that the imposition of a fiscal food tax could help prevent 1000 deaths a year in the UK, but Kennedy and Offutt (2000) debated the effect of such a tax on food choice and focused on the negative impact that such taxes have on the poor. Leicester and Windmeijer (2004) modeled the impact of a fat tax on nutrients purchased as well as the financial implications. Across all income groups, the amount of nutrients purchased would change little between those with high-income and those with low-income because the amount of fat, sodium and cholesterol consumed does not vary much between the different income groups. However, they also found that the impact of an average "fat tax" across the income quintiles would result in the very poorest 2 percent of the population spending 0.7 percent of their total income on the fat tax, while those in the middle-income brackets would pay around 0.25 percent of their total income, and the richest would pay less than 0.1 percent of their income. They concluded, "[T]he very poorest perhaps consume slightly less fat and cholesterol, but they also have particularly low-incomes such that even a small tax would constitute a fairly high average tax rate."

The principle of such a tax is often based on discouraging potentially negative behaviors without any corresponding promotion or subsidy of desired healthy ones. Further, the focus of indirect taxes and subsidies is often on the symptoms as opposed to the causes of such a relationship. We know that low-income equates with poor nutrition and that increasing income results in an improvement in nutrition status up to a certain tipping point; for example, there is evidence of a relationship between income levels and fruit consumption, albeit an indirect one (Pomperleau, Lock, Knai, & McKee, 2005). Food poverty/security may be a symptom of income inequality, and indirect taxes may not influence the primary determinant.

In the long-term, the real issue is one of income maintenance and the reduction of absolute poverty. This can only be achieved by equalizing incomes (or access to resources) in a context of eco-friendly consumption, economic stability and environmental sustainability (Barling, Lang, & Caraher, 2001; Carr-Hill & Lintott, 2003). Proposals to break the cycle of poverty through full employment (Diderichsen, 2002) are not environmentally sustainable because they require ever increasing use of energy, and not desirable because full employment would require reliance on employment that is undesirable to most and does not generate welfare (Carr-Hill & Lintott, 2003; Hirsch, 1977).

2.3.1. What are the Purposes of a Taxation Policy on Goods?

Broadly, taxes on goods can be applied in two ways. First, taxes on goods can influence behavior by encouraging healthy or discouraging unhealthy consumer choices. In reality, a combination of taxes to discourage specific behaviors and subsidies to encourage desired behaviors is required to effect change. Second, a less frequently used approach involves targeting changes at a structural level, as in a tax on growers and manufacturers, to influence the growing and production of certain goods (e.g., fruit and vegetables) or to discourage the production of others (e.g., tobacco). There are few examples of taxation at a structural level. Perhaps the most obvious is smoking in both the developed and developing worlds (Jha & Chaloupka, 2000). Revenues from taxation on cigarettes is used as a subsidy to help shift agricultural policies away from growing tobacco to alternative cash crops and help open up markets.

Both of these approaches act to influence behavior at different levels; the latter upstream at the level of production and the former downstream at that of individual choice. Governments do use taxation at the structural level to subsidize agricultural production but put little emphasis on health impacts. In fact, the subsidies often encourage the production of unhealthy or at least unwanted food and goods, such as the case with the Common Agricultural Policy of the European Union or the US approach to agricultural subsidies (Dahlgren, Nordgren, & Whitehead, 1997; Lock & McKee, 2005; Nestle, 2002).

In practical terms, taxes on goods are not usually set at a sufficiently high level to discourage behavioral choice, while subsidies even at quite a low level can encourage "better" behavior. The neo-liberal market economy favors the application of choice, and taxes on goods or services are seen as barriers to such choice. Governments often adopt a middle ground, introducing taxes high enough to make it clear that something is being done but not high enough to discourage behavior. This has led to a compromise with hypothecated revenues from taxes on goods or services being used to fund health promotion or social marketing campaigns. In the arena of food there are numerous examples of such policies at regional or state levels (Caraher & Cowburn, 2005).

2.4. Smoking, Food and Alcohol

It is worth asking why taxes on smoking have been partially successful and other areas, such as alcohol and unhealthy food, less successful. Successes in the US, Australia and Ireland on smoking have resulted from a complex interaction of factors, chief among which are the growing evidence of the addictive nature of cigarette smoking and the health impacts of tobacco, the effects of passive smoking on children and workers, the success of public health advocacy, which alerts and gains the support of the public by basing the messages on more social as opposed to health agendas, and the fact that it has become harder to argue for smoking as either a right or entitlement (see Gilmore, 2005). Alcohol often draws attention and there are indications that the economic costs of alcohol can be as great as that of tobacco, taxes on alcohol have not had the same impact as taxes on tobacco (Cave & Godfrey, 2005). The costs of poor nutrition, obesity and low physical activity for Europe are also higher than those due to smoking (World Health Organization, 2000). Analysis suggests strategies to promote healthy eating and dietary change are among the most cost-effective methods of preventing cardiovascular disease (Brunner, Cohen, & Toon, 2001). Yet, because food occupies the realms of both necessity and luxury, agreements over taxation are harder to reach.

Taxing goods and services to influence behaviors should be approached with caution. As the price people are willing to pay for a good depends on its significance in their life, whether addictive or habitual, the role and social significance of a good/service in everyday life should be included as part of the equation. In other words, social costs, not just economic and financial costs, must be factored in. It is easier to influence attitudes when people do not feel personally involved and to reinforce behaviors that already exist. For example, it is easier to convince those who already eat fruit to expand their range of fruit intake than to persuade those who do not eat fruit to begin. Taxing treat foods such as chocolate is rarely successful, as consumers regard these goods as a luxury and therefore feel personally involved with them (Caraher & Landon, 2006). There are examples, particularly at a sub-regional levels and in specific settings (such as schools), of taxation on certain foods (carbonated and sugared beverages) being applied (see Caraher & Cowburn, 2005, for examples of selective taxation approaches; see Popkin, Armstrong, Bray, Caballero, Frei, & Willett, 2006, for a discussion of carbonated beverages).

As the market economy becomes more globalized, TNCs resist the imposition of indirect taxes on consumer goods such as food and alcohol. Even when taxes are levied on goods as in sales taxes like the value added tax (VAT) or a general service tax (GST), the mechanisms are so convoluted that their use as an influence on health behavior at a macrosocial level is unclear (see Caraher & Cowburn, 2005, for some examples). Indirect taxes are generally regressive; the tax burden is the same for all, but the poor end up spending a greater percentage of their incomes on necessities such as food and housing.

3. Taxation, Welfare, and Principles of Operation – From Public to Private Goods

In this section we set out a discussion of the underlying principles of goods and services as in public/private utilities, rights/entitlements and hidden and externalized costs. Taxation is seen as a means of providing welfare or public systems where services and systems could not be effectively provided by the family and community (e.g., schooling), of filling in gaps in family and community provision and/or support, and of encouraging existing family or community behaviors, as in the area of child rearing, through child benefits.

It has become fashionable to regard taxation and public services as barriers to growth and development. Believers argue that taxation disincentivizes individuals to work hard and that public services funded from taxation prevent the private sector from offering cheaper and more efficient services. Oxfam (2006) offers another perspective: For developing countries (low- and middle-income), raising and investing taxation revenues in essential services is key to growth. Such approaches are in fact a contribution to the overall wealth of a country, as infant and childhood mortality are cut, and a healthy workforce is more likely to lead to reductions in inequality within a country or region.

On a global level, the Millennium Development Goals on health, education, water and sanitation require an extra US$47 billion a year; this compares with US$4 billion spent on pet food and US$1 trillion on armaments Taxation revenues used to fund public services such as education or health may in fact save people money as compared with tax cuts to buy these services in the private sector. Countries with rising high-growth, such as China and India, are at the forefront of the process of introducing neo-liberal reform to their economies, but progress in reducing child-hood mortality has slowed. For example, in China in recent years there have been moves to phase out free health care and replace it with health insurance and for-profit hospitals. This has resulted in household health expense increases of forty percent, with detrimental impacts on other spending, such as food, as well . Overall, progress in tackling infant mortality has slowed (French, 2006; Oxfam, 2006). In contrast, countries such as Vietnam and Bangladesh, which have lower incomes but continue to invest tax revenue in public services, are more successful in lowering their child-hood mortality rates (United Nations Development Program, 2005).

3.1. Welfare Systems and Public Services

Revenues from taxation are traditionally directed toward welfare systems and public services, divided generally between insurance based systems (Bismarckian) and universal provision (Beveridge). Within these broad categories are a range of operating philosophies, from conservative welfare (where the system upholds the *status quo*), through liberal welfare (an emphasis on market based social insurance), to social democratic regimes (where the focus is on universalism and equity) (Cochrane & Clarke, 1997). In many systems, public health services are universal as there are many threats to public health beyond individual risk. For example, achieving maximum immunization coverage is seen as a public good that justifies funding from the public purse. The Beveridge vision in the UK involved tackling the five great giants of want, disease, ignorance, squalor and idleness though the British Welfare State, funded mainly through general taxation (Timmins, 1995).

The philosophy favored may influence the ways in which welfare is managed and taxation revenues spent. Within conservative welfare schemes, benefit levels may be set be set below minimum wage levels in order to encourage work and tax money allocated to education viewed as a contribution to the economy. In contrast, in a system informed by social democratic principles, benefit levels may be set at a level to enable people to partake in the norms of that society and education viewed as a right with additional benefits, especially for women. Within either system, some benefits are means-tested, where those falling below a threshold are entitled to help in the form of loans or grants rather than benefits (Cochrane & Clarke, 1997; Diderichsen, 2002).

3.2. Public and Private Utilities and Goods

Economists use the terms public goods and private goods to distinguish between goods that are purely private affairs and subject to market demands and those that have a wider community benefit. In reality many goods cross the boundary between private and public and may do so for different groups in society; the relative position of the boundary may affect different sets of goods. The concept of a "Public Good for Health" (PGfH) has relatively new application in the health arena and draws on the older notion of "Public Goods" (PGs) (Kaul, Grunberg, & Stern, 1999). The assumption behind a public good is that human well-being requires both public and private goods. Public goods have in the past tended to be outside the market and heavily regulated. They are goods that are accessible to the public and have universal value, even if they are privately owned in whole or in part. Public goods should be non-rivalrous – everyone must be able to benefit from the good once it has been produced – and non-exclusive – none can be excluded from accessing them (Sandler, 1992). Public goods in the global economy can cross countries, people and generations and include the environment and publicly owned infrastructures, such as schools and hospitals.

Increasingly, public utilities such as water, sewerage and electricity are now subject to market forces, and progressively more have become private utilities (Coles & Wallace, 2005; Human Development Report, 2005; Water Aid, 2005). Even where there is extensive regulation of private activity in public utilities, this is increasingly being challenged and subjugated to private rights and the right of private enterprise to locate the issues within a consumer – as opposed to a citizenship -framework.

International agreements have relegated the common good to one dominated by market principles so that the "free market" and the lowering of tax burdens are guiding principles instead of the public utility of goods or services (Sen, 1997). This is despite the fact that aid agencies such as the World Bank and Department for International Development (DFID), whose funding of course depends on taxation, now put poverty alleviation as their principal aim. Indeed, many of the proposed global trade controls, such as those emerging from the Doha round, are collapsing under both the inability of the developed world to agree on a way forward and the opposition from the developing world/aid agencies and non-governmental lobbies. TNCs, often larger in financial terms than nation states, argue for lower levels of corporate tax (de Soto, 2000; Soros, 1998), while nation states are – at least to some limited extent – trying to protect their citizens' health. The TNCs are responding by including more and more corporate social responsibility programs in their portfolios, whether in terms of fair trade or ecological approaches; however, they do so in ways that help increase their turnover and, therefore, their eventual potential for extracting surplus value from the poor.

There is a move from an era where taxation (whether direct or indirect) was used to fund public utilities to one where the indirect taxation is the focus of market reforms. In the past there was a concern with contagion and infectious diseases, albeit with a certain selfishness or recognition of self interest, in that using public words to prevent disease spread was seen as beneficial. This is perhaps not different from today where the containment and treatment of diseases – whether the rise in diet related non-communicable diseases) or the treatment of HIV infection in the developing world – are as influenced by the realization that poor population health is a detriment to the presumed never-ending economic growth as by a sense of injustice. Improving population health is seen as a contribution to growth in both social and economic terms (Mackenbach, Bakker, Sihto, & Diderichsen, 2002; Oxfam 2006). Indeed, the Global Fund to fight AIDS, Tuberculosis, and Malaria is aimed at controlling those conditions that are likely to affect the economically active population and, therefore, the global capacity to care and sustain children and older people (see Department for International Development (DFID), 2006).

3.3. Entitlements and Rights

Welfare systems and access to them are dictated by the entitlement that one has to them. We have seen shifts from the use of direct taxation for public health commensurate with the privatization of public goods. This has altered the emphasis from one of public rights to one based on benevolence, leading to what Sen (1981; 1997) has called the "entitlement dilemma."

In many high- and middle-income countries, access to potable water is increasingly a feature of individual rights as opposed to a public (health) right. For example, Sen (1981) has argued that food shortages (famines) are rarely caused by lack of food but by the abilities and entitlements necessary to access that food; food shortages occur when a society allows some to go without. He asserts that it "is the characteristic of some people not having enough food to eat. It is not the characteristic of there not being enough food to eat."

This is an important distinction as, in the old global order, the nation state had a commitment to citizens to ensure entitlement however it was manifested (for instance in food welfare schemes or even philanthropy). Now in the development of economies there is a danger that social contracts based on the concept of citizenship are being replaced with market reforms and protective legislation designed to benefit consumers (see Alexander, 2005; Coles & Wallace, 2005; Water Aid, 2006). At an international level, there are a number of conventions and documents that state the right of a population to a healthy diet; among them are the Universal Declaration of Human Rights from 1948 and the 1989 Convention on the Rights of the Child. Few national governments have translated these statements into national laws or realized the right to a healthy diet as an entitlement. Only two countries, Brazil and South Africa, have placed the "right to food" in their constitutions. The South African Constitution contains three references to food and nutrition rights as well as requirements to legislate such rights. Fome Zero in Brazil is a national zero hunger policy and is institutionalized at both national and program policy levels.

The new global order owes no such allegiance to its customers. We believe a similar situation will arise where these new rights will define the ability to access potable water; the next series of global conflicts will be over water (Water Aid, 2005, 2006). The issue of entitlement also affects the use and distribution of taxation revenues; if a welfare system is based on the "greater good," then presumably there will be some distribution (and entitlement) to taxation revenues along these lines.

3.4. Hidden and External Costs

The epidemiologic transition that occurs as countries move from developing (low and middle-income) to developed (high-income) status comes with the commensurate problem of having to change existing public health and health care practice to partake in the global economy. The key requirements of globalization for those wishing to "join the club" are a lowering of trade barriers and meeting quality standards of the rich world. Allied to these is the lowering of tax burdens on both individuals and corporations in the belief that such taxes are barriers to economic growth. For decades, the neo-liberal economic perspective has promoted a view that health would gain from greater wealth, which in turn would be driven by trade liberalization, reduction and privatization of the state, and encouragement of private enterprise. The basic principle behind this is that wealth will trickle down, and thus, there will be less need for the welfare state. While many campaigns and organizations developed their expertise in relation to national governments and the rights of citizenship, the new world order of TNCs demands a new way of dealing with the issues. There is, however, a countervailing tendency in terms of the aid agency emphasis on "good governance," which has effectively taken up the anti-corruption campaigns of Transparency International (www.transparancy.org).

The problem is that the development of global governance comes with hidden costs, burdens at the national and individual level within nation states, which may be difficult to recognize and address. Lower rates of income tax come with associated but unaccounted for increases in health care costs and environmental degradation, with greater costs for low and middle-income countries (McMichael, 2001; Oxfam, 2006). For example, lowering taxes and grant subsidies to food growers and producers results in more production of food at cheaper prices. However, the food is often unhealthy and the production damages the environment through increased use of pesticides and food traveling greater distances (Griffiths, 2003). The developing world shoulders much of the burden, while the countries of the developed world have the advantage of cheap goods without the associated costs of over production and pollution (Pretty, et al., 2000).

On a global scale, since the development of the 1994 General Agreement on Tariffs and Trade (GATT), nation states have adopted the neo-liberal mindset that market rigors will yield improved food security by reducing protection and import tariffs (Hertz, 2001). This almost certainly means one or more of three things: first, that taxes are spent elsewhere as in cleaning up the effects of cheap food; second, that no extra taxes are imposed to account for this degradation, and/or third, the degradation of the environment is accepted as the price of growth. All of these are hidden externalities. The point is not that trade should be discouraged but that that such developments should work for the benefit of the poor and that these externalities should be factored into the equation.

4. A Question of Global Taxation for Public Health

At a global level the issue of taxation has not been seriously addressed as an area of public health concern. Whilst the amount of global aid is rising, funding from some national governments to the World Health Organization and some global programs are in doubt. Thus, despite the emphasis on the Millennium Development Goals, funding of some otherwise useful and effective programs have been influenced by political considerations, e.g., the provision of funds by US agencies to The International Planned Parenthood Federation. While endowments to fund global public health programs from private donors such as the Bill and Melinda Gates Foundation and Warren Buffet are welcome, they continue to treat the symptoms and not the root causes of health inequality. Such aid contributions and relief measures need to be balanced with others that tackle corruption and make trade work for the poor (DFID, 2006). Public services funded from taxation can also be major contributors to growth and economic development.

Further, though communicable diseases remain important in an increasingly interconnected world, it is often forgotten that globalization of the economy is now partially responsible for hastening the epidemiologic transition. Popkin (1998) has shown that small changes in the price of fats on the global market can have major implications for whole populations; in the case of China, a drop of the price of oils on the world market by one per cent resulted in a doubling of energy intake from fat (displacing carbohydrates) between 1952 and 1992, as well as an increase in the energy intake from animal protein in the same period. None of this is countered by subsidies for health foods at the point of sale; the major benefits are for producers and manufacturers of processed food products.

4.1. Foreign Direct Investment

Again, an example from the food sector shows the role of foreign direct investment in low- and middle-income countries: TNCs contribute to the nutrition transition by controlling the food manufacturing market and encouraging a move from traditional foods to low priced processed foods high in salt, fat and sugar (Hawkes, 2005). Such developments are encouraged by the lack of controls and taxation on such foreign investment and by global policies and national governments wanting to promote investment and therefore reluctant to tax foreign investors. Food can be produced in countries with low labor and overhead costs and then transported for many thousands of miles. Though production and shipping create external hidden costs as noted in Section 3.4., they do not contribute in real terms to these costs and food can be sold in the developed world at prices that would be impossible if the products were grown and manufactured there.

There has been growing consensus on "green taxes," which are levied to contribute to maintenance of the environment. Estonia has just introduced an eco-tax, whereby the Baltic state will reduce personal income tax and levy increasing taxes on polluting industries, fossil fuels and the use of non renewable natural resources over a ten year period (see www.eea.europa.eu for further details).

4.2. Financial Markets and Global Speculation

It is not just goods and services that are traded on the world market, but money flows based on speculation. TNCs account for 70 percent of world trade, much of which is untaxed and unregulated as it occurs outside of national boundaries. Financial speculation at a global level means that benefits do not accrue to communities, individuals or nation states.

Currency speculators trade over US$1.8 trillion dollars each day across national borders. Most of this is speculative and does not involve the movement of goods. James Tobin (1978), a Nobel laureate economist, was the first to propose a simple sales tax on currency trades across borders. Tobin Taxes could be enacted by national legislatures but require multilateral cooperation to be effectively enforced. Each trade would be taxed at 0.1 to 0.25 percent of volume (about 10 to 25 cents per one hundred US dollars). This would discourage frequent short-term currency trades, currently about 90 percent speculative, but leave long-term productive investments mostly unaffected. This would raise an estimated US$100–$300 billion per year and make it possible to meet urgent global health and environmental concerns, including disease and poverty. A side effect would be the strengthening of national economies and more money flows at this level (see www.ceedweb.org/iirp/factsheet.htm for more detail on Tobin taxes). The same principle can be applied to money flows for the raising of revenues to fund global public health programs.

4.3. Voluntary Taxation to Fight Global Poverty

If global taxes seem far-fetched, there are some examples of interim solutions, such as taxation on luxuries to fund disease and poverty work in Africa. What is unorthodox may become orthodox given advocacy and public concern. France has been campaigning for an international air tax to help fight global poverty, and this issue was raised at the World Economic Forum in Switzerland in January 2005. The airline industry opposed the tax, and another option of a tax on jet fuel was rejected. Equally, a number of countries, including the US, do not support the idea. Despite this, roughly a dozen countries have now agreed to the introduction of what is being called an "international solidarity contribution" to help fight AIDS, tuberculosis, and malaria in Africa. From small beginnings there may come major acceptance of taxation as an investment in and means to serve the public good.

5. Current Developments in Taxation and Public Health

Some debates focus on the approaches to influencing healthy behavior; for example, in the UK early drafts of a report referred to the use of taxation as a direct influence on lifestyle behaviors and the effect of monetary distributive policies (The Cabinet Office, 2004). However, the proposals were omitted from the final version (Halpern, Bates, Beales, & Heathfield, 2004) because of industry lobbying and the feeling among politicians that taxes to influence behavior would be unpopular.

This leads us to outline two dominant trends in taxation and public health policy that are symptoms of a move away from direct taxation. The first is to use taxation as an influence on issues of choice and availability by taxing certain goods or services. The second trend is to identify hypothecated revenues and use them for the funding of public health practice. This is apparent in the areas of smoking and alcohol prevention and, to a lesser extent, in the realm of food and nutrition.

The first option is employed as a direct influence on lifestyle choices and is most commonly used for substances that are deleterious to health, such as tobacco (Jha & Chaloupka, 2000). In the UK the government has explicitly rejected this approach in relation to alcohol harm reduction despite overwhelming evidence that it helps reduce alcohol consumption and related family violence and road accidents (Institute of Alcohol Studies, 2006). Similarly, even for those foodstuffs high in salt, fat and sugar, the application of taxes is disparate and inconsistent (Caraher, 2003; Caraher & Cowburn, 2005). They are often applied, in our experience, within sub-regional or closed contexts such as schools or workplaces, missing the opportunity to change behaviors at the macrosocial level.

The second option, using identified taxation revenues to fund public health and health promotion activities, is becoming increasingly popular. This is understandable as we are in a time of crisis in funding for health systems and public health, This option guarantees income, however small. In France the government has introduced legal measures to require health warnings on advertisements for high sugar and high salt foods. If advertisers do not cooperate with this measure, they must pay a 1.5 percent tax to finance health promotion activities (Caraher, Landon, & Dalmeny, 2006; EU Food Law, 2004). In a review of social marketing campaigns from the UK, similar proposals include running public health campaigns from hypothecated taxes or levies on specific goods or services such as advertising of foods (National Social Marketing Centre, 2006). In Thailand, early successes in the area of tobacco control have resulted in the TNCs fighting back and threatening the achievements of the anti-smoking coalition. This has led to the proposal for a "Health Promotion Act, which would challenge the tobacco industry with a hypothecated excise tax dedicated to health awareness campaigns" (Chantornvong & McCargo, 2001).

The three examples above avoid the use of tax as a direct influence on macrosocial influences, instead favoring a soft approach to fund health promotion or social marketing type programs. For some, this is a reflection of the political reality. Our is that hypothecated taxes for specific activities cannot hope to compete with the private sector in terms of their reach or spending. Social marketing or health promotion campaigns reliant on hypothecated tax revenues are a drop in the ocean compared to what the private sector has at its disposal. In addition, the taxation of goods such as cigarettes ensures revenues when spending is high; if these campaigns are successful, fewer hypothecated revenues are available, thus leading to a reduction in revenues available for public health work.

6. Conclusions

The use of taxation as a means of addressing the determination of health needs to be redressed and become a key plank of public health policy. However, the use of taxation as major influence on macrosocial determinants comes with a caveat. The use of taxation in low-income or developing nations as a direct means of redistribution will be minimal without economic growth to raise basic income levels or support the raising of taxation revenues. Still, its utility as a tool to promote public services that contribute to health and economic well-being is beyond argument. In middle to high-income countries, the best way to reduce poverty is to use taxation as one method among many to achieve redistribution (Beblavy & Mizsei, 2006).

Public health increasingly fails to see taxation as a means to address inequality and macrosocial determinants; a notable exception is the area of childhood poverty. Work in the areas of tobacco control and food taxation suggest that there is a move to use the revenues from indirect taxes on goods and, increasingly, services to fund public health interventions. However, the impact that redistribution through taxation can have on macrosocial determinants is largely ignored.

Taxation needs to work alongside moves towards eco-friendly consumption and environmental sustainability to produce healthy societies. It needs to be aligned to benefits (or entitlements) as a means of influencing macrosocial determinants and reducing long-term continuous poverty. In low-income countries it is clear that taxation used to fund public services can contribute to health enhancement and economic development; for example, monies directed towards continuing and extending education for young women has an impact on pregnancy and HIV rates. Therefore, subsidizing school feeding systems from tax revenues targeted at young people in the developing world have additive effects.

There is a need to develop taxation systems that recognize the public good and to which the community and the private sector contribute as an investment (Fee, 1993).

While hypothecated taxes and philanthropy clearly have a role to play in helping fund public health programs at a macrosocial level, the continuation and long-term sustainability of such programs needs to be balanced with revenues from direct taxation or other sources.

Using hypothecated taxes as a means of funding health promotion campaigns should be seriously questioned from the point of view of both whom they serve and their effectiveness: They can be part of a whole package of measures but cannot be effective on their own. It seems to us that the use of hypothecated taxation to fund social marketing and health promotion campaigns is seriously flawed except perhaps as a short-term measure in the early stages of a program. There is a need for longer-term and core funding supported by fiscal measures such as redistribution of income to address poverty. In this respect, it is essential that any such programs adopt a lobbying approach to public health advocacy (Chapman & Lupton, 1994).

Further, there is a need to look for ways of using taxation to fund global public health work. While many may eschew the notion of a global tax as fanciful, we point out that in the global business community many are calling for regulation. Soros (1998) indicates that there is a need to regulate and govern global society if it is intended to continue as an "open society"; developments in the Middle and Near East since the September 11, 2001 terrorist attaks make this glaringly obvious. Douthwaite (1996) and Gray (1998) both point out the limits of unregulated global capitalism. They argue that an open society is dependent on regulation and taxation, and contributions by industry should be part of this continuing development. Also, concern with the spread of diet related non-communicable diseases, especially obesity, has shifted the policy landscape and allowed the topic of taxation of foods to be reintroduced and discussed. The food and advertising industries are developing social programs, public private partnerships and corporate social responsibility programs to deflect attention from taxation (JP Morgan, 2003; UBS Warburg, 2002).

Finally, a word of caution: Wealth creation approaches based on neo-liberal economic agendas and outdated notions of full employment are not ecologically sustainable. Western style capitalism does not work everywhere and brings its own problems (de Soto, 2000). Unlike the approach by Sachs (2005), which focuses on the global economic production of wealth, we maintain such approaches must be tempered by taxation systems that ensure redistribution and address inequality. These should work alongside and be integrated with development aid.

Taxation needs to be understood as key in efforts to influence population health, and it should be designed to have the maximum possible impact on the health status of the poor.

References

Acheson, D. (1998). *Independent inquiry into inequalities in health report*. London: The Stationery Office.

Alexander, N. (2005). *The roles of the IMF, The World Bank and the WTO in liberalization and privatization of the water services sector*. Maryland: Citizens Network on Essential Services.

Barling, D., Lang, T., & Caraher, M. (2001). Social policy and the environment: Towards a new model. In M. Cahill & T. Fitzpatrick (Eds.), *Environmental issues and social welfare*. Oxford: Blackwell.

Beblavy, M., & Mizsei, K. (2006). Make spurious poverty statistics history. *Development & Transition, 4*, 4.

Brunner, E., Cohen, D., & Toon, L. (2001). Cost effectiveness of cardiovascular disease prevention strategies: A perspective on EU food based dietary guidelines. *Public Health Nutrition, 4*(2B), 711–715.

The Cabinet Office. (2004). *Personal responsibility and changing behaviour: The state of knowledge and its implications for public policy*. London: The Cabinet Office Prime Minister's Strategy Unit.

Canadian Association of Food Banks. (2003). *HungerCount 2003: "Something has to give": Food banks filling the policy gap in Canada*. Toronto: Canadian Association of Food Banks.

Caraher, M. (2003). Food protest and the New Activism. In S. John & S. Thomson (Eds.), *New activism and the corporate response*. Basingstoke: Palmgrave.

Caraher, M., & Coveney, J. (2004). Public health nutrition and food policy. *Public Health Nutrition, 7*(5), 591–598.

Caraher, M., & Cowburn, G. (2005). Taxing food: Implications for public health nutrition. *Public Health Nutrition, 8*(8), 1242–1249.

Caraher, M., & Landon, J. (2006). The impact of advertising on food choice: The social context of advertising. In R. Shepherd & M. Ratts (Eds.), *The psychology of food choice*. Wallingford, Oxfordshire: CABI.

Caraher, M., Landon. J., & Dalmeny, K, (2006). TV advertising and children: Lessons from policy development. *Public Health Nutrition, 9*(5), 596–605.

Carr-Hill, R. A. (1987). The inequalities in health debate: A critical review of the issues. *Journal of Social Policy, 16*(4), 509–542.

Carr-Hill, R. A. (1990). Being statistical with the truth. *Radical Statistics Newsletter, 47*, 18–20.

Carr-Hill, R. A., & Lintott, J. (2003). *Consumption jobs and the environment*. London: Macmillan.

Cave, J., & Godfrey, C. (2005). *Economics of addiction and drugs: A review commissioned by Office of Science and Technology*. London: Office of Science and Technology.

Chamberlayne, P. (1992). Income maintenance and institutional forms: A comparison of France, West Germany, Italy and Britain 1945–90. *Policy and Politics, 20*(2), 299–318.

Chantornvong, S., & McCargo, D. (2001). Political economy of tobacco control in Thailand. *Tobacco Control, 10*(1), 48–54.

Chapman, S., & Lupton, D. (1994) The Fight for Public Health; Principles and Practice of Media Advocacy. BMJ Publishing Group, London.

Cobb, C. W., & Cobb, J. B. (1994). *The green national product*. Lanham, Maryland: University Press of America.

Cochrane, A., & Clarke, J. (1997). *Comparing welfare states: Britain in international context*. London: Sage.

Coles, A., & Wallace, T. (Eds.). (2005). *Gender, water and development*. Oxford: Berg.

Dahlgren, G., Nordgren, P., & Whitehead, M. (Eds.). (1997). *Health impact of the common agricultural policy, policy report for the national institute of public health*. Stockholm: National Institute of Public Health.

Daly, H., & Cobb, J. B. (1990). *For the common good*. London: Green Print.

Deacon, B., Ollila, E., Koivusalo, M., & Stubbs, P. (2003). *Global social governance: Themes and prospects*. Helsinki: Ministry for Foreign Affairs of Finland.

Department for International Development. (DFID). (2006). *Eliminating world poverty.* London: DFID.

de Soto, H. (2000). *The mystery of capital; Why capitalism triumphs in the west and fails everywhere else.* London: Black Swan.

Diderichsen, F. (2002). Impact of income maintenance policies. In J. Mackenbach & M. Bakker (Eds.), *Reducing inequalities in health: A European perspective.* London: Routledge.

Douthwaite, R. (1996). *Short circuit: Strengthening local economies for security in an unstable world.* London: The New Economics Foundation.

Dowler, E., Turner, S., & Dobson, B. (2001). *Poverty bites: Food, health and poor families.* London: Child Poverty Action Group.

EU Food Law. (2004). French agency favours ban on TV adverts aimed at children. *EU Food Law, 175*(July 16), 1.

Fee, E. (1993). Public health past and present: A shared social vision. In G. Rosen (Ed.), *A history of public health (expanded version).* Baltimore: The John Hopkins University Press.

French, H. (2006, January 14). Wealth grows but health care withers in China. *New York Times;* Accessed online March 31st 2006 <http://*www.nytimes.* com/2006/01/14/international/asia/14health.html?ex=1294894800&en=d0cb13755ea14446&ei=5088&partner=rssnyt&emc=rss>.

Galbraith, J. K. (1958). *The affluent society.* London: Pelican Books.

Gilmore, N. (2005). *Cleaning the air: The battle over the smoking ban.* Dublin: Liberties Press.

Gravelle, H. (1998). How much of the relation between population mortality and unequal distribution of income is a statistical artefact? *British Medical Journal, 316,* 382–385.

Gray, J. (1998). *False dawn: The delusions of global capitalism.* London: Granta.

Griffiths, P. (2003). *The economist's tale: A consultant encounters hunger and the world bank.* London: Zed Books.

Halpern, D., Bates, C., with Beales, G., & Heathfield, A. (2004). *Personal responsibility and changing behaviour: The state of knowledge and its implications for public policy.* London: Cabinet Office, Prime Minister's Strategy Unit.

Hawkes, C. (2005). The role of foreign direct investment in the nutrition transition. *Public Health Nutrition, 8*(4), 357–365.

Hertz, N. (2001). *The silent takeover: Global capitalism and the death of democracy.* London: William Heinemann.

Hirsch, D. (2006). *What will it take to end child poverty? Firing on all cylinders.* York: Joseph Rowntree Foundation.

Hirsch, F. (1997). *Social limits to growth.* London: Routledgge & Kegan Paul.

Howard, M. (2004). *Tax credits: One year on.* London: Child Poverty Action Group.

Human Development Report. (2005). *International co-operation at a crossroads; Aid, trade and security in an unequal world.* New York: UNDP

Institute of Alcohol Studies. (2006). *Alcohol: Tax, price and public health.* Cambridge: Institute of Alcohol Studies.

Jackson, T., & Marks, N. (1994). *Measuring sustainable economic welfare – A pilot index: 1950–1990.* Stockholm: Stockholm Environment Institute.

Jackson, T., & Marks, N. (1999). Consumption, sustainable welfare and human needs – with reference to UK expenditure patterns between 1954 and 1994. *Ecological Economics, 28,* 421–441.

Jha, P., & Chaloupka, F. (2000). *Tobacco control in developing countries*. Oxford: Oxford University Press.

Kaul, I., Grunberg I., & Stern, M. A. (1999). Defining global public goods. In I. Kaul, I. Grunberg, & M. A. Stern (Eds.), *Global public goods: International cooperation in the 21st century*. Oxford: Oxford University Press / United Nations Development Programme.

Kennedy, E., & Offutt, S. (2000). Commentary: Alternative nutrition outcomes using a fiscal food policy. *British Medical Journal, 320*, 305–309.

Lee, K. (2003). *Globalization and health: An Introduction*. London: Palgrave.

Lee, K., Buse, K., & Fustukian, S. (2002). *Health policy in a globalising world*. Cambridge: Cambridge University Press.

Leicester, A., & Windmeijer, F. (2004). *The "fat tax": Economic incentives to reduce obesity*. London: Institute for Fiscal Studies.

Lock, K., & McKee, M. (2005). Commentary: Will Europe's agricultural policy damage progress on cardiovascular disease? *British Medical Journal, 23*(331), 188–189.

Mackenbach, J. P., Bakker, M. J., Sihto, M., & Diderichsen, F. (2002). Strategies to reduce socioeconomic inequalities in health. In J. Mackenbach & M. Bakker (Eds.), *Reducing inequalities in health: A European perspective*. London: Routledge.

Marmot, M. (1999). *The social determinants of health*. Oxford: Oxford University Press.

Marmot, M. (2001). *Inequalities in health: The role of nutrition*. The Caroline Walker Trust Lecture 2001. London: The Caroline Walker Trust.

Marmot, M. (2005). *Status syndrome: How your social standing directly affects your health*. London: Bloomsbury.

Marmot, M., & Wilkinson, R. (Eds.). (2006). *Social determinants of health*. 2nd edition. Oxford: Oxford University Press.

Marshall, T. (2000). Exploring a fiscal food policy: The case of diet and ischemic heart disease. *British Medical Journal, 320*, 301–305.

McMichael, T. (2001). *Human frontiers, environments and disease: Past patterns, uncertain futures*. Cambridge: Cambridge University Press.

Morgan, J. P. (2003). *Food manufacturing: Obesity the big issue*. London: JP Morgan European Equity Research.

National Social Marketing Centre. (2006). *It's our health: Realising the potential of effective social marketing*. London: National Consumer Council.

Nestle, M. (2002). *Food politics: How the food industry influences nutrition and health*. Berkeley, CA: California State University Press.

Ollila, E. (2003). *Global health-related public private partnerships and the United Nations*. Helsinki: Ministry for Foreign Affairs of Finland.

Oxfam. (2006). *In the public interest: Health, education and water and sanitation for all*. Oxford: Oxfam.

Pieterse, J. N. (1998). My paradigm or yours? Alternative development, post development, reflexive development. *Development and Change, 29*, 343–373

Pomperleau, J., Lock, K., Knai, C., & McKee, M. (2005). *Effectiveness of programmes and interventions promotion fruit and vegetables*. Geneva: World Health Organization.

Popkin, B. (1998). The nutrition transition and its health implications in lower-income countries. *Public Health Nutrition, 1*(1), 5–21.

Popkin, B. M., Armstrong, L. E., Bray, G. M., Caballero, B., Frei, B., & Willett, W. C. (2006). A new proposed guidance system for beverage consumption in the United States. *American Journal of Clinical Nutrition, 83*(3), 529–542.

Pretty, J., Brett, C., Hine, R. E., Mason C. F., Morison, J. I. L., Raven, H., et al. (2000). An assessment of the total external costs of UK agriculture. *Agricultural Systems, 65*, 113–136.

Riches, G. (2002). Food banks and food securty: Welfare reform, human rights and social policy. *Social Policy and Administration, 36*(6), 648–663.

Sachs, G. (2005). *The end of poverty: How we can make it happen in our lifetime*. London: Penguin Books.

Sandler, T. (1992). *Collective action: Theory and applications*. Ann Arbor: University of Michigan Press.

Scanlan, J. P. (2006). Measuring health inequalities. Presentation at the 5th International Conference on Health Economics, Management and Policy, Athens Greece (June 5–7, 2006).

Sen, A. (1997). *Inequality re-examined*. Oxford: Oxford University Press.

Sen, A. (1981). *Poverty and famines*. Oxford: Oxford University Press.

Soros, G. (1998). *The crisis of global capitalism: Open society endangered*. London: Little, Brown and Company.

Stewart-Brown, S. (2000). What causes social inequalities: Why is this question taboo? *Critical Public Health, 10*(2), 233–242.

Thompson, E. P. (1993). *Customs in common: Studies in traditional popular culture*. New York: The New Press.

Timmins, N. (1995). *The five giants: A biography of the Welfare State*. London: Fontana.

Tobin, J. (1978). A proposal for international monetary reform. *Eastern Economic Journal*, July-October 1978, 153–159.

Townsend, P., Davidson, N., & Whitehead, M. (1988). *Inequalities in health: The black report & the health divide*. Harmondsworth: Penguin.

UBS Warburg. (2002). *Global equity research: Absolute risk of obesity*. London: UBS Warburg.

United Nations Development Programme. (2005). *Human development report 2005: International cooperation at a crossroads; Aid, trade and security in an unequal world*. New York: United Nations Development Project.

Water Aid. (2005). *Getting to boiling point: Turning up the heat on water and sanitation*. London: Water Aid.

Water Aid. (2006). *Bridging the gap: Citizens' action for accountability in water and sanitation*. London: Water Aid.

Whiteford, P., Mendelson, M., & Millar, J. (2003). *Timing it right; Tax credits and how to respond to income changes*. York: Joseph Rowntree Foundation.

Wilkinson, R. (2005). *The impact of inequality: How to make sick societies healthier*. London: Routledge.

World Health Organization. (2000). *Food and nutrition action plan for Europe, August 2000*. Copenhagen: WHO European Regional Office.

Chapter 11
Patent Law and Policy

Aaron S. Kesselheim and Jerry Avorn

1. Introduction: Patents and Intellectual Property

Patents are government-issued monopolies on intellectual property that provide their owners a legal means to prevent others from unauthorized production or usage of their inventions for a set period of time. The promise of receiving a patent has served for many centuries as an important tool to promote innovation. However, concern has grown recently over whether in the public health context such promotion of innovation has come to pose unacceptable hurdles to access.

Controversies have erupted over whether patents are sought and awarded to protect aspects of medical research that are not truly novel, are improperly used to manipulate health care costs or limit access to vital treatments, or are extended past their proper termination point, preventing needed discoveries from entering the public domain. As a result, a central question regarding the relationship of patents and the public health is how to continue to encourage innovation while avoiding the problems that can emerge from the effect of monopolies on population health.

In this chapter, we briefly review the basic legal properties of patents and their application to the field of public health and health care. We then highlight four major arenas in which patents affect public health: health care costs, access to therapeutics and other medical technologies, the practice of medicine, and the development of new medical innovations. Finally, we suggest several strategies that can be applied to the field of intellectual property so that the patenting system can better promote public health.

2. US and International Patent Law

2.1. US Patenting Requirements

In the United States, the Constitution permits Congress to pass laws to "promote the progress of science and the useful arts." The American Patent Act, which dates back to 1790, sets forth a number of basic requirements that an invention must meet to qualify for intellectual property protection. For example, an invention must be novel, be non-obvious to a person of ordinary skill in the appropriate field, and have some utility. It must also be within a proper category, which the Patent Act defines as a "process, machine, manufacture, or composition of matter." The wide breadth of this definition was reinforced in the 1980 Supreme Court case of *Diamond v. Chakrabarty*, involving the patentability of a microbe into which an inventor had inserted a special DNA plasmid. The court ruled that the Patent Act covered "anything under the sun made by man," including this single-celled living organism.

A patent is classically thought of as a *quid pro quo* between the inventor and society. On the one hand, the government provides the inventor with monopoly control over the innovation, which might otherwise be illegal, for a limited time. In return, inventors must fully explain their discoveries in systematized patent documents, which then become part of the public domain and can help inspire other inventions. The patent document must therefore be clear, include enough information to enable colleagues to make and use the invention, and show the public the best mode the inventors considered for making their inventions work. Officers at the US Patent and Trademark Office (USPTO) evaluate patent documents and determine if the described inventions meet the requirements in the Patent Act and are worthy of a patent. Currently, a patent monopoly can last for up to twenty years from the date the inventor officially submits the application to the USPTO. This monopoly power, however, can have a negative impact on public health, especially if patent holders restrict dissemination of their inventions or raise prices such that patients have difficulty accessing or affording important health care-related products.

2.2. International Patent Laws and Treaties

Across the world, the extent of intellectual property rights protection granted by governments, such as criteria for patenting and patent length, has historically varied widely. This caused some international tension, as manufacturers in wealthier nations, such as the United States and Japan, felt subject to illegal copying from manufacturers based in countries where intellectual property protections were more lenient.

This tension has been particularly acute in the field of health care. As recently as the 1980s, over fifty countries – most in the developing world, but a few in the developed world as well – did not confer patent protection on pharmaceuticals. The government of India, for example, chose to exclude drug products from its 1970 patent law, deciding that providing low-cost pharmaceutical agents to its population was more important than providing incentives to create new agents (Barton, 2004).

In 1995, the Agreement on Trade-Related Aspects of Intellectual Property Rights (TRIPs) aimed to standardize intellectual property protections in the international community. This accord among countries in the World Trade Organization (WTO) established a general understanding that novel, non-obvious, and useful inventions in all fields of technology could be patented and set down a framework for respecting patent rights granted by other WTO members. Wealthier countries agreed to open their markets to agriculture and other exports. As a result, a nation such as India was obliged to recognize other nations' intellectual property rights and faced higher costs for pharmaceutical products patented in other countries.

The TRIPs agreement contained a number of exceptions specifically addressing public health. It excluded from covered subject matter all diagnostic, therapeutic, and surgical techniques describing ways of treating humans or animals, as well as inventions "the prevention of whose commercial exploitation is necessary to protect" public health. It also allowed member states, under extreme circumstances, to authorize compulsory licenses of patented items. This legal mechanism permits governments to unilaterally set down terms for manufacturing and selling products without the authorization of the patent owner. In 2001, WTO member states attempted to clarify the compulsory license provision in the Doha Declaration, which recognized that public health crises "can represent a national emergency" sufficient to allow such licenses to be granted.

3. Effects of Patents on Public Health

Patented innovations have long helped shape the practice of medicine and have had a substantial impact on health in a number of different ways. Technological innovation in sanitation and agriculture has been critical to improving the health of populations, and patents on health care-related discoveries have played an increasingly central role in pharmaceutical development. In modern times, new therapeutic modalities, such as prescription drugs, vaccines, diagnostic tools, and medical equipment, are all invariably developed under the auspices of patent protection.

Health care-related patents swelled in number during the 1980s, as medical researchers pursued the molecular and genetic basis of disease and identified more potential targets for therapeutic products and diagnostic tools. In the United States, a number of legal and social factors emerged concurrently to facilitate this patenting explosion. Patent disputes were centralized in a special appeals court, the Federal Circuit Court of Appeals, which took a liberal view of the limits of patenting and allowed inventors to push the envelope by upholding increasingly broad patents (Jaffe & Lerner, 2004). Additionally, starting in 1983, Congress changed the structure of the USPTO so that applicants' fees helped pay for patent examiners' salaries, which helped speed the patent approval process (Jaffe & Lerner, 2004).

By the late 1990s, however, some began to question the social good of the large numbers of patents being granted in the field of health care. Inventors worldwide held the intellectual property patent rights to more than 25,000 DNA-based patents (Cook-Deegan & McCormack, 2001); however, these basic elements of life were critical as targets and building blocks for future research to determine the biochemical basis of disease states and develop new treatments. Some observers predicted that granting these intellectual property rights to different parties could create an "anticommons" such that the "proliferation of intellectual property rights upstream may be stifling life-saving innovations further downstream in the course of research and product development" (Heller & Eisenberg, 1998). Other commentators documented the ways in which pharmaceutical companies have used loopholes in the patent and drug regulatory system to derive substantial profits after expiration of the intellectual property protection on their products (Kesselheim, Fischer, & Avorn, 2006). In this section, we discuss four different ways that patents can interact with public health by affecting health care costs, access to essential therapeutic products, the practice of medicine, and research and technological development in the health care industry.

3.1. Patents and Drug Costs

More than nearly every other industrial sector, patents are integral to the development of pharmaceutical products (Cohen, Nelson, & Walsh, 2000). Some have argued that patents provide necessary incentives for investment in drug research because of the high cost of developing new drugs and the relative ease of producing chemically similar or identical copies. In addition, the functional duration of patent protection is usually less than the full twenty-year patent term because pharmaceutical manufacturers usually apply for patents early in the drug discovery process, often years before completing the clinical trials necessary for marketing approval in most countries.

As a result, pharmaceutical companies charge high prices for new products, depending on the health care system in which they operate. Nearly all industrialized countries other than the US negotiate the prices that will be paid, but prescription drug costs still account for a substantial and growing portion of health care expenditures. The problem is even more acute in the United States because of the absence of governmental participation in drug prices. In 2004, total US prescription drug spending exceeded $200 billion and accounted for about 11% of total health expenditures; a rise to 14.5% is expected by 2012 (Heffler et al., 2003).

There is growing evidence that improper use of patents has helped inflate prescription drug costs even further. When patent monopoly ends, other companies can enter the pharmaceutical market with lower cost generic alternatives to brand-name drugs, which enable private payers and government programs to control costs (Fischer & Avorn, 2004; Haas, Phillips, Gerstenberger, & Seger, 2005). However, market exclusivity of pharmaceutical products can be extended inappropriately to blocking these cost savings.

One primary means used to extend market exclusivity is known as "patent evergreening." To supplement patents on innovative active ingredients, brand-name manufacturers apply for patents on peripheral features of products, including aspects of their formulation, metabolites, or method of administration. This process can delay generic copies from reaching the marketplace, sometimes for years. A report from the US Federal Trade Commission (FTC) detailed numerous instances in which brand-name manufacturers maintained their market exclusivity by listing improper or invalid patents with the Food and Drug Administration (FTC, 2002).

For example, in the case of the proton-pump inhibitor omeprazole (Prilosec), the basic US patent expired in April 2001, including time restored to the length of patent under federal law due to the regulatory process. Before a generic alternative could be marketed, however, its manufacturer claimed that prospective generic manufacturers infringed patents on Prilosec's coating that protected their brand-name product until 2007. This process delayed the marketing of generic omeprazole by nearly two years until 2003.

Prilosec's manufacturer also separated the drug's two isomers and obtained a new patent on the s-isomer (esomeprazole, marketed as a new, improved product called Nexium). During the Prilosec legal process, Nexium was vigorously promoted as the newest proton-pump inhibitor. Physicians' use of Nexium or Prilosec over delayed generic alternatives has led to many millions of dollars of extra spending by government and private payers on prescription drugs (Kesselheim et al., 2006).

It is vital to respect basic intellectual property rights in drug development to help protect innovation. However, inappropriate extension of such rights, combined with reduced generic substitution, can lead to excessive costs and can have a number of effects on the public health. Prescription drug costs have strained government health care budgets, and publicly-funded health insurance programs such as Medicaid have been forced to restrict eligibility or introduce policies such as cost-sharing. Studies have shown that such policies can cause patients to avoid even essential medications and lead to more adverse events (Tamblyn et al., 2001). Further, manufacturers' focus on extending patent terms and protecting revenues from older products may also divert resources from research into new products (Kesselheim & Avorn, 2005). A recent US government study documented the decrease in pharmaceutical development by examining reduced numbers of innovative products on the market in recent years (Congressional Budget Office, 2006).

3.2. Access Issues

One of the most compelling arguments supporting the use of patents to protect intellectual property has been their potential to encourage widespread proliferation of innovations because inventors can use the power of the government to prevent illegal copying. In some cases, however, patent-holders have been criticized for using their patent monopolies to restrict dissemination of technology, and patents have been particularly implicated in poor health outcomes in less developed countries.

Patents can hinder access to new health technologies when patent-holders either choose not to allow others to use their inventions or cannot negotiate contracts with licensees. For instance, the company that holds the patent on the BRCA-1 gene test for a type of hereditary breast cancer requires all tests be done in its Utah laboratories. Thus, testing is unavailable to consumers who cannot access sophisticated academic centers that can arrange for long-distance transfer of blood samples (Butler & Goodman, 2001). Similarly, licensing enforcement practices by the holder of the patent on the hemochromatosis gene have prevented many laboratories from offering the gene test to consumers (Merz, Kriss, Leonard, & Cho, 2002).

In extreme cases, patents can be used to drive a new health care technology off the market entirely, sometimes even in the case of patents held by the non-profit sector. Researchers at Fred Hutchinson Cancer Center developed a novel cell separation technology based on antibodies to a CD34 antigen meant to improve outcomes in patients undergoing bone marrow transplantation. However, researchers at Johns Hopkins University had a broad patent covering the CD34 antigen; a court found that the Hutchinson-developed device infringed the patent, even though it was independently created and involved a different binding mechanism. Though the Hopkins product was not yet available to patients, the patent drove the Hutchinson-developed device off the market (Bar-Shalom & Cook-Deegan, 2002).

The most substantial access issue in terms of magnitude of public health impact is the effect of patents on the international availability of basic medical therapies, particularly pharmaceutical products. Aggressive enforcement of patents in poor countries can limit distribution of drugs to treat diseases such as tuberculosis and cancer (Pecoul, Chirac, Trouiller, & Pinel, 1999), although other factors provide substantial barriers as well (Attaran & Gillespie-White, 2001).

A pressing current concern is the potential for patents to limit access to HIV drugs for AIDS patients in poor regions such as sub-Saharan Africa. Before the TRIPs agreement, HIV medications patented in industrialized nations could be produced by generic manufacturers in countries such as India and then sold to poorer countries at markedly reduced prices. The TRIPs agreement, however, forced many countries to adopt international patenting standards and cease production of these less costly generic drugs. Though certain exceptions allowed production of drugs for public health crises, these exceptions remain contentious because of the many bureaucratic steps required to implement them (Pollock & Price, 2003). In addition, these exceptions can allow importation of patented drugs for domestic use, but not necessarily allow their export, so poorer countries without domestic production capacity may be unable to find a willing trade partner to supply them with needed medications.

As a result, patent-protected second-line treatments for resistant varieties of HIV are largely unavailable in the developing world. Pharmaceutical manufacturers have feared that the lower-priced copies produced in poorer countries will find their way into the lucrative markets of wealthier nations. Brazil, which has an ambitious domestic HIV treatment plan, reported spending 63% of its AIDS drug budget on three patent-protected medications. Ultimately, it used the threat of imposing a compulsory license to negotiate price reductions with one manufacturer on its combination anti-retroviral lopinavir/ritonavir (Kaletra) (Okie, 2006).

3.3. Patents and Medical Practices

Patents can affect population health by influencing the delivery of care by health care professionals. Patents over basic medical practices, such as making a diagnosis or treating a patient in a certain way, are particularly controversial. These patents are similar to business method patents, such as Amazon.com's "one-click" method of shopping, and have been increasing in popularity in health care. Medical processes are not considered patentable subject matter in nearly 80 countries (and are excluded from the TRIPs agreement). In the US, rather than making medical practices unpatentable, amendments to the Patent Act in 1996 deprived patent holders of remedies against health care practitioners. Under new Section 287(c), a court can hold that physicians infringed a patent but cannot order them to pay damages or stop using the process.

Still, numerous exceptions to Section 287(c) allow patents on medical practices to affect the delivery of healthcare. Such patents may be enforceable if they involve a patented drug or device. For example, a process patent granted in 2004 covers combination therapy of rheumatoid arthritis using two different classes of known medications (a TNF-alpha antagonist and cyclosporin). As long as either drug is under patent protection, the patent could be enforced. In a recent case, a laboratory testing company was found to have infringed a patent on a process for diagnosing a vitamin deficiency on the basis of an elevated blood homocysteine level because it published materials alerting physicians to the biochemical association between vitamin deficiencies and homocysteine (Kesselheim & Mello, 2006).

These kinds of patents threaten to prevent dissemination of important medical information and may impact physicians' practice of medicine. As a result of the homocysteine patent case, the educational papers distributed by the laboratory testing company were withdrawn from the market. Medical process patents also can intervene in the physician-patient relationship if physicians are concerned that their actions might infringe someone else's intellectual property, and they can be used to increase the costs of health care, especially if different treatment pathways are associated with licensing fees before they can be promoted publicly.

3.4. Medical Research Patents

A final way patents can affect public health is through their influence on the field of medical research. In the US, the Bayh-Dole Act of 1980 allowed private institutions to pursue patents on government-funded research, and some university researchers were able to turn patented biotechnology into substantial profits (Eisenberg, 1996). The model example of this situation was a group of patents held by Stanford University on a gene splicing technique, which it licensed broadly. The proprietary technology soon became the industry standard, and Stanford reaped hundreds of millions of dollars in revenue from their patent licenses.

Over the subsequent two decades, other research universities set up technology transfer offices and encouraged their employees to pursue patents on research outcomes. Unlike the Stanford case, however, many of these initiatives did not lead to new revenue streams and ended up losing money for the university (Sobolski, Barton, & Emanuel, 2005). This has been attributed in part to the high legal costs of negotiation and the small number of patents that become profitable end products.

The overlapping licenses and agreements required for using patents can create a "patent thicket," which has been defined as a "dense web of overlapping intellectual property rights that a company must hack its way through" to develop and commercialize new technology (Shapiro, 2001). This thicket raises the cost of collaborative research or can make it impossible altogether. For example, the company that owns a broad patent on the BRCA-1 gene has refused to license it, preventing others from improving the relatively insensitive test (Bosch, 2004).

The perceived importance of patents in the medical research and development community and the commercialization of some elements of the non-profit research setting have also helped influence the type of research that is pursued. Development of effective treatments for diseases prevalent in low-income countries, such as malaria and other tropical infectious diseases, have lagged behind maladies more common in the developed world. The patent system has been implicated in society's inability to stimulate innovation in this area of public health. Some have argued that research has focused on public health problems in regions with strong intellectual property protections because innovators may be able to garner a better return on their investment (Troullier et al., 2002).

Finally, patenting within the medical research community can raise ethical dilemmas for scientists. In a study of information dissemination practices among life sciences investigators, filing a patent application was the leading reason for withholding data for 6 months or more (Blumenthal, Campbell, Anderson, Causino, & Louis, 1997). Similarly, a survey of life science companies found that many required universities to keep research results secret even beyond the period needed to file a patent application (Blumenthal, Causino, Campbell, & Louis, 1996).

As a result, the growing push to patent early-stage research technology can raise the costs of technological innovation and prevent efficient dissemination of ideas critical to achieving public health-related goals. However, discouraging upstream patenting entirely can allow for-profit companies to use technology developed in university settings, often funded by government grants, to create successful products and gain windfall profits. In this setting, the public may in essence be paying twice for medical innovation (Avorn, 2004). In the case of selective cyclooxygenase-2 (COX-2) inhibitors such as celecoxib, a number of critical discoveries were made and patented at the University of Rochester during the 1990s. Pharmacia, as well as a number of other pharmaceutical companies, used the screening methods identified to find a workable selective COX-2 inhibitor, and Pfizer (which had purchased Pharmacia) marketed the product as Celebrex and garnered nearly $3 billion in annual sales worldwide (Kesselheim & Avorn, 2005).

The primary goal of patent reform in the upcoming years will be to balance the importance of creating incentives to innovate with the need to ensure that patents are not used to harm the public health by inflating medical costs, hindering access to medical products, improperly restricting medical practices, or complicating medical research. In the next section, we will examine some policies aimed at reforming the patent system with these goals in mind.

4. Patent System Reforms to Promote Public Health

4.1. Regulatory Reforms

In recent years, there have been some indications that the trend towards increased health care-related patenting in the 1980s and 1990s is slowly reversing course. The USPTO, for example, has shown signs that it is re-thinking its permissive policies regarding patenting of biochemical products. The agency recently tightened its utility requirement to prevent patenting of small DNA sequences with unclear functional significance. The Federal Circuit and other courts have also taken a somewhat more critical view of overly broad patents on biochemical tools. Finally, more researchers are placing health-care related discoveries in the public domain, foregoing patent protection altogether.

Nevertheless, these incremental steps may not change the medical patenting environment significantly enough. A number of other strategies have been suggested to reform the management of government-sponsored monopolies of intellectual property to protect public health, patient care, and medical research. For example, noting that brand-name pharmaceutical companies' strategies have "prevented the availability of more generic drugs," the FTC proposed changes to the patent registration system to ensure that improperly obtained or duplicative patents do not extend the effective market exclusivity of brand-name products (FTC, 2002). The FTC is also scrutinizing agreements between brand-name and generic companies to ensure that they do not restrain trade by keeping generics off the market (FTC, 2002). Such critical examination of patents by government regulators can help combat the excesses of patent evergreening. If the original length of intellectual property protection on a given drug were more effectively enforced, pharmaceutical companies could continue to make appropriate revenues on true medical innovations throughout the patent life (Avorn, 2005; Kesselheim & Avorn, 2005).

In extreme cases, the principle of eminent domain allows governments to step in and take over privately held property for the greater good. We have argued that if excessive pricing of an innovative drug for cancer or AIDS makes the treatment unavailable to poor patients, this could qualify as a threat to public health and justify invoking eminent domain to ensure access. A general standard should be developed to define when the risk of damage to the public's health is substantial enough to take such a step (Kesselheim & Avorn, 2006).

4.2. Legislative Reforms

The basic laws authorizing patents can also be adjusted to help counteract certain negative effects on public health. As we discussed in Section 3.3, with the growth of certain medical process patents in the US, physicians could be forced to enter into licensing agreements or otherwise inhibited from using their best medical judgment. To address this, Section 287(c) could be extended to make medical processes using patented drugs and devices unpatentable. This would bring the

US into harmony with the European Patent Convention and other countries. Under such a rule, a novel process for purifying a new pharmaceutical product for human use would be patentable – thereby promoting the discovery of novel compounds – but the ways physicians used the product would not be.

Legislative reform could also help support international access to patented agents. The Bayh-Dole Act allows the government to retain "march in" rights to any patent developed with federal funds if the patent holder sets too strict limits on use of its discovery. This means that the government could assume control of the patent and dictate the licensing terms. In the past, there have been efforts to encourage the government to "march in" when pharmaceutical manufacturers threaten to raise prices on products high enough to make them unavailable to low-income patients (Love, 2004), but the government has never exercised these rights. If the Bayh-Dole Act was amended to allow the government to become a more active participant earlier in the intellectual property development process, public agencies could help evaluate the appropriateness of patenting publicly funded research that might inhibit future innovation. Alternatively, the government could modify the Bayh-Dole Act to encourage the licensing of such rights in the international community by, for example, including a mandatory license for third world countries to use drug products derived from government-financed innovation (Rai & Eisenberg, 2003). It may also be helpful to change the patent review process to allow consumer representatives to challenge some patents and thus allow courts to weigh the inventiveness of a product against its public health implications (Kesselheim & Avorn, 2006).

4.3. Market Reforms

Some have proposed market reforms to address patenting dilemmas. Better management of patents by inventors based in academic research centers may improve international access to needed therapies. This means that, since much of the basic research that lays the groundwork for successful medical products occurs in academic settings, universities could be more proactive in negotiating licenses of their intellectual property to for-profit companies. Licensing agreements could be formulated to require that pharmaceutical products based on university-developed research be made available to low- and middle-income countries at greatly reduced prices (Kapczynski, Chaifetz, Katz, & Benkler, 2005). Leaders in science, law, and public health have signed a consensus policy statement supporting this approach (Universities Allied for Essential Medicine, 2006). Similar public-private cooperative arrangements that promote investment in research and development while protecting intellectual property have been suggested as a way to improve drug development for neglected infectious diseases in lower income countries (Grabowski, 2002).

An alternative model for pharmaceutical companies has emerged as well. The Institute for OneWorld Health has become a successful non-profit pharmaceutical manufacturer, having introduced an effective treatment for visceral leishmaniasis in underserved markets in India. Leveraging its non-profit status may allow the

Institute to promote research and cooperative licensing agreements for future products to treat diseases prevalent in the developing world, such as malaria and Chagas' disease, that might not be targeted by traditional for-profit manufacturers (Hale, Woo & Lipton, 2005).

Market-based strategies can also help alleviate the problems a "patent thicket" poses to medical research. Patent pools are frequently employed in fields such as computer science, where numerous manufacturers contribute to producing one integrated product. These pools assign market-value licensing rates to a range of products, making them available without requiring individual negotiation with each party claiming intellectual property rights in different steps of complex research processes (Levin, 2002). If patent pools were popularized in the health care industry, they could lower transaction costs and promote cooperation while allowing a reasonable royalty on intellectual property (Andrews, 2002).

5. Conclusion

While patents in health care are useful means of encouraging innovation, they can also increase costs, hinder access to diagnostic and therapeutic products, distort clinical practice, and complicate progress in medical research. In each of these domains, the central policy goal remains trying to balance the legitimate use of patents in supporting innovation with preventing their improper use and the resultant negative impact on public health.

References

Andrews, L. B. (2002). Genes and patent policy: Rethinking intellectual property rights. *Nature Reviews Genetics, 3*, 803–808.

Attaran, A., & Gillespie-White, L. (2001). Do patents for antiretroviral drugs constrain access to AIDS treatment in Africa? *Journal of the American Medical Association, 286*, 1886–1892.

Avorn, J. (2004). *Powerful medicines: The benefits, risks, and costs of prescription drugs.* New York: Alfred A. Knopf.

Avorn, J. (2005). Sending pharma better signals. *Science, 309*, 669.

Bar-Shalom, A., & Cook-Deegan, R. (2002). Patents and innovation in cancer therapeutics: Lessons from CellPro. *Milbank Quarterly, 80*, 637–676.

Barton, J. H. (2004). TRIPS and the global pharmaceutical market. *Health Affairs, 23*, 146–154.

Blumenthal, D., Campbell, E. G., Anderson, M. S., Causino, N., & Louis, K. S. (1997). Withholding research results in academic life science. *Journal of the American Medical Association, 277*, 1224–1228.

Blumenthal, D., Causino, N., Campbell, E., & Louis, K. S. (1996). Relationships between academic institutions and industry in the life sciences—an industry survey. *New England Journal of Medicine, 334*, 368–373.

Bosch, X. (2004). Myriad loses rights to breast cancer gene patent. *Lancet, 363*, 1780.

Butler, D., & Goodman, S. (2001). French researchers take a stand against cancer gene patent. *Nature, 413,* 95–96.

Cohen, W. M., Nelson, R. R., & Walsh J. P. (2000). Protecting their intellectual assets: Appropriability conditions and why U.S. manufacturing firms patent (or not). National Bureau of Economic Research Working Paper No. 7552.

Congressional Budget Office. (2006). *Research and development in the pharmaceutical industry.* (October, 2006); http://www.cbo.gov/ftpdocs/76xx/doc7615/10–02-DrugR-D.pdf.

Cook-Deegan, R. M., & McCormack, S. J. (2001). Patents, secrecy and DNA. *Science, 293,* 217.

Eisenberg, R. S. (1996). Public research and private development: Patents and technology transfer in government-sponsored research. *Virginia Law Review, 82,* 1663–727.

Federal Trade Commission. (2002). *Generic drug entry prior to patent expiration.* (July, 2002); http://www.ftc.gov/os/2002/07/genericdrugstudy.pdf

Fischer, M. A., & Avorn, J. (2004). Economic implications of evidence-based prescribing for hypertension: Can better care cost less? *Journal of the American Medical Association, 291,* 1850–1856.

Grabowski, H. (2002). Patents, innovation and access to new pharmaceuticals. *Journal of International Economic Law, 5,* 849–860.

Haas, J. S., Phillips, K. A., Gerstenberger, E. P., & Seger A. C. (2005). Potential savings from substituting generic drugs for brand-name drugs: Medical expenditure panel survey 1997–2000. *Annals of Internal Medicine, 142,* 891–897.

Hale, V. G., Woo, K., & Lipton H. L. (2005). Oxymoron no more: The potential of non-profit drug companies to deliver on the promise of medicines for the developing world. *Health Affairs, 24,* 1057–1064.

Heffler, S., Smith, S., Keehan, S., Clemens, M. K., Won, G., & Zezza, M. (2003). Health spending projections for 2002–2012. *Health Affairs,* (Supplemental Web Exclusive), W3 – 54–65.

Heller, M. A., & Eisenberg, R. S. (1998). Can patents deter innovation? The anticommons in biomedical research. *Science, 280,* 698–701.

Jaffe, A. B., & Lerner, J (2004). *Innovation and its discontents.* Princeton, NJ: Princeton University Press.

Kapczynski, A., Chaifetz, S., Katz, Z., & Benkler, Y. (2005). Addressing global health inequities: An open licensing approach for university innovations. *Berkeley Technology Law Journal, 20,* 1031–114.

Kesselheim, A. S., & Avorn, J. (2005). University-based science and biotechnology products: Defining the boundaries of intellectual property. *Journal of the American Medical Association, 293,* 850–854.

Kesselheim, A. S., & Avorn, J. (2006). Biomedical patents and the public health. Is there a role for eminent domain? *Journal of the American Medical Association, 295,* 434–437.

Kesselheim, A. S., Fischer, M. A., & Avorn, J. (2006). Extensions of intellectual property rights and delayed adoption of generic drugs: Effects on Medicaid expenditures. *Health Affairs, 25,* 1637–1647.

Kesselheim, A. S., & Mello, M. M. (2006). Medical process patents – monopolizing the delivery of health care. *New England Journal of Medicine, 355,* 2036–2041.

Levin, R. C. (2002). *FTC/DOJ joint hearings on competition and intellectual property law.* Washington, DC: Federal Trade Commission.

Love, J. (2004). NIH meeting on Norvir/Ritonavir march-in request. (May 25, 2004); http://www.essentialinventions.org/legal/norvir/may25nihjamie.pdf.

Merz, J. F., Kriss, A. G., Leonard, D. G., & Cho, M. K. (2002). Diagnostic testing fails the test. *Nature, 415,* 577–579.

Okie, S. (2006). Fighting HIV – lessons from Brazil. *New England Journal of Medicine, 354,* 1977–1981.

Pecoul, B., Chirac, P., Trouiller, P., & Pinel, J. (1999). Access to essential drugs in poor countries: A lost battle? *Journal of the American Medical Association, 281,* 361–367.

Pollock, A. M., & Price, D. (2003). New deal from the World Trade Organisation. *British Medical Journal, 327,* 571–572.

Rai, A. K., & Eisenberg, R. S. (2003). The public domain: Bayh-Dole reform and the progress of biomedicine. *Law & Contemporary Problems, 66,* 288–313.

Shapiro, C. (2001). Navigating the patent thicket: Cross licenses, patent pools and standard-setting. In A. Jaffe, J. Lerner, & S. Stern (Eds.), *Innovation policy and the economy.* volume I. Cambridge, MA: MIT Press.

Sobolski, G. K., Barton, J. H., & Emanuel, E. J. (2005). Technology licensing: Lessons from the US experience. *Journal of the American Medical Association, 294,* 3137–3140.

Tamblyn, R., Laprise, R., Hanley, J. A., Abrahamowicz, M., Scott, S., Mayo, N., et al. (2001). Adverse events associated with prescription drug cost-sharing among poor and elderly persons. *Journal of the American Medical Association, 285,* 421–429.

Troullier, P., Olliaro, P., Torreele, E., Orbinski, J., Laing, R., & Ford, N. (2002). Drug development for neglected disease: A deficient market and public-health policy failure. *Lancet, 359,* 2188–2194.

Universities Allied for Essential Medicine. (2006). Philadelphia consensus statement on university policy for health-related innovations. (2006); http://www.essentialmedicine.org/cs/wp-content/uploads/2006/10/philadelphiaconsensusstatement.pdf

Chapter 12
Migration

Sana Loue and Sandro Galea

1. Background

1.1. Defining Migration

Migration has been defined as:

"the physical transition of an individual or a group from one society to another. This transition usually involves abandoning one social setting and entering a different one" (Eisenstadt, 1955)

"a relatively permanent moving away of . . . migrants, from one geographical location to another, preceded by decision-making on the part of the migrants on the basis of a hierarchically ordered set of values or valued ends and resulting in changes in the interactional set of migrants" (Mangalam, 1968)

"a permanent or semipermanent change of residence" (Lee, 1966)

Accordingly, migration refers to movement both within and across national borders. It encompasses internal migrants, such as agricultural workers, and immigrants, regardless of the manner or legality of their entry into a country. Importantly, it occurs as the result of a decision-making process undertaken by individuals that is premised on a set of values that may or may not be explicit. It is not only the movement of populations that affects health, but also the context in which that movement occurs. This chapter focuses on health issues arising in the context of population movement and the macrosocial factors that underlie that movement.

In 1990 migrants accounted for 15 percent of the population of 52 countries (Council of Europe, 2001). Estimates suggest that currently 175 million people, or 2.9 percent of the world's population, live either permanently or temporarily outside of their countries of origin (International Organization for Migration, 2003) and that by the year 2050, the number of international migrants will approach 250 million (International Labour Office, International Organization for Migration, and the Office of the United Nations High Commissioner for Human Rights [ILO, IOM, & OHCHR], 2001). These figures include migrant workers, permanent immigrants, and those who are seeking asylum or refugee status. The estimates do not include individuals who migrate across borders illegally, known variously as "illegal," "undocumented," or "irregular" (World Health Organization, 2003); such individuals may migrate themselves; may be trafficked, a process that involves coercion or deception; or may be smuggled, meaning that their entry has been facilitated by others for profit (ILO, IOM, & OHCHR, 2001). Consequently, the figures underestimate the magnitude of migration and its demographic impact in various regions of the world (Council of Europe, 2000).

Individuals may migrate from one area to another for any number of reasons. Circumstances at the point of origin that may "push" individuals to leave include poverty, unemployment, persecution, internal civil strife, a change in government or regime, and/or natural disasters such as hurricanes. Individuals may feel a "pull" towards the intended destination as a result of perceived employment prospects, the ability to reunify with other family members, expectations of a better economic and/or political situation, freedom from persecution, and/or a safe haven from the ravages of manmade or natural disasters. Distinctions have been made between those immigrants who are "voluntary," such as students, tourists, and migrant workers, and those who are "forced" to migrate as a result of displacement due to internal conflict, environmental disaster, famine, or development projects (Loughna, n.d.).

The health of migrating individuals and groups, whether documented/regular or undocumented/irregular, voluntary or forced, may be shaped by each stage of the migration process. During the period preceding migration ("pre-migration stage"), before individuals have physically left their countries of origin, individuals have formed beliefs about health, illness, disease, treatment, and expectations of care that they will carry with them to their intended destinations. They may also have developed chronic or infectious diseases that they will bring with them. During the process of migration itself ("peri-migration"), individuals will be affected by the conditions that they confront and the experiences that they undergo during this process. Contrast, for example, how the health of two individuals may be differentially affected where one enters into the US legally as a corporate executive traveling as a first class passenger on an international airline and the second flees internal political turmoil and genocide in his country by paying smugglers to facilitate his escape through war-torn territories.

It is important to note, however, that the impact of factors identified at one stage of the migration process often have repercussions well into subsequent phases of migration. As an example, severe poverty during pre-migration affects individual and group health during this phase, but it also has implications for the manner of migration, the health risks associated with peri-migration, and the health conditions that may persist or ensue post-migration. Further, during the peri- and post-migration phases, the migration of individuals and groups may impact the health of the individuals with whom they come into contact. For instance, migrants with active tuberculosis can potentially transmit the disease to others, such as during the course of airline travel. Undiagnosed and untreated, they may further transmit the infection following their arrival to their new country. Similarly, those who were inadvertently exposed during their air travel may develop active infection and transmit it to others. Less frequently considered, but no less important, is the impact of the individuals' departure on the health of the populations that they have left, as in the case of health professionals' emigration to more developed countries.

In this chapter, we utilize the framework of pre-, peri-, and post-migration stages to explore the impact of migration on population health. Within each phase of migration, we examine the historical, geographical, socioeconomic, cultural, and political contexts that frame the interplay of migration and health. Table 12.1 provides a summary of some of the factors that are encompassed within each domain. Although we explore a number of these within each context and stage of migration, it is beyond the scope of this chapter to provide a detailed examination of all such factors. We utilize trafficking as a case example to explore the intersectionality of the various factors throughout the migration process and their resulting health effects. Finally, we provide a series of recommendations intended to improve the well-being of migrant populations and the communities in which they reside.

2. Pre-Migration

2.1. Historical Context

The effects of history may affect individuals' health before, during, and following immigration. Several scholars, for instance, have noted the impact of Jewish and Zionist history on individuals who wish to migrate from Israel (Knafo & Yaari, 1997). The historical culture may affect both their ability to emigrate, the stress that they feel during the process, and their mental health following migration:

"In their homeland they would be called a *yored,* a derogatory nickname meaning "one who descends by leaving Israel," thereby shattering the basic tenets of Zionism. This is in contrast to *oleh,* one who ascends by immigration to Israel. The *yored* is perceived as a selfish and weak person, a failure and a traitor" (Knafo & Yaari, 1997).

Yet another example is provided by India and Pakistan. Many Indian Muslims within particular states of India are more likely to marry Pakistani Muslims than other Indian Muslims because they believe that those from Pakistan are more culturally and ethnically similar to themselves (Majumder & Jolly, 2003). The closing of the border between Pakistan and India in December 2001, following an attack on the Indian Parliament, prevented Indian Muslims from marrying and prevented cross-border families from joining each other. The closing of the border brought about severe emotional pain for those who have been separated from family members.

2.2. Geographical Context

The cross-border utilization of health care on the US-Mexico border exemplifies the importance of the geographical context in which migration occurs and the

TABLE 12.1. Features of migration that may influence population health

Context	Pre-migration stage	Peri-migration stage	Post-migration stage
Historical	History of settlement; formation of cross-border families due to political divisions of territories, e.g. India and Pakistan, Mexico and the US; political tensions between countries	History of migration across certain borders and attendant challenges in place to prevent migration, e.g., US-Mexico border	Extent to which receiving country has historically accepted immigrants
Geographical	Natural disasters, such as floods and hurricanes, resulting in disruption of health-related services, sewage, water supplies, etc.	Natural barriers, e.g. oceans, mountains, deserts, resulting in injury from exposure to elements	Geographical isolation, e.g. rural areas; rapid influx of migrants from rural to urban areas and resulting inadequacy of sewage systems, utilities, and health services; importation of disease from country of origin
Socioeconomic	High prevalence of poverty and unemployment; poor employment and economic prospects	Extent and nature of law enforcement efforts	Level of economy of receiving country; employment opportunities; extent to which ethnic economic networks have been developed
Cultural	Gender norms; health and illness beliefs; value of women and children	Gender norms; language	Gender norms; cultural differences between sending and receiving countries; extent to which homo-ethnic networks exist in receiving country; extent to which immigrants adapt norms of receiving culture and retain norms of original culture
Political	Armed conflict; political tensions between countries	Extent and nature of law enforcement efforts; armed conflict	Level of xenophobia, racism and discrimination in receiving country

relationship between migration, health, and health service utilization. A study conducted among individuals residing in relatively rural, isolated areas along the US-Mexico border found that a large proportion traveled into Mexico for primary care services and for the purchase of prescription medications (Parchman, 2002). Individuals without health insurance and who spoke Spanish were more likely to utilize these cross-border services. Increasingly, health insurance companies in California are offering to pay for the health care services that their US resident insurees obtain in Mexico (Geis, 2005), further reflecting the benefits that geography may bring.

The geographical context may, however, portend disaster as well. The capacity of an area to survive and recover from the effects of a natural disaster is associated with the magnitude of destruction in the specific area and the socioeconomic conditions that prevail there at the time of the disaster (Martine, 1999). Hurricane Mitch is considered to have been the most powerful hurricane to hit Central America and the Caribbean during the last two centuries. The after effects of the storm included a lack of access to drinking water, sanitation, and the deterioration in conditions in health centers, as well as increases in the rates of infectious diseases. The storm's impact fell disproportionately on poor individuals, who suffered a high rate of mortality and were forced to flee their homes. Researchers observed an increase in sexual abuse, sexually transmitted diseases, and unwanted pregnancies as a result of both the diversion of health care services to deal with the emergency and the poor conditions that prevailed in places of shelter (Martine, 1999).

Natural disasters do not occur in a vacuum but within a cultural and socioeconomic context. Their ill effects often fall disproportionately on women, who bear the majority of responsibility for child care and other community and family responsibilities, and on the poor, who may live in more geographically vulnerable areas and less stable housing structures (Hannan, 2002). Because of gender-related constraints, such as lack of decision-making authority, lack of financial and physical capital, and presence of cultural norms relating to mobility, women may be unable to act on advance warnings of the approaching natural disaster. Natural disasters may result in men's migration due to the loss of jobs locally, leading to an increase in *de facto* female-headed households. Women may be forced to spend an increased proportion of their time each day queuing for supplies such as water and food, forcing children to assume the responsibility to care for each other and for any surviving animals, as well as attend to other household tasks (Hannan, 2002).

2.3. Socioeconomic Context

Professionals constitute the largest proportion of economic migrants, and a sizable number of them are health care professionals (World Health Organization, 2003). Although migration is a personal decision, it is heavily influenced by the socioeconomic realities and the lack of opportunities for career advancement in the countries of origin (Bach, 2003).

The importance of the pre-migration socioeconomic context as both a "push" and "pull" factor is reflected in the numbers of health professionals who have left their native countries. Ghana has reported a 72.9% vacancy level for physicians in specialty areas, and Malawi reported a 52.9% vacancy level for nurses (World Health Organization, 2003). Over 70% of graduating nurses in the Philippines leave their country each year, contributing to the annual outflow of 15,000 nurses who migrate to over 30 countries (Adversario, 2003). It has been estimated that there are currently 30,000 unfilled nursing positions in the Philippines due to the emigration of nurses to other countries and the in-country funding shortages (Organisation for Economic Co-operation and Development, 2003).

Many physicians and nurses trained in India also choose to leave their home country to practice their profession elsewhere (Hindu Business Line, 2002; Khadria, 2002). In part, this decision may be premised on the expectation of larger incomes and increased material acquisition associated with life in Western industrialized nations (Mullan, 2006). However, it may also be attributable to the availability of more advanced medical technology and the existence of less chaotic commercial systems in the countries of intended migration (Mullan, 2006).

2.4. Cultural Context

"Culture" has been defined as "a common heritage or set of beliefs, norms, and values" (United States Department of Health and Human Services, 1999). Such a definition gives the impression that culture is something that is static and that resides in the individual, however common the particular values may be. Rather,

" . . . culture is constituted by, and in turn constitutes, local worlds of everyday experience. That is to say, culture is built up ("realized") out of the everyday patterns of daily life activities – common sense, communication with others, and the routine rhythms and rituals of community life that are taken for granted – which reciprocally reflect the patterning downward of social relations by shared symbolic apparatuses – language, aesthetic sensibility, and core value orientations conveyed by master metaphors. In these local worlds, experience is an interpersonal flow of communication, interaction, and negotiation—that is, it is social, not individual—which centers on agreement and contestation about what is most at stake and how that which is at stake is to be sought and gained. Gender, age cohort, social role and status, and personal desire all inflect this small universe in different ways. The upshot is culture in the making, in the processes that generate action and that justify practices. Thus the locus of culture is not the mind of the isolated person, but the interconnected body/self of groups: families, work settings, networks, whole communities." (Kleinman, 1996).

This definition underscores both that culture is a system shared by members of a defined group. Culture consists of elements that comprise "everyday patterns of daily life activities," such as language, diet, patterns of social interaction, health and illness beliefs, religious and spiritual beliefs and traditions, manners of dress, and gender roles, among others. When individuals emigrate from one country to another, they do not leave these aspects of their lives at the border. Rather, they carry their beliefs, knowledge, and practices with them to their new homeland where, to varying degrees, they may preserve, modify, or eliminate them from their every day lives. Consider as an example the impact of health beliefs of several immigrant groups and the impact of such beliefs on illness detection and health care seeking behavior.

In absolute numbers, immigrants from the Philippines and Mexico are the two largest immigrant groups in the United States to develop tuberculosis (TB) (Zuber, McKenna, Binkin, Onorato, & Castro, 1997). Findings from focus groups conducted with Filipino immigrants in California and Hawaii indicate that participants attributed TB to environmental causes, such as cigarettes, alcohol, and unsanitary conditions; to imbalances of the body resulting from overwork, poor nutrition, worrying, and family problems and inheritance; and to contagion through touch, air, and shared utensils (Yamada, Caballero, Matsunaga, Agustin, & Magana, 1999). Although respondents perceived tuberculosis as highly contagious, they believed that medical treatment was not always necessary. In addition to modern medicine, they believed that this highly stigmatizing disease could be treated through improved diet, smoking cessation, improved sanitation, restoration of the body's balance, and the use of traditional medicines. Vietnamese focus group participants in a study based in Orange County, California, drew distinctions between transmissible physical TB, which was found to be similar to Western biomedical knowledge of TB, and non-transmissible psychological TB, characterized by fatigue, lethargy, and a loss of appetite (Houston, Harada, & Makinodan, 2002). These pre-existing conceptualizations of disease and illness may have adversely impacted infected individuals' ability to identify and respond appropriately to illness symptoms that require immediate care and that signal disease transmissibility. As a result, others around them may be at increased risk of disease transmission and the individuals themselves may be at increased risk of adverse consequences resulting from infection.

It is not surprising, therefore, that between 1985 and 1994, 98% of the 3,364 cases of TB reported among Asians in Los Angeles County, California, were among immigrants (Makinodan et al., 1999). The rate per 100,000 foreign-born Asians living in Los Angeles County was 162.1, compared to 2.6 per 100,000 among US-born Asians. In 1997, 39 percent of all TB cases nationally were reported to have occurred in foreign-born persons (Centers for Disease Control and Prevention, 1998). Although these data relate to individuals post-migration, after they have arrived in the US, it is likely that a substantial proportion of these persons had tuberculosis prior to their departure from their countries. Pre-existing health beliefs or availability of screening and care services may have contributed to interpretation of premigration symptoms and disease detection only post-migration.

2.5. Political Context

Political conflict often brings about resulting economic hardship, dislocation, and ill health effects. The disruption occasioned by political factors occurs within a cultural and socioeconomic context, resulting in a disproportionate impact on more vulnerable segments of the society in which it occurs.

Armed conflict may bring military conscription of males within a household, leaving women to cope with decreasing access to food, health care, and other basic goods and services (El Jack, 2003). As communities break down during this process, women may become increasingly vulnerable to domestic violence (United Nations, 2002). Women may be forced to trade sexual "favors" for needed food supplies, leading to an increased risk for HIV and other sexually transmitted infections (Benjamin, 2001; Smith, 2002). Following the cessation of the conflict, the women may be seen as prostitutes who willingly provided these services and may be marginalized by their families and communities as a result. They may be further victimized by increasing violence from their surviving male partners, who suffer from guilt and anger at their own inability to protect them (El Jack, 2002).

The political context in which migration occurs may result in health effects in a much less dramatic way as well. Consider, for instance, the political context of TB control efforts associated with immigration. It has been estimated that over one-third of the world's population is currently infected with TB (World Health Organization, 2006); a single untreated person can infect between 10 and 15 people a year (World Health Organization, 2005b). The disease kills more people every year than any other infectious disease; in fact, someone dies of tuberculosis every 15 seconds (World Health Organization, 2005a,b). There are annually approximately 9 million new cases of tuberculosis and 2 million deaths attributable to tuberculosis worldwide, despite the availability of affordable, effective treatment (Jong-wook, 2006). The vast majority of incident cases occur in various parts of Africa, Asia, and newly formed states of the former Soviet Union. There is a 1 percent rise in tuberculosis cases worldwide each year and an increasing incidence worldwide of drug-resistant tuberculosis (Centers for Disease Control and Prevention, 2006; Jong-wook, 2006; World Health Organization, 2002, 2006). The increasing rates of TB are associated with poverty, an increase in HIV prevalence, falling living standards, and failing public health systems (Almeida & Thomas, 1996; World Health Organization, 2002).

These pre-migration circumstances may be exacerbated prior to migration as the result of inadequate attempts by destination countries to protect their citizens from disease transmission post-migration. As an example, US immigration law excludes from legal entry those seeking admission who have active tuberculosis infection. However, TB screening, to be conducted in the home country by US government-authorized physicians ("panel physicians") prior to the commencement of physical migration, is required primarily for those seeking to immigrate permanently, such as lawful permanent residents ("green card" holders), asylees, refugees, and several other specified groups. The screening requirement does not apply to the vast majority of foreign-born individuals seeking admission to the US each year, such as tourists, students, and business-persons here temporarily. Those who enter illegally circumvent these and all other procedures required for admission. Consequently, the findings of a recent study of culture-positive TB patients in the Dallas-Ft. Worth metroplex area of Texas should not be surprising. Researchers found that a greater proportion of nonimmigrants had multi-drug resistant TB and were HIV-positive, compared to those with permanent resident status (Weis et al., 2001). Similar issues confront other countries, where a large proportion of incident cases of tuberculosis may be attributable to unscreened immigrants arriving from regions of the world that are characterized by a high prevalence of tuberculosis (Aebischer-Perone, Bovier, Pichonnaz, Rochat, & Loutan, 2005).

Even when screening is required, its effectuation may be problematic; inadequacies in the screening process may lead to further health problems during peri- and post-migration. A study among Tibetan immigrants in Minneapolis from 1992 to 1994 found that despite initial screening by US-authorized physicians in India prior to immigration to the US, 51% of the chest radiographs were abnormal (Truong et al., 1997). A comparison with the results from the chest radiograph evaluations conducted in India indicated that 79% of the Tibetans had unchanged readings, and 21% showed evidence of potentially progressive TB. In yet another instance, despite the screening by US government-authorized physicians and treatment administered through a US-monitored TB treatment program in a Thailand refugee camp, between 2004 and the present, 50 Hmong refugees arrived in the US with active TB infection. Five of the 30 individuals who migrated to California were found to be multi-drug resistant (MDR), and of these, at least one had acquired MDR-TB as the result of inappropriate treatment prescribed in this US-monitored treatment program (Centers for Disease Control and Prevention, 2005). Four of the five individuals arrived in California highly infectious, having traveled from their home country to the US via airplane, with the potential to infect others during transit (peri-migration) and following arrival in the US (post-migration).

The process of screening would-be migrants on the basis of health and the issues associated with such screening are not unique to the United States. It has been estimated that at least 60 countries now screen foreign-born visitors for HIV prior to entry across their borders, despite the lack of any evidence to indicate that HIV-infected immigrants create additional risk to native-born populations (World Health Organization, 1994, 2003).

3. Peri-Migration

3.1. Historical Context

Historical context inevitably shapes the conditions under which migration is carried out. There have been numerous historic examples of dramatic and large scale movement between countries that were, to a large extent, facilitated by the host country; think, for example, of western European migration to the United States in the latter part of the 19th century. Conversely, however, historic precedent and circumstance can also conspire to make peri-migration circumstances treacherous and potentially harmful to migrants. For example, the history of migration between the Mexico-US border is fraught with the effects of the two countries' political relations and with the fluctuating views of the US on acceptance or rejection of migrants. By the latter half of the 20th century and the early 21st century, the Mexico-US border had become a near militarized zone, with tremendous effort being expended by the US to control the border and to minimize migration across the border. This has increasingly forced those attempting border crossing to adopt dangerous routes, associated with greater mortality and morbidity.

3.2. Geographical Context

Geographical factors may heighten the health risks of individuals intending to migrate. For example, the current circumstance of migration from Mexico into the US, as part of an increasingly hostile historic trajectory of rejection of possible migrants, as summarized above, involves navigating through polluted waterways, crossing through large desert areas, or traversing major high-volume, high-speed freeways. Not surprisingly, then, increased numbers of injuries and deaths have been reported in recent years among individuals attempting to cross into the United States illegally through the southern border areas of California, Arizona, New Mexico, and Texas. The morbidity and mortality associated with this migration process result from dehydration or hypothermia in the deserts, drownings in waterways, and injuries sustained by smuggled individuals during high speed car maneuvers by traffickers avoiding arrest by law enforcement officers (Cooper, 2005; Franklin, 2005; Marosi, 2005; Schleicher, 2005). The increased health risks associated with the geography of these illegal crossings is further heightened by smugglers' disregard for human life and their focus on economic gain, for instance in May 2003, 17 undocumented immigrants from Mexico and Central America were found asphyxiated in a tractor-trailer holding approximately 100 people that had been abandoned by smugglers in south Texas (Madigan, 2003; Romero, 2003); increasing hostility directed against would-be immigrants by populations along the border; and paramilitary law enforcement activities by civilian groups, such as the Minuteman, that assert their right to bear arms and defend the country from entrants (Schleicher, 2005).

Oceans also present barriers to immigration and may entail increased health risks.. In one example, the Honduran-registered ship, *Golden Venture*, ran aground off the Rockaway Peninsula in Queens, New York, after failing in its attempt to rendezvous with smaller ships to deliver its 289 Chinese passengers illegally to shore (McFadden, 1993). Ten of the passengers died from hypothermia or drowning. Others disappeared after receiving treatment at local hospitals (McFadden, 1993) and some were taken into custody by the immigration authorities.

3.3. Socioeconomic Context

The socioeconomic status within countries that are traversed may indirectly impact the migration process. For instance, individuals who are fleeing their homelands for a place of safety may have to traverse several countries before they reach their intended destination. The intending immigrants may be subjected to violent attacks associated with robbery. Such attacks against individuals crossing the border have, for instance, been documented at the US-Mexico border (Coronado & Orrenius, 2005).

3.4. Cultural Context

Relatively little has been written relating to the impact of culture on the actual process of migration, as distinct from pre-migration, when the individual is in his or her homeland, and post-migration, following the individual's arrival at his or her final destination. It is conceivable, however, that cultural factors may be relevant to this period and its health effects.

Gender norms may impact the migration experience. Women who migrate to a country illegally may be victimized en route more easily than men. Women may have been socialized to seek protection from men, some of whom may not be trustworthy figures. Language differences between those who are migrating and individuals with whom they come into contact may reduce the immigrants' ability to obtain legitimate assistance or to utilize services that may be available.

3.5. Political Context

Individuals who are forcibly displaced during periods of armed conflict may experience significant health effects even as they are in the process of internal migration. Women may be forced to serve in rape camps or provide the occupying forces with sexual services in exchange for food and protection (El Jack, 2003). A study of the effect of forced migration on HIV prevalence in Rwanda found that post-war, the HIV seroprevalence in both rural and urban areas was 11 percent, in contrast with the pre-war level of 1 percent in rural areas (where 95 percent of the population had lived) and 10 percent among pregnant women in urban areas (UNAIDS, 1998). HIV seroprevalence among those who had lived in refugee camps in Tanzania or Zaire was 9 percent, representing a 6- to 8-fold increase in the rates of HIV in the rural areas from which they had been displaced.

Individuals who traverse through one or more countries in their attempts to leave their homeland for their destination country may experience health effects in the intermediate country as a result of the existing political climate. As an example, individuals escaping from violence in their homeland in Central America who intend to seek refuge in Canada must travel through the United States. Recently, there have been efforts in the United States to increase the level of assistance from local police to enforce immigration laws. This would require that local law enforcement officers detain individuals suspected of being in the United States illegally and notify appropriate immigration authorities (Seghetti, Viña, & Ester, 2004). This could result in an erosion of public safety because individuals who are victims of or witnesses to crimes may be unwilling to reports these incidents to the police for fear of being arrested (American Civil Liberties Union, 2003).

4. Post-Migration

4.1. Historical Context

There is some suggestion in the literature that addiction to various substances has been internationalized as the result of migration. Substances traditionally or frequently used in countries of origin have been brought to the new homeland for use or sale. As an example, coca, originally produced and used extensively in Brazil and Peru before the Inca empire, is now widely used in the United States. Smoking tobacco had been grown in the tropical and subtropical regions of the Americas. It was later cultivated by the Spaniards in Santo Domingo, by the Portuguese in Brazil, and by the British in Virginia. Merchants then exported it to European nations. Opium and hashish, once used widely throughout various Asian countries, came to the Americas both via Europe and directly across the Pacific (Berlinguer, 1993).

Various diseases have "migrated" from their places of origin with their hosts to become diseases within the country of immigration. Examples include the introduction of influenza into Santo Domingo by the Spanish in 1493 (Guerra, 1993), the introduction of syphilis from the Americas following the return of Columbus and his crew to Naples in 1494 (Berlinguer, 1993; Curtin, 1993), and the introduction of smallpox into the Americas in 1510 from Africa through the illegal slave trade (Henige, 1986; Lipschutz, 1966; Naranjo, 1992).

4.2. Geographical Context

Although significant research has addressed the geographical context post-migration, relatively little of that research has examined its health implications. The settlement of foreign-born persons in the United States provides an example of the geographical context post-migration and its interplay with other factors.

Approximately 72 percent of foreign-born persons arriving in the US between 1970 and 1980 migrated to six states. One out of every four settled in California (Isserman, 1993). Specific settlement patterns have been linked to various migrant groups. Ninety percent of Mexicans appear to settle in only three states: California, Texas, and Illinois. Twenty-seven percent of European immigrants settle in New York and New Jersey, while almost 40 percent of Asian immigrants to the United States travel to California.

These apparent concentrations of individuals from the same nation is believed to be a function of a desire of displaced persons to recovery their "community," whether in a physical or in a social sense (Shami, 1993). Successive contingents of immigrants from the same country of origin may join already-established communities, where they may be more likely to find employment and mutual support (Allen & Turner, 1996; Portes & Rumbaut, 1990).

4.3. Socioeconomic Context

The economic realities within the countries receiving migrants clearly affect immigrants' ability to obtain needed medical care. As an example, although applicants for asylum in the UK theoretically have free access to the National Health Service, research suggests that there exists a scarcity of government-funded resources for asylum seekers. (Connelly & Schweiger, 2000; Ramsey & Turner, 1993; Woodhead, 2000). Similar difficulties confront undocumented immigrants in Australia, Germany, Spain, and Switzerland (Harris & Telfer, 2001; Scott, 2004; Torres & Sanz, 2000). In Sweden, undocumented immigrants, known as *gömda*, are eligible for only "immediate health care," which refers to urgent care at a hospital emergency department and generally excludes primary health care and maternity care (Medecins Sans Frontieres, 2006). When *gömda* are able to access care, they are confronted with significantly higher charges for the services than would be charged to Swedish nationals. There may be significant interplay between these socioeconomic realities and political factors. In a 2005 study involving 102 *gömda*, 67 percent of the respondents reported a high or very high risk of being arrested if they were to present to a hospital, and this fear deterred them from seeking medical care and treatment for both chronic conditions, such as asthma, and infectious disease, such as tuberculosis (Medecins Sans Frontieres, 2006).

4.4. Cultural Context

Some have suggested that the psychological health of immigrants depends to a large degree on the magnitude of the cultural differences that exists between their country of origin and their adopted country, as well as the extent to which social networks have already been established by others who have immigrated from the same homeland (Akhtar, 1999). "Intramural refueling," whereby new immigrants are supported by a "homo-ethnic community" of co-nationals, occurs through visits to ethnic markets, participation in religious and cultural events, and attendance at cultural and religious centers (Akhtar, 1999).

Immigrants' health may also be affected as they adopt, to varying degrees, behaviors and perspectives of their adopted country's culture. This process of acculturation is "a long-term fluid process in which individuals simultaneously move along at least two cultural continua (or dimensions) and whereby individuals learn and/or modify certain aspects of the new culture and of their culture of origin" (Marin & Gamba, 1996).

As an example, immigrants to Israel display a decreased rate of pancreatic and stomach cancer as compared to their non-immigrating counterparts (Iscovich & Howe, 1998). This has been attributed to post-migration increased consumption of fruits and vegetables and decreased ingestion of highly salted, smoked, and preserved meats. Exposure to a "diabetogenic environment" following immigration has been linked to an increase of type I diabetes among Ethiopian and Yemenite immigrants to Israel (Weintrob et al., 2001; Zung et al., 2004).

Studies of HIV risk within the United States have consistently found that immigrants who are less acculturated to US culture have lower levels of knowledge about HIV risk (Shedlin, Decena, & Oliver-Velez, 2005). However, research suggests that as individuals become more familiar with US norms relating to sexual behavior and substance use, they are more likely to adopt risky behaviors, such as increased substance use and an increased number of sexual partners (Marin & Flores, 1994).

4.5. Political Context

Stigma, racism, xenophobia, and/or discrimination may affect the health of migratory populations (ILO, IOM, & OHCHR, 2001). As an example of a discriminatory action that is both racist and stigmatizing, a hospital located in Texas near the US-Mexico border was alleged to have security personnel wear uniforms similar to those of the US Border Patrol in an effort to discourage Latinos from utilizing hospital services (Perez, 2003). Such an action could well affect immigrants' willingness to access care, regardless of their legal status.

Fear of immigrants may lead to discrimination, which may provide an unspoken motivation for further political actions that may impact the health of the immigrant population and, oftentimes inadvertently, the native population as well. Reforms to the immigration and welfare laws of the United States provide an excellent example of how fears of immigrants and their economic impact may serve as the underlying basis for political action.

On August 22, 1996, the US Congress passed the Personal Responsibility and Work Opportunity Reform Act (PRWORA) and the Illegal Immigration Reform and Responsibility Act (IIRAIRA). PRWORA created two classes of immigrants for the purpose of determining eligibility for publicly funded benefits, including medical care deemed to be of a nonemergency nature, such as prenatal care. The national implementation of this restrictive legislation followed the 1994 attempt of California voters to implement Proposition 187, which would have barred undocumented individuals from utilizing publicly funded benefits, including Medicaid (Palinkas & Arciniega, 1999; Ziv & Lo, 1995). Unlike the California legislation, which was enjoined by the California Supreme Court as unconstitutional, the federal law was successfully implemented.

Pursuant to this federal legislation, immigrants who obtained their legal permanent resident status prior to August 22, 1996, the date of the law's enactment, were to be known as "qualified aliens." Individuals who obtained their legal permanent resident status after the date of enactment were to be classified as "nonqualified aliens." Such individuals were largely ineligible to receive publicly funded benefits, including Medicaid-funded services, for a period of five years following their receipt of their legal status. Exceptions were created for certain classes of immigrants, including refugees, asylum seekers, immigrants with 40 quarters of qualifying work history, and noncitizens who had served in the United States military. Somewhat later, an exception was created for specified noncitizens whose need for publicly funded medical care was attributable to domestic violence. Nonqualified aliens were subject to a deeming requirement, whereby the income of the US citizen or permanent resident individual(s) who sponsored them for immigration would be considered in calculating eligibility for the benefit.

In addition to the restrictions that were imposed on the receipt of benefits by certain legally immigrated individuals, the federal legislation specified that states may not provide nonemergency services to nonqualified aliens, including undocumented persons, without first passing new state legislation providing for the use of state funding for this coverage. Relatively few states have passed such legislation; in those that have, benefits are generally available to only a few, specified classes of particularly disadvantaged and/or vulnerable nonqualified immigrants, such as the disabled, the elderly, victims of torture, pregnant women, and children (National Immigration Law Center, 2002).

The impact of restrictive legislation such as Proposition 187, PRWORA, and IIRAIRA on immigrants' utilization of health services and the health of immigrant communities remains somewhat unclear. Asch and colleagues (1998) reported that the passage of Proposition 187 in California may have discouraged immigrants in Los Angeles County from seeking screening and/or early treatment for tuberculosis infection. Legislation that increases the fear of detection by immigration authorities may exacerbate delays in seeking care for tuberculosis (Asch, Leake, & Gelberg, 1994). Such delays have implications for not only the immigrants who are directly impacted by the legislation, but for others in their communities, as well, due to the manner of tuberculosis transmission.

The passage of Proposition 187 was also found to be associated with a decrease in new walk-in patients at an ophthalmology clinic at a major public inner-city hospital in Los Angeles County (Marx et al., 1996) and a decrease in patients at an STD clinic (Hu et al., 1995). However, Loue and colleagues (2005) found no statistically significant difference in time between onset of gynecological illness and seeking of care or length of time between seeking care and receipt of care among women of Mexican ethnicity of varying immigration status in San Diego County. Another study of immigrants of various nationalities, languages, and immigration status in Cuyahoga County, Ohio, similarly found no effect of the reform laws on immigrants' ability to access care (Loue, Faust, & Bunce, 2000). A high proportion of respondents in this latter study, however, had entered the US as refugees, and as such, they were not subject to the restrictions on their receipt of publicly funded health care.

The effort by the US House of Representatives in 2006 to reform U.S. immigration law has the potential to exacerbate delays in seeking treatment by both documented and undocumented persons and, consequently, may inadvertently facilitate the transmission of communicable diseases in the destination communities. The Border Protection, Antiterrorism, and Illegal Immigration Control Act of 2005, if adopted in its current form, would criminalize the presence of any individual who has entered the country illegally and establish minimum prison sentences for those convicted of being in the country illegally (Sensenbrenner, 2005). Such a provision would likely intensify individuals' fear of detection, leading to increased delays in seeking treatment (Asch et al., 1994). Confinement in prison is also likely to facilitate disease transmission, in view of the substandard medical care that prevails in many of these facilities (Bone et al., 2000).

Reliance on international law as a basis for the provision of medical care to undocumented/irregular migrants is likely to prove futile. Only two international treaties expressly recognize the rights of such persons to health care: the Convention on Migrant Workers (1990) and the Rural Workers' Organizations Convention (1975). Additionally, although the International Convention on the Protection of the Rights of All Migrant Workers and Members of Their Families (1990) assures all immigrant workers and their families the right to emergency medical care, regardless of their legal status, it does not provide for follow-up care or disease prevention for undocumented/irregular persons. Additionally, these treaties are not self-executing, meaning that the signatory countries must take further action within their own borders to implement the treaty provisions.

5. A Case Study of Intersectionality: Trafficking

Trafficking has been defined in a number of ways through various protocols and conventions, as indicated in Table 12.2, below. Although the trafficking of women and children is often associated with sexual exploitation, trafficking does not always result in involuntary sex work. Individuals may be drafted into involuntary servitude in factories, domestic situations, sweat shops, and other commercial enterprises. The lack of international consensus regarding the definition of trafficking limits the effectiveness of international collaborative efforts to halt trafficking in human beings and to protect the health of those who are victimized.

As can be seen from Table 12.2, the concept of trafficking overlaps with that of illegal migration. Some individuals may actively enlist the aid of traffickers to cross into another country. The individuals may be motivated by any number of reasons, such as a search for economic opportunities, flight from persecution and/or torture, or reunification with family members who migrated previously. Regardless of their motive, the trafficked individuals may be caught up in a small- or large-scale enterprise that focuses on the trafficking of human beings as commodities.

5.1. Pre-Migration

5.1.1. The Legal Landscape and Implications for Health

Governments and agencies have adopted varying approaches to trafficking, which have been classified into six distinct perspectives (Foundation of Women's Forum, citing Marjan Wijers, Foundation Against Trafficking in Women, 1998) based upon their views towards trafficking, immigration, and sex work. The perspective that is ultimately adopted by a government or agency may have implications during the pre-, peri-, and/or post-migration phases for the health of both the

TABLE 12.2. Definitions of trafficking.

Use of Definition	Definition of Trafficking
Archivantikul, 1998	A child who is recruited and transported from one place to another across a a national border, legally or illegally, with or without the child's consent, usually but not always organized by an intermediary: parents, family member, teacher, procurer, or local authority. At the destination, the child is coerced or semi-forced (by deceptive information) to engage in activities under exploitative and abusive conditions.
Bangladesh National Women Lawyers Association	All acts involved in the recruitment and/or transport of a woman (or child) within and across national borders for work or services (or marriage) by-means of violence or threat of violence, abuse of authority or dominant position, debt bondage, deception or other forms of coercion (Ali, 1996).
Consultation Workshop of the Resistance Network, Bangladesh, 1999	Trafficking in women consists of all acts involved in the procurement, transportation, forced movement, and/or selling and buying of women within and/or across borders by fraudulent means, deception, coercion, direct and/or indirect threats, abuse of authority, for the purpose of placing a woman against her will without her consent in exploitative and abusive situations such as forced prostitution, forced marriage, bonded and forced labour, begging, organ trade, etc. Trafficking in children consists of all acts involved in the procurement, transportation, forced movement, and/or selling and buying of children within and/or across borders by fraudulent means, deception, coercion, direct and/or indirect threats, abuse of authority, for the purpose of placing a child against his or her will without consent in exploitative and abusive situations, such as commercial sexual abuse, forced marriage, bonded and forced labour, begging, camel jockeying and other sports, organ trade, etc.
Global Alliance against Trafficking in Women	All acts involved in the recruitment and/or transportation of a woman within and across national borders for work or services by means of violence or threat of violence, abuse of authority or dominant position, debt-bondage, deception or other forms of coercion (Archivantikul, 1998).
International Office of Migration (1999)	Trafficking occurs when a migrant is illicitly recruited and/or moved for the purpose of economically or otherwise exploiting the migrant, under conditions that violate their fundamental human rights.
United Nations' Protocol to Prevent, Suppress, and Punish Trafficking in Persons, Especially Women and Children	The recruitment, transportation, transfer, harbouring or receipt of persons, by means of the threat or use of force or other forms of coercion, of abduction, of fraud, of deception, of the abuse of power or of a position of vulnerability . . . or of the giving or receiving of payments or benefits to achieve the consent of a person having control over another person, for the purpose of exploitation. Exploitation shall include, at a minimum, the exploitation of the prostitution of others or other forms of sexual exploitation . . . forced labour or services, slavery or practices similar to slavery, servitude, or the removal of organs (United Nations Office for Drug Control and Crime Prevention, 2000).
US Agency for International Development	The recruitment of girls/women by means of violence or threat, debt bondage, deception or coercion to act as sex workers under menace of penalty and for which the individual has not offered themselves voluntarily (Gazi et al., 2001, quoting Matt Friedman)
US President's Interagency Council on Women	All acts involved in the recruitment, transport, harboring, or sale of persons within national or across international borders through deception or fraud, coercion or force, or debt bondage for purposes of placing persons in situations of forced labor or services, such as forced prostitution or sexual services, domestic servitude, or other forms of slavery-like practices

persons who have been trafficked and individuals with whom they come into contact. These approaches are explicated below:

(a) The moral approach views trafficking as an evil that must be controlled. This approach focuses on the punishment of all parties involved, which may result in the stigmatization and punishment of the victims, as well as the perpetrators.

(b) The criminal approach seeks to improve international police cooperation and increase the effectiveness of prosecutions. This approach subordinates the interests of the trafficked women and children and may result in women being indicted for prostitution and/or illegal entry into the country (Foundation of Women's Forum, citing Marjan Wijers, Foundation Against Trafficking in Women, 1998).

(c) The immigration perspective seeks stricter control of national boundaries and may also seek to regulate marriage between citizens and foreigners. The interests of the state are paramount. Individuals who are voluntarily trafficked may be identified as illegal immigrants and dealt with as illegal entrants pursuant to a country's immigration laws. As an example, although US immigration law offers some potential recourse for individuals who have been involuntarily trafficked and forced into sex work, the interests of the government in controlling the illegal activity are clearly dominant. A maximum of 5,000 "T" visas are available each year to individuals who are or who have been the victim of a severe form of trafficking in persons, are physically present in the United States or various territories, are under the age of 15 or have complied with any reasonable request for assistance in the investigation or prosecution of trafficking, and would suffer extreme hardship involving unusual or severe harm upon removal from the United States (Victims of Trafficking and Violence Protection Act, 2000). This visa allows the individual to remain in the United States only for a temporary period of time. Additionally, even though the issuance of the visa is based on the individual's cooperation in the investigation or prosecution of the trafficking, witness protection is not generally provided to the trafficked individual. The benefit is potentially available only to those who have been involuntarily brought into the country; this does not encompass individuals who were voluntarily smuggled, even though they may have been victimized by their smugglers. Alternatively, a "U" visa, which also allows an individual to remain in the United States only temporarily, is potentially available to up to 10,000 persons each year who have suffered substantial physical or mental abuse as a result of having been the victim of trafficking or various other enumerated offenses; possesses information about the crime; and are, have been, or are likely to be helpful to law enforcement authorities in the investigation or prosecution of the crime, which must have been in violation of US law or committed in the US or a designated territory or possession (Victims of Trafficking and Violence Protection Act, 2000). Again, witness protection is generally unavailable.

(d) The human rights perspective sees prostitution itself or conditions under which women engage in commercial sex work (deceit, abuse, violence, etc.) as violative of human rights.

(e) The public order approach views trafficking as a problem of public order and/ or public health and focuses on control, such as that effectuated through medical examinations, as a solution.

(f) The labor perspective holds that trafficking in women is the result of women's relatively low social and economic status and advocates the establishment of increased economic rights and opportunities for women as a solution (Foundation of Women's Forum, 1998, citing Marjan Wijers, Foundation Against Trafficking in Women).

Only the public order approach is explicitly concerned with the health of those who are trafficked and the communities to which the trafficked persons arrive. While the human rights perspective is concerned with the conditions of commercial sex work and, accordingly, the health implications of such, the remaining approaches focus on issues related to economic, political, and legal concerns; the associated health issues do not warrant attention within these schema.

5.1.2. Other Pre-Migration Factors

Numerous factors, outlined in Table 12.3, may underlie the voluntary or involuntary trafficking of individuals. During the pre-migration stage of the trafficking

TABLE 12.3. Pre-migration factors influencing the incidence of trafficking in women and children.

Factor	Examples
Historical context	Formation of cross-border families due to political divisions between nations, e.g. U.S-Mexico, Pakistan-India, and frequent cross-border traffic for commercial reasons (Gazi et al., 2001)
Geographical context	Natural disasters such as flooding or drought, leading to increased poverty, separation of families and search for employment (Gazi et al., 2001)
Socioeconomic context	High prevalence of poverty leading to search for employment outside of country, sale of children by families; high prevalence of female-headed households; low levels of education limiting economic opportunities (Gazi et al., 2001); difficulty accessing the formal labor market in country of immigration (International Organization for Migration, 2003)
Cultural context	Cultural norms promoting early and arranged marriage of girls; vulnerability of women to abuse/sale by relatives due to dissatisfaction with bridal dowry (Nagi, 1993); stigma and ostracism of women who have been deserted or divorced by their husbands; mores dictating female dependency on men; desire of migrant men abroad for sex workers with common cultural and linguistic background (Gazi et al., 2001); sexual harassment and demanded sexual favors in the workplace making payment for sex a desirable alternative (Foundation of Women's Forum, 1998)
Political context	Collapse of the Soviet Union with resulting economic hardships and dislocation (Cwikel et al., 2004; Foundation of Women's Forum, 1998); corruption of law enforcement personnel, facilitating trafficking; lack of shelter and support for women in distress (Gazi et al., 2001); illegality of prostitution and probable prosecution and/or deportation of trafficking victims for legal and/or immigration violations (International Organization for Migration, 2003)

process, the situations of those who will be trafficked are often characterized by poverty or disrupted relationships (Zimmerman et al., 2003).

5.2. Peri-Migration

The peri-migration stage spans the period from the individual's voluntary or involuntary departure with a trafficker to his or her arrival at the destination. During this stage, individuals may experience a variety of adverse health consequences, including accidental or intentional injury, communicable disease, hypothermia, and even death. These conditions may result from the process of immigration itself, which is often effectuated through reliance on dangerous modes of transportation that have been designed to evade discovery.

5.3. Post-Migration

The post-migration stage begins when the individual arrives at the location where he or she is put to work. The period extends through custody by legal authorities, if that should occur, and/or integration into the destination site and re-integration upon return to the country of origin.

During this period, the individual may be the target of coercion, violence, exploitation, debt-bondage, or other forms of abuse. He or she may be subjected to physical violence, deprivation of food, human contact, and valued items. The individual may be held in solitary confinement, forced to use drugs and/or alcohol, and deprived of earnings. Adverse health consequences may include traumatic injury, depression, posttraumatic stress disorder, unwanted pregnancy, sexually transmitted infections, and involuntary sterilization (World Health Organization, 2003). During custody by law enforcement authorities, individuals are rarely provided with health assistance, and the conditions in which they are held are often inadequate.

Consider, as an example, the situation of those held in forced labor in the United States. Forced labor has been found to exist in at least 90 cities and is most prevalent in five sectors of the economy: prostitution and sex services (Luna & Tran, 2004; McCormick & Zamora, 2000; Pacenti, 1998; United States Department of Justice, 2003b), domestic service, agriculture (Greenhouse, 2002; United States Department of Justice, 2002, 2003a; Viotti, 2003), factory/sweatshop work, and restaurant and hotel work. Forced labor operations are concentrated in the states of California, Florida, New York, and Texas. Between 2000 and 2005, the press reported 131 cases of forced labor involving 19,254 men, women, and children, most of whom were immigrants (Free the Slaves and the Human Rights Center of the University of California, Berkeley, 2005). Although victims of forced labor came from 39 countries as of December 2003, the majority came from China, Mexico, and Vietnam (Free the Slaves and the Human Rights Center of the University of California, Berkeley, 2005).

The trafficking of human beings for the purpose of forced labor continues due to a variety of factors that exist at the US destination. In the case of forced labor in the sex industries, these conditions include ties to organized crime; the absence of safe, legal, and timely mechanisms for immigration to the US; and a demand for cheap sexual services (Free the Slaves and the Human Rights Center of the University of California, Berkeley, 2005). A desire for cheap services similarly drives the demand for forced labor in the domestic, agricultural, and factory service sectors. In addition, within the domestic and agricultural sectors, legal protections for workers are weak, and there is inadequate monitoring of work conditions. Manufacturers may operate within the informal economy and attempt to evade the enforcement of US labor laws.

The largest concentrations of trafficking survivors who have received federal assistance are located in California, Oklahoma, Texas, and New York (United States Department of Justice, 2004). The majority of these individuals are originally from India, Vietnam, Indonesia, Tonga, Zambia, and Thailand (United States Department of Justice, 2004). Reports from survivors detail forced prostitution, the commercial exploitation of children, and the use by captors of violent beatings, withdrawal of food, and attacks by dogs as means of exerting control (Free the Slaves and the Human Rights Center of the University of California, Berkeley, 2005). Although the health effects of these conditions have not been well-documented, it is believed that survivors suffer from a broad range of adverse health effects that include physical injury and disability from beatings, post-traumatic stress disorder and other mental health conditions, and infectious diseases that include hepatitis B and C, HIV, and other sexually transmitted diseases (Free the Slaves and the Human Rights Center of the University of California, Berkeley, 2005).

6. Future Directions

A substantial body of literature exists pertaining to the health status of immigrants in their adopted countries, the differences in health status existing between those who have migrated and those who remained in their countries of origin, and risk factors for specific illnesses and syndromes within immigrant populations. However, relatively little research has focused on the health effects resulting from the interplay of macrosocial factors within the context of migration. Even for human trafficking, which has been the focus of substantial research efforts, we know little about this interaction during the actual transit process.

This chapter provides a framework for the conduct of such research throughout the process of migration, beginning prior to the point of departure (pre-migration), through the transit period (peri-migration), until arrival at the destination country (post-migration). Examples have been provided to demonstrate the interplay of migration with various macrosocial factors to ultimately impact, either directly or indirectly, the health of the migrating individuals or those with whom they come into contact. We suggest that this framework can be used to guide further research into the influence of particular elements of the immigration experience and circumstance. This will allow greater understanding of the impact that migration has on population health (of both host and country of origin) and will help to illuminate possible avenues for intervention.

References

Adversario, S. (2003). Nurses' exodus making health system ill. Inter press service. Manilla, Philippines (May 15, 2003); http://www.ipsnews.net.

Aebischer-Perone, S., Bovier, P., Pichonnaz, C., Rochat, T., & Loutan, L. (2005). Tuberculosis in undocumented migrants, Geneva [letter]. *Emerging Infectious Diseases* *11*(2), 351–352.

Akhtar, S. (1999). *Immigration and identity: Turmoil, treatment, and transformation.* Northvale, NJ: Jason Aronson Publishers.

Ali, S. (1996). Trafficking in Commercial Sexual Exploitation in Prostitution and Other Intolerable Forms of Child Labour in Bangladesh: Country Report. Dhaka: Bangladesh National Women Lawyers Association.

Allen, J. P., & Turner, E. (1996). Spatial patterns of immigrant assimilation. *Professional Geographer, 48,* 140–155.

Almeida, M. D., & Thomas, J. E. (1996). Nutritional consequences of migration. *Scandinavian Journal of Nutrition, 40*(2 Supplement 31), 119–121.

American Civil Liberties Union. (2003). ACLU statement on H.R. 2671, the "Clear law Enforcement for Criminal Alien Removal (CLEAR) Act of 2003" before the House Subcommittee on Immigration, Border Security and Claims. New York (October 1, 2003); http://www.aclu.org/immigrants/gen/11793leg20031001.html.

Archivantikul, K. (1998). *Trafficking in children for labour exploitation including child prostitution in the Mekong Sub-Region (dissertation).* Bangkok, Thailand: Institute for Population and Social Research, Mahidol University.

Asch, S., Leake, B., Abderson, R., & Gelberg, L. (1998). Why do symptomatic patients delay obtaining care for tuberculosis? *American Journal of Respiratory and Critical Care Medicine, 157,* 1244–1248.

Asch, S., Leake, B., & Genlberg, L. (1994). Does fear of immigration authorities deter tuberculosis patients from seeking care? *Western Journal of Medicine, 161*(4), 373–376.

Bach, S. (2003). *International migration of health workers: Labour and social issues.* Geneva: International Labour Office.

Benjamin, J. A. (2001). Conflict, post-conflict, and HIV/AIDS – the gender connections: Women, war and HIV/AIDS: West Africa and the Great Lakes. Women's Commission for Refugee Women and Children. (March 8, 2001); http://www.rhrc.org/resources/sti/benjamin.html.

Berlinguer, G. (1993). The interchange of disease and health between the old and new worlds. *International Journal of Health Services, 23,* 703–715.

Bone, A., Aerts, A., Grzemska, M., Kimerling, M., Levy, M., Portaels F., et al. (2000). *Tuberculosis control in prisons: A manual for programme managers.* Geneva, Switzerland: World Health Organization, International Committee of the Red Cross.

Centers for Disease Control and Prevention. (1998). Recommendations for prevention and control of tuberculosis among foreign-born persons: Report of the Working Group on Tuberculosis among Foreign-Born Persons. *Morbidity and Mortality Weekly Report, 47,* 1–26.

Centers for Disease Control and Prevention. (2005). Multidrug-resistant tuberculosis in Hmong refugees resettling from Thailand into the United States, 2004–2005. *Morbidity and Mortality Weekly Report, 54,* 741–744.

Centers for Disease Control and Prevention. (2006). Emergence of mycobacterium tuberculosis with extensive resistance to second-line drugs—worldwide, 2002–2004. *Morbidity and Mortality Weekly Report, 55*, 301–305.

Connelly, J., & Schweiger, M. (2000). The health risks of the UK's new Asylum Act: The health of asylum seekers must be closely monitored by service providers. *British Medical Journal, 321*, 5–6.

Cooper, M. (2005, May 24). Twelve die on the US border. *The Nation.*

Coronado, R., & Orrenius, P. M. (2005). *The effect of undocumented immigration and border enforcement on crime rates along the U.S.-Mexico border.* El Paso, Texas: Federal Reserve Bank of Dallas.

Council of Europe, Parliamentary Assembly. (2001). Health conditions of migrants and refugees in Europe: Report of the Committee on Migration, Refugees and Demography. (March 14, 2001);
http://www.refugeelawreader.org/686/Recommendation_1503_2001_on_Health_Conditions_of_Migrants_and_Refugees_in_Europe.pdf.

Curtin, P. D. (1993). Disease exchange across the tropical Atlantic. *History, Philosophy and Life Science, 15*, 329–356.

Cwikel, J., Chudakov, B., Paikin, M., Agmon, K., & Belmaker, R.H. (2004). Trafficked female sex workers awaiting deportation: Comparison with brothel workers. Archives of Women's Mental Health 7: 243–249

Eisenstadt, S. N. (1955). *The absorption of immigrants.* Glencoe, Il: Free Press.

El Jack, A. (2002). Gender perspectives on the management of small arms and light weapons in the Sudan. In V. Farr & K. Gebre-Wold (Eds.). *Gender perspectives on small arms and light weapons: Regional and international concerns, Brief 24.* Bonn: Bonn International Center for Conversion.

El Jack, A. (2003). *Gender and armed conflict: Overview report.* Brighton, UK: Institute of Development Studies, University of Sussex.

Foundation of Women's Forum/Stiftelsen Kvinnoforum / Northvegr Félag. *(1998). Trafficking in women for the purpose of sexual exploitation: Mapping the situation and existing organisations in Baelarus, Russia, the Baltic and Nordic States.* Stockholm, Sweden: Foundation of Women's Forum/Stiftelsen Kvinnoforum.

Franklin, S. (2005, August 24). Opportunity—and death—await migrants at U.S. border. *Chicago Tribune.*

Free the Slaves, & Human Rights Center of the University of Berkeley, California (2005). Hidden slaves: Forced labor in the United States. *Berkeley Journal of International Law, 23*, 47–110.

Gazi, R., Chowdhury, Z.H., Alam, S. M. N., Chowdhury, E., Ahmed, F., & Begum, S. (2001). *Trafficking of women and children in Bangladesh: An overview.* Dhaka, Bangladesh: ICDDR,B: Centre for Health and Population Research.

Geis, S. (2005, November 6). Passport to health care at lower cost to patient. *Washington Post*, p. A03.

Greenhouse, S. (2002, June 21). Migrant-camp operators face forced labor charges. *New York Times.*

Guerra, F. (1993). The European-American exchange. *History, Philosophy and Life Sciences 15*, 313–327.

Hannan, C. (2002). Mainstreaming gender perspectives in environmental management and mitigation of natural disasters. Presented at United Nations Division for the Advancement of Women and the NGO Committee on the Status of Women, 46th Session of the Commission on the Status of Women, United Nations. (January 17, 2002); http://www.un.org/womenwatch/osagi/pdf/presnat%20disaster.PDF.

Harris, M. F., & Telfer, B. L. (2001). The health needs of asylum seekers living in the community. *The Medical Journal of Australia, 175*, 589–592.

Henige, D. (1986). When did smallpox reach the New World (and why does it matter?). In A. E. Lovejoy (Ed.), *Africans in bondage*. Madison, WI: University of Wisconsin.

Hindu Business Line. (2002). U.S. hospitals scouting for Indian nurses. Bangalore (August 2, 2002); http://blonnet.com/bline/2002/08/03/stories/2002080302191700.htm.

Houston, R. K., Harada, N., & Makinodan, T. (2002). Development of a culturally sensitive educational intervention program to reduce the high incidence of tuberculosis among foreign-born Vietnamese. *Ethnicity and Disease, 7*(4), 255–265.

Hu, Y., Donovan, S., Ford, W., Courtney, K., Rulnick, S., & Richwald, S. (1995). The impact of Proposition 187 on the use of public health services by undocumented immigrants in Los Angeles County [abstract 1008]. 123rd Meeting of the American Public Health Association Meeting.

International Convention on the Elimination of All Forms of Racial Discrimination. (1965). G.A. res. 2106 (XX), Annex, 20 U.N. GAOR Supp. (No. 14) at 47, U.N. Doc. A/6014 (1966), 660 U.N.T.S. 195, *entered into force* Jan. 4, 1969.

International Labour Office, International Organization for Migration, Office of the United Nations High Commissioner for Human Rights. (2001). International migration, racism, discrimination, and xenophobia. Geneva: United Nations.

International Organisation for Migration. (2003). *World migration report*. Geneva: International Organisation for Migration.

Iscovich, J., & Howe, G. R. (1998). Cancer incidence patterns (1972–91) among migrants from the Soviet Union to Israel. *Cancer Causes and Control, 9*, 29–36.

Isserman, A. M. (1993). United States immigration policy and the industrial heartland: Laws, origins, settlement patterns and economic consequences. *Urban Studies, 30*, 237–265.

Jong-wook, L. (2006). *Global plan to stop TB*. Geneva, Switzerland: World Health Organization.

Khadria, B. (2002). Skilled labour migration from developing countries: Study of India. [International Migration Papers No. 49]. Geneva: International Labour Organisation.

Kleinman, A. (1996). How is culture important for DSM-IV? In J. E. Mezzich, A. Kleinman, H. Fabrega, Jr., & D. L. Parron (Eds.), *Culture & psychiatric diagnosis: A DSM-IV perspective*. Washington, DC: American Psychiatric Press, Inc.

Knafo, D., & Yaari, A. (1997). Leaving the promised land: Israeli immigrants in the United States. In P. Elovitz & C. Khan (Eds.), Chapters in immigrant experiences. Madison, NJ: Fairleigh Dickinson.

Lee, E. (1966). A theory of migration. *Demography, 3*, 47–57.

Lipschutz, A. (1996). La despoblacion de las Indias despues de la conquista. *America Indigena, 26*, 229–247.

Loue, S., Cooper, M., & Lloyd, L. S. (2005). Welfare and immigration reform and use of prenatal care among women of Mexican ethnicity in San Diego, California. *Journal of Immigrant Health, 7*(1), 37–44.

Loue, S., Faust, M., & Bunce, A. (2000). The effect of immigration and welfare reform legislation on immigrants' access to health care, Cuyahoga and Lorain Counties. *Journal of Immigrant Health, 2*, 23–30.

Loughna, S. (n.d.). What is forced migration? Oxford, UK; http://www.forcedmigration.org/whatisfm.htm.

Luna, C., & Tran, M. (2004, February 13). Arrest in sex slave case. *Los Angeles Times*.

Madigan, N. (2003, May 17). 2nd group of trapped people is found in a truck in Texas. *New York Times*, p. A13.

Majumder, S., & Jolly, A. (2003, June 6). Muslims look to end misery of separation. *BBC News.*

Makinodan, T., Liu, J., Yumo, E., Knowles, L. K., Davidson, P. T., & Harada, N. (1999). Profile of tuberculosis among foreign-born Asians residing in Los Angeles County, California, 1985–1994. *Asian American Pacific Islander Journal of Health, 7*(1), 38–46.

Mangalam, J. J. (1968). *Human migration: A guide to migration literature in English 1955–1962.* Lexington, KY: University of Kentucky.

Marin, B. V., & Flores, E. (1994). Acculturation, sexual behavior, and alcohol use among Latinas. *International Journal of the Addictions, 29,* 1101–1114.

Marin, G., & Gamba, R. J. (1996). A new measurement of acculturation for Hispanics: The Bidimensional Acculturation Scale for Hispanics. *Hispanic Journal of Behavioral Sciences, 18,* 297–316.

Marosi, R. (2005, October 1). Border crossing deaths set a 12-month record. *Los Angeles Times.*

Martine, G. (1999). Population, poverty and vulnerability: Mitigating the effects of natural disasters, Part I. (December, 1999); http://www.fao.org/sd/wpdirect/wpan0042.htm.

Marx, J. L., Thach, A. B., Grayson, G., Lowry, L. P., Lopez, P. F., & Lee, P. P. (1996). The effects of California Proposition 187 on an ophthalmology clinic utilization at an inner-city urban hospital. *Ophthalmology, 103,* 847–851.

McCormick, E., & Zamora, J.H. (2000, February 13). Slave trade still alive in US: Exploited women, children trafficked from poorest nations. *San Francisco Examiner.*

McFadden, R. D. (1993, June 7). Smuggled to New York: The overview—7 die as crowded immigrant ship grounds off Queens. *New York Times.*

Medecins Sans Frontieres. (2006). *Experiences of Gömda in Sweden: Exclusion from health care for immigrants living without legal status.* Stockholm, Sweden: Medecins Sans Frontieres.

Mullan, F. (2006). Doctors for the world: Indian physician emigration. *Health Affairs, 25,* 380–393.

Nagi, B. S. (1993). *Child marriage in India.* New Delhi, India: Mittal Publications.

Naranjo, P. (1992). Epidemic hecatomb in the new world. *Allergy Proceedings, 13,* 237–241.

National Immigration Law Center. (2002). *Guide to immigrant eligibility for federal programs.* Los Angeles, California: National Immigration Law Center.

Organisation for Economic Co-operation and Development. (2003). *Trends in international migration: Annual report, 2002 Edition.* Paris: Organisation for Economic Co-operation and Development.

Pacenti, J. (1998, February 25). Enslaved women in Florida ring. *Laredo Morning Times,* p. 2A.

Palinkas, L. A., & Arciniega, J. L. (1999). Immigration reform and the health of Latino immigrants in California. *Journal of Immigrant Health, 1,* 19–30.

Parchman, M. (2002). *Cross-border utilization of health care on the U.S.-Mexico border.* Washington, DC: Unpublished presentation at the 2002 Annual Meeting of the Academy for Health Services Research and Health Policy.

Perez, T. E. (2003). The civil rights dimension of racial and ethnic disparities. In B. D. Smedley, A. Y. Stith, & A. R. Nelson, (Eds.), *Unequal treatment: confronting racial and ethnic disparities in health care.* Washington, DC: National Academies Press.

Personal Responsibility and Work Opportunity Reconciliation Act. (1996). Public Law Number 104–193.

Portes, A., & Rumbaut, R. G. (1990). *Immigrant America: A portrait*. Berkeley, CA: University of California Press.

Ramsey, R., & Turner, S. (1993). Refugees' health needs. *British Journal of General Practice, 43*, 480–481.

Romero, S. (2003, May 16). Scene of horror and despair in trailer. *New York Times*, p. A20.

Schleicher, A. (2005, April 6). Civilian military patrol U.S.-Mexico border. Public Broadcast Service.

Scott, P. (2004). Undocumented migrants in Germany and Britain: The human "rights" and "wrongs" regarding access to health care. *Electronic Journal of Sociology*. (2004); http://www.sociology.org/content/2004/tier2/scott.html.

Seghetti, L. M., Viña, S. R., & Ester, K. (2004). *Enforcing immigration law: The role of state and local law enforcement*. Washington, DC: Congressional Research Service, Library of Congress.

Sensenbrenner, J. (2005). Border protection, antiterrorism, and Illegal immigration control act of 2005. H.R. 4437, 109th Cong. United States House of Representatives.

Shami, S. (1993). The social implications of population displacement and resettlement: An overview with a focus on the Arab Middle East. *International Migration Review, 27*, 4–33.

Shedlin, M. G., Decena, C. U., & Oliver-Velez, D. (2005). Initial acculturation and HIV risk among new Hispanic immigrants. *Journal of the National Medical Association, 97*(7 supplement), 32S–37S.

Smith, A. (2002). *HIV/AIDS and emergencies: Analysis and recommendations for practice*. London: Overseas Development Institute.

Torres, A. M., & Sanz, B. (2000). Health care provision for illegal immigrants: Should public health be concerned? *Journal of Epidemiology and Community Health, 54*, 478–479.

Truong, D. H., Hedemark, L. L., Mickman, J. K., Mosher, L. B., Dietrich, S. E., & Lowry, P. W. (1997). Tuberculosis among Tibetan immigrants from India and Nepal in Minnesota, 1992–1995. *Journal of the American Medical Association, 277*(9), 735–738.

UNAIDS. (1998). *AIDS epidemic update: December 1998*. Geneva, Switzerland: UNAIDS and World Health Organization.

United Nations. (2002). *Women, peace, and security*. Geneva: United Nations.

United Nations Office for Drug Control and Crime Prevention. (2000). *The protocol to prevent, suppress, and punish trafficking in persons, especially women and children*. Geneva: United Nations.

United States Department of Health and Human Services. (1999). *Mental health: A report of the Surgeon General*. Rockville, MD: United States Department of Health and Human Services.

United States Department of Justice. (2002). Six indicted in conspiracy for trafficking and holding migrant workers in conditions of forced labor in New York. Washington, DC (June 19, 2002); http://www.usdoj.gov/opa/pr/2002/June/02_crt_360.htm

United States Department of Justice. (2003a). Jury convicts New Hampshire couple of forced labor. Washington, DC (September 2, 2003); http://www.usdoj.gov/opa/pr/2003/September/03_crt_481.htm

United States Department of Justice. (2003b). Leader of Ukrainian alien smuggling operation sentenced to 17–1/2 years in federal prison. (March 10, 2003); http://www.usdoj.gov/usao/cac/pr2003/041.htm.

United States Department of Justice. (2004). Report to Congress from Attorney John Ashcroft on U.S. government efforts to combat trafficking in persons in fiscal year 2003. Washington, DC; http://www.usdoj.gov/ag/speeches/2004/050104agreporttocongresstvprav10.pdf

Victims of Trafficking and Violence Protection Act. (2000). Pub. L. No. 106–386, Div. A; 114 Stat. 1464, Oct. 28.

Viotti, V. (2003, June 14). Waipahu man accused of human trafficking. *Honolulu Advertiser.*

Weintrob, N., Sprecher, E., Israel, S., Pinhas-Hamiel, O., Kwon, O.J., Bloch, K., et al. (2001). Type I diabetes environmental factors and correspondence analysis of HLA class II genes in the Yemenite Jewish community in Israel. *Diabetes Care, 24*(4), 650.

Weis, S. E., Moonan, P. K., Pogoda, J. M., Turk, L., King, B., Freeman-Thompson, S., et al. (2001). Tuberculosis in the foreign-born population of Tarrant County, Texas by immigration status. *American Journal of Respiratory Critical Care Medicine, 164*, 953–957.

Woodhead, D. (2000). *The health and wellbeing of asylum seekers and refugees.* London: King's Fund.

World Health Organization. (1994). Report of the preparatory meeting for a consultation on long-term travel restrictions and HIV/AIDS, Global Programme on AIDS, October 4–6, Geneva, Switzerland.

World Health Organization. (2002). *WHO Report 2002: Global tuberculosis control.* Geneva: World Health Organization.

World Health Organization. (2003). *International migration, health, & human rights.* Geneva: World Health Organization.

World Health Organization. (2005a). *Genes and human disease.* Geneva: World Health Organization.

World Health Organization. (2005b). *Stop TB Partnership: Annual report 2004.* Geneva: World Health Organization.

World Health Organization. (2006). *Fact sheet no. 104: Tuberculosis.* Geneva: World Health Organization.

World Health Organization. (2006). *The world health report 2006: Working together for health.* Switzerland: World Health Organization.

Yamada, S., Caballero, J., Matsunaga, D. S., Augustin, G., & Magana, M. (1999). Attitudes towards tuberculosis in immigrants from the Philippines to the United States. *Family Medicine, 31*(7), 477–482.

Yamamoto, J., Niem, T.T., Nguyen, D., & Snodgrass, L. (1989). Post traumatic stress disorder in Vietnamese refugees. Unpublished manuscript, University of California Los Angeles, School of Medicine, Neuropsychiatric Institute.

Zimmerman, C., Yun, K., Schvab, I., Watts, C., Trappolin, L., Treppete, M., et al. (2003). *The health risks and consequences of trafficking in women and adolescents. Findings from a European study.* London: London School of Hygiene & Tropical Medicine (LSHTM).

Ziv, T. A., & Lo, B. (1995). Denial of care to illegal immigrants, Proposition 187 in California. *New England Journal of Medicine, 332*(16), 1095–1098.

Zuber, P. L. F., McKenna, M. T., Binkin, N. J., Onorato, I. M., & Castro, K. (1997). Long-term risk of tuberculosis among foreign-born people in the United States. *Journal of the American Medical Association, 278*, 304–307.

Zung, A., Elizur, M., Weintrob, N., Bistritzer, T., Hanukoglu, A., Zadik, Z., et al. (2004). Type I diabetes in Jewish Ethiopian immigrants in Israel: HLA class II immunogenetics and contribution of new environment. *Human Immunology, 65*(12), 1463–1468.

Chapter 13
Mass Media

K. Viswanath, Shoba Ramanadhan, and Emily Z. Kontos

1. Introduction

Mass media are among the most important mechanisms of integration into a society and its culture. They offer information, entertainment, persuasion, and cultural transmission. For good or ill, media help define our worldviews, knowledge, and behaviors as individuals and our actions as social actors. Often, the impact of media is discussed in the context of individuals; however, media both influence and are influenced by social groups, institutions, and social contexts such as neighborhoods, communities and nation-states.

Mass media are influential because of their extensive reach and the cumulative effects of exposure to media messages over time. Media institutions are organized and structured to reach the largest number of people at the same time with similar messages. Thus, media have power that is arguably unrivalled by other institutions, even family or religious organizations. Media influence on our worldviews in the realms of religion, politics, family, education, and health spans across both personal and public lives. Impacts on population health can occur either through deliberate efforts by public health agencies to communicate about risks, prevention and treatments, or through routine use of media for news or entertainment.

Clearly, an understanding of media influence on population health requires a delineation of both how media shape individual health and social context as well as the macrosocial forces that shape that influence. Additionally, a focus on media impact on social actors and public policy is imperative. This chapter provides an overview of how media influence population health by (a) identifying the four broad ways in which health communication can influence public health, (b) defining mass media and describing the organization and structure of mass media, (c) discussing examples of effects of mass media exposure on public health, and (d) delineating the relationship between communication inequalities and health disparities. The chapter closes with a brief discussion of the implications for public health practice and policy.

2. Why Communication Matters for Health

As mentioned above, media can affect population health through proactive communication efforts by public health institutions or through regular media use for news or entertainment. It is possible to categorize the mechanisms by which this occurs through the four functions of communication in health: informational, instrumental, social control and communal (Viswanath, 2006). Media and other channels serve the *informational* function by providing information about various aspects of health along the prevention-treatment continuum, promoting awareness and knowledge. These functions are routinely performed when news stories cover discovery of new drugs, novel treatments, or even risk factors. Local television news programs often have segments providing snippets of information and "tips" on various health issues. Both routine use of media as well purposive information seeking may lead to information gain by the audience. The literature clearly documents individuals' abilities to develop ideas about health while using the media (Hornik, 2002a; Institute of Medicine & Committee on Communication for Behavior Change in the 21st Century: Improving the Health of Diverse Populations, 2002; Robinson & Levy, 1986; Tichenor, Donohue, & Olien, 1980; Viswanath & Finnegan, 2002).

Both in times of crises as well as in ordinary times, media provide information that allows for action, characterized as the *instrumental* function. This has also been called "mobilizing information" by some (Lemert, 1981). In a health application, it may include announcement of dates, times, and places for screening, vaccination, or free clinics. Alternately, media may alert the public to contamination of local drinking water supply, levels of heat and humidity, or food contamination and provide advice on preventive actions. The instrumental function of media offers information that is practical and directly leads to action on the part of the audience.

The *social control* function of media has been well-documented (Demers & Viswanath, 1999; Gitlin, 2003; Tichenor, Donohue, & Olien, 1980). In this case, media define the parameters of debate, social norms and acceptable behaviors. The social control function has been a critical function in health promotion, for example, in changing social norms around binge drinking (Wechsler, Nelson, Lee, Seibring, Lewis, & Keeling, 2003), discouraging tobacco use (Gilpin, Emery, White, & Pierce, 2003), or encouraging seatbelt use. The social control function includes elements of coercion, though media typically soften the coercion through ideological acceptance.

Last, the *communal function* of media includes building a sense of community, social connectedness, norms of reciprocity, and access to social capital (Berkman, 1986; Demers, 1996; Friedland & McLeod, 1999; Kawachi, 1999; Kawachi & Berkman, 2000; Putnam, 2000; Viswanath, Randolph Steele, & Finnegan, 2006). Media use, particularly of local media, engenders a spirit of connectedness and identification with the local community, allowing for social action in pursuit of health.

3. What are Mass Media and How do They Work?

Understanding of the role of media in public health necessitates a precise definition of what media are. Mass media are organizations explicitly structured and organized to create, or gather, generate, and disseminate, news and entertainment through such different media as print, radio, television, the Internet, and more recently, through new technologies such as iPods and cell phones. Unlike other communication interactions, communication among family members or friends, for example, mass media refer explicitly to *organized* entities that generate and disseminate information.

Two features are worth noting here. One, the term "mass media" is somewhat misleading as it may imply anonymous organizations disseminating information to vast undifferentiated audiences, information that is often a product of creativity by artists. In reality, mass media are like any industry, with well-defined organizational structure, logic, rules, and processes. Of course, certain processes and structures are unique to the media, but like any other for-profit corporate entity, media are subject to the economic logic of generating a product efficiently and making profits.

Two, it is more fruitful and accurate to discuss the "mass media industry," taking into account the ecology of media, to understand the nature of ultimate products such as news, entertainment (movies, television shows, features), advertisements, and public relations output, including news releases and corporate communications outreach to external audiences (Ettema & Whitney, 1994). This calls for an "institutional conception" of mass media, in which different segments of the communication industry exist in a symbiotic relationship and interact with each other to market products to different audiences (Ettema & Whitney, 1994). For example, the delivery of news, irrespective of channels of delivery –newspaper, television and the Internet – requires the collaboration and cooperation among generators of news, such as spokespersons of government organizations and agencies (e.g. department of public health), public relations agencies or spokespersons (e.g. media relations department of a beverage company), reporters and editors within the news medium, and advertisers and advertising agencies who subsidize the production of media by buying space and time. That is, while the consumer of news is important and vital, news itself is a product of a sophisticated organization of different media industries.

Given the tremendous complexity, it is easy to despair on how to "capture" the media industry and understand its influence on population health. For the purposes of this chapter, we focus on media products, such as news and entertainment (movies and television), generated within well-defined organizations with clear hierarchies, rules and processes.

3.1. Mass Media Organizations: Structure, Occupational Practices and Routines

The impact of media on health is primarily due to the resonance of the symbolic nature of their products with contemporary culture. It is therefore critical to develop an appreciation for the organizational and corporate context in which the media products are generated in order to understand how they could in turn influence public health.

Specialization of function and structure is a particularly important characteristic of media organizations. News media are organized into editorial and business divisions, with the editorial side focusing on news and the business side focusing on advertising and marketing. Television may have additional sections focusing on procuring entertainment. The structure of other agencies, such as public relations and advertising, is also specialized by functions such as client service, creative departments to develop the products, and media selection and placement, among others. In short, the sociological study of the media industry offers a sound understanding of the organization of routines that could potentially influence the output – news, entertainment and advertising.

Within the media organizations, despite the seemingly creative nature of their products (TV shows, for example), the occupational routines are well defined and designed to generate the media products efficiently. The occupational practices of journalists, a well-studied area of media sociology (Shoemaker & Reese, 1996), serve as a good illustration of this approach. Newsrooms are organized to collect information, package it, and disseminate it in the form of news stories. News collection is organized along a "beat system," either along geographic lines, such as the White House, the office of the Surgeon General, the National Institutes of Health or the local department of public health, or along subject areas, such as crime, health, sports, or a combination. Depending on the size of the news organization or the market, each beat may have a reporter or a group of reporters who gather information. Often, in smaller media, a reporter may cover more than one beat or act as a "generalist," covering a variety of stories. Thus, specialization is a function of size. News stories written by reporters are copy edited by copy desk personnel who customize them and truncate them to fit the day's news "budget" (allocation of space or time). The newsrooms are supervised by managing editors of different types. This structure and specialization of functions lend a degree of predictability and certainty to what could be an unpredictable environment, making the process efficient and routine. For example, while the specific topic of the news may vary on a given day, such as bird flu, influenza or food contamination, the local department of health beat is always certain to provide some information on health to the reporters. Some have characterized this as "information subsidy" (Fishman, 1980; Gandy, 1982).

Another practice worth noting is how journalists "operationalize" objectivity, an ideal they strive to achieve while covering news. Given the difficulty in achieving this ideal while working under deadline constraints, journalists often report on two sides of an issue, conveying an impression of fairness (Tuchman, 1978). Often, this effort to provide both sides of the story unintentionally leads to equal weighting of two contrasting interpretations of an issue, irrespective of the weight of evidence. In this way, tobacco companies have been able to capitalize on raising doubts on harmful effects of smoking and other tobacco control measures despite overwhelming scientific evidence against tobacco use.

Reliance on institutionalized sources may similarly influence how an issue is "framed" in the media. News sources can influence framing by offering their version or interpretation, sometimes quite successfully, as in the case of tobacco companies explained above. How issues are framed in the news may ultimately impact how news audiences may think and act (Iyengar & Kinder, 1987).

3.2. Media as Market-Based and Profit Driven Organizations

Mass media rely on two major sources of revenue to sustain them: subscription services and advertising. Even when media rely on subscriptions, such as newspapers, magazines, and cable and satellite services, they still rely heavily on subsidy from advertising to keep the cost of their products low.

For example, according to the industry trade magazine, *Advertising Age*, the total revenue for marketing communications for the year 2005 in the United States was $24.38 billion, including spending on public relations, interactive marketing, online advertising, and marketing promotions. *Advertising Age* also reports that traditional boundaries between conventional advertising and marketing communications have become porous, with advertisers using a variety of media and channels to reach their target audience.

The influence of advertising on population health can never be overemphasized. The influence of advertising on media and audience may occur in three ways. First, advertising has a direct influence on consumer behavior through promotion of products such as tobacco ($154.6 million in 2005) (Advertising Age, 2006), alcohol ($2.2 billion in 2005) (Advertising Age, 2006), leading fast food chains ($2.2 billion in 2004) (Institute of Medicine, 2005), sugar sweetened beverages ($556.6 million in 2004) (Institute of Medicine, 2005), and direct to consumer advertising (DTCA) of drugs ($3.2 billion in 2003) (IMS Health, 2006). Second, advertising indirectly may alter audience perceptions about health or behaviors that influence health such as consumption of certain food products or drugs or lifestyles and may counter the effect of health campaigns. Third, advertising subsidizes the production of media content that may or may not be conducive to health, such as *Prevention Magazine* or *Cigar Afficianado*.

Such reliance on advertising demands a precise account of the audience attending to the media. This need has led to a reliance on social sciences to systematically track and measure audience use of media, and a group of companies have successfully drawn upon and contributed to social science measurement. For example, competition among television stations for advertising dollars led to the emergence of the ratings industry, dominated by Nielsen Media Research, which uses well-honed social science techniques to track audience television viewing patterns and report those patterns by standard demographics such as age and gender. Print-based media rely on companies such as Simmons Market Research Bureau or Mediamark Research Incorporated to gather readership data (Sissors & Bumba, 1989). More recently, several efforts are being made to measure the "eyeballs," or visitors, to different Internet websites. Thus, web analytics or metrics measure the behavior of visitors to a particular website, with especial interest in which aspects of the website encourage people to make a purchase (Almind & Ingwersen, 1997).

4. News Media Influence on Public Health

Health is increasingly an important focus for news media, and attention to health in news has been steadily increasing over the last twenty-five years, particularly on topics such as tobacco/smoking, HIV/AIDS, and obesity (Viswanath, 2006). The increase in health coverage in the news media is also reflected in high attention by the public to health topics in different media (Viswanath, 2006). News may influence population health through all four functions stated in Section 2.0: informational, instrumental, social control, and communal.

News media play an important role in defining health issues and in disseminating the latest biomedical findings to the American public (McCombs & Ghanem, 2001; Reese, Gandy, & Grant, 2001; Schwartz & Woloshin, 2002; Tichenor et al., 1980). Further, they are a major source of health information for patients and health care providers (Meissner, Potosky, & Convissor, 1992; Phillips, Kanter, Bednarczyk, & Tastad, 1991; Ward, Morrison, & Schreiber, 1982; Yanovitzky & Blitz, 2000).

Sustained attention to issues in the media leads the audience to perceive that issue as important. The power of news media lie in their capacity to amplify and draw attention to public health topics, such as threats and new medical developments, thus potentially influencing the priorities people place on issues (McCombs & Ghanem, 2001; Tichenor et al., 1980; Viswanath, 2005). This is the "agenda setting" effect of media.

Media provide arguments (Noelle-Neumann, 1984) or "frame" issues for the public (Entman, 1993; Pan & Kosicki, 2001). Therefore, news is not mere neutral delivery of "topics" but an articulation of "points of view" about health issues. For example, second hand smoke has been framed as both harmful to innocent bystanders who choose not to smoke as well as an issue of individual rights. Initiatives to tax cigarettes have been framed both as an unfair burden and regressive taxation as well as an effective tool for tobacco control. News frames are a product of struggle between "frame sponsors," such as tobacco companies and tobacco control advocates, and the reporters who try to write a story under a deadline while attempting to be objective. Over time, some frames may gain greater currency over others; however, though a majority of audience may accept leading frames, there is seldom a monopoly of frames.

Finally, while the power of the media lies in its capacity to amplify an issue and reach large audiences, it is limited by the reliance of reporters on established news sources such as spokespersons for agencies of powerful institutions, including the government and corporations. Sources partially influence *what* is covered and *how* it is covered. The relationship between reporters and sources is symbiotic – each relying on the other with the ultimate aim of making the information public from their point of view. This is not to imply reporters are mere conduits for the sources or that the relationship is free of tension. On the contrary, the interaction is not always smooth, and the relationship endures amidst the stresses and strains of any professional relationship.

4.1. News Media and Public Health Activism

Most attention in public health focuses on a gradual, linear, and planned change that is orderly and seldom confrontational. The emphasis is often on social cohesion and collaboration. However, the use of conflict and confrontation to bring about changes in public policies and society that affect population health are not uncommon and are often quite effective. Indeed, activism on public health problems such as smoking, drunk driving, and HIV/AIDS, among others, has contributed significantly to changes in public health policy and practice.

Participants in social movements need three resources to push their cause on to the public agenda: people, money, and legitimacy (McCarthy & Wolfson, 1996). Activists use a variety of strategies and tactics to attract attention, to seek legitimacy, generate public outrage and draw sympathy to their causes. Media are considered an important resource because they help in communicating with followers, in facilitating recruitment, in articulating definitions of social problems, and in neutralizing arguments of the opposition (McCarthy & Wolfson, 1996; Molotch, 1979). Mass media, particularly news media, have played a critical role in public health activism by drawing public attention to the problem, framing issues, and amplifying frames, which in turn may have influenced public opinion and policy outcomes.

It is usually agreed that mainstream media reception of social movements is seldom supportive, often derisive, and sometimes indifferent. Given that social movements challenge the *status quo*, and given media's rather symbiotic reliance on established interests, it is not surprising that media coverage is less hospitable to these causes. As we reviewed earlier, newsgathering is routinized and structured, relying on established groups for a steady supply of information (Tuchman, 1978). Activists, by definition, are outside the establishment; therefore, they may not be a part of a regular beat unless they attract reporters' attention. For this reason, activists choose a variety of tactics to attract media attention, such as chaining themselves to doctors' offices or federal agencies (AIDS, ACT-UP), displaying car wrecks (MADD), protesting at public meetings (AIDS), and "rating the states" (RTS) on the strength of drunk driving laws in different states (MADD). Drama is a critical ingredient in attracting media attention (Hilgartner & Bosk, 1988). In addition, it is possible that the morale of members of the social movement groups improves when they see their cause getting attention, though it may also depend on how the movement is being portrayed.

It is not possible to provide a more complete treatment of social activism and media advocacy (Wallack & Dorfman, 1996) and its influence on population health in this piece, but suffice it to say that media coverage of movements to promote healthy change depends on: (a) the degree of acceptance of the cause and the social groups affected by mainstream society, (b) the ethnic and racial makeup of the groups affected, (c) the social power of affected groups, and (d) the target of the activism, whether it is the corporate sector or the public sector. More systematic exploration is needed in this area.

5. Media Effects and Public Health Outcomes: Some Examples

The effects of media on health often are unintentional and adventitious, though it is equally likely that health or illness could be of explicit focus in some media. Whether intentional or not, the impact of mass media on public health has been a source of considerable attention and controversy in the public arena, particularly when it comes to impact of entertainment programs on "vulnerable audiences," such as children. Major areas of contention include portrayals of sexuality on television and effects on teen sex behavior, media portrayal of violence and its effects on cognitions and behaviors of adults and children, and portrayals of cigarette smoking in movies and effects on children, as well as television and its role in obesity.

5.1. Teen Sex Behavior

Teens may be exposed to two different forms of sexual content in media. First, sexual behaviors can be "embedded" within the content or storyline, such as in television soap operas or in sexually suggestive advertisements in magazines. Second, teens can also be exposed to "sexually explicit media," typically referred to as pornography. These portrayals often provide young people with powerful messages concerning how to be sexual, why to have sex, and appropriate sequences of sexual activities (Malamuth & Impett, 2001). Correlational and, to a lesser extent, experimental data on exposure to both types of content has been shown to affect young people's judgments and attitudes regarding sexual behaviors (i.e., premarital and extramarital sex) and possibly to influence their sexual behaviors (Brown & Newcomer, 1991; Bryant & Rockwell, 1994). Some theorize that what is portrayed in the media and what may be left out (i.e., caring, mutual respect) may 1) affect interpretations, perceptions, perceived norms and other cognitive/emotional processes; 2) teach novel modes of behavior; 3) facilitate already learned behaviors; and/or 4) strengthen or weaken inhibitions concerning forms of sexual behavior (Hogben & Byrne, 1998).

5.2. Cigarette Smoking in Movies and Children

Teens account for nearly one-third of all movie admissions, and unlike in real life, smoking rates in movies have not changed since 1960 (Roberts, Henriksen, & Christenson, 1999). Almost all top grossing films over the past few decades have contained tobacco use, and some even have portrayed greater smoking rates than the US average (Hazan, Lipton, & Glantz, 1994). Additionally, children's G-rated movies contain an alarming amount of smoking scenes. A review of 50 G-rated animated feature films released between 1937 and 1997 found that more than half portrayed one or more instances of tobacco use, including all seven films released in 1996 and 1997 (Goldstein, Sobel, & Newman, 1999). Evidence shows that portrayal of smoking in movies could potentially lead to smoking initiation among youth (Sargent, Beach, Adachi-Mejia, Gibson, Titus-Ernstoff, Carusi, Swain, Heatherton, & Dalton, 2005).

5.3. Mental Health

Studies consistently show that both entertainment and news media provide overwhelmingly dramatic and distorted images of mental illness that emphasize dangerousness, criminality, and unpredictability (Corrigan, Watson, Gracia, Slopen, Rasinski, & Hall, 2005; Coverdale, Nairn, & Claasen, 2002; Nairn, Coverdale, & Claasen, 2001). They also model negative reactions to the mentally ill, including fear, rejection, derision, and ridicule (Francis, Pirkis, Blood, Dunt, Burgess, Morley, Stewart, & Putnis, 2004; Lauber, Nordt, Falcato, & Rossler, 2004). The consequences of negative media images for people who have a mental illness are profound. They impair self-esteem, help-seeking behaviors, medication adherence, and overall recovery (Nairn & Coverdale, 2005; Pirkis, Blood, Francis, & McCallum, 2006).

5.4. Television and Obesity

A vast and growing body of work reports a moderate association between television viewing and obesity, particularly among children (Coon, Goldberg, Rogers, & Tucker, 2001; Gortmaker, Must, Sobol, Peterson, Colditz, & Dietz, 1996). Two hypothesized mechanisms may be offered as explanations for this relationship. One involves television's influence on diet, and the other deals with television's effect on physical activity (see Figure 13.1).

Television can influence diet in a number of ways. Heavy viewing can increase the potential for exposure to heavily advertised food products that are high in calories and sugars (Kuribayashi, Roberts, & Johnson, 2001). Heavy exposure could increase the salience of the advertised goods (Shaw & McCombs, 1977) and increase their desirability (Shrum, O'Guinn, Semenik, & Faber, 1991). Media exposure in fact may "prime" the audience member by providing social cues and suggestions and framing issues related to diet, physical appearance, and obesity, leading to behavior in consonance with media messages (Iyengar & Kinder, 1987).

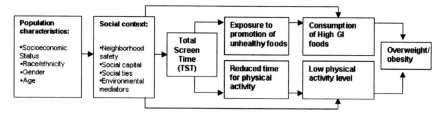

FIGURE 13.1. Conceptual model: Pathways to obesity

Additionally, the power of "narratives" in entertainment genre absorbs the attention of the audience and may make them more accepting of mediated messages (Green & Brock, 2000). It is also possible that snacking increases while watching television, although these data are based on parent reports on children (Coon et al., 2001; Matheson, Killen, Wang, Varady, & Robinson, 2004; Stroebele & de Castro, 2004).

It is also argued that time spent viewing television displaces time spent on physical activity (Andersen, Crespo, Bartlett, Cheskin, & Pratt, 1998; Ariza, Chen, Binns, & Christoffel, 2004; Dietz & Gortmaker, 1985; Taras, Sallis, Patterson, Nader, & Nelson, 1989). Another possibility is that heavy exposure to television programs, especially violent content, may lead to an overestimation of crime and violence in the real world (Gerbner, Gross, Morgan, Signorielli, & Shanahan, 2002; Shanahan & Morgan, 1999). The "fear of crime" engendered by heavy television viewing could deter the viewer from engaging in any physical activity outside the home, thus potentially leading to more television viewing and a sedentary life. Studies testing the "theories of neighborhood disorder" suggest that a heightened fear of crime in the neighborhood could influence physical activity (King, Stokols, Talen, Brassington, & Killingsworth, 2002).

Despite the overwhelming number of studies that posit a relationship between television and obesity, there are many limitations that warrant a more systematic and empirical scrutiny. One, most studies that link television viewing with obesity have used self-reported "time spent with TV" as a measure of exposure, which fails to capture exposure to the actual content or to time spent with computers and other media. Two, a majority of studies asserting the role of television in obesity have focused on children. Three, few studies, if any, take into account of an important contingent condition – neighborhood environment – that could moderate the effect of television on obesity (Doob & Macdonald, 1979; Hirsch, 1980; Shrum & Darmanin, 1998). That is, the relationship between television and fear of crime could be based in reality if the viewer lives in a neighborhood that is less safe (King et al., 2002). If so, neighborhood conditions could compel someone to stay home and watch TV rather than engage in activity outside home. This may be a particular problem with resource-poor neighborhoods with high crime, where staying home and watching TV is safer and a cheaper form of entertainment compared to going out and engaging in other leisure time activities. Finally, the role of social class that is tied to both television use and residential location has been neglected in the literature.

5.5. Media Violence

A heavily studied area of entertainment media effects on audience health cognitions and behavior is in relation to violence. The negative impact of entertainment media, particularly on children, has a long history in media studies starting in the 1930s (Wartella & Reeves, 1985). The Payne Fund studies, 1928–33, collectively examined the impact of movies on children. They concluded that media are one among many other sources of influence that include the church, parents, school, peers, and "street life." Subsequently, attention of scholars, activists, and policy makers have focused on the effects of comics, television and now the Internet. Several congressional committees and the Surgeon General have looked into the effects of violent media on children (Rowland, 1983).

In general, it is reasonable to infer a casual connection between exposure to mediated violence on television, films, and video games and aggressive behavior in *some* children (Anderson & Bushman, 2001; Paik & Comstock, 1994). The evidence comes from a variety of studies that include longitudinal, cross-sectional, and laboratory and field experiments (Anderson & Bushman, 2002). While short-term exposure to media violence could result in aggressive cognitions and emotions, some evidence suggests a relationship between "frequent" exposure to violence in childhood and subsequent aggression "later in life" (Anderson, Berkowitz, Donnerstein, Huesmann, Johnson, Linz, Malamuth, & Wartella, 2003). Researchers explain that it is possible that watching violent content in the media may "prime" aggressive thoughts and emotions, potentially desensitizing the audience to violence and reducing inhibitions. There is inconsistent evidence whether parental mediation and supervision could reduce the effects of exposure to media violence.

Violence in the media, especially televised violence, has also been shown to have a social control effect on large populations. A number of studies suggest that heavy exposure to television "cultivates" a distorted worldview (Gerbner et al., 2002). That is, a heavy viewer of television is more likely to think that the world of television is a reflection of the reality of daily life. The theory of the "cultivation" effect of television has generated heated debate over the degree of relationship and causality, as well as several alternative explanations. The weight of the evidence and reviews, however, suggest at least a modest cultivation effect.

The cumulative impact on public perceptions and public health could be profound. As mentioned in Section 5.4, the perception that they are likely to be victims of violence may potentially deter people from engaging in physical activity in their immediate neighborhoods. Other outcomes of cultivation effects include acceptance of harsher corrections policies and greater acceptance of restrictions on civil liberties.

These examples of media effects suggest that entertainment media such as television, movies, and videogames may have an influential impact on population health and must be central to any study of influence of media on population health.

6. Health Disparities and Communication Inequalities: The Structural Influence Model

Thus far, we have discussed the ways in which media work and specified mechanisms and outcomes of importance for public health. We now move to a more enduring concern for students of population health: how the media can exacerbate or reduce health disparities. It is widely accepted that certain population subgroups face a disproportionate burden from chronic diseases compared to other groups. These differences between different social classes and racial and ethnic groups span the prevention, treatment, and survivorship continuum and a variety of health areas (Kawachi & Kroenke, 2006; Paltoo & Chu, 2004; Ries, Eisner, Kosary, Hankey, Miller, Clegg, Mariotto, Feuer, & Edwards, 2004), diabetes, obesity and CVD among others (Institute of Medicine, 2003).

Health disparities researchers have identified a variety of factors, "social determinants," that are potentially linked to and lead to health disparities. Social determinants influencing health disparities include social cohesion, social class or socioeconomic status (SES), social networks, work environment and life transition, neighborhood and residential conditions, and social policies (Galea & Vilahov, 2005; Kaplan, 2004; Kawachi & Berkman, 2000; Krieger, 2005; Phelan, Link, Diez-Roux, Kawachi, & Levin, 2004). The large and growing body of work on health disparities has struggled to identify the precise mechanisms through which different levels of social determinants influence individual health (Kaplan, 2004). A more complete explanation should connect the distal factors to more proximal factors that affect population health .

We argue that inequalities in communication could offer one potent explanation for inequalities in health. Drawing on the Structural Influence Model of Health Communication (SIM), we suggest that communication may play a role in linking SES, resources, and final health outcomes (see Figure 13.2). This model is based on the premise that control of communication is power and that whoever has the capacity to generate, access, use, and distribute information enjoys social power and the advantages that accrue from it (Tichenor et al., 1980; Viswanath & Demers, 1999).

Our model posits that health outcomes and health disparities could be explained by understanding how structural determinants, such as socioeconomic status, and geography, and mediating mechanisms, such as gender, age, and social networks, lead to differential communication outcomes, such as access to and use of information channels, attention to health content, recall of information, knowledge and comprehension, and a capacity to act on relevant information among individuals. Structural antecedents such as SES and geography influence both the information environment and resources for consumption. Thus, they lead to differential communication behaviors that in turn may affect actions along the public health continuum, including knowledge, prevention, detection and treatment, survivorship, and quality of life. Health disparities, therefore, could potentially be explained by inequalities along the communication continuum, resulting in a cumulative effect on ultimate health outcomes.

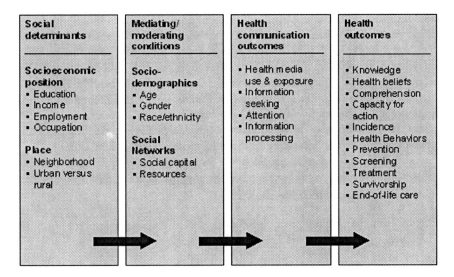

Social determinants	Mediating/ moderating conditions	Health communication outcomes	Health outcomes
Socioeconomic position • Education • Income • Employment • Occupation **Place** • Neighborhood • Urban versus rural	**Socio-demographics** • Age • Gender • Race/ethnicity **Social Networks** • Social capital • Resources	• Health media use & exposure • Information seeking • Attention • Information processing	• Knowledge • Health beliefs • Comprehension • Capacity for action • Incidence • Health Behaviors • Prevention • Screening • Treatment • Survivorship • End-of-life care

FIGURE 13.2. Structural Influence Model (SIM) and health communication

6.1. Communication Inequalities and Health Disparities

"Communication inequality" may be defined as differences among social classes in the generation, manipulation, and distribution of information at the group level and differences in access to and ability to take advantage of information at the individual level (Viswanath, 2006). For example, many indicators of SES, education, income, employment, and occupation are related to the use of and exposure to media and information channels, which in turn are related to health knowledge (Viswanath, 2005, 2006; Viswanath, Breen, Meissner, Moser, Hesse, Steele, & Rakowski, 2006). The data from National Cancer Institute's Health Information National Trends Survey (HINTS) tellingly demonstrate differential access and exposure to information services such as cable or satellite TV and the Internet among different social groups (Viswanath, 2006).

Similarly, attention to health information and one's ability to process it is influenced by SES. For example, there are differences in the degree of attention people from different education and income groups pay to media content. At the same time, according to data from HINTS, there are no differences among various racial and ethnic groups in the amount of self-reported attention to health information in diverse media. This suggests strong interest in health information among all racial and ethnic groups, despite differential access.

Last, there are major differences among social groups in their ability to act on information and take advantage of it. The navigation of the health system and the organization of medical care place a considerable burden on low SES groups. Issues such as language, culture, and social status may interfere with having a positive experience with the system (Cooper & Roter, 2003). There are differences in what people learn from the mass media as well as the advantages that accrue from public health communication campaigns (Hornik, 2002b; Viswanath & Finnegan, 2002). An unintended effect is that, absent some conditions, advantages from increased availability of information accrues to higher SES groups compared to lower SES groups, a phenomenon characterized as "knowledge gap" (Gaziano, 1983; Tichenor et al., 1980; Viswanath & Finnegan, 1996). However, carefully designed public health interventions have been successful in reducing smoking among adults and teens, increasing seat belt use, reducing Sudden Infant Death Syndrome (SIDS), and increasing mammography use (Hornik, 2002a,b).

The key point is that inequalities in communication reflect inequalities in health and may offer one potent explanation for why, despite improving population health, some groups are not benefiting.

7. Implications for Public Health Practice

Clearly, media are integral to population health and contribute to both healthy as well as unhealthy practices. The power of the media to influence public health stems not only from purposive uses of media for health or against health, but also from routine uses of media for purposes other than health. Similar to other institutions of social integration, such as the family, church, or school, media play a role in shaping what we know about health and illness, how we know, and what we can do about it. However, media is differentiated by its overwhelming reach and ubiquity, which dominates our lives as few institutions can or do.

It is these features – ubiquity, reach, widespread use – that make the study of media in public health so vital and so exciting. It is important to remember that in addition to media's ability to amplify discussion of a given topic and provide frames within which audiences receive information, media are typically for-profit institutions that rely on advertising for financial support and on sources for information. Lastly, we must acknowledge the tension between First Amendment rights and public health goals, tension that will inform any efforts to regulate media content in the interest of public health. Two areas in which this comes into play are the limited regulations regarding advertising to children and the portrayal of risk-taking behaviors such as alcohol abuse and risky sexual activity.

Some generalizations are comfortably drawn. One, media contribute to knowledge, beliefs and behaviors about health both for good and ill. Two, media may be successfully used to promote health through media-based campaigns. Three, media influence spans across different levels of social determinants of health from individuals to social institutions and social policies. Four, there are inequalities in communication that appear to contribute to health disparities.

While these issues are clear, some questions remain. One, how does routine use of media influence health? This question is important because unlike strategic use of media that focuses on health, it is difficult to intervene in programs to which people routinely attend. Two, what are the influences of media at different levels of social determinants that influence individual health? Finally, the media landscape is changing dramatically. The range of information delivery systems, including the Internet and cell phones, offers tremendous opportunities as well as challenges in understanding how they influence health.

An understanding of and appreciation for the complex role of mass media in population health could be extremely valuable to students of public health given the powerful role media play in the contemporary information environment. More specifically, an understanding of how media work and the environment in which media operate will be helpful in intervening with mass media. Even as we focus on health education to promote health and prevent disease, major social changes are more likely to be possible if we work through mass media organizations. Changes due to information revolution are more likely to have a wider impact, albeit with the caveat that the impact may not benefit everyone unless social power and equitable distribution of resources are taken into account. Indeed, the information revolution may end up as a pyrrhic victory if it only widens the disparities in health instead of bridging them. How we address these questions may ultimately shape how we address the larger role of social determinants in health.

Endnotes

i. This section draws on Viswanath, K., Breen, N., Meissner, H., Moser, R. P., Hesse, B., Steele, W. R., & Rakowski, W. (2006). Cancer knowledge and disparities in the information age. *Journal of Health Communication, 11* (Supplement 1), 1–17. which provides a more extensive and elaborate treatment of the communication inequalities and health disparities.

References

Advertising Age. (2006). Domestic ad spending by category, 2006 Edition. New York (June 23, 2006); http://adage.com/datacenter/article?article_id = 110123.

Almind, T. C., & Ingwersen, P. (1997). Informetric analyses on the World Wide Web: Methodological approaches to "webometrics". *Journal of Documentation, 53*(4), 404–426.

Andersen, R. E., Crespo, C. J., Bartlett, S. J., Cheskin, L. J., & Pratt, M. (1998). Relationship of physical activity and television watching with body weight and level of fatness among children: Results from the Third National Health and Nutrition Examination Survey. *Journal of the American Medical Association, 279*(12), 938–942.

Anderson, C. A., & Bushman, B. J. (2001). Effects of violent video games on aggressive behavior, aggressive cognition, aggressive affect, physiological arousal, and prosocial behavior: A meta-analytic review of the scientific literature. *Psychological Science, 12*(5), 353–359.

Anderson, C. A., & Bushman, B. J. (2002). Psychology. The effects of media violence on society. *Science, 295*(5564), 2377–2379.

Anderson, C. A., Berkowitz, L., Donnerstein, E., Huesmann, L. R., Johnson, J. D., Linz, D., et al. (2003). The influence of media violence on youth *Psychological Science* (Supplement S), 81–110.

Ariza, A. J., Chen, E. H., Binns, H. J., & Christoffel, K. K. (2004). Risk factors for overweight in five- to six-year-old Hispanic-American children: A pilot study. *Journal of Urban Health, 81*(1), 150–161.

Berkman, L. F. (1986). Social networks, support, and health: Taking the next step forward. *American Journal of Epidemiology, 123*(4), 559–562.

Brown, J. D., & Newcomer, S. F. (1991). Television viewing and adolescents' sexual behavior. *Journal of Homosexuality, 21*(1–2), 77–91.

Bryant, J., & Rockwell, S. (1994). Effects of massive exposure to sexually oriented prime-time television programming on adolescents' moral judgment. In D. Zillmann, J. Bryant, & A. Huston (Eds.), *Media, children, and the family*. Hillsdale, NJ: Lawrence Erlbaum.

Coon, K. A., Goldberg, J., Rogers, B. L., & Tucker, K. L. (2001). Relationships between use of television during meals and children's food consumption patterns. *Pediatrics, 107*(1), E7.

Cooper, L., & Roter, D. (2003). Patient-provider communication: The effect of race and ethnicity on process and outcomes of healthcare. In B. Smedley, A. Stith, & A. Nelson (Eds.), *Unequal treatment: Confronting racial and ethnic disparities in healthcare*. Washington, DC: National Academies Press.

Corrigan, P. W., Watson, A. C., Gracia, G., Slopen, N., Rasinski, K., & Hall, L. L. (2005). Newspaper stories as measures of structural stigma. *Psychiatric Services, 56*(5), 551–556.

Coverdale, J., Nairn, R., & Claasen, D. (2002). Depictions of mental illness in print media: a prospective national sample. *The Australian and New Zealand Journal of Psychiatry, 36*(5), 697–700.

Demers, D. (1996). Does personal experience in a community increase or decrease newspaper reading? *Journalism & Mass Communication Quarterly, 73*(2), 304–318.

Demers, D., & Viswanath, K. (Eds.). (1999). *Mass media, social control and social change: A macrosocial perspective*. Ames, IA: Iowa State University Press.

Dietz, W. H., Jr., & Gortmaker, S. L. (1985). Do we fatten our children at the television set? Obesity and television viewing in children and adolescents. *Pediatrics, 75*(5), 807–812.

Doob, A., & Macdonald, G. (1979). Television viewing and fear of victimization: Is the relationship causal? *Journal of Personality and Social Psychology, 37*(2), 170–179.

Entman, R. M. (1993). Framing – toward clarification of a fractured paradigm. *Journal of Communication, 43*(4), 51–58.

Ettema, J. S., & Whitney, D. C. (Eds.). (1994). *Audiencemaking: How the media create the audience*. Volume 22. Thousand Oaks: Sage Publications.

Fishman, M. (1980). *Manufacturing the news*. Austin, TX: University of Texas Press.

Francis, C., Pirkis, J., Blood, R. W., Dunt, D., Burgess, P., Morley, B., et al. (2004). The portrayal of mental health and illness in Australian non-fiction media. *The Australian and New Zealand Journal of Psychiatry, 38*(7), 541–546.

Friedland, L. A., & McLeod, J. M. (1999). Community integration and mass media: A reconsideration. In D. Demers & K. Viswanath (Eds.), *Mass media, social control & social change: A macrosocial perspective*. Ames, IA: Iowa State University Press.

Galea, S., & Vilahov, D. (2005). *Handbook of urban health: Populations, methods, and practice*. New York: Springer.

Gandy, O. H. (1982). *Beyond agenda setting: Information subsidies and public policy*. Norwood, NJ: Ablex Publishing.

Gaziano, C. (1983). The knowledge gap – an analytical review of media effects. *Communication Research, 10*(4), 447–486.

Gerbner, G., Gross, L., Morgan, M., Signorielli, N., & Shanahan, J. (2002). Growing up with television: Cultivation processes. In J. Bryant & D. Zillman (Eds.), *Media effects: Advances in theory research*. 2nd edition. Mahwah, NJ: Lawrence Erlbaum.

Gilpin, E. A., Emery, S., White, M. M., & Pierce, J. P. (2003). Changes in youth smoking participation in California in the 1990s. *Cancer Causes & Control, 14*(10), 985–993.

Gitlin, T. (2003). *The whole world is watching: Mass media in the making & unmaking of the New Left*. Berkeley: University of California Press.

Goldstein, A. O., Sobel, R. A., & Newman, G. R. (1999). Tobacco and alcohol use in G-rated children's animated films. *Journal of the American Medical Association, 281*(12), 1131–1136.

Gortmaker, S. L., Must, A., Sobol, A. M., Peterson, K., Colditz, G. A., & Dietz, W. H. (1996). Television viewing as a cause of increasing obesity among children in the United States, 1986–1990. *Archives of Pediatrics & Adolescent Medicine, 150*(4), 356–362.

Green, M. C., & Brock, T. C. (2000). The role of transportation in the persuasiveness of public narratives. *Journal of Personality and Social Psychology, 79*(5), 701–721.

Hazan, A. R., Lipton, H. L., & Glantz, S. A. (1994). Popular films do not reflect current tobacco use. *American Journal of Public Health, 84*(6), 998–1000.

Hilgartner, S., & Bosk, C. L. (1988). The rise and fall of social problems – a public arenas model. *American Journal of Sociology, 94*(1), 53–78.

Hirsch, P. (1980). The scary world of the nonviewer and other anomalies: A reanalysis of Gerbner et al.'s findings on cultivation analysis. *Communication Research, 7*, 403–456.

Hogben, M., & Byrne, D. (1998). Using social learning theory to explain individual difference in human sexuality. *Journal of Sex Research, 35*(1), 58–71.

Hornik, R. (2002a). Public health communication: Making sense of contradictory evidence. In R. Hornik (Ed.), *Public health communication: Evidence for behavior change*. New York: Lawrence Erlbaum.

Hornik, R. (Ed.). (2002b). *Public health communication: Evidence for behavior change*. New York: Lawrence Erlbaum.

IMS Health. (2006). IMS 2005 annual report. (2006); http://www.imshealth.com/vgn/images/portal/cit_40000873/62/45/77617933IMS2005 AR.pdf.

Institute of Medicine. (2003). *Unequal treatment: Confronting racial and ethnic disparities in health care*. Washington, DC: National Academies Press.

Institute of Medicine. (2005). *Food marketing to children and youth: Threat or opportunity?* Washington, DC: National Academies Press.

Institute of Medicine, & Committee on Communication for Behavior Change in the 21st Century: Improving the Health of Diverse Populations. (2002). *Speaking of health: Assessing health communication strategies for diverse populations*. Washington, DC: National Academies Press.

Iyengar, S., & Kinder, D. R. (1987). *News that matters: Television and American opinion*. Chicago, IL: University of Chicago Press.

Kaplan, G. A. (2004). What's wrong with social epidemiology, and how can we make it better? *Epidemiologic Reviews, 26*, 124–135.

Kawachi, I. (1999). Social capital and community effects on population and individual health. *Annals of the New York Academy of Sciences, 896*, 120–130.

Kawachi, I., & Berkman, L. (2000). Social cohesion, social capital, and health. In L. Berkman & I. Kawachi (Eds.), *Social epidemiology*. New York: Oxford University Press.

Kawachi, I., & Kroenke, C. (2006). Socioeconomic disparities in cancer incidence and mortality. In D. Schottenfeld & J. F. J. Fraumeni (Eds.), *Cancer epidemiology and prevention*. 3rd edition. New York: Oxford University Press.

King, A. C., Stokols, D., Talen, E., Brassington, G. S., & Killingsworth, R. (2002). Theoretical approaches to the promotion of physical activity: Forging a transdisciplinary paradigm. *American Journal of Preventive Medicine, 23*(2 Supplement), 15–25.

Krieger, N. (2005). Defining and investigating social disparities in cancer: Critical issues. *Cancer Causes & Control, 16*(1), 5–14.

Kuribayashi, A., Roberts, M. C., & Johnson, R. J. (2001). Actual nutritional information of products advertised to children and adults on Saturday. *Children's Health Care, 30*(4), 309–322.

Lauber, C., Nordt, C., Falcato, L., & Rossler, W. (2004). Factors influencing social distance toward people with mental illness. *Community Mental Health Journal, 40*(3), 265–274.

Lemert, J. B. (1981). *Does mass communication change public opinion after all? A new approach to effects analysis.* Chicago: Nelson-Hall.

Malamuth, N. M., & Impett, E. A. (2001). Research on sex in the media: What do we know about effects on children and adolescents? In D. Singer & J. Singer (Eds.), *Handbook of children and the media.* Thousand Oaks, CA: Sage Publications.

Matheson, D. M., Killen, J. D., Wang, Y., Varady, A., & Robinson, T. N. (2004). Children's food consumption during television viewing. *American Journal of Clinical Nutrition, 79*(6), 1088–1094.

McCarthy, J. D., & Wolfson, M. (1996). Resource mobilization by local social movement social organizations. *American Sociological Review, 61*, 1070–1088.

McCombs, M. E., & Ghanem, S. I. (2001). The convergence of agenda setting and framing. In S. D. Reese, O. H. Gandy, & A. E. Grant (Eds.), *Framing public life: Perspectives on media and our understanding of the social world.* Mahwah, NJ: Lawrence Erlbaum.

Meissner, H. I., Potosky, A. L., & Convissor, R. (1992). How sources of health information relate to knowledge and use of cancer screening exams. *Journal of Community Health, 17*(3), 153–165.

Molotch, H. (1979). Media and movements. In M. N. Zald & J. D. McCarthy (Eds.), *The dynamics of social movements: Resource mobilization, social control and social tactics.* Cambridge, MA: Winthrop Publishers.

Nairn, R., & Coverdale, J. (2005). People never see us living well: An appraisal of the personal stories about mental illness in a prospective print media sample. *Australian and New Zealand Journal of Psychiatry, 39*(4), 281–287.

Nairn, R., Coverdale, J., & Claasen, D. (2001). From source material to news story in New Zealand print media: A prospective study of the stigmatizing processes in depicting mental illness. *Australian and New Zealand Journal of Psychiatry, 35*(5), 654–659.

Noelle-Neumann, E. (1984). *The spiral of silence: Public opinion – our second skin.* Chicago, IL: University of Chicago Press.

Paik, H., & Comstock, G. (1994). The effects of television violence on anti-social behavior. *Communication Research, 21*(4), 516–546.

Paltoo, D. N., & Chu, K. C. (2004). Patterns in cancer incidence among American Indians/ Alaska natives, United States, 1992–1999. *Public Health Reports, 119*(4), 443–451.

Pan, Z., & Kosicki, G. M. (2001). Framing as a strategic action in public deliberation. In S. D. Reese, O. H. Gandy, & A. E. Grant (Eds.), *Framing public life: Perspectives on media and our understanding of the social world .* Mahwah, NJ: Lawrence Erlbaum.

Phelan, J. C., Link, B. G., Diez-Roux, A., Kawachi, I., & Levin, B. (2004). "Fundamental causes" of social inequalities in mortality: A test of the theory. *Journal of Health and Social Behavior, 45*(3), 265–285.

Phillips, D. P., Kanter, E. J., Bednarczyk, B., & Tastad, P. L. (1991). Importance of the lay press in the transmission of medical knowledge to the scientific community. *New England Journal of Medicine, 325*(16), 1180–1183.

Pirkis, J., Blood, R. W., Francis, C., & McCallum, K. (2006). On-screen portrayals of mental illness: Extent, nature, and impacts. *Journal of Health Communication, 11*(5), 523–541.

Putnam, R. (2000). *Bowling alone: The collapse and revival of the American community*. New York: Simon & Schuster.

Reese, S. D., Gandy, O. H., & Grant, A. E. (Eds.). (2001). *Framing public life: Perspectives on media and our understanding of the social world*. Mahwah, NJ: Lawrence Erlbaum Associates.

Ries, L. A. G., Eisner, M. P., Kosary, C. L., Hankey, B. F., Miller, B. A., Clegg, L., et al. (Eds.). (2004). *SEER cancer statistics review, 1975 – 2001*. Bethesda, MD: National Cancer Institute.

Roberts, D., Henriksen, L., & Christenson, P. (1999). *Substance use in popular movies and music*. Washington, DC: Office of National Drug Control Policy.

Robinson, J. P., & Levy, M. (1986). *The main source: Learning from television news*. Beverly Hills, CA: Sage Publications.

Rowland, W. D. (1983). *The politics of TV violence: Policy uses of communication research*. Beverly Hills: Sage Publications.

Sargent, J. D., Beach, M. L., Adachi-Mejia, A. M., Gibson, J. J., Titus-Ernstoff, L. T., Carusi, C. P., et al. (2005). Exposure to movie smoking: its relation to smoking initiation among US adolescents. *Pediatrics, 116*(5), 1183–1191.

Schwartz, L. M., & Woloshin, S. (2002). News media coverage of screening mammography for women in their 40s and tamoxifen for primary prevention of breast cancer. *Journal of the American Medical Association, 287*(23), 3136–3142.

Shanahan, J., & Morgan, M. (1999). *Television and its viewers: Cultivation theory and research*. Cambridge, UK: Cambridge University Press.

Shaw, D., & McCombs, M. (Eds.). (1977). *The emergence of American political issues*. St. Paul, MN: West.

Shoemaker, P., & Reese, S. (1996). *Mediating the message: Theories of influences on mass media content*. 2nd edition. New York: Longman.

Shrum, L. J., & Darmanin, V. (1998). Understanding the effects of television consumption on judgments of crime risk: The impact of direct experience and type of judgment. In K. Machleit & M. Campbell (Eds.), *Society for Consumer Psychology 1998 Winter Conference Proceedings*.

Shrum, L. J., O'Guinn, T. C., Semenik, R. J., & Faber, R. J. (1991). Processes and effects in the construction of normative consumer beliefs: The role of television. In R. H. Hollman & M. R. Solomon (Eds.), *Advances in consumer research*. Provo, UT: Association for Consumer Research.

Sissors, J., & Bumba, L. (1989). *Advertising media planning*. 3rd edition. Lincolnwood, IL: NTC Business Books.

Stroebele, N., & de Castro, J. M. (2004). Television viewing is associated with an increase in meal frequency in humans. *Appetite, 42*(1), 111–113.

Taras, H. L., Sallis, J. F., Patterson, T. L., Nader, P. R., & Nelson, J. A. (1989). Television's influence on children's diet and physical activity. *Journal of Developmental and Behavioral Pediatrics, 10*(4), 176–180.

Tichenor, P. J., Donohue, G. A., & Olien, C. N. (1980). *Community conflict and the press*. Newbury Park, CA: Sage Publications.

Tuchman, G. (1978). *Making news: A study in the construction of reality*. New York: Free Press.

Viswanath, K. (2005). The communications revolution and cancer control. *Nature Reviews Cancer, 5*(10), 828–835.

Viswanath, K. (2006). Public communications and its role in reducing and eliminating health disparities. In G. E. Thomson, F. Mitchell, & M. B. Williams (Eds.), *Examining *the health disparities research plan of the national institutes of health: Unfinished business.*. Washington, DC: Institute of Medicine.

Viswanath, K., & Finnegan, J. R. (1996). The knowledge gap hypothesis: Twenty five years later. In B. Burleson (Ed.), *Communication yearbook 19*. Thousand Oaks, CA: Sage Publications.

Viswanath, K., & Demers, D. (1999). Mass media from a macrosocial perspective. In D. Demers & K. Viswanath (Eds.), *Mass media, social control and social change: A macrosocial perspective*. Ames, IA: Iowa State University Press.

Viswanath, K., & Finnegan, J. R. (2002). Community health campaigns and secular trends: Insights from the Minnesota Heart Health Program and Community Trials in Heart Disease Prevention. In R. Hornik (Ed.), *Public health communication: Evidence for behavior change*. New York: Lawrence Erlbaum.

Viswanath, K., Breen, N., Meissner, H., Moser, R. P., Hesse, B., Steele, W. R., et al. (2006). Cancer knowledge and disparities in the information age. *Journal of Health Communication, 11*(Supplement 1), 1–17.

Viswanath, K., Randolph Steele, W., & Finnegan, J. (2006). Social capital and health: Civic engagement, community size, and recall of health messages. *American Journal of Public Health, 96*(8), 1456–1461.

Wallack, L., & Dorfman, L. (1996). Media advocacy: a strategy for advancing policy and promoting health. *Health Education Quarterly, 23*(3), 293–317.

Ward, G. W., Morrison, W., & Schreiber, G. (1982). Pilot study of health professionals' awareness and opinions of the hypertension information in the mass media they use. *Public Health Reports, 97*(2), 113–115.

Wartella, E., & Reeves, B. (1985). Historical trends in research on children and the media – 1900–1960. *Journal of Communication, 35*(2), 118–133.

Wechsler, H., Nelson, T. F., Lee, J. E., Seibring, M., Lewis, C., & Keeling, R. P. (2003). Perception and reality: A national evaluation of social norms marketing interventions to reduce college students' heavy alcohol use. *Journal of Studies on Alcohol, 64*(4), 484–494.

Yanovitzky, I., & Blitz, C. L. (2000). Effect of media coverage and physician advice on utilization of breast cancer screening by women 40 years and older. *Journal of Health Communication, 5*(2), 117–134.

Chapter 14
Integrative Chapter: Macrosocial Determinants of Population Health

Sandro Galea

The first section of this book includes eleven chapters each of which discusses one macrosocial determinant of population health. The factors covered by these chapters encompass a broad range of intellectual concerns—ranging from regulations and legal frameworks (global governance, patent law and policy), to overarching global phenomena (globalization, migration, urbanization, the media), to a specific consideration of the role of economic, political, and corporate policies and practices. These chapters also, to some extent, bring to bear different disciplinary lenses on the topic of their concern. Although the overall approach is epidemiologic, concerned with the determination of health and disease, economics, sociology, and health policy perspectives, among others, all play an important role in shaping the content of these chapters. In some respects however, these chapters are alike in as many ways as they are diverse. I offer here a brief discussion of the principal common themes that emerge from these chapters in order to suggest how the intellectual concerns raised in these chapters can illuminate future inquiry.

The abiding theme underlying the preceding eleven chapters is clearly that the factors discussed somehow influence the health of populations. I use the word "somehow" judiciously in this context and come back to it in my second point below. Although easy to forget in the context of a book that explicitly sets out to consider the macrosocial determination of population health, the observation that processes as diverse as global governance, migration, and taxation all play a role in influencing health is a remarkable observation. Most academic and policy thinkers concerned with these processes and factors on a day-to-day basis are not particularly thinking about health, but rather of the many other ramifications and implications of these factors. Clearly taxation has important implications for government functioning and is a subject of intense political and policy debate. Urbanization occasions much concern about urban form and drives discussion about how cities can best be designed or modified to accommodate the ever-increasing population burden they face, particularly in the developing world. However, these chapters, while not ignoring the important political, sociological, and ecological role of these macrosocial factors show us that these factors are also linked to health and that in some respects a concern with population health may be the only common theme linking such diverse macrosocial processes. These chapters offer convincing arguments why those of us interested in improving population health may want to consider the role played by these macrosocial factors, and conversely, why those concerned with these macrosocial processes may want to keep health considerations in mind. As elegantly put in Chapter 8, considering the role of macroeconomics, "Treasury secretaries do not consult the nation's health experts before changing interest rates and endorsing fiscal policy. This chapter has discussed at least one reason why this might need to be reconsidered." All these chapters to some extent center around this point.

These chapters also summarize the long intellectual history that has considered and in many cases explained why these macrosocial factors may indeed influence health. This point is made most clearly in the lively historic discussion provided in Chapter 5 that considers the role of political economic systems. However, while there may have been historic interest and intellectual focus on these issues, that interest has waxed and waned over time and certainly has not held up long enough or cogently enough to move thinking about macrosocial determination of the health of populations into the mainstream of either public health and medicine or, conversely, to move thinking about population health into the mainstream of politics, economics, or cultural and civic enterprises. The chapters are one small attempt to change this state of affairs.

There is little doubt that the topics that concern these preceding eleven chapters may be appropriately termed "macrosocial". These chapters consider processes and phenomena for which there exist no individual analogs. For example, as Chapter 9 makes clear, culture has little meaning when applied to any one individual, but is a product of the social interaction of many. These factors manifest at a social scale that is at least a group concern, and indeed, most of the factors discussed here are best considered and understood within a broader global context. Similarly, these chapters clearly suggest that the influence of these factors best may be understood with respect to their impact on the health of populations rather than on the health of individuals. The health of populations, as discussed in the first chapter, is very much a reflection of processes and social interactions that go beyond individual pathogenesis. In some respects the chapters in this book tell us little about individual risk and may have limited appeal to those concerned only with the determination of their own health or of the health of their own particular patient or client. Rather, these chapters suggest how complicated global processes set in motion mechanisms that influence national risk behaviors, the presence or absence of environmental exposures, and the social environment within which individuals live their lives and in so doing how these macrosocial factors determine rates of health indicators in populations.

The preceding chapters then present arguments, rooted in theoretical (and in some cases historical) perspectives and an understanding of the nature of the macrosocial factors being discussed, to suggest why these macrosocial factors may shape the health of populations. These chapters, in various forms shaped by their particular disciplinary orientation, also offer plausible mechanisms suggesting how it is that these factors do indeed shape the health of populations. This is presented very explicitly, for example, in Chapter 2, concerned with globalization. The authors offer an explicit mechanistic framework and provide examples suggesting how globalization may influence particular population health indicators. However, as these chapters consider their topics in detail, a gulf readily emerges between the mechanisms that plausibly link macrosocial factors and health and the evidence that buttresses the links being suggested. Several authors call explicitly for future empiric research that may test, and confirm or refute, the mechanisms being posited as a way to improve our understanding of the determination of population health being suggested in these chapters. Therefore, if these chapters all suggest that *somehow* the factors discussed here do indeed shape population health our understanding of how they exactly do this is by and large still informed speculation with relatively little data to buttress our claim of *determination*. In some respects these chapters make a convincing case for why macrosocial factors *may* determine population health. But clarifying *how* will require a concerted effort to pose clear deterministic hypotheses, as some of these chapters do, and to test them empirically.

It is perhaps not surprising that the evidence here lags behind the theory. We might argue that our theory itself is nascent; this book represents one attempt to push that theory forward and to push the authors, and the readers, to consider the determination of health from the perspective of macrosocial determination. Clearly, our next step forward needs to be the generation of empiric evidence that brings greater clarity to the issues raised in these preceding chapters. With that in mind the next section of this book presents five chapters that concern themselves explicitly with the methodologic challenges and opportunities that must be considered to do just that.

Section II
Methods

Chapter 15
Identifying Causal Ecologic Effects on Health: A Methodological Assessment

S. V. Subramanian, M. Maria Glymour, and Ichiro Kawachi

1. Introduction

Although ecologic factors may have tremendous importance for population health (Kawachi & Berkman, 2003; Kawachi & Subramanian, 2007), identifying ecologic effects poses critical methodological challenges. With the exception of surveillance research aimed at monitoring health disparities (Krieger, Chen, Waterman, Rehkopf, & Subramanian, 2005; Subramanian, Chen, Rehkopf, Waterman, & Krieger, 2006a,b), quantitative contextual studies typically focus on causality; for instance, establishing how much a particular context (e.g., a neighborhood) improves or worsens residents' health outcomes. Most studies, however, fail to explicitly define the causal ecologic estimand, with regards to "units", "treatments", and "potential outcomes". This is partly because even these basic definitions are not straightforward for studies interested in estimating causal ecologic effects (Raudenbush & Willms, 1995; Rubin, Stuart, & Zanutto, 2004). For instance, when estimating the ecological influence of neighborhoods, should the units be neighborhoods or the individuals residing in the neighborhood? Should the outcomes focus on individual values or neighborhood-level averages? Furthermore, are we interested in the treatment effect of a specific neighborhood characteristic, such as services or amenities, or in the overall neighborhood effect?

This chapter considers the prospects and pitfalls in identifying ecologic or contextual effects with observational data and offers a methodological assessment of the research estimating ecological effects on health outcomes. We begin by defining the causal effect for ecologic variables, distinguishing between common and specific ecological effects. We then discuss the role of multilevel modeling in identifying such effects and clarify the assumptions for these analyses. Following from this, we review the key threats to causal inference for ecologic effects and discuss approaches aimed at strengthening the identification of neighborhood effects on health. Throughout the chapter, we use the term "neighborhoods" as one realization of a context or ecology, but the issues raised are equally applicable to identifying other ecological effects, such as those associated with schools, clinics, communities, states, etc. We also use the term "treatment", not from the limited perspective of a randomized experiment, but to reflect the general motivation where a researcher is interested in a causal, rather than a descriptive, effect of a variable of interest.

2. Defining a Causal Ecologic Effect

Consider an individual i living in neighborhood j, characterized by presence of fast-food outlets T. We hypothesize that T (measured at the level of neighborhoods) *causes* an increase in the BMI of individual i. The units at which potential outcomes are measured are, thus, individuals (i), while the treatment (T) is observed at the level of neighborhood (j), such that all individuals within a neighborhood are exposed to the same treatment (T_j). When we say there is a ecologic effect of living in neighborhoods where $T_j = 1$ on the BMI of individual i_1, we mean either of the following:

1. Changing T from 1 to 0 in neighborhood $j = 1$ would decrease the BMI of resident i living in that neighborhood (conversely, changing T from 0 to 1 in neighborhood $j = 1$ would increase i's BMI); or
2. If individual i is moved to a new neighborhood $j = 2$ with $T = 1$, she will have a higher BMI than if she is moved to a new neighborhood $j = 3$ where $T = 0$.

   In the above characterization, the primary interest is on a specific aspect of the neighborhood, i.e., presence of fast-food outlets in a neighborhood. We refer to this as the specific ecologic effect (SEE) of an ecologic variable.

   One can, however, additionally hypothesize an overall neighborhood effect without necessarily specifying *why* some neighborhoods are beneficial or harmful; this we refer to as the common ecologic effect (CEE) of higher-level units, e.g., neighborhoods. This would entail introducing a variant to the scenario proposed in (2) as follows:
3. If individual i is moved to a new neighborhood $j = 2$ (with no information on T), his BMI will be different (although we do not know if it will be higher or lower) than if he is moved to some other neighborhood, say $j = 3$.

Such generic neighborhood effects are useful for two reasons. First, recognizing that neighborhoods matter is often a first step in identifying the specific influential neighborhood characteristic. Second, neighborhood influences on health are likely to be mediated through multiple characteristics and synergistic interactions of several neighborhood elements, as opposed to a single exposure. As such, CEE may be important in an intrinsic sense (Sampson & Morenoff, 2002). The common neighborhood effect would include the consequences of being placed in a different environment with different opportunity structures *as well as* different neighbors or residents. Assigning an individual to Neighborhood *A* rather than neighborhood *B* may have very different consequences than increasing the level of a specific characteristic (e.g., services, amenities, employment opportunities) in the individual's current neighborhood; in the latter situation, the individual retains all her current neighbors.

The basic idea of a causal neighborhood effect, therefore, is that if one were to change specific neighborhood characteristic(s) or the neighborhood setting but change nothing about the individual in question, one would expect, on average, a change in the individual's health. In recent years, the analytical framework used to estimate neighborhood effects (CEE or SEE) on individual health outcomes have typically used some variant of "multilevel models" (Raudenbush & Bryk, 2002; Goldstein, 2003). Multilevel models have proved extremely valuable in advancing our understanding of the potential importance of ecologies for health, besides providing an appropriate statistical framework for analyzing the nested structure of the data (Subramanian, Jones, & Duncan, 2003; Subramanian, 2004; Moon, Subramanian, Jones, Duncan, & Twigg, 2005). We turn to contrasting a typical multilevel study compared to other possible study types.

3. Multilevel Framework: A Necessity for Understanding Ecologic Effects

Figure 15.1 identifies a typology of designs for data collection and analyses (Blakely & Woodward, 2000; Kawachi & Subramanian 2006) where the rows indicate the level or unit at which the outcome variable is being measured (i.e., at the

		Exposure	
		t	T
Outcome	y	$\{y,t\}$ Traditional risk factor study	$\{y,T\}$ Contextual study
	Y	$\{Y,t\}^{(A)}$	$\{Y,T\}$ Ecological study

FIGURE 15.1. Typology of studies.

Note: (A) This type of study is impossible to specify as it stands. Practically speaking, it will either take the form of $\{Y,T\}$, i.e., ecological study, where T will now simply be central tendency of t, or, if dis-aggregation of Y is possible so that we can observe y, then it will be equivalent to $\{y,t\}$.

individual level (y) or the aggregate, or ecological, level (Y)), and the columns indicate whether the treatment is being measured at the individual level (t) or the ecological level (T). Study-type$^{\{y,t\}}$ is most commonly encountered when the researcher aims to link treatment measured at the individual level (e.g., diet) to individual health outcomes (e.g., BMI). Study-type$^{\{y,t\}}$ not only ignores ecological effects (either implicitly or explicitly), but with its individualistic focus, resonates with the notion of health as solely a matter of individual responsibility (Moon et al., 2005). Conversely, study-type$^{\{Y,T\}}$ – referred to as an "ecological study" – may seem intuitively appropriate for research on population health and ecological exposures. However, study-type$^{\{Y,T\}}$ conflates the genuinely ecological and the "aggregate," or compositional (Moon et al., 2005), and precludes the possibility of testing heterogeneous contextual effects on different types of individuals.

Ecological effects reflect predictors and associated mechanisms operating solely at the contextual level. The search for such measures and their scientific validation and assessment is an area of active research (Raudenbush, 2003). Aggregate effects, in contrast, equate the effect of a neighborhood with the sum of the individual effects associated with the people living within the neighborhood. In this situation, the interpretative question becomes particularly relevant. If common membership of a neighborhood by a set of individuals brings about an effect that is over and above those resulting from individual characteristics, then there may indeed be an ecological effect (i.e., the whole may be more than the sum of its parts). If this is not the case, then it is individual factors that matter, not ecological effects. For example, if we find that average levels of BMI tend to be higher in neighborhoods with a higher proportion of impoverished residents, such an observation does not, by itself, provide insight into the causal question of interest, i.e., does living in high-poverty neighborhoods increase individual residents' BMI compared to living in a low-poverty neighborhood? Any association between neighborhood average poverty and neighborhood average BMI might simply be due to individual poverty leading to higher individual BMI.

Answering the above question requires a study-type$^{\{y,T\}}$, in which an ecological exposure (*e.g.*, proportion in poverty) is linked to an individual outcome (BMI). A more complete representation would be type$^{\{y,x,T\}}$, whereby we have an individual outcome, individual confounders (x), and ecologic exposure, reflecting a multilevel structure of individuals nested within ecologies. When the ecological exposure is an aggregate measure of individual characteristics, such as percent poverty, it is obvious that information on both individual poverty and neighborhood percent poverty is required to test for an ecological effect. However, multilevel data are essential even if the ecological variable is a structural feature such as neighborhood presence of fast food outlets because people with individual level disadvantage are likely to be overrepresented in places with structural risk factors.

A fundamental motivation for study-type$^{\{y,x,T\}}$ is to distinguish "neighborhood differences in health" from "the difference a neighborhood makes to individual health outcomes" (Moon et al., 2005). Stated differently, ecological effects on the individual outcome can only be ascertained after individual factors that reflect the composition of the neighborhood have been controlled. Indeed, compositional explanations for ecological variations in health are common, to paraphrase the methodologist Gary King, "if we really understood [health variations], we would not need to know much of contextual effects" (King, 1997). This is an important challenge for researchers interested in understanding ecologic effects. It nonetheless makes intuitive sense to test for the possibility of ecological effects, besides anticipating that the impact of individual level, compositional factors may vary by context. Thus, unless contextual variables are considered, their direct effects and any indirect mediation through compositional variables remain unidentified. Moreover, composition itself has an intrinsic ecologic dimension; the very fact that individual (compositional) factors may "explain" ecologic variations serves as a reminder that the real understanding of ecologic effects is complex. The multilevel framework with its simultaneous examination of the characteristics of the individuals at one level and the context or ecologies in which they are located at another level offers a comprehensive framework for understanding the ways in which places can affect people (contextual) or, alternatively, people can affect places (composition).

In the presence of multilevel data, as described above, there are substantive as well as technical reasons to use multilevel statistical models to analyze such data (Goldstein, 2003; Raudenbush & Bryk, 2002). We shall not review the basic principles of multilevel modeling here, as they have been described elsewhere in the context of health research (Blakely & Subramanian, 2006; Moon et al., 2005; Subramanian et al., 2003), but we provide a brief overview of the type of models invoked for identifying ecologic effects.

4. Multilevel Analytic Models

Multilevel statistical models incorporate parameters for individual and ecologic effects, parameters for individual and ecologic variable effects, and parameters that apportion the variation in the outcomes to different levels (individuals versus ecologies) (Subramanian et al., 2003; Subramanian, 2004). We present the multilevel model specification for the two types of ecologic effects: the CEE and the SEE.

4.1. Common Ecologic Effects (CEE)

Consider the model:

$$y_{ij} = \beta_0 + \boldsymbol{\beta} x_{ij} + (u_{0j} + e_{0ij}) \tag{1}$$

where y_{ij} is the health outcome (e.g., BMI) for individual i in neighborhood j; x is a vector of continuous and categorical individual covariates (e.g., age, sex, socioeconomic status) for that individual; u_{0j} is the random displacement for neighborhood j, assumed to be normally distributed with a mean of zero and variance σ_{u0}^2; and e_{0ij} is the individual- or the level-1 residual, assumed to be identically, independently, and normally distributed with mean zero and a variance

σ_{e0}^2. In model (1) the regression and variance parameters take on the following interpretations: β_0 (associated with a constant x_{0ij}, which is a set of 1s, and therefore, not written) is the average BMI for referenced individuals across all neighborhoods; β is a vector of regression coefficients associated with the vector of individual covariates; σ_{u0}^2 represents the between-neighborhood variation in BMI, conditional on individual (compositional) covariates on BMI; and σ_{e0}^2 represents the between-individual within-neighborhood variation. The presence of more than one residual term (or the structure of the random part more generally) distinguishes the multilevel model from the standard linear regression models or analysis of variance models (Goldstein, 2003). The underlying random structure (variance-covariance matrix, represented as Ω) of model (1) is typically specified as: $Var[u_{0j}] \sim N(0, \sigma_{u0}^2)$; $Var[e_{0ij}] \sim N(0, \sigma_{e0}^2)$; and $Cov[u_{0j}, e_{0ij}] = 0$. Model (1) is usually referred to as the "random-intercepts" or "variance components" model, since it allows us to partition variation according to the different levels, with the variance in y_{ij} being the sum of σ_{u0}^2 and σ_{e0}^2. This in turn also allows us to ascertain the degree of similarity between two randomly chosen individuals within a

neighborhood, expressed as $\rho = \dfrac{\sigma_{u0}^2}{\sigma_{u0}^2 + \sigma_{e0}^2}$ (Goldstein, 2003).

Note that model (1) estimates a variance based on the observed sample of neighborhoods. While this is important to establish the overall importance of neighborhoods as a unit or level, another quantity of interest may pertain to estimating whether living in neighborhood $j = 1$, as compared to neighborhood $j = 3$, for example, predicts a different BMI, conditional on compositional influences of covariates. Given model (1), we can estimate for each level-2 unit: $\hat{u}_{0j} = E(u_{0j} | Y, \hat{\beta}, \hat{\Omega})$. The quantity $\hat{u}_{0j}$ are referred to as "estimated" or "predicted" residuals, or using Bayesian terminology, as "posterior" residual estimates, and are calculated

as $\hat{u}_{0j} = r_j \times \dfrac{\sigma_{u0}^2}{\sigma_{u0}^2 + \sigma_{e0}^2/n_j}$ where σ_{u0}^2 and σ_{e0}^2 are as defined above, r_j is the mean

of the individual-level raw residuals for neighborhood j, and n_j is the number of individuals within each neighborhood j. This formula for $\hat{u}_{0j}$ uses the level-1 and level-2 variances and the number of people observed in neighborhood j to scale the observed level-2 residual (r_j). As the level-1 variance declines or the sample size increases, the scale factor approaches 1, and thus estimated $\hat{u}_{0j}$ approaches r_j.

These neighborhood-level residuals are "random variables with a distribution whose parameter values tell us about the variation among the level-2 units" (Goldstein, 2003). Another interpretation is that each $\hat{u}_{0j}$ estimates neighborhood j's departure from expected mean outcome. This interpretation is premised on the assumption that each neighborhood belongs to a population of neighborhoods, and the distribution of the population provides information about plausible values for neighborhood j (Goldstein, 2003). For a neighborhood with only a few individuals, we can obtain more precise estimates by combining the population and neighborhood-specific observations than if we were to ignore the population membership assumption and use only the information from that neighborhood.

When the estimated residuals at higher-level units are of interest in their own right, we need to provide standard errors, interval estimates, and significance tests as well as point estimates for them (Goldstein, 2003). Contrasting these estimates between different neighborhoods can be used to estimate the CEE, while the distribution of u_{0j} (summarized as σ_{u0}^2) gives a sense of the plausible magnitude of the CEEs.

4.2. Specific Ecologic Effects (SEE)

Model (1) estimated neighborhood effects and differences in the outcome through σ_{u0}^2, and $\hat{u}_{0j}$ but did not consider any specific neighborhood exposures that could have induced the neighborhood differences. Rather, specific exposures (e.g., presence of fast-food outlets) were conceived to be the unobservable part of the neighborhood effect that remains after the contributions of observed individual's background and characteristics are removed. Model (2) considers the specific effect of a neighborhood exposure T_j, coded as 1 if the neighborhood j has fast-food outlets, 0 otherwise:

$$y_{ij} = \beta_0 + \boldsymbol{\beta} \mathbf{x}_{ij} + \alpha T_j \, (u_{0j} + e_{0ij}) \tag{2}$$

where the additional parameter α provides the average change in BMI in neighborhoods with fast food outlets, conditional on the effect of individual covariates, with σ_{u0}^2 estimating the residual variation in neighborhoods after accounting for the observed neighborhood exposure and individual covariates. If aspects of neighborhood environment other than T_j (and aspects of individuals other than x_{ij}) influence BMI, then we expect σ_{u0}^2 to be non-zero. In other words, these differences may be due to neighborhood composition with respect to unmeasured individual characteristics or unmeasured neighborhood exposures. In the neighborhood effects specified in models (1) and (2), we assume uniform effects of neighborhoods or neighborhood characteristics on individual BMI. In other words, we assume that CEE and SEE do not vary across different population groups, but this can be easily incorporated through what are referred to as "random-slopes" and "cross-level interaction" models, respectively (Blakely & Subramanian, 2006; Subramanian et al., 2003).

4.3. Modeling CEE: Fixed or Random?

It is worth drawing parallels between a multilevel or a random-effects model (1) and the conventional OLS or fixed-effects regression model. Consider the fixed-effects model, whereby the neighborhood effect (CEE) is estimated by including a dummy for each neighborhood, as shown below:

$$y_{ij} = \beta_0 + \boldsymbol{\beta} \mathbf{x}_{ij} + \boldsymbol{\beta} N_j + (e_{0ij}) \tag{3}$$

where N_j is a vector of dummy variables for $N - 1$ neighborhoods. The key difference between the fixed- and the random-effects approach to modeling contexts is that while the fixed part coefficients are estimated separately, the random part differentials (u_{0j}) are conceptualized as coming from a distribution (Goldstein, 2003). This conceptualization results in three practical benefits (Jones & Bullen, 1994):

1. *pooling information* between neighborhoods, whereby all the information in the data being used in the combined estimation of the fixed and random part; in particular, the overall regression terms are based on the information for all neighborhoods;
2. *borrowing strength*, whereby neighborhood-specific relations that are imprecisely estimated benefit from the information for other neighborhoods; and
3. *precision-weighted estimation*, whereby unreliable neighborhood-specific fixed estimates are differentially down-weighted or shrunk toward the overall city-wide estimate. A reliably estimated within-neighborhood relation will be largely immune to this shrinkage.

The random-effects and the fixed-effects estimates for each neighborhood, meanwhile, are related (Jones & Bullen, 1994). The neighborhood-specific random intercept (β_{0j}) in a multilevel model is a weighted combination of the specific neighborhood coefficient in a fixed-effects model (β_{0j}^*) and the overall multilevel intercept (β_0) in the following way: $\beta_{0j} = w_j \beta_{0j}^* + (1 - w_j)\beta_0$; the overall multilevel intercept is a weighted average of all the fixed intercepts: $\beta_0 = (\Sigma w_j \beta_{0j}^*)/\Sigma w_j$. Each neighborhood weight is the ratio of the true between-neighborhood parameter variance to the total variance, which additionally includes sampling variance resulting from observing a sample from the neighborhood. Consequently, the weights represent the reliability or precision of the fixed terms: $w_j = \dfrac{\sigma_{u0}^2}{v_j^2 + \sigma_{u0}^2}$ where the random sampling variance of the fixed parameter is $v_j^2 = \dfrac{\sigma_e^2}{n_j}$, with n_j being the number of observations within each neighborhood. Indeed, this is exactly similar to the weights discussed in the Section 4.1. When there are genuine differences between the neighborhoods and the sample sizes within a neighborhood are large, the sampling variance will be small in comparison to the total variance. As a result, the associated weight will be close to 1, with the fixed neighborhood effect being reliably estimated, and the random effect neighborhood estimate will be close to the fixed neighborhood effect. As the sampling variance increases, however, the weight will be less than 1, and the multilevel estimate will increasingly be influenced by the overall intercept based on pooling across neighborhoods. Shrinkage estimates allow the data to determine an appropriate compromise between specific estimates for different neighborhoods and the overall fixed estimate that pools information across places over the entire sample (Jones & Bullen 1994).

Importantly, the fixed-effects approach to modeling neighborhood differences using cross-sectional data is *not* a choice for a typical multilevel research question, where there is an intrinsic interest in an exposure measured at the level of neighborhood, such as the one specified in model (2); in such instances, a multilevel modeling approach is a necessity. This is because the dummy variables associated with the neighborhoods (measuring the fixed-effects of each neighborhood) and the neighborhood exposure is perfectly confounded and, as such, the latter is not identifiable (Fielding, 2004). Thus, the fixed-effects specification to understand neighborhood differences is unsuitable for the sort of complex questions which multilevel modeling can address.

4.4. Exploiting the Flexibility of Multilevel Models to Incorporating "Realistic" Complexity

Current implementations of multilevel models have generally failed to exploit the full capabilities of the analytical framework (Leyland, 2005; Moon et al., 2005; Subramanian, 2004). Much, if not all, of the current research linking neighborhoods and health is cross-sectional and assumes a hierarchical structure of individuals nested within neighborhoods. This simplistic scenario ignores, for instance, the possibility that an individual might move several times and, therefore reflect neighborhood effects drawn from several contexts or that other competing contexts (e.g., schools, workplaces, hospital settings) may simultaneously contribute to contextual effects.

Figure 15.2 provides a visual illustration of one complex, but realistic, multilevel structure for neighborhoods and health research, where time measurements (level 1) are nested within individuals (level 2), who are in turn nested within neighborhoods (level 3). Importantly, individuals are assigned different weights for the time spent in each neighborhood. For example, individual 25 moved from neighborhood 1 to neighborhood 25 during the time period t1-t2, spending 20 percent of her time in neighborhood 1 and 80 percent in her new neighborhood. This multiple membership design would allow control of changing context as well as changing composition. Such designs could be extended to incorporate memberships to additional contexts, such as workplaces or schools. The design can also be extended to enable consideration of weighted effects of proximate

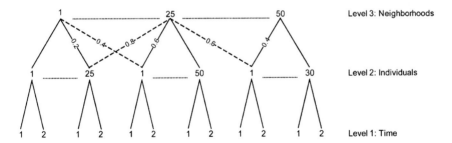

FIGURE 15.2. Multilevel structure of repeated measurements of individuals over time across neighborhoods, with individuals having multiple membership to different neighborhoods across the time span.

Source: (Subramanian, 2004)

contexts (Langford, Bentham, & McDonald 1998). Therefore, for example, the geographic distribution of disease can be seen not only as a matter of composition and the immediate context in which an outcome occurs, but also as a consequence of the impact of nearby contexts, with nearer areas being more influential than more distant ones. While such analyses require high-quality longitudinal and context-referenced data, models that incorporate such "realistic complexity" (Best, Spiegelhalter, Thomas, & Brayne, 1996) are likely to improve our understanding of true neighborhood effects.

While the foregoing discussion provides a sound rationale to adopt a multilevel analytic approach for modeling ecologic effects, this approach obviously does not overcome the limitations intrinsic to any observational study design, single-level or multilevel. Recent discussions on identifying causal ecologic effects (Oakes, 2004) inappropriately conflates issues of study design with the relevance of multilevel models. The critical challenge for identifying neighborhood effects arises from the use of observational (and often cross-sectional) study design and not from the use of any specific analytic technique. Arguably, multilevel models are appropriate analytical techniques for understanding ecologic effects, regardless of whether the data were generated through observation or were a result of an experiment (Subramanian, 2004). Using a counterfactual causal framework, we now discuss the challenges in identifying ecologic effects in non-experimental or observational data settings.

5. Identifying Ecologic Effects: A Causal Counterfactual Perspective

While the original articulation of counterfactual perspectives of causality was undertaken in experimental research (Winship & Morgan, 1999), the counterfactual framework (also referred to as the "potential outcomes" or Rubin Causal Model (RCM)) has been formalized and extended to non-experimental and observational research context, mainly by Donald Rubin (Rubin, 1974, 1978, 2004). According to RCM, the causal effect of any exposure on a person is defined as the difference in the outcome between the world in which the subject receives the treatment and the counterfactual world in which the same individual receives a different exposure value (such as no treatment).

Consider estimating the effect of living in a neighborhood with fast food outlets ($T_j = 1$) compared to living in a neighborhood without fast food outlets ($T_j = 0$) on the BMI (y) of individual i. To directly obtain such an estimate, we would need information on i's BMI when i is a resident of the neighborhood that is exposed to the treatment (denoted $y_i^{T=1}$) and i's BMI when i is a resident of the neighborhood that is not exposed to the treatment ($y_i^{T=0}$), or the control. The "fundamental problem of causal inference" (Holland, 1986), therefore, is that only one of these potential outcomes, $y_i^{T=1}$ or $y_i^{T=0}$, can be observed for individual i. Consequently, identifying causal effects constitutes a "missing data" problem, with half of the potential outcomes missing (Little & Rubin, 2003). Because either outcome is observable in theory, however, one can define the causal effect as the difference (Δ_i) between the two potential outcomes in the treatment (y_i^T) and control (y_i^C) state (Winship & Morgan, 1999).

The target quantities of interest typically are population average treatment effect, i.e., $\bar{y}^T$ (the average or expected value of y_i^T for all individuals had they been exposed to the treatment neighborhoods) and $\bar{y}^C$ (the average or expected value of y_i^C for all individuals had they been exposed to the control neighborhoods). The population average treatment effect is then

$$\bar{\Delta} = \bar{y}^T - \bar{y}^C \tag{4}$$

The two values y_i^T and y_i^C are, however, never observed for the same individuals, so neither $\bar{y}^T$ nor $\bar{y}^C$ can be calculated, but $\bar{y}^T$ and $\bar{y}^C$ can potentially be *estimated*. The aim is to construct from observational data consistent estimates of $\bar{y}^T$ and $\bar{y}^C$ in order obtain a consistent estimate of $\bar{\Delta}$.

This is accomplished in the following manner. Let $\bar{y}^T_{i \epsilon T}$ be the expected value of y_i^T for all individuals in the population who are assigned to the treatment group for observation, and let $\bar{y}^C_{i \epsilon C}$ be the expected value of $\bar{y}^C$ for all individuals in the population who are assigned to the control group for observation. Both these quantities can be calculated and thus effectively estimated by their sample analogs, the mean of y_i for those actually assigned to the treatment and the mean of y_i for those actually assigned to the control (Winship & Morgan, 1999). The standard estimator for the average treatment effect is the difference between these two estimated means:

$$\hat{\bar{\Delta}} = \hat{\bar{y}}^T_{i \epsilon T} - \hat{\bar{y}}^C_{i \epsilon C} \tag{5}$$

where the hats on all three terms signify that they are the sample analog estimators (sample means) of the expectations defined above (Winship & Morgan, 1999). More fundamentally, each sampled individual can be used only once to estimate *either* $\bar{y}^T_{i \epsilon T}$ *or* $\bar{y}^C_{i \epsilon C}$ in equation (5) (Winship & Morgan, 1999).

Consequently, the way in which individuals are assigned (or assign themselves) to the treatment and control groups determines how effectively the standard estimator $\hat{\bar{\Delta}}$ estimates the true or the causal average treatment effect $\bar{\Delta}$. If the outcomes of those who were exposed do not represent the outcomes those in the control group would have had if they had been exposed, the effect estimate will be biased. The goal of most estimators, therefore, is to eliminate the bias resulting from inherent differences (observed and unobserved) between the treatment and control neighborhoods.

A sufficient condition to eliminate the bias is that treatment assignment T_j be independent of the potential outcome distributions of y_i^T and y_i^C. The cleanest way to achieve this independence is through random assignment to the treatment (the cornerstone of RCTs). By definition, observational data are not generated by an explicit randomization scheme, and in most instances treatment assignment will be correlated with the potential outcome variables. The standard estimator thus may yield biased and inconsistent estimates of the true average treatment effect in the population. We briefly discuss the key sources of biases to identifying causal ecologic effects.

5.1. Sources of Bias for Average Treatments Effects

Suppose we find that individuals living in neighborhoods with fast food outlets have higher BMI compared to individuals living in neighborhoods with no fast food outlets. This observation can mean that living in a neighborhood with fast food outlets caused increases in BMI, i.e., the neighborhood BMI difference represents a true causal average treatment effect. Alternatively, it may also mean that individuals living in neighborhoods that have fast food outlets would have had a higher BMI regardless of their exposure to fast food outlets (e.g., because they have a preference for eating calorie-dense foods, which they obtain from other outlets). Specifically, there are three arguments for why those who are exposed to risky neighborhoods may be inherently different from those who are not.

1. *Reverse causation:* What if people choose to move to a particular neighborhood – for example, one with no fast food outlets – and they do so *because* of an existing health status (i.e., they are lean and wish to remain so). This would imply reverse causation, whereby the outcome status drives the extent to which exposure is experienced. Under such a situation, the model with BMI as an outcome and presence of fast food outlets in the neighborhood as the treatment or exposure give biased estimates.

2. *Unobserved confounding:* Bias in the treatment effects can also occur because of the presence of unobserved common causes of neighborhood-level exposures and health outcomes. For example, it is plausible that the decision of fast food franchises to open in particular neighborhoods occurs in response to the "tastes" of local residents. In this instance, "taste for fatty food" would be an unobserved variable that is related to both the location of fast food outlets (exposure) as well as high BMI (outcome).

3. *Covariate balance:* A third bias in the treatment effects estimates can arise if the covariates are mis-specified. This can easily happen if the individual or neighborhood covariate distributions in the treatment neighborhoods (those with fast food outlets) are substantially different from those in the control neighborhoods (those without fast food outlets). In such instances, the estimation of the treatment effects conditional on covariates may not provide a comprehensive adjustment. With little overlap in the covariate values between the treatment and control neighborhoods, the estimated effect for each covariate must be extrapolated and becomes unreliable. Consider individual poverty as an observed confounder of the relationship between presence of fast food outlets in neighborhood and individual BMI, such that individual poverty is related to living in neighborhoods with fast food outlets *and* individual poverty also directly affects BMI. Suppose that in the observed data, there are no poor people living in neighborhoods without fast food outlets (and no non-poor people living in neighborhood with fast food outlets). It is then impossible to estimate the treatment effect "conditional" on poverty. Reliable estimates can only be made where covariate distributions overlap (Rubin, 2004).

4. *Treatment heterogeneity:* If treatment effects are heterogeneous (i.e., the potential effects of treatment may differ for the treatment and control groups), that too may bias the practical relevance of average treatment effects. That is, living in neighborhoods with fast food outlets may adversely affect the BMI of those who actually lived in such neighborhoods even if such exposure would have been innocuous for those who actually lived in neighborhoods without fast food outlets. Of course, it is equally plausible that the treatment has no effect on those who were actually treated but would have been harmful for those who were actually not treated. For example, individuals may only be willing to live in neighborhoods with lots of fast food joints if they believe they can resist the greasy temptations. In this scenario, while the average treatment effect would be biased, the effect of treatment on the treated would be a consistent estimate. The plausibility of heterogeneous treatment effects is specific to social and biological background for each research question. Furthermore, such "treatment heterogeneity" can be of substantive importance in its own right.

Having outlined the key sources of bias, we now discuss methodological approaches that may offer an improved scientific basis for a causal interpretation of ecologic effects and may provide insights into the challenges of identifying ecologic effects in the context of observational data. We conduct this review by using the perspective of Directed Acyclic Graphs (DAGs).

6. Directed Acyclic Graphs (DAGS)

DAGs provide convenient tools for determining the assumptions under which a proposed analysis would identify a causal effect of interest (Greenland & Pearl, 1999; Hernán & Hernandez-Diaz, 2002; Pearl, 2000). Researchers frequently use causal diagrams to visually represent assumptions about causal relations among exposures, outcomes, and covariates. Because causal relations typically manifest as statistical associations, a formalization of these drawings allows us to encode in a diagram the statistical independences entailed by any set of causal assumptions. The statistical dependencies amongst the variables can also be read off a causal DAG under additional assumptions. Figure 15.3 introduces some essential terminology and describes the rules for drawing causal DAGs (see Greenland & Pearl, 1999; Pearl, 2000; Glymour, 2006 for more comprehensive introductions and references).

Here we discuss how analyses for ecologic effects fit with the DAG framework for causal inference. Specifically, quantitative analyses aimed at identifying causal effects can exploit one of three approaches: "the back-door criterion", which involves adjusting for all common causes of the exposure and the outcome; "the front-door criterion", which is premised on measuring an un-confounded mediator along every pathway linking the exposure and the outcome; or "instrumental variables" (e.g., experiments and natural experiments).

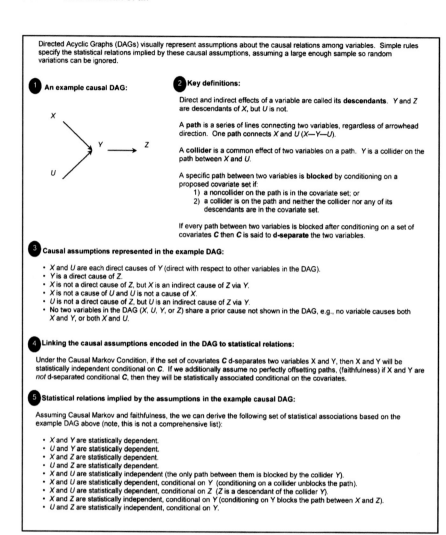

FIGURE 15.3. An overview of Directed Acyclic Graphs.

6.1. The Back-Door Criterion

A set of variables **Z** fulfills the back-door criterion relative to X and Y, if no variable in **Z** is a descendant of X and **Z** blocks every path between X and Y that contains an arrow into X (Pearl, 2000). If **Z** fulfills the back-door criterion, then it is sufficient to identify the causal effect of X on Y. The first element of the back-door criterion – no variable in **Z** is a descendant of X – fits with the general intuition that one ought not adjust for variables influenced by the exposure of interest. The second element specifies that paths induced by common prior causes of X and Y (i.e., "back-door" paths, which have arrows pointing into X) must be blocked in order to identify the effect of *X* on *Y*. Epidemiologic research focusing on identifying causal effects from observational data typically exploits the back-door criterion, for example, by using various forms of covariate adjustment, restriction, stratification, or matching. A major contribution of multilevel models can be conceptualized as improving the likelihood that we have fulfilled the back-door criterion. For example, a completely crude ANOVA or a null multilevel model can be thought of as implicitly assuming the model in Figure 15.4(a), in which neighborhood influences the value of outcome *Y*.

6.1.1. Fulfilling the Back-Door Criterion Using Regression Adjustment

The model presented in figure 15.4(a) may be considered unsatisfactory, however, because people with characteristics that put their health at risk may move into different neighborhoods than people with health advantages. Thus, we believe that individual

(a) Is neighborhood statistically associated with outcome Y?

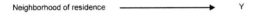

(b) Is neighborhood statistically associated with outcome Y conditional on individual traits

believed to influence Y and neighborhood of residence?

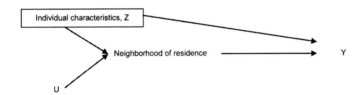

(c) Is neighborhood statistically associated with outcome Y conditional on Z and putative

mediator "neighborhood poverty"?

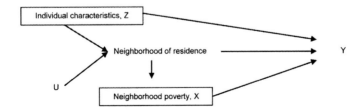

FIGURE 15.4. Graphical illustration of the use of Directed Acyclic Graphs (DAGs) for understanding ecologic effects using the back-door criterion.

characteristics influence both neighborhood of residence and the outcome variable, producing a spurious relationship between neighborhood and the outcome (as in Figure 15.4(b)). In DAG terminology, we consider individual traits Z to be a variable on a back-door path between X and Y, so we adjust for Z. In the remainder of this section, we use the convention of placing boxes around variables in a DAG to indicate that we are interested in a model conditioning on that variable. In Figure 15.4(b), we also include an unmeasured cause of neighborhood of residence (U) and assume that U does not directly affect Y. Under the assumptions in Figure 15.4(b), conditioning on Z would be sufficient to identify the effect of neighborhood of residence on the outcome. If we were to add, however, a direct effect from U to Y, analyses adjusting for Z could of course not estimate the causal neighborhood effect. If neighborhood of residence predicts health even after adjusting for individual traits, we may want to assess whether a specific characteristic of neighborhoods accounts for this association. As in Figure 15.4(c), we conceptualize the effect of neighborhood on outcome Y to be mediated by a specific neighborhood characteristic.

To integrate this distinction with the earlier discussion, the path from neighborhood of residence to Y in Figure 15.4(b) corresponds to the neighborhood CEE discussed earlier; the path from neighborhood poverty to Y in Figure 15.4 (c) corresponds to the SEE for neighborhood poverty. We estimate both the effect of a specific neighborhood characteristic on the outcome and whether the neighborhood predicts the outcome in a model conditional on that neighborhood characteristic.

Neighborhood characteristics that are "structural" or "intrinsic" (e.g., high density of fast food outlets) are often preferred to neighborhood characteristics that are based on aggregating individual characteristics (e.g., percent poverty). Part of the appeal of using intrinsic or structural neighborhood characteristics as the exposure, instead of aggregated individual traits, is that individual characteristics are less likely influence to influence structural features of a neighborhood and thus less likely to confound the neighborhood effect estimate. For example, individual poverty does not directly cause zoning laws permitting dense aggregation of fast food outlets. Nevertheless, individual income may indirectly influence even structural neighborhood characteristics: poor people may select to live in neighborhoods with high density of fast food outlets (the rents may be lower), and poor people may be at a disadvantage for implementing and enforcing zoning laws keeping out fast food stores. Thus, although intrinsic neighborhood characteristics may be less vulnerable to individual level confounding than aggregated traits, they are not immune to such biases.

In summary, we can think of efforts to account for neighborhood composition as attempts to block back door paths between neighborhood and outcomes. One critique of efforts to identify neighborhood effects is that it is impossible to adequately model the variables that block the back-door paths. For example, it is argued that people living in deprived neighborhoods are almost entirely non-comparable to people living in advantaged neighborhoods with respect to individual-level determinants of health outcomes (Oakes, 2004). If individual level SES and neighborhood SES were completely collinear, then it would certainly not be possible to disentangle neighborhood from individual effects. This is a testable proposition, however. One approach to address this concern is to use matching.

6.1.2. Fulfilling the Back-Door Criterion Using Matching or Propensity Scores

Matching methods enable observational data to replicate two key features of randomized experiments (Rosenbaum & Rubin, 1983; Rubin, 2004). First, the study is done on groups of units that are similar with respect to observed covariates. Second, the study is "designed" in a way that treated and control units are matched *without* using the outcome variable. Prior to analyzing the outcome, the matched samples are assessed for covariate overlap ("balance") to ensure that, within each matched group, treatment assignment looks as if it could have arisen from a randomized experiment, where treatment assignment probability is a function of observed covariates. If a covariate balance is impossible using matching methods, researchers should conclude that reliable causal inferences cannot be drawn from the existing data without invoking unrealistic assumptions to justify ambitious extrapolations.

Ideally, one could match control groups to treatment groups by matching exactly on all observed covariates, such that each treatment-control pair has the same values on all observed covariates; this is known as "exact matching". In practice, however, this may not be feasible, especially when the dimensionality of the covariate is set is very high (e.g., when there are several relevant covariates or some covariates are continuous). An alternative means of matching is to match treatment and control groups on a summary measure based on a joint function of all covariates. The goal is to estimate the probability of a subject being exposed to a treatment, known as the propensity score, conditional on all observed covariates (Rosenbaum & Rubin, 1983; Rubin, 1997a,b). Researchers can also combine exact and propensity score-based matching, and matching can also be done as a pre-processing step before conducting modeling (Ho, Imai, King, & Stuart, 2007).

In randomized experiments the true propensity scores, or the probability that a particular subject will receive the treatment, is known (in a balanced 2-arm trial $p = 0.5$). In observational studies, the propensity scores must be estimated from the data, often using a logit or a probit model. Rosenbaum and Rubin (1983), who coined the term "propensity score", show that sub-classification, pair matching, and model-based adjustment for the propensity score all lead to unbiased estimates of the treatment effect when the treatment assignment is correctly modeled (Rosenbaum & Rubin, 1983). The general method is relatively simple (Rubin, 1997a,b). First, a regression model using all observed covariates to predict whether an individual receives the treatment is estimated. Second, the predicted probabilities of receiving the treatment (the propensity scores) are estimated from the first stage model. Third, treated subjects are matched to controls based on their propensity scores, using any of several matching algorithms. Unmatched observations are excluded from further analyses. Fourth, observed covariates are checked for balance. Finally, treated and control groups are compared on the outcome. Alternatively, a regression model can be estimated on the "matched" sample, predicting the outcome with the treatment variable and controlling matched covariates. Incorrect specification of the treatment model (stage 1), e.g., by including variables affected by the treatment or outcome, omitting an important confounder, or mis-specifying the functional form, can invalidate the propensity score adjusted effect estimates. When all the assumptions for regression analysis are met, particularly correct functional form and well-supported data, propensity score matching alone offers little advantage over traditional regression models.

Figure 15.5 brings an explicitly multilevel perspective to propensity models (PM), where rows present the unit at which the treatment is observed (individual (t) or neighborhood (T)) and the columns indicate level (individual (x) and neighborhood (X))) at which covariates are measured. The critical substantive question for a model where the treatment is at the neighborhood level is whether the matching should be done based on a vector of individual covariates (PM^{III}), neighborhood covariates (PM^{IV}, 1), or both (PM^{IV}, 2).

Ideally, one should consider Pr $(T = 1| x, X)$(PM^{IV}, 2) where the propensity to receive the treatment is a function of observed individual and neighborhood covariates. Consider implementing the PM^{III} $(T = 1| x)$, where the probability that neighborhood treatment $= 1$ is estimated conditional on individual observed covariates. Because the treatment cannot vary within a neighborhood (between individuals), we need to consider T as an individual treatment (i.e., replicate the same value of T for every individual in an area). As such, the model would be indistinguishable from Pr $(t = 1| x)$, a situation when treatment is at the individual level (PM^{I}). The treatment, strictly speaking, is, observed at the neighborhood level, but this may present a serious difficulty with respect to precision, as the number of neighborhoods in the study will be smaller than the n for individuals.

The difficulties posed by small samples of neighborhoods are exacerbated because neighborhood risk factors often coexist: Neighborhoods with one harmful exposure tend to have other potentially harmful exposures as well. As a result,

		Covariate	
		Individual (x)	Neighborhood (X)
Treatment	Individual (t)	PM^{I} 1. $\Pr(t=1|x)$	PM^{II} 1. $\Pr(t=1|x,u_j)$ 2. $\Pr(t=1|x,X,u_j)$ 3. $\Pr(t=1|x,X)$
	Neighborhood (T)	PM^{III} 1. $\Pr(T=1|x)$	PM^{IV} 1. $\Pr(T=1|X)$ 2. $\Pr(T=1|x,X)$

FIGURE 15.5. Multilevel perspective on propensity score models.

it is often very difficult to disentangle which neighborhood characteristic is driving health outcomes. In some cases, the neighborhood characteristics may interact with one another (so that any one of them alone would be sufficient to cause ill health or so that all are required simultaneously). Such correlations reduce the effective sample size, rendering it very difficult to identify the independent effect of each neighborhood characteristic. This highlights the importance of considering both the CEE and the SEE. In the above situation, the SEE for a potentially very harmful neighborhood trait T could approach zero in some strata, for example, if most neighborhoods with T = 1 also had some other harmful trait Z = 1, and Z alone was sufficient to create bad outcomes. This phenomenon would not affect the CEE.

A limitation of the propensity score approach and other matching strategies is that they are entirely based on observed covariates. Sensitivity analyses can help define bounds for the effect estimates under a plausible range of unobserved confounding. In a recent analysis, Harding (2003) examined how the point estimates and confidence intervals for a neighborhood exposure (neighborhood poverty on teenage pregnancy and school drop out) changed under combinations of unobserved confounder influence on the outcome and treatment (Harding, 2003). Such a strategy pushes researchers to quantify a plausible range of "unobservables". Consider the example outlined in Figure 15.4(c), but imagine we believed some unmeasured individual characteristics influenced both neighborhood of residence and the outcome Y (i.e., some elements of the vector Z were unmeasured). We might adopt a sensitivity analysis to calculate the bias that would be introduced under a range of relationships between the putative individual level confounders and the neighborhood poverty and the individual level confounders and the outcome. We now turn to two approaches to causal inference that may be used when all of the confounders of the treatment and outcome have *not* been measured.

6.2. The Front Door Criterion

A set of variables M satisfies the front-door criterion relative to X and Y if: M intercepts all directed paths from X to Y, there is no back-door path from X to any member of M, and all back door paths from M to Y are blocked by X (Pearl, 2000). In other words, if M includes a variable on every pathway linking X and Y and all the common causes of variables in M and Y operate via X, then M fulfills the front-door criterion (Figure 15.6).

Conceptually, the front-door criterion can be used because the effects of X on each individual mediator (e.g., M_1 and M_2 in Figure 15.6) are unconfounded, and the relationships between the individual mediators and Y are unconfounded *conditional on* X. Each element in the pathway between X and Y can be identified, and thus the entire effect of X on Y can be identified. Satisfying the front-door criterion is difficult because one rarely has unconfounded, measured mediators along every pathway between an exposure and outcome of interest. Because the front door criterion is quite different than the conventional approaches, however, it may be a promising way to solve apparently intractable identification problems (Winship & Morgan, 1999; Winship & Harding, in press).

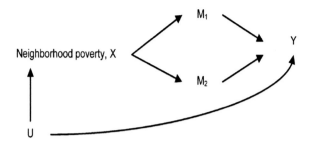

FIGURE 15.6. Graphical illustration of the use of Directed Acyclic Graphs (DAGs) for understanding ecologic effects using the front-door criterion. The crucial assumptions are that all paths between the exposure of interest X and the outcome include measured mediators (M_1 and M_2) and that there is no direct arrow from an unmeasured cause of the outcome (U) into the measured mediators (all paths from the confounder to the mediators pass through X).

6.3. Instrumental Variables

Instrumental variables (IV) are useful when collecting data on a comprehensive list of possible confounders is quite impractical. No matter how long the list of measured covariates, it is never as long as the list of potential confounders. Certain confounders can never be observed. For instance, "taste for fatty food" may confound the relationship between BMI and presence of fast food outlets in neighborhoods, but such preferences are quite challenging, if not impossible, to measure.

Instrumental variables have been defined in econometric terms (Angrist, Imbens, & Rubin, 1996), in terms of counterfactuals, and by using DAGs (Pearl, 2000). The intuition for instrumental variables is the same as the intuition for randomized trials. In fact, trials can be thought of as a special case of instrumental variables, a case in which we feel particularly confident that the assumptions for a valid instrument have been met (Greenland, 2000). Instrumental variable estimation with naturally occurring instruments, such as natural experiments or policy discontinuities, are more typical in econometrics (Angrist et al., 1996). Figures 15.7(a)–15.7(f) contrast graphical structures with valid and invalid instruments.

Figure 15.7(a) graphically describes the threat posed by unmeasured confounders (U) (e.g., taste for junk food) for the effect of treatment (T) (e.g., presence of fast food outlets) on individual outcome (y) (e.g., BMI). Figure 15.7(b) introduces an IV (Z) (e.g., proximity to schools) as a solution to remove the bias in the association between T and y caused by U. We hypothesize that the instrumental variable (Z) influences exposure (T) but has no direct effect on y (other than through induced changes in values of T) and shares no common causes with y. In our example, we propose that fast food outlets tend to locate near schools, and thus, an individual's proximity to a school probably influences their proximity to fast outlets in the neighborhood. However, living near a school should not affect individual BMI through any pathway other than the presence of fast outlets in the neighborhood.

(a) Notion of unobserved confounder (U)

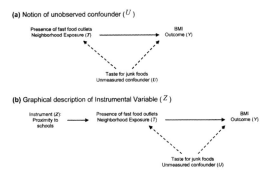

(b) Graphical description of Instrumental Variable (Z)

(c) Invalid instrument, due to a "direct path from Z to y"

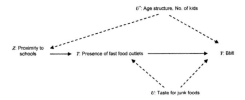

(d) Invalid instrument, due to a "path from Z to U"

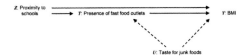

(e) Invalid instrument, due to the "common prior cause for Z and y"

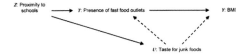

(f) Invalid instrument, due to direct effect from T to Z, so unmeasured common causes of T and Y are also unmeasured causes of Z and Y.

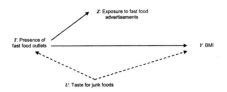

FIGURE 15.7. Graphical illustration of valid and invalid Instrumental Variables (IV) in the presence of an unmeasured confounder.

6.3.1. Challenges to IV Analysis

Except for cases when intentional randomization is possible, it is not easy to identify convincing instrumental variables. We present four examples of invalid instruments (which do not avoid the bias induced by unmeasured confounders). If there is a *direct* path from proximity to schools (Z) to individual BMI (y) that is not mediated by fast food outlets, then Z would be an invalid instrument (Figure 15.7(c)). Similarly if there is a path from Z to U (the unmeasured confounder, "taste for junk foods"), then that too would make Z an invalid instrument (Figure 15.7(d)). In the presence of a common prior cause U^* of Z and y, then Z would be an invalid instrument. For instance, age structure of the neighborhood or number of families with school-going children in the neighborhood is likely to determine the presence of schools and may also influence BMI (Figure 15.7(e)). It is important that the instrument affects the exposure of interest, not vice versa. For example, "exposure to fast food advertising" is not likely to be a valid instrument for presence of fast food outlets in the neighborhood (Figure 15.7(f)). Living in a neighborhood with a number of fast food outlets likely causes one to be exposed to the advertisements which accompany such places, but all of the unmeasured factors that confound the association between neighborhood presence of fast food outlets and the outcome will also confound the association between exposure to advertising and the outcome. Conceptually, the cleanest instrument is a randomized trial, and it is plain that some completely external assignment mechanism for the instrument is needed.

Most prior IV work focuses on finding instruments for the effects of individual-level exposures on individual level outcomes. In this research, ecological variables, such as state policies, are often used as instruments to estimate the effect of an individual-level exposure on an individual level outcome (Currie & Gruber, 1996; Ettner, 1997). These administrative policies and other ecological variables that are sometimes used as instruments to estimate individual level effects may themselves be the exposures of interest for researchers working on contextual effects. In fact, if there are truly contextual effects, not mediated by the individual level variables, such place-level characteristics may not be valid instruments for the individual level exposure. For example, consider using state unemployment rate is an instrument for the effect of individual unemployment on health on the grounds that state unemployment rate influences each residents' own chances of being unemployed but is uncorrelated with any individual's personal skills or talents that would make him or her more likely to be unemployed. However, if living in a place with high unemployment rates has a directly harmful (or beneficial) effect on individuals that is not mediated by their own employment status (e.g., due to psychological anxiety about potential job loss or to divestment in public goods because all the extra money is being spent on unemployment insurance), then this is not a valid instrument.

Identifying a convincing natural experiment is even more difficult when the exposure of interest is a neighborhood characteristic. The work of Cutler and Glaeser (1997) and Hoxby (2000) is notable for clever use of ecological characteristics such as rivers (which affected formation of school district boundaries) as instruments for ecological exposures, specifically school-choice options and residential segregation. Acemoglu and Angrist (1999) attempted to use two instruments – month of birth at the individual level and state compulsory schooling law at the ecological level – to disentangle the effects of one's own education from the effects of living in a highly educated community. This approach is quite challenging because confidence bounds for instrumental variable effect estimates are inflated (in inverse proportion to the association between the instrument and the exposure).

Efforts to identify valid instrumental variables for neighborhood effects might focus on potential natural experiments, such as arrival or departure of major employers, market dominance of discriminatory versus non-discriminatory lenders and insurers, rent stabilization programs, or placement of low-income housing complexes. The possibility of identifying truly ecological effects (not mediated by individual SES) depends on measuring individual level social position and blocking this pathway in the analyses. Convincing stories will almost certainly require longitudinal data. Interrupted time-series designs or quasi-experiments hold some promise. Cummins and colleagues (2005) reported a prospective, quasi-experiment in a deprived Scottish community where the researchers were able to assess dietary intakes among 412 adults before and after the opening of a large supermarket. They concluded that fruit and vegetable consumption did not change over follow-up in response to the intervention. However, before hastening to the conclusion that local availability of fruits and vegetables does not matter for maintaining a healthy diet, we need to be cautious about drawing firm conclusions from what was effectively an experiment with a sample size of 1.

The most devastating critique of an IV analysis is that the instrument is not valid because it either directly affects the outcome or it has a common prior cause with the outcome. If the instrument derives from an ecological variable, these concerns are especially pertinent. The weaker the instrument (that is, the smaller the effect of the instrument on exposure), the greater is the dependence of the IV estimate on the assumption of a valid instrument. Because of the way that IV effect estimates are typically calculated, small biases are inflated in inverse proportion to the association between the instrument and the exposure (Z and T in Figure 15.7). Even a small association between the instrument and the outcome that is not mediated by the exposure of interest can produce serious biases in IV effect estimates for the exposure. For this reason, criticisms of the validity of the instrument must be taken seriously, even if they hypothesize fairly small relationships.

Sample size poses an additional challenge in applying IV methods in the context of natural experiments. Because IV analyses identify causal effects based on changes in the subgroup of the population whose exposure was affected by the instrument, the effective sample size for the analysis is much smaller than the actual sample size. As a result, the confidence intervals for IV effect estimates are often very wide. Using instruments with a greater effect on the exposure or increasing the sample size can tighten confidence intervals. Because of the potential for bias in weak instruments, finding "better" natural experiments (that is, instruments that have a large effect on the exposure of interest or are unequivocally valid) is generally preferable to increasing the sample size.

Furthermore, conventional IV estimates do not estimate the population average causal effect. They specifically estimate the effect of the exposure on people whose exposure was influenced by the instrument (sometimes called cooperators). If treatment effects are homogeneous, this equals the population average causal effect. If treatment effects differ across population substrata, the specific estimates available from IVs may be an advantage or a disadvantage, depending on the question and the instrument. For example, the effect of exposure on cooperators may be of greater interest than the effect on those who avoided the exposure. For many social exposures, there is every reason to suspect heterogeneous treatment effects.

A general criticism of IV estimates is that it is impossible to identify the particular subpopulation to which the causal effect estimate applies – those whose exposure was affected by the instrument. For any one person, we observe the level of exposure they received given the value the instrument actually took but not the level of exposure they would have received had the instrument taken on a different value. Although we know the IV effect estimate is the causal effect among cooperators, we generally have no way to identify who in a population is a cooperator.

A more prosaic challenge in interpreting IV estimates from natural experiments is to understand what the instrument represents, that is, what precisely is the exposure that is influenced by the instrument? This may be especially challenging for instruments for contextual variables. For example, if we use proximity to schools as an instrument for residence near fast food outlets, we might ask, is there anything unusual about the types of fast food outlets that locate near schools?

7. Randomized Experiments

Although most of this chapter focuses on observational studies, it is also helpful to consider experiments. Defining the ideal experiments to identify neighborhood effects serves to highlight the limitations of observational studies and therefore potential approaches to addressing such limitations. Furthermore, many of the data collection and analysis issues in observational multilevel studies are also relevant in experimental studies.

Two types of experiments can be conceptualized for identifying ecologic effects. One approach would randomly assign individuals to different neighborhoods, e.g., neighborhoods with or without fast food outlets or with high or low poverty rates, and assess any health differences that emerge between residents assigned to different types of neighborhoods. These experiments are referred to as "mobility experiments", and the *Gatreaux* (Rosenbaum, 1995) and the *Moving to Opportunity* (MTO) (Katz, Kling,& Liebman, 2001) studies provide the only experimental investigation of neighborhood effects on socioeconomic and health outcomes (although *Gatreaux* was technically quasi-experimental).

For instance, as a part of the MTO Project (Kling, 2000), between 1994 and 1997, 4248 families living in public housing in Baltimore, Boston, Chicago,

Los Angeles, and New York were randomly assigned to (1) receive a housing voucher that could be used to move to a low poverty neighborhood along with mobility counseling; (2) receive a housing voucher with no geographic restrictions; or (3) be included in the control group (no new assistance, but continued eligibility for public housing). In 2002, one adult from each family was interviewed regarding five domains: economic self-sufficiency, mental health, physical health, risky behavior, and education. Significant beneficial effects were observed for adult mental health outcome and physical health associated with BMI (Katz et al., 2001). The experiment also found evidence for treatment heterogeneity such that the health outcomes improved for girls in the experimental group relative to control but were in some cases worse for boys in the experimental group compared to control. These results underscore the need to develop and test theoretical perspectives on treatment heterogeneity (Kling, Liebman, & Katz, 2005).

MTO has been criticized because the design randomized families to move to low poverty neighborhoods rather than randomizing neighborhoods to poverty reduction programs. Moving families may not identify the specific effect of neighborhood poverty if individuals have ties to their neighborhoods that influence their well-being independently of the poverty rate of the neighborhood. The consequences of breaking those ties – whether they are harmful (e.g., gang ties) or beneficial (e.g., trusted neighbors) – could swamp the consequences of changing individual exposure to a high poverty community. Such interventions are sometimes called "fat-hand": The clumsy intervening hand has altered more than the specific causal agent of interest. If this is the case, it does not speak to the causal effect (or non-effect) of neighborhood poverty level. Comparing movers to non-movers is not an adequate way to estimate the effect of neighborhood poverty because it also changes social connections. The causal structure would look like that in Figure 15.7(c), in which the instrument (randomization to a housing voucher) influences the health outcome via a pathway not mediated by neighborhood poverty, specifically, breaking social connections in the original neighborhood. To handle this problem, we would either have to leave people in the neighborhoods where they had long resided but change the poverty level in that neighborhood, or compare families who moved to different types of neighborhoods, e.g., low poverty versus high poverty communities.

Similarly, it is often difficult to intervene specifically on one neighborhood characteristic and not affect numerous other neighborhood characteristics. High crime neighborhoods will likely have greater levels of social distrust; therefore, it may be difficult to disentangle these effects. However, if it is impossible to change one neighborhood characteristic without changing other neighborhood characteristics, the causal effect of isolated interventions may not be of much public health interest anyway.

Another instance in which the effects of moving people might diverge from changing the neighborhood could occur if the characteristic of interest is an aggregate characteristic of neighborhood residents. If so, moving an individual to a new neighborhood actually changes the exposure in the new neighborhood.

It is tempting to assume this affect would be trivial, but that need not be the case. For example, the well-being of neighborhood residents may be driven by the very poorest residents, and the transplants might be quite a bit more impoverished than even the worst-off of the current residents. For many mechanisms, a small minority may have disproportionate influence, for better or worse.

Another frequently raised issue has been the relatively low take-up rates of the treatment in the study population. Nonetheless, the MTO results present some important challenges to neighborhood effects research because effect estimates are generally more modest than the results from observational studies (and, for boys, in the opposite direction). In addition to a direct treatment effect estimate, one of the most important questions that we might hope to answer with MTO results is to what extent the observational studies of neighborhoods are biased. We need to address this because the observational studies can be used for a much wider range of exposure characterizations and much more diverse samples than even the most ambitious randomized trial. If the observational results are reliable, they are thus likely to help us learn more useful information about neighborhood effects. However, if they are unreliable, we need to understand this in interpreting such studies.

The MTO study authors directly addressed this question by treating MTO as an observational follow-up study and comparing their effect estimates from this approach to the effect estimates when they used the randomization. They concluded that the results suggested very complicated selection processes prevailed in observational data, making causal effect estimates from observational data quite challenging. However, it will also be invaluable to directly compare MTO results to other observational studies using comparable causal contrasts. For example, if we follow individuals in an observational study who move from high to low poverty communities, do we see their outcomes improve? Which outcomes and how long after the move do improvements appear? Such analyses can give plausible ranges for input parameters in sensitivity analyses such as that exploited by Harding (2003).

A second type of experiment for identifying ecologic effects would involve randomly assigning neighborhoods certain desirable characteristics (such as closing down fast food outlets or observing the opening of a new supermarket) and evaluating the change before and after the intervention. This type of experiment poses two challenges. First, there is the difficulty of disentangling secular trends from effects of the intervention, so it is important to have comparison neighborhoods that do not receive the intervention or receive it on a delayed schedule. Secondly, the sample size requirements are very demanding for reliably estimating any effects, since the number of neighborhoods that would be part of the treatment and control group would be much lower than the number of individuals in these groups. For example, suppose we observe the opening of supermarkets in 10 communities and compare the impact on residents' intake of fresh fruits and vegetables to those living in 10 control communities without a supermarket. Regardless of the size of each community, the effective n is only 20. The "small" sample size is a concern that is intrinsic to all study designs with an interest estimating ecologic effects – experimental, quasi-experimental, or purely observational.

A final point to add is that experiments and natural experiments are useful only to the extent that assignment of the exposure was effectively randomized, i.e., is independent of the potential outcomes. If the opening of a new supermarket in a neighborhood reflects the underlying preferences of residents (or example, they lobbied for one to open), then we are "back to square one" with respect to the problems of selection and endogeneity.

8. Conclusions

In this chapter, we focused our discussion on the methodological assessment of research on ecologic effects. We undertook this assessment from the objective of estimating "causal" as opposed to "descriptive" ecologic effects and highlighted the challenges confronting researchers in accomplishing this task in observational studies. We did not address issues related to measurement of ecologies (Raudenbush, 2003; Sampson & Morenoff, 2002; Mujahid, Diez Roux, Morenoff, & Raghunathan, 2007), which represent an important challenge (as well as opportunity) for researchers interested in modeling ecologic effects. How we measure ecologies can be important for interpreting the causal effect. For instance, if the ecologic variable is based on aggregating individual information, this may suggest the presence of correlated or collective effects (Macintyre, 1997; Manski, 1993), as opposed to measures that are uniquely observed and measured at the ecologic level, suggesting contextual or exogenous effects (Macintyre, 1997; Manski, 1993). Defining the estimand in the former may be somewhat more challenging than in the latter.

While researchers should exercise caution when estimating ecological causal effects using observational data, the challenges are similar to the perennial difficulties in observational epidemiology. It is encouraging to note in a review comparing observational studies and randomized controlled trials between 1984 and 1998 for a same outcome and exposure, the authors found little evidence that estimates of treatment effects in observational studies were consistently larger than or qualitatively different from those obtained in the randomized controlled trials (Benson & Hartz, 2000). Moreover, even the results from MTO suggest causal effects of neighborhoods for risk of obesity and a range of mental health outcomes, although they also highlight the importance of examining heterogeneous treatment effects in future research (Katz et al., 2001). Furthermore, while experiments provide valuable knowledge on the magnitude and presence of causal effects, ideal experimental designs are rarely feasible for neighborhood and health studies due to high cost, difficulty of implementation, restrictiveness of the sample (typically low income people), self-selection of participants in the intervention, the impossibility of manipulating every potentially relevant neighborhood characteristic, etc. Observational study designs are likely to be more practical and may sometimes provide a qualitatively better source of understanding for diverse ecologic effects. Because of the tremendous difficulty of implementing neighborhood experiments, a primary analysis goal for the few convincing experiments available should be to test for and quantify the magnitude of factors that may confound observational studies.

In summary, we have discussed two types of ecologic effects and emphasized the importance of clearly defining the causal contrast of interest in any proposed analysis. Multilevel models can potentially be applied to estimate either CEEs or SEEs, but with observational data, both types of estimates are vulnerable to bias due to selection effects or heterogeneous treatment effects. We have highlighted some areas where we believe future efforts should focus to advance our understanding of neighborhood effects: modeling complex, multiple membership models; improving control of measured confounders using matching and propensity score techniques; advancing approaches exploiting instrumental variables; and conducting experiments and natural experiments to directly assess neighborhood effects and to quantify potential biases in observational studies. By incorporating the methods and approaches from economics, geography, and sociology (among other disciplines) into public health, research on ecologic effects is poised to make a quantum leap in causal inference as well as usefulness for policy.

References

Acemoglu, D., & Angrist, J. D. (1999). *How large are the social returns to education? Evidence from compulsory schooling laws.* NBER Working Paper Series Working Paper 7444.

Angrist, J. D., Imbens, G. W., & Rubin, D. B. (1996). Identification of causal effects using instrumental variables. *Journal of the American Statistical Association, 91,* 444–55.

Benson, K., & Hartz, A. J. (2000). A comparison of observational studies and randomized controlled trials. *New England Journal of Medicine, 342*(25), 1878–1886.

Best, N. G., Spiegelhalter, D. J., Thomas, A., & Brayne, C. E. G. (1996). Bayesian analysis of realistically complex models. *Journal of Royal Statistical Society A, 159,* 232–342.

Blakely, T. A., & Subramanian, S. V. (2006). Multilevel studies. Methods for social epidemiology. In J. M. Oakes & J. S. Kaufman (Eds.), *Methods in social epidemiology.* New York: Jossey-Bass/Wiley.

Blakely, T. A., & Woodward, A. J. (2000). Ecological effects in multi-level studies. *Journal of Epidemiology and Community Health, 54,* 367–374.

Cummins, S., Petticrew, M., Higgins, C., Findlay, A., Sparks, L. (2005). Large scale food retailing as an intervention for diet and health: Quasi-experimental evaluation of a natural experiment. *Journal of Epidemiology and Community Health, 59*(12), 1035–1040.

Currie, J., Gruber, J. (1996). Saving babies: The efficacy and cost of recent changes in the Medicaid eligibility of pregnant women. *Journal of Political Economy CIV, 104*(6), 1256–1296.

Cutler, D. M., Glaeser, E. L. (1997). Are ghettos good or bad? *Quarterly Journal of Economics 112*(3), 827–872.

Ettner, S. L. (1997). Measuring the human cost of a weak economy: Does unemployment lead to alcohol abuse? *Social Science & Medicine, 44*(2), 251–60.

Fielding, A. (2004). The role of the Hausman Test and whether higher level effects should be treated as random or fixed. *Multilevel Modeling Newsletter, 16*(2), 3–9.

Glymour, M. (2006). Using causal diagrams to understand common problems in social epidemiology. In J. M. Oakes & J. S. Kaufman (Eds.), *Methods in social epidemiology*. New York: Jossey-Bass/Wiley.

Goldstein, H. (2003). *Multilevel statistical models*. London: Arnold.

Greenland, S. (2000). An introduction to instrumental variables for epidemiologists. *International Journal of Epidemiology*, 29, 722–9.

Greenland, S., & Pearl, J. (1999). Causal diagrams for epidemiologic research. *Epidemiology, 10*(1), 37–48.

Harding, D. J. (2003). Counterfactual models of neighborhood effects: The effect of neighborhood poverty on dropping out and teenage pregnancy. *American Journal of Sociology, 109*(3), 676–719.

Hernán, M. A., & Hernandez-Diaz, S. (2002). Causal knowledge as a prerequisite for confounding evaluation: An application to birth defects epidemiology. *American Journal of Epidemiology, 155*(2), 176–184.

Ho, D. E., Imai, K., King, G., & Stuart, E. A. (2007, in press). Matching as nonparametric preprocessing for reducing model dependence in parametric causal inference. *Political Analysis*.

Holland, P. W. (1986). Statistics and causal inference (with discussion and rejoinder). *Journal of the American Statistical Association, 81*, 945–970.

Hoxby, C. M. (2000). Does competition among public schools benefit students and taxpayers? *American Economic Review, 90*(5), 1209–1238.

Jones, K., & Bullen, N. (1994). Contextual models of urban house prices: A comparison of fixed- and random-coefficient models developed by expansion. *Economic Geography, 70*, 252–272.

Katz, L. F., Kling, J., & Liebman, J. (2001). Moving to opportunity in Boston: Early impacts of a housing mobility program. *Quarterly Journal of Economics 116*(2), 607–654.

Kawachi, I., & Berkman, L. F. (Eds.), (2003). *Neighborhoods and health*. New York: Oxford University Press.

Kawachi, I., & Subramanian, S. V. (2006). Measuring and modeling the social and geographic context of trauma: A multilevel modeling approach. *Journal of Traumatic Stress, 19*(2), 195–203.

Kawachi, I., & Subramanian, S. V. (2007). Neighborhood influences on health. *Journal of Epidemiology and Community Health,61*(1), 3–4.

King, G. (1997). *A solution to the ecological inference problem: Reconstructing individual behavior from aggregate data*. Princeton: Princeton University Press.

Kling, J. (2000). *Moving to opportunity research*. Washington, DC (April 30, 2006); http://www.nber.org/~kling/mto/

Kling, J. R., Liebman, J. B., & Katz, L. F. (2005). *Experimental analysis of neighborhood effects*. Cambridge, MA: National Bureau of Economic Research.

Krieger, N., Chen, J. T., Waterman, P. D., Rehkopf, D. H., & Subramanian, S. V. (2005). Painting a truer picture of US socioeconomic and racial/ethnic health inequalities: The Public Health Disparities Geocoding Project. *American Journal of Public Health, 95*(2), 312–323.

Langford, I. H., Bentham, G., & McDonald, A. L. (1998). Multilevel modeling of geographically aggregated health data: A case study on malignant melanoma mortality and UV exposure in the European Community. *Statistics in Medicine, 17*(1), 41–57.

Leyland, A. H. (2005). Assessing the impact of mobility on health: Implications for life course epidemiology. *Journal of Epidemiology and Community Health, 59*, 90–91.

Little, R. J., & Rubin, D. B. (2003). *Statistical analysis with missing data*. New York: John Wiley & Sons.

Macintyre, S. (1997). What are the spatial effects and how can we measure them? In A. Dale (Ed.), *Exploiting national surveys and census data: The role of locality and spatial effects*. Manchester: Faculty of Economic and Social Studies, University of Manchester.

Manski, C. F. (1993). Identification problems in social sciences. *Sociological Methodology, 23*, 1–56.

Moon, G., Subramanian, S. V., Jones, K., Duncan, C., & Twigg, L. (2005). Area-based studies and the evaluation of multilevel influences on health outcomes. In A. Bowling & S. Ebrahim (Eds.), *Handbook of health research methods: Investigation, measurement and analysis*. Berkshire, England: Open University Press.

Mujahid, M., Diez Roux, A., Morenoff, J., & Raghunathan./ T. (2007). Assessing the measurement properties of neighborhood scales: from psychometrics to ecometrics. *Amercian Journal of Epidemiology, 165*(8), 858–867

Oakes, M. (2004). The (mis)estimation of neighborhood effects: Causal inference for a practicable social epidemiology. *Social Science and Medicine, 58*, 1929–1952.

Pearl, J. (2000). *Causality*. Cambridge, UK: Cambridge University Press.

Raudenbush, S., & Bryk, A. (2002). *Hierarchical linear models: Applications and data analysis methods*. Thousand Oaks, CA: Sage Publications.

Raudenbush, S. W. (2003). The quantitative assessment of neighborhood social environment. In I. Kawachi & L. F. Berkman (Eds.), *Neighborhoods and health*. New York: Oxford University Press.

Raudenbush, S. W., & Willms, J. D. (1995). The estimation of school effects. *Journal of Educational and Behavioral Statistics, 20*(4), 307–335.

Rosenbaum, J. (1995). Changing the geography of opportunity by expanding residential choice: Lessons from the Gautreaux program. *Housing Policy Debate, 6*, 231–269.

Rosenbaum, P. R., & Rubin, D. B. (1983). The central role of the propensity score in observational studies for causal effects. *Biometrika, 70*, 41–55.

Rubin, D. B. (1974). Estimating causal effects of treatments in randomized and non-randomized studies. *Journal of Educational Psychology, 66*, 688–701.

Rubin, D. B. (1978). Bayesian inference for causal effects: The role of randomization. *Annals of Statistics, 6*, 34–58.

Rubin, D. B. (1997a). Estimating causal effects from large data sets using propensity scores. *Annals of Internal Medicine, 127*, 757–763.

Rubin, D. B. (1997b). Practical implications of the modes of statistical inference for causal effects and the critical role of the assignment mechanism. *Biometrics, 47*, 1213–1234.

Rubin, D. B. (2004). Teaching statistical inference for causal effects in experiments and observational studies. *Journal of Educational and Behavioral Statistics, 29*(3), 343–367.

Rubin, D. B., Stuart, E. A., & Zanutto, E. L. (2004). A potential outcomes view of value-added assessment in education. *Journal of Educational and Behavioral Statistics, 29*(1), 103–116.

Sampson, R. J., & Morenoff, J. D. (2002). Assessing neighborhood effects: Social processes and new directions in research. *Annual Review of Sociology, 28*, 443–478.

Subramanian, S. V. (2004). Multilevel methods, theory and analysis. In N. Anderson (Ed.), *Encyclopedia on health and behavior*. Thousand Oaks, CA: Sage Publications.

Subramanian, S. V., Chen, J. T., Rehkopf, D. H., Waterman, P. D., & Krieger, N. (2006a). Comparing individual and area-based socioeconomic measures for the surveillance of health disparities: A multilevel analysis of Massachusetts (US) births, 1988–92. *American Journal of Epidemiology, 164*(9), 823–834.

Subramanian, S. V., Chen, J. T., Rehkopf, D. H., Waterman, P. D., & Krieger, N. (2006b). Subramanian et. al. Respond to Think conceptually, act cautiously. *American Journal of Epidemiology, 164*(9), 841–844.

Subramanian, S. V., Jones, K., & Duncan, C. (2003). Multilevel methods for public health research. In I. Kawachi & L. F. Berkman (Eds.), *Neighborhoods and health*. New York: Oxford University Press.

Winship, C., & Morgan, S. L. (1999). The estimation of causal effects from observational data. *Annual Review of Sociology, 25*, 659–706.

Chapter 16
Ecological Studies

Sarah Curtis and Steven Cummins

1. Introduction

Ecological studies examine health determinants and outcomes for groups rather than for individuals, so they can be considered essential for macrosocial level investigations. In this chapter we consider the scope and potential of ecological approaches, some key principles of study design, and the direction of new methodological developments in this field. We begin by considering the nature of ecological analyses of both health outcomes and their determinants, how these differ from analyses that solely focus on individuals, and why an ecological approach is important for understanding macrosocial determinants of health and action to improve public health.

2. The Scope and Potential of Ecological Approaches

Ecological studies analyze aggregated or grouped data (Last, 2001). These grouped data can be defined according to geographical setting or social or demographic category, as well as (in longitudinal studies) for different periods of time. Data for ecologic studies may be derived from individuals as well as their social or physical environments. Although many ecological studies are concerned with medically diagnosed conditions, many also focus on health related behaviors or on "health status" as defined by non-medical criteria, such as self-reports of functional capacity, quality of life and well-being. Ecological studies often involve multi-disciplinary research. Groups of people in ecological studies are often defined in terms of membership of socially defined categories, or physical location in specified areas, and social and geographic theory helps us to understand why the health of these groups varies. In this chapter we discuss ecological studies of health variation primarily from a geographical perspective but will also draw on ideas and examples from epidemiology and other disciplines.

Health geography is concerned in part with why *places* are important for human health (Curtis, 2004); for instance, this chapter focuses particularly on ecological studies for which neighborhood and geographic location define the population groupings. Some of the earliest ecological strategies for examining "medical geography" date back at least as far as ancient Greek ideas about "airs, waters and ground" and their significance for human health (Barrett, 2000; Meade & Earickson, 2000). Present day methods employ sophisticated statistical techniques to analyze group-level variation in health and health determinants at varying "scales" in populations. They sometimes also involve the integration of epidemiological statistical techniques with advanced Geographical Information Systems (GIS) (Cromley & McLafferty, 2002). Though this chapter focuses mainly on statistical approaches, qualitative methodologies have an important contribution to make in ecological studies as well.

Ecological studies are the most obvious method to use if one is interested in establishing the significance of environmental factors in individual health. For example, geographers, epidemiologists and sociologists argue that the area where a person lives and the community s/he belongs to are important for her/his health, and there is a large body of theoretical and empirical research literature which outlines the role of "neighbourhood effects" in generating health inequalities (Curtis, 2004; Curtis & Jones, 1998; Diez-Roux, 1998; Jones & Moon, 1987, 1993; Kearns, 1993; Macintyre, Maciver, & Soomans, 1993). Concern with the ecological factors shaping health is shared by those working in environmental epidemiology. Examples include research on climatic factors (see Bentham & Langford, 2001; Epstein, 1998, 2005; Haines, Kovats, Campbell-Lendrum, & Corvalan, 2006; Keatinge & Donaldson, 2004) and pollution and environmental quality (see Hodgson, Nieuwenhuijsen, Hansell, Shepperd, Flute, Staples, Elliott, & Jarup, 2004; Jerrett, Burnett, Kanaroglou, Eyles, Finkelstein, Giovis, & Brook, 2001).

Group level analysis of health outcomes does not allow us to predict with certainty the health of an individual within the group, but it does provide a powerful way of examining the risks and burden of diseases across whole populations. Authors such as Rose (1992) have made a case for a population based strategy for preventive medicine because it focuses on aspects of health variation that are of greatest collective importance and thus may enable more effective and efficient investment of resources. Ecological research also sometimes demonstrates that similar types of individuals may vary in terms of health risks and determinants, depending on their setting or social group. Thus, particular policies, intervention strategies and treatments may not be equally effective or appropriate in all settings, even though, at the personal level, they may be targeted at apparently similar individuals (Curtis, 2004).

Debates about ecological factors that are important for health also figure in policy for health promotion and sustainability, for example, in relation to urban design and regeneration programs; public environmental health measures, such as water fluoridation; health education campaigns; and national or local health systems (Brown, Grootjans, Ritchie, Townsend, & Verrinder, 2005; Curtis, 2004; Macintyre, 1999). Furthermore, there has been much interest in the health significance of the collective characteristics of whole communities, such as social cohesion or shared sense of trust, which are regarded as dimensions of social capital (Kawachi, Kennedy, & Glass, 1999; Kawachi, Kim, Coutts, & Subramanian, 2004; Subramanian, Lochner, & Kawachi, 2003; Veenstra, 2000). As we will see below, however, it is often difficult to make a clear theoretical and empirical case for completely independent health determinants that operate either at the level of the individual person or at the level of the ecological context in which an individual is situated. Ecological research is much more concerned with the interactions between individuals (with varying attributes) and aspects of their social and physical environment (which may also vary from one setting to another).

Thus the scope of ecological research is quite broad, and it comprises more than simply a suite of technical research methods. We refer below to ecological "approaches" to reflect the theoretical and conceptual stance crucial to understanding the methodological and analytical techniques adopted for collecting and analyzing information. We are not able to cover all aspects of ecological method in this chapter so we summarize selected aspects of technical methods that are applicable to ecological studies and focus on principles that are important to avoid confounding of ecological research findings. We begin by considering the limitations of using aggregate data, particularly the problem of the "ecological fallacy."

3. The Ecological and the Atomistic Fallacies

Where detailed data on individuals are not available (due either to confidentiality restrictions or absence of information), it may be possible to obtain information on groups of people from routine sources such as population censuses, mortality registers and aggregated health service statistics. In such situations, ecological studies may provide the only feasible way to examine how health outcomes are associated with other population variables. However, ecological research is sometimes criticized because of concerns about the "ecological fallacy" – wrongly attributing information and relationships observed at the aggregate level to individuals (Susser, 1994). This is also sometimes referred to as the "sociologistic fallacy" because it may involve "essentializing" or "stereotyping" by projecting information relating to a whole social or demographic group onto its individual members (Diez Roux, 2002).

The ecological fallacy is a danger in studies that use data on populations aggregated to geographical (or other) units and is especially likely to be problematic when we describe groups using information that is originally observed at the individual level. Thus, for example, in areas with large concentrations of socioeconomically deprived populations (which are therefore, on average, poor areas), not all residents will be poor. If we tried to predict one individual's socioeconomic status from the average of the area in which s/he lives, we would under- or over- estimate in many cases. Even for variables that are originally measured at the ecological level (e.g., air pollution or temperature levels across geographical areas), the observations may be from one or more point sources (e.g. observation stations), and we may only be able to estimate conditions over the wider area. Individuals within these areas may also vary in exposure and susceptibility to environmental factors.

The most serious cases of the ecological fallacy might lead to erroneous attribution of disease causation and risk. For example, cardiovascular diseases were once referred to as "diseases of affluence," since the incidence of mortality from these conditions is more common in rich rather than poor nations. However, within wealthy countries, poor populations and poor neighborhoods are frequently found to have the highest prevalence of cardiovascular disease and are often the slowest to respond to public health campaigns to reduce related illness and death (Bryce, Curtis, & Mohan, 1994). Similarly, when considering risks of an infectious disease, we may summarize the risk for an area using information on infection rates across the entire population, but individual risk will vary according to immune status, exposure factors and other individual characteristics. One illustration of this complexity is a study of tuberculosis incidence among children in Leeds, UK (Parslow, El-Shimy, Cundall, & McKinney, 2001). The rates of infection varied by ethnic group, with South Asian children (from the Indian subcontinent), particularly girls, having much higher incidence than average for the population of children in the city as a whole.

Commentators have often dismissed the utility of an ecological approach on the basis of the arguments outlined above or have accepted ecologic studies as simply "hypothesis generating" rather than confirmatory. However, ecological studies are important in order to avoid the "atomistic fallacy", also termed the "individualistic" or "psychologistic" fallacy (Diez Roux, 2002; Schwartz, 1994). This fallacy occurs as a result of over-emphasizing risk and causal processes operating at the individual and under-emphasizing the ecological component. For example, work on the increasing global obesity epidemic has suggested that traditional individual risk factors, such as genetic endowment, as well as social and psychological factors, are inadequate in explaining the increasing prevalence of obesity. Instead, it has been proposed that ecological features of the external "obesogenic environment" promote excessive energy intake and reduced energy expenditure (Egger & Swinburn, 1997).

Despite our warnings above, ecologic studies can be used to demonstrate plausible causal ecological processes that may influence population health (Ebrahim, 2005; Ebrahim & Davey Smith, 1998). For example, work on the Russian mortality crisis using aggregated data illustrated that the increase in mortality rates between 1987 and 1994 was predominantly due to alcohol-related diseases. This increase most likely reflected a combination of historical and contemporary factors affecting society at the ecological level, including governmental and fiscal actions (the reversal of the Russian government's anti-alcohol campaign in 1985, the end of state monopoly on alcohol imports and sales, and a reduction in the unit cost of alcohol) (Leon, Chenet, Shkolnikov, Zakharov, Shapiro, Rakhmanova, Vassin, & McKee, 1997; Shkolnikov, McKee, & Leon, 2001).

4. The (Impossible) Distinction Between Context and Composition

Though many epidemiological studies treat individual and ecological risks and processes as separate, there are theoretical and methodological problems with such an approach. In recent years, epidemiological techniques have often aimed to establish statistically significant independent health effects of context (attributes and processes at the ecological, group level) and composition (attributes of the individual people that make up the group) (see Section 12.0.) This approach raises some quite complex questions of cross-level confounding.

Oakes (2004) argues, for example, that it is very difficult through statistical modeling to distinguish the (compositional) causal effects of individual attributes that vary by neighborhood due to selective sorting of individuals into neighborhoods with varying conditions from the (contextual) causal effects of neighborhood conditions on health of individuals. This is because individuals are not randomly allocated to areas, areas influence individual attributes and are not statistically independent, it is not necessarily correct to extrapolate relationships which apply in one area, with a given set of conditions, to other areas which have different combinations of individual and area attributes, and one could not theoretically test whether the same group of people would have different health if they were in a different neighborhood because it is impossible to transfer individuals between neighborhoods without changing the contextual attributes of the neighborhoods.

Oakes suggests that these problems could be addressed theoretically by a more careful interpretation of the causal pathways through which neighborhood effects may operate and empirically by more use of methods that help to explain and test causal relationships. Qualitative methods, for instance, can demonstrate through intensive examination the factors that shape individual experience. Also, causal relationships can be tested using randomized community trials in which the impact of interventions modifying neighborhood conditions are evaluated against data from areas where such interventions are not being implemented. Further, these problems call for a focus on the modeling of interactions between individual and ecological level variables. There is further discussion of some of these methods below.

5. Confounding Due to Auto-Correlation of Measured and Unmeasured Ecological Variables

Another common problem in ecological research (as for research on individuals) is isolating the influence of ecological factors that are closely correlated with each other. Kaufman and Kaufman (2001) use an example based on data from the National Longitudinal Mortality Study (NLMS) in the USA to expound on approaches to modeling complex causal pathways in studies of individual and environmental variables that relate to health outcomes. They point out that evidence about the association between specific factors and health outcomes needs to be interpreted very carefully, bearing in mind the various ways in which other measured or unmeasured covariates may influence either the factor of interest or the health outcome.

Most epidemiological studies attempt to control for the important covariates (confounding factors). However, the conventional strategy of standardizing for these confounding factors is not always effective, especially if the covariates cannot be measured or are multi-dimensional or if there are complex relationships between the factor of interest, the outcome, and the confounding covariate. For instance, in an analysis of the differences in survival rates for people grouped by educational level, age, and sex, Kaufman and Kaufman show that parental income is a possible confounder of the relationship between educational level and mortality. They demonstrate that there are a number of different possible combinations of causal pathways by which parental income, educational attainment, and mortality might be related and that these are difficult to disentangle using standard statistical modeling techniques. Furthermore, they show that these associations may vary throughout the lifecourse.

It is extremely difficult to eradicate all possible errors in research design that are due to failure to include ecological variables pertinent to health variation. However, there are some strategies that can be helpful in dealing with these problems of intra-correlation, auto-correlation and complex causal relationships. We consider some strategies below.

6. Defining the Ecological Unit of Analysis

In research on individuals, it is relatively easy to identify the person as the unit of analysis; however, in ecological research there is much more uncertainty over what the appropriate "units" of analysis should be. There are many different ways of grouping individuals – socially, spatially, demographically and biologically – and the choice of categories will depend on the conceptual model, as well as more pragmatic issues of data availability. Thus, ecological researchers must make decisions on category and area definitions and cope with multiple scales and classification systems that may relate to each other in complex ways.

Defining groups for ecological study is often theoretically complex and can be quite variable between different studies. This is an especially important consideration when comparing the results of different investigations. For many of the macrosocial determinants of health, the methods of measurement and classification generally available at present are quite crude, and this may be a source of weakness in ecological research. For social and geographical analyses, for example, this is illustrated by problems of defining ethnic and socioeconomic categories in the population. Ethnicity may be important as an individual variable relating to health, but the ethnic profile of a population may also be important as an ecological variable. For example, research suggests that "ethnic density" (neighborhood concentration of individuals belonging to a particular ethnic group) may be important for health (Fagg, Curtis, Stansfeld, & Congdon, 2006; Halpern & Nazroo, 2000; Neeleman, Wilson-Jones, & Wessely, 2005; Subramanian, Acevedo-Garcia, & Osypuk, 2005).

Several authors have argued that it is unhelpful to study health variation by ethnic or racial group without a clear theoretical rationale for the research (Ahmad, 1993; Bhopal, 1997; Nazroo, 1998). Controlling for socio-economic position is important when considering racial or ethnic groups that are highly differentiated in terms of material and economic factors. Karlsen and Nazroo (2000) provide a theoretical framework for interpreting ethnicity in terms of socioeconomic position, cultural identity, and race. The framework requires criteria relating to nationality, racial type and genetic origin, expressions of traditional social or cultural affiliation, community participation in social networks that reinforce ethnic groups, and racialization due to discrimination and racial abuse. While the use of surveys may provide opportunities to collect detailed ethnic background information, many studies use small area data derived from population censuses, which are based on very simplified categories of racial or ethnic classification, and individual data from hospital and medical records, which are also frequently limited and simplified. Such simplified categories are only very approximate ways of distinguishing ethnic categories, and such classifications are becoming progressively more convoluted as they are modified to incorporate information about individuals from mixed racial or ethnic backgrounds.

For ecological studies that use geographically defined groups, there are questions over how to define the relevant "places." For example, we may be concerned with residential neighborhoods, socio-geographical communities, or places of work or recreation. These are often defined in terms of standard administrative boundaries (particularly those used for small area census statistics or postal districting). Administrative zones are convenient because they often correspond to areas for which information is routinely available, but they may not always delineate socio-geographical divisions that are relevant for describing the socioeconomic environment. This limitation has been termed the "modifiable unit area problem."

Developments in Geographical Information Systems (GIS) make it possible to combine information in more flexible and analytically powerful ways, and these techniques overcome some of the constraints of the modifiable unit area problem by allowing analysis of clusters of disease or of other socio-demographic phenomena that do not fall neatly within administrative zones (for introductory reviews of these methods, see Cromley, 2003; Cromley & McLafferty, 2002; Ricketts, 2003). To an extent, GIS techniques help us to move beyond the constraints of studying ecological variability in health and health determinants solely in terms of differences between administrative areas.

In contrast, some studies suggest that conventional administrative zones may be quite effective proxies for "natural" socio-geographical units in ecological analyses of health variation at the neighborhood level. For example, in their research in Montreal, Canada, Ross, Tremblay, & Graham, (2004) found that analyses using geographical data for administrative units from the population census predicted health outcomes as powerfully as measures calculated for "natural" (defined using GIS) geographical units.

Even more challenging for ecological research is that the complex time-space paths of individuals, both over their lifecourse and from day to day, mean that the places and settings that contribute to their health may be very diverse and widely dispersed. It is not very realistic to define the ecological factors impinging on a person in terms of a single, geographically bounded small area. In modern society, with social and economic networks supported by advanced communication technologies, individuals may even be influenced by settings and social groups with which they have no physical contact.

Thus, ecological variables important for human health are often difficult to measure quantitatively. There is a danger that, in concentrating on those that are easier to measure, we will ignore others that are not so amenable to empirical operationalization as statistical indicators but are of equal, or greater, importance for individuals and for societies. Further, places and settings are socially constructed in ways that are difficult to grasp using statistical data and Geographical Information Systems but may be important for health and wellbeing (Cummins, Curtis, Diez Roux, & Macintyre, in press). This means that a range of qualitative, as well as quantitative, methods are needed to help us understand the relationships between individuals and their environment.

7. Strategies for the Measurement of Health and Health Determinants at the Group Level and Problems of Cross-Level Confounding

The measurement of population health at the ecological level often presents a challenge in itself. Some population censuses (as in the UK) have introduced questions on self reported health, but this information is relatively rare. Researchers in many countries have to rely on data drawn from health service activity records, which are imperfect indicators of health of the population, or try to extrapolate from sample survey data, which may not be available for all areas of the country or at sufficiently fine levels of resolution to adequately define neighborhoods.

Measuring macrosocial health determinants is also problematic. Thus, for example, some commentators have argued that research on neighborhood effects on health relies too heavily on small area census data in measuring aspects of the social environment. While variables derived from the census are certainly useful predictors of health variation, they tend to be restricted to certain dimensions of socioeconomic conditions, such as demographic composition, housing and household amenities, and employment (Cummins, McIntyre, Davidson, & Ellaway, 2005).

Similarly, quantitative research on social capital and health is severely hampered by lack of adequate indicators of local level conditions such as social cohesion, trust, or practical support. Some studies of social capital and health use the same survey to produce both individual data on health predictors and also, in aggregated form, to describe the perceived social conditions in areas where the sample of individuals were living. For example, Weitzman and Kawachi (2000) comment on their use of this method in a study that related binge drinking among individual students to measures of perceived social capital aggregated to the level of the university campus where the students studied. This approach raises questions over whether the sources of individual and ecological data are sufficiently independent or whether they may be subject to same source bias.

Research to improve the repertoire of ecological variables that can be used to describe macrosocial health determinants at the community level includes that reported by Cummins et al. (2005) who compiled over 280 variables relating to material and social conditions in districts of England and Scotland. However, the researchers also commented on the difficulty of obtaining information on some aspects of the environment in a systematic form across the whole country. Further, there have been efforts in the UK and other countries to collate indicators of socioeconomic conditions that not only draw on a wider range of routine sources but are also collected more frequently and are therefore more regularly updated than census data (Noble, Wright, Dibben, Smith, McLennan, Anttila, Barnes, Mokhtar, Noble, Avenell, Gardner, Covizzi, & Lloyd, 2004).

Apart from the problem of availability of suitable data, the construction of composite indicators poses further methodological problems. For example, caution is necessary when combining information from measures with very different statistical distributions. Ecological measures of phenomena that are very unevenly distributed in space will produce skewed distributions. One particular example is measures of concentrations of racial or ethnic minority populations, which tend to be spatially concentrated in certain urban areas of the UK and the USA and very sparsely distributed in some other areas. When combining variables to make composite indicators, it is therefore necessary to standardize the variance of the components. One common strategy is the use of zscore transformations (see Curtis, Copeland, Fagg, Congdon, Almog, & Fitzpatrick, 2006).

There are also issues of whether and how to weight the different components of composite indicators of social environmental factors. Quite commonly, researchers use principal component analysis or similar data reduction techniques to produce summary measures and weightings of variables that reflect the covariance among the components in statistical terms. This approach was used, for example, by Noble et al. (2004) to produce indicators on various dimensions of deprivation for small areas in England. Cummins et al. (2005) also used principal component analysis to reduce a large data set on area conditions to 11 factors representing theoretically and empirically salient dimensions of the environment; these included quality of the residential environment, facilities for recreation, facilities giving access to money and the means of exchange. Others have used expert opinions to produce weightings. For example, Jarman (1983) combined variables that were selected and weighted on the basis of a survey of the views of general practitioners to produce a well known indicator of small areas in England needing general practitioner services.

Problems of measurement are also important for ecological studies concerned with physical environmental factors. For example, (Martuzzi, Kryzanowski, & Bertollini, 2003) discuss the complications of drawing conclusions from research on air pollution and respiratory illness. They summarize some of the challenges faced in order to provide more conclusive information for health impact assessment, including issues over the validity of using average data and extrapolating risks over large populations; poor reliability of some measures; problems of how to treat multiple pollutants; whether or not response to varying exposure shows a linear pattern; and problems of attribution and measurement of exposure over time. Research in environmental epidemiology often has to use information on pollution from monitors at specific spatial locations to estimate pollution over a wider area. Wakefield (2004) discusses the use of exposure surfaces, calculated using GIS techniques, rather than ecological designs based on geographically bounded area units. These impute the spatial distribution of exposures between observation sites, producing results similar to topological contour maps.

Varying exposure over time is another major issue for research on how health is influenced by environment. The growing emphasis on lifecourse perspectives in research on health variation (Graham, 2000) has demonstrated the contribution of cumulative health related experiences throughout life to health inequalities and has shown the value of longitudinal study designs. Although a good deal of ecological research is cross sectional, it is likely that the health of populations has been influenced by ecological conditions in the past as well as by their current environment. For example, Curtis et al. (2003) linked data from the Longitudinal Study in England to information from a GIS database on historical socioeconomic conditions in the 1930s, to demonstrate that self reported illness and mortality among older adults in the 1980s was partly related to conditions in their areas of residence 40 years earlier.

The issue of mobility of populations is a major question that is often overlooked in cross sectional ecological analyses. It is particularly important because movement of individuals between geographical areas or socioeconomic groups may be differentiated according to health status (Boyle, Gattrel, & Duke-Williams, 1999; Boyle, Norman, & Rees, 2002). Since inward and outward migration rates vary geographically, the effects of health-selective migration are not consistent from one area to another. Rogerson and Han (2002) illustrate an approach to comparing mortality in different areas, which controls for migration effects by adjusting area mortality rates in relation to information on local rates of inward and outward migration.

Failure to take into account population turnover and change can result in fallacious conclusions, which is especially of concern for analyses that inform policy decisions. For example, arguments that area regeneration projects result in improvements in population health often fail to consider that poor, unhealthy populations may be displaced by the gentrification effects associated with regeneration and that the improved health in the area may result from healthier populations moving in to replace them (Curtis, 2004).

8. How Small Can a Micro Group be?

Increasingly, ecological studies are aiming to examine variability in hierarchically structured data sets which classify people into smaller (and often more local) categories, as well as into larger (regional or national) groupings. The advantages of small geographical groupings of rather small populations (e.g., neighborhoods) are that ecological conditions will generally vary less over small areas than large ones, and there will be more variation between the spatial units than within them. This means that small areas are better for differentiating ecological conditions and analyzing the range of variability in macrosocial conditions that can be measured at the level of local neighborhoods.

However, area indicators provide statistically more reliable comparisons of health among population groups when the numbers on which they are based are large. In cases of rare illnesses or low mortality rates, conventional aggregated measures for small areas or population groups will be less reliable statistically. It may also be necessary to use approaches suitable for situations where a significant number of the ecological units have zero events of death or illness. This has often been a problem, for example, in studies comparing sparsely populated rural areas (with indicators based on small numbers) with urban areas (that are more densely populated and therefore have a greater absolute number of health events to analyze). Conventional statistical approaches have either excluded aggregations with very few cases or combined them together to make larger units or groups; however, these solutions can introduce bias through the inadequate representation of some sample units. Bayesian methods for smoothing data on health outcomes based on small counts are now being used widely for research of this type (for a comprehensive discussion see Congdon, 2001). By "borrowing strength" from the entire data set to inform inferences about sample units with few or no cases of the outcome of interest, these methods allow us to use ecological data more effectively.

9. Is Bigger Better? The Potentials and Limitations of Meta-Analyses and Research on Macro-Level Ecological Processes

Epidemiological research often requires large samples in order to test the relationships between health outcomes and a range of risk factors. When resources are limited, research designs may be too small (statistically underpowered) to allow such analysis or may not be distributed widely enough geographically to cover the full range of possible risk factors. One solution to the problem of underpowered or unrepresentative research designs for ecological study is to group together sets of data from different studies, often from different regions or even different countries. For those interested in macrosocial health determinants, this strategy may also offer exciting possibilities to examine the impacts of very different ecological settings on health variation. However, for some of the reasons already discussed, it can be very challenging to combine data sets collected under such varying conditions; simply aggregating data and findings from different regional studies can be quite problematic. This is not only an issue for ecological studies, since it also calls into question, for example, strategies for multi-center drug trials on individuals.

Apart from the need to generate large samples for international meta-analyses in epidemiology and clinical science, there are strong theoretical motivations for considering macrosocial health determinants operating at the global level (e.g. Kickbusch & de Leeuw, 1999). The spatial patterning of health is not dependent just on local process but also extra-local policies and relations that have varying effects at multiple scales. Ecological studies that aim to incorporate information on global processes raise methodological issues about how to research processes operating at a very broad scale (e.g., for international regions, continents, or the whole world). The most fundamental problem is that the macro-social determinants may be variably constructed and interpreted between societies, so it may be very difficult to make meaningful comparisons. A lively debate has developed, for example, around Wilkinson's (1996) work on whether inequality of wealth at the national scale is more important than average wealth for health variation among high income countries. One point of discussion concerns the several alternative measures of inequality, which may not all produce similar analytical results (discussed for example, by Mackenbach & Kunst, 1997).

In order to produce consistently measured data that make international comparisons possible, it is often necessary to use indicators that are defined in relatively simple terms and can be collected in all the participating countries. These often take the form of "tracer" indicators and international "common data sets." For instance, (Torsheim, Currie, Boyce, Kalnins, Overpeck, & Haugland, 2004) analyzed data on 125,000 young people in a multi-national survey conducted in 29 European and North American countries. In order to measure socio-economic conditions, this study used a "family affluence scale," which combined data on car ownership, having one's own bedroom, and the number of holidays away from home. This indicator of social affluence/deprivation was associated with self-rated health reported in the study. The authors were able to use these data to show that self rated poor health varied among individuals, and also at the level of the schools where the students had been sampled and the countries where they lived.

There is a long established field of epidemiologic research that seeks to predict the regional and global spread of epidemics. Such disease diffusion modeling incorporates information on mixed contagious-hierarchical diffusion (see Trevelyan, Smallman-Raynor, & Cliff, 2005). Diffusion of diseases through human populations (including world wide pandemics) progresses through a combination of contagious diffusion, spreading to populations that are physically close to the initial point of infection, and hierarchical diffusion, transferring between major centers of human activity that may be very distant from each other. Thus, the size and relative socioeconomic significance of settlements is as important as the geographical proximity of one to another. Human innovations and communications of all types (including diseases) may transfer over long distances, between "high ranking" global cities more quickly than they spread to smaller settlements that are nearer. A simple measure of national and global city rank is population size, and many disease diffusion models include this factor because diseases are often transmitted across the world most rapidly among the largest urban centers (Gatrell, 2002; Löytenen & Arbona, 1996). In contrast, the most influential global cities are not necessarily the largest in terms of population size. Alternative indicators of global "rank" may aim to measure, for example, rates of international travel, levels of electronic communication, and the relative concentration of multinational corporate interests.

Studies of global level macrosocial determinants of health also raise questions of how to include information on the geographically variable impacts of the processes involved. The fact that certain macrosocial processes (such as global circuits of capital, and global economic systems, for example) operate internationally does not mean that they impact in the same way on all places. One example from a large literature on the variable impact of globalizing economies is Taylor and Derudder (2004), who suggest that European cities are particularly "porous" to some global processes, compared with cities in the US. Taylor and Derudder's paper is one of many studies using data on "advanced producer" service industries. There is potential to use such indicators of global ranking of cities more widely in research on global processes in public health.

10. Approaches to Spatial Auto-Correlation and Confounding Covariates

In ecological studies of macrosocial health determinants based on geographical areas, some further aspects of statistical analyses should be considered. Two particular issues relate to spatial auto-correlation and cross-level confounding.

Spatial auto-correlation occurs where variability in conditions for each areal unit in the analysis is not independent of conditions in other areas in the sample. In geographical studies, it is common, for example, to find that similar small areas are clustered together and that conditions in one area influence conditions in other places within the region studied. Independence is assumed in some conventional methods of regression analysis, and so appropriate techniques for ecological analysis should control for spatial auto-correlation (Cliff & Ord, 1981). Methods to control for spatial auto-correlation may incorporate information about correlation of areas on a contiguity basis (using information for each small area about the other areas with which it shares a boundary) or in terms of proximity (using data on the distances between areas in the sample). For a detailed discussion, including methods using empirical Bayes solutions, see Cressie, (1992); (Pascutto, Wakefield, Best, Richardson, Bernardinelli, Staines, & Elliott, 2000); Stern and Cressie (1999).

A further issue is whether and how to standardize for potentially confounding covariates. A range of indicators are used to assess both health outcomes and ecological conditions, and the choice of appropriate measures will depend on the aims of the study. Health outcomes in the population may be measured in terms of absolute (unstandardized) numbers of health events, which provide an indicator of the total burden of mortality or morbidity; crude morbidity or mortality rates normally calculated relative to a person-years denominator, which corresponds to the size of the population at risk over a given time period, giving an indication of comparative levels of mortality that controls for population size but not for demographic structure; and directly or indirectly age and/or sex standardized rate or ratios measures, which provide comparative indicators controlling for differences in demographic structure of the population as well as its size.

Methods of standardization for the composition of populations within ecological units are crucial to questions of cross-level confounding, mentioned in the previous section. This is explained very well by Greenland (2002), who shows that even if ecological level relationships are the main focus of interest, we need to consider individual level relationships within areas because of issues relating to the underlying structure of the regression models (i.e., this is not just a problem of random error or sampling variation). Greenland discusses the problem of "information lost during aggregation" (Greenland, 2001: 1344). Greenland argues that when a health outcome depends on individual factors as well as contextual environmental factors, in order to identify contextual effects it is important to be able to control for differences in the outcome for different population subgroups within each area. Some of this within-area, between-group variation might be attributable to area effects, but it might equally be due to the influence of individual attributes, such as age and sex differences in susceptibility to illness, or the influence of individual socioeconomic conditions. Greenland also demonstrates that it would be possible for significant ecological associations to be masked by confounding effects due to differences among groups of individuals within the areas.

Ecological studies often use indirect standardization to produce standardized mortality ratios (in order to compare health outcomes between areas, allowing for individual differences in risk – e.g., standardization by age and sex) and then examine how these standardized rates vary in relation to environmental variables. Greenland argues that direct standardization is preferable; however, this is usually not possible since it requires breakdowns of the health outcome variable by each sociodemographic subgroup within the areas being studied, and these are rarely available. Alternatively, Greenland suggests that one would ideally use separate information on the ecological exposure variable for each sociodemographic group within each area in the analysis, but again, such detailed data on environmental exposure is rarely available.

11. How to Attribute Health Variation to Ecological Factors: The Potential of Natural Experiments

Ecological research raises serious questions about the feasibility of classic case-control methodology. As Diez Roux (2003) notes, ecological randomized experimental designs have a set of methodological and practical problems that are not easy to surmount. This is because many of the major ecological determinants of health (such as new housing and neighborhood service infrastructure) are not amenable to randomization for practical or political reasons and because sample size requirements within trial designs are cost-prohibitive (Habicht, Victora, & Vaughan, 1999; Kirkwood, Cousens, Victora, & Zoysa, 1997; Petticrew, Cummins, Ferrell, Finday, Higgins, Hoy, Kearns, & Sparks, 2005).

However, we noted above that authors such as Oakes (2004) consider that randomized community trials have good potential to advance research on the macrosocial determinants of health, and research designs incorporating some aspects of controlled trials may be feasible. Prospective quasi-experimental evaluations of natural experiments may solve many of the practical problems associated with true ecological experimental trial designs and provide much more convincing evidence for causality than straight-forward, single-site observational studies (Millward, Kelly, & Nutbeam, 2001). Natural experiments are studies "where the researcher cannot control or withhold the allocation of an intervention to particular neighborhoods or communities of interest, but where natural variation in allocation occurs" (Pettigrew et al., 2005). This often applies to area-based interventions intended to reduce health inequalities or even interventions where changes in health are not the intended outcome. For example, a recent study evaluated the effects of the development of a large food hypermarket in a deprived and previously under-served area of Glasgow, UK, on individual fruit and vegetable consumption, (Cummins, Pettigrew et al., 2005). The researchers took the opportunity to study naturally occurring large-scale food retail changes using a before and after controlled design that also included information on communities that were not affected by the new developments. Though not a true randomized controlled trial and suffering from limitations in statistical power, this quasi-experimental approach may provide better evidence for ecological effects than straightforward observational cross sectional ecological studies. Another example (Thomas, Evans, Huxley, Gately, & Rogers, 2005) also used a longitudinal, controlled research design to compare changes in residents' mental health before and after implementation of a housing improvement scheme, both in the intervention zone and in a non-intervention area.

12. Linking the Individual and the Group Perspectives: Multi-Level Models

Major developments in statistical modeling aim to tackle the complexity of ecological research incorporating information about both micro and macrosocial determinants. The application of multilevel modeling (or hierarchical modeling) to ecological research on human health has now become something of an industry in geography, as well as in epidemiology, and has considerably advanced our thinking about the importance of ecological effects vis-à-vis individual risk factors for health. Detailed discussion of these methods as they relate to ecological research in health includes, for example, (Duncan, Jones, & Moon, 1993, 1998); Duncan and Jones (2000); Diez-Roux (2002); Jones (2005); Blakely and Subramanian (2005).

Duncan et al. (1993, 1998) and Diez Roux (2002) respectively provide accessible explanations for non-statisticians and a glossary of terms relating to multilevel methods. These are suited for data comprising information on individuals or small groups (level 1 data) that are nested within at least one set of larger groups or areas (level 2, level 3, etc.). Hierarchical models allow for hierarchical clustering at more than one level; an example would be individuals grouped in neighborhoods that are located in regions, producing a three-level model. In longitudinal data sets with repeated measures of the same individuals at different time points, multilevel models can also be used to examine time trends by interpreting time as one of the variable levels. These models require a sufficient number of the level 1 observations within each of the level 2 groups for meaningful analysis, so they may not be very suitable for a sample of individuals that is sparsely distributed across groups. Multilevel modeling is intended for data sets with a reasonably large (e.g., 12 or more) higher level clusters. Where a sample is distributed among a small number of groups, other techniques, such as analysis of variance, may be more suitable. Researchers considering multilevel modeling in health geography should also be clear whether they are interested in variation associated with being in a particular place (in which case the place of interest should be specified as a categorical variable) or whether they are concerned about variation across places generally (in which case place may be specified as a level).

Blakely and Subramanian (2005) point out that multilevel models are useful when (a) there is clustering of effects in areas, time periods, or social groups; (b) there are causal processes thought to operate at an aggregate level; and (c) there is an interest in variability of relationships across areas or groups, as well as in average patterns of association. Multilevel models are useful in these situations because they permit decomposition of the variance in a health outcome of interest into level 1 variance and variance at level 2 or at higher levels. Where there is significant variance at level 2, this has often been taken to indicate that contextual factors are important for health. It is also possible to introduce explanatory variables (parameters) representing risk factors at each level to test their relevance to the health outcome.

Multilevel models are quite flexible and can also be used for situations where individuals can be simultaneously attributed to more than one set of higher level groupings that are not completely nested hierarchically. For example, individuals might be grouped according to their residential areas and their workplace, but the neighborhood and workplace ecological units are unlikely to be hierarchically nested. Workplaces will draw employees from many different areas, and residents from each area will work in many different locations. In this type of situation, cross-classified structures (individuals belong to non-nested ecological units) can also be specified in multilevel models. (For an example concerning electoral geography, see Jones, Gould, & Watt, 1992). Multilevel modeling has also advanced in ways that make it applicable to outcome data that do not correspond either to normal or conventional Poisson distributions, which is very often the case for information on health outcomes (Browne, Subramanian, Jones, & Goldstein, 2005).

Although multilevel models seem to offer the possibility of distinguishing compositional and contextual effects, the interpretation may not in fact be straightforward. Blakely and Subramanian (2005) argue that even if spatial variation in health is found to be significant predominantly at level 1 (i.e., due local population composition resulting from concentration of individuals with certain characteristics in particular areas), this does not mean that macrosocial determinants are irrelevant. There may still be macro-level processes that explain why the individuals are geographically clustered. Thus, the explanation may be ecological even if the phenomenon seems to be individual. Blakely and Subramanian (2005) also join with other authors already cited to point out other potential sources of "error" in ecological studies that might make it difficult to interpret multi-level models. These include the possibility that there may be insufficient variation in the ecological variable to detect an effect, even though the ecological condition is important for health. As with all analyses using samples, selection bias may influence the results (in ecological terms, for example, the places selected may be unrepresentative of places generally). There are also potential problems of mis-specification and measurement (for example, individuals may be attributed to the wrong areas, or the area characteristics may have been inaccurately assessed).

Perhaps more problematic to determine, however, is whether multilevel modeling is theoretically appropriate, since it distinguishes between individual level and ecological level variation in health and thus implies that health determinants operate specifically at one level or another. Critics are now questioning whether we really need many more studies to establish whether health variation has independent individual and ecological components; some suggest that we need to concentrate more on multilevel models that explore the interactions between individual and ecological effects and help us to distinguish causal pathways more effectively (Cummins et al., in press). We may in future see more studies that combine multilevel modeling with Bayesian techniques (Congdon, 2001; Curtis et al., 2003) and also with approaches such as structural equation modeling (Der, 2002; Stafford, Cummins, Sacker, Wiggins, & Macintyre, in press).

13. There's Nothing So Practical as a Good Theory

We conclude this chapter by emphasizing the need for methodological and theoretical development in ecological research to advance hand in hand. Some critics lament that ecological epidemiological research has advanced more quickly in terms of methods (particularly statistical and geo-informatic techniques) than in terms of sound theory on which to base analyses. It is important to select methods that fit soundly with the theoretical structures being advanced in ecological studies. Authors such as (Potvin, Gendron, Bilodeau, & Chabot, 2005) and (McQueen, Kickbusch, Potvin, Balbo, Abel, & Pelikan, 2007) argue that social theory, as well as epidemiological perspectives, is important to make public health more sensitive to macrosocial health determinants.

An important aspect of theory building in ecological research on health involves the specification of causal pathways that are thought to account for the associations revealed in empirical studies. This may be most readily advanced using qualitative methods to produce a rich picture of individual experiences of particular settings rather than through more extensive statistical analyses. Researchers are increasingly using mixed methods that combine statistical and qualitative strategies. This issue of establishing causal relationships is developed in more detail in the following chapter.

We have tried to demonstrate above that there are some profound theoretical issues to be addressed in terms of the construction of ecological units of analysis. Because ecological research often works with information organized for social groups or for administratively defined geographical areas, these units of analysis are often determined socially and politically rather than scientifically. We have argued that the definition and interpretation of ecological units can have important implications for ecological methods. Good ecological research will always aim to be reflexive about the strategies used to structure research designs and to offer clear explanations for the ecological frameworks that it uses.

References

Ahmad, W. (Ed.). (1993). *"Race" and health in contemporary Britain.* Buckingham: Open University Press.

Barrett, F. (2000). *Disease and geography: The History of an idea.* Toronto: Atkinson College, Department of Geography.

Bentham, G., & Langford, I. (2001). Environmental temperatures and the incidence of food poisoning in England and Wales. *International Journal of Biometeorology, 45*(1), 22–26

Bhopal, R. (1997). Is research into ethnicity and health racist, unsound or important science? *British Medical Journal, 314*(7096), 1751–1756.

Blakely T., & Subramanian, S. V. (2005). Multilevel studies. In M. Oakes & J. Kaufman (Eds.), *Methods for social epidemiology. San Francisco: Jossey Bass.*

Brown, V., Grootjans, J., Ritchie, J., Townsend, M., & Verrinder, G. (2005). *Sustainability and health: Supporting global ecological integrity in public health.* Sterling, VA: Earthscan.

Browne, W. J., Subramanian, S. V., Jones, K., & Goldstein, H. (2005). Variance partitioning in multilevel logistic models that exhibit over-dispersion. *Journal of the Royal Statistical Society Series A, 168*(3), 599–613

Boyle, P., Gattrel, A., & Duke-Williams, O. (1999). The effect on morbidity of variability in deprivation and population stability in England and Wales: An investigation at small area level. *Social Science & Medicine, 49,* 791–799.

Boyle, P., Norman, P., & Rees, P. (2002). Does migration exaggerate the relationship between material deprivation and long term illness? A Scottish analysis. *Social Science & Medicine, 55,* 21–31

Bryce, C., Curtis, S., & Mohan, J. (1994). Coronary heart disease: Trends in spatial inequalities and implications for health care planning in England. *Social Science & Medicine, 38*(5), 677–690.

Cliff, A., & Ord, J. (1981). *Spatial processes, models and applications*. London: Pion.

Congdon, P. (2001). *Bayesian statistical modelling*. Chichester: Wiley.

Cressie, N. (1992). Smoothing regional maps using empirical Bayes predictors. *Geographical Analysis, 24*(1), 75–95.

Cromley, E. (2003). GIS and disease. *Annual Review of Public Health, 24*, 7–24.

Cromley, E., & McLafferty, S. (2002). *GIS and public health*. New York: Guildford Press.

Cummins, S., Curtis, S., Diez-Roux, A., & Macintyre, S. (in press). Understanding and representing "place" in health research: A relational approach. *Social Science & Medicine*.

Cummins, S., McIntyre, S., Davidson, S., & Ellaway, A. (2005). Measuring neighbourhood social and material context; Generation and interpretation of ecological data from routine and non-routine sources. *Health & Place, 11*, 249–260.

Curtis, S. (2004). *Health and inequality: Geographical perspectives*. London: Sage.

Curtis, S., & Jones, I. R. (1998). Is there a place for geography in the analysis of health inequality? *Sociology of Health and Illness, 20*(5), 645–672.

Curtis, S., Southall, H, Congdon, P., & Dodgeon, B. (2003). Area effects on health variation over the life-course: Analysis of the longitudinal study sample in England using new data on area of residence in childhood. *Social Science & Medicine, 58*, 57–74.

Curtis, S., Copeland, A., Fagg, J., Congdon, P., Almog, M., & Fitzpatrick, J., (2006). The ecological relationship between deprivation, social isolation and rates of hospital admission for acute psychiatric care; A comparison of London and New York City. *Health & Place, 12*(1), 19–37.

Der, G. (2002). Structural equation modelling in epidemiology: Some problems and prospects. *International Journal of Epidemiology, 31*, 1199–1200.

Diez Roux, A. (1998). Bringing back context into epidemiology: Variables and fallacies in multilevel analysis. *American Journal of Public Health, 88*(2), 222–216.

Diez Roux, A. (2002). A glossary for multi-level analysis. *Journal of Epidemiology and Community Health, 56*, 588–594.

Diez Roux, A.V. (2003). Residential environments and cardiovascular disease risk. *Journal of Urban health , 80*(4), 569–589.

Duncan, C., & Jones, K. (2000). Using multilevel models to model heterogeneity: Potential and pitfalls. *Geographical Analysis, 32*(4), 279–305.

Duncan, C., Jones, K., & Moon, G. (1993). Do places matter – a multilevel analysis of regional variations in health-related behaviour in Britain. *Social Science & Medicine, 37*(6), 725–733.

Duncan, C., Jones, K., & Moon, G. (1998). Context, composition and heterogeneity: Using multilevel models in health research. *Social Science & Medicine, 46*(1), 97–117.

Ebrahim, S. (2005). Socioeconomic position (again), causes and confounding. *International Journal of Epidemiology, 34*(2), 237–238.

Ebrahim, S., & Davey Smith, G. (1998). Ecological studies are a poor means of testing aetiological hypotheses. *British Medical Journal, 317*(7159), 678–678.

Egger, B., & Swinburn, G. (1997). An ecological approach to the obesity pandemic. *British Medical Journal, 315*, 477–480.

Epstein, P. R. (1998). Climate, ecology, and human health. *Infectious Diseases in Clinical Practice, 7*(Supplement 3), S100–S116.

Epstein, P. R. (2005). Climate change and human health. *New England Journal of Medicine, 353* (14), 1433–1436.

Fagg, J., Curtis, S., Stansfeld, S., & Congdon, P. (2006). Psychological distress among adolescents, and its relationship to individual, family and area characteristics; Evidence from East London, UK. *Social Science & Medicine,. 63*(3), 636–648

Gatrell, A. (2002). *Geographies of health.* Oxford: Blackwells.

Graham, H. (2000). The challenge of health inequalities. In H. Graham (Ed.), *Understanding health inequalities.* Buckingham: Open University Press.

Greenland, S. (2001). Ecologic versus individual-level sources of bias in ecologic estimates of contextual health effects. *International Journal of Epidemiology, 30*(6), 1343–1350.

Greenland, S. (2002). A review of multilevel theory for ecologic analyses. *Statistics in Medicine, 21,* 389–395.

Habicht, J., Victora, C. G., & Vaughan, J. P. (1999). Evaluation designs for adequacy, plausibility and probability of public health programme performance and impact. *International Journal of Epidemiology, 28,* 10–18.

Haines, A., Kovats, R. S., Campbell-Lendrum, D., & Corvalan, C. (2006). Harben Lecture – Climate change and human health: Impacts, vulnerability, and mitigation. *Lancet, 367*(9528), 2101–2109

Halpern, D., & Nazroo, J. (2000). The ethnic density effect: Results from a national community survey of England and Wales. *International Journal of Social Psychiatry, 46*(1), 34–46.

Hodgson, S., Nieuwenhuijsen, M. J., Hansell, A., Shepperd, S., Flute, T., Staples, B., et al. (2004). Excess risk of kidney disease in a population living near industrial plants. *Occupational and Environmental Medicine, 61*(8), 717–719.

Jarman, B. (1983). Identification of underprivileged areas. *British Medical Journal, 286*(6379), 1705–1709.

Jerrett, M., Burnett, R., Kanaroglou, P., Eyles, J., Finkelstein, N., Giovis, C., et al. (2001). A GIS – environmental justice analysis of particulate air pollution in Hamilton, Canada. *Environment and Planning A, 33*(6), 955–973.

Jones, K. (2005). Methodology and epistemology of multilevel analysis: Approaches from different social sciences. *Environment and Planning B – Planning and Design, 32*(6), 926–928.

Jones, K., Gould, M. I., & Watt, R. (1992). Multiple contexts as cross-classified models: The labour vote in the British General Election of 1992. *Geographical Analysis, 30*(1), 65–93.

Jones, K., & Moon, G. (1987). *Health, disease and society: An introduction to medical geography.* London: Routledge & Kegan Paul.

Jones, K., & Moon, G. (1993). Medical geography: Taking space seriously. *Progress in Human Geography, 17*(4), 515–524.

Karlsen, S., & Nazroo, J. (2000). Identity and structure: Rethinking ethnic inequalities and health. In H. Graham (Ed.), *Understanding health inequalities.* Buckingham: Open University.

Kaufman, J., & Kaufman, S. (2001). Assessment of structured socioeconomic effects on health. *Epidemiology, 12,* 157–167.

Kawachi, I., Kennedy, B., & Glass, R. (1999). Social capital and self-rated health: A contextual analysis. *American Journal of Public Health, 89,* 1187–1193.

Kawachi, I., Kim, D., Coutts, A., & Subramanian, S. V. (2004). Health by association? Social capital, social theory, and the political economy of public health – Commentary: Reconciling the three accounts of social capital. *International Journal of Epidemiology, 33*(4), 682–690.

Kearns, R. (1993). Place and health: Toward a reformed medical geography. *Professional Geographer, 45,* 139–147.

Keatinge, W., & Donaldson, G. (2004). The impact of global warming on health and mortality. *Southern Medical Journal, 97*(11), 1093–1099.

Kickbusch, I., & de Leeuw, E. (1999). Global public health; Revisiting public policy at the global level. *Health Promotion International, 14*(4), 285–288.

Kirkwood, B., Cousens, S., Victora, C. G., & Zoysa, I. (1997). Issues in the design and interpretation of studies to evaluate the impact of community-based interventions. *Tropical Medicine & International Health, 2*(11), 1022–1029

Last, J. (2001). *A dictionary of epidemiology.* 4th edition. Oxford: Oxford University Press.

Leon, D. A., Chenet, L., Shkolnikov, V. M., Zakharov, S., Shapiro, J., Rakhmanova, G., et al. (1997). Huge variation in Russian mortality rates 1984–94: Artefact, alcohol, or what? *Lancet, 350*(9075), 383–388.

Löytenen, M., & Arbona, S. (1996). Forecasting the AIDS epidemic in Puerto Rico. *Social Science & Medicine, 42*(7), 997–1010.

Macintyre, S. (1999). Geographical inequalities in mortality, morbidity and health related behaviour in England. In D. Gordon, M. Shaw, D. Dorling, & G. Davey Smith (1999). *Inequalities in health: The evidence presented to the independent inquiry into inequalities in health, chaired by Sir Donald Acheson.* Bristol: Policy Press.

Macintyre, S., Maciver, S., & Soomans, A. (1993). Area, class and health: Should we be focusing in places or people. *Journal of Social Policy, 22*(2), 213–234.

Mackenbach, J., & Kunst, A. (1997). Measuring the magnitude of socio-economic inequalities in health: An overview of available measures illustrated with two examples from Europe. *Social Science & Medicine, 44*(6), 757–771.

Martuzzi, M., Kryzanowski, M., & Bertollini, R. (2003). Health impact assessment of air pollution: Providing further evidence for public health action. *European Respiratory Journal, 31*(supplement 40), 86s–91s.

McQueen, D., Kickbusch, I., Potvin, L., Balbo, L, Abel, T., & Pelikan, J. (2007). *Health and modernity: The role of theory in health promotion.* New York: Springer.

Meade, M., & Earickson, R. (2000). *Medical geography.* 2nd edition. New York: Guilford.

Millward, L., Kelly, M., & Nutbeam, D. (2001). *Public health intervention research: The evidence.* London: Health Development Agency.

Nazroo, J. (1998). Genetic, cultural or socio-economic vulnerability? Explaining ethnic inequalities in health. In M. Bartley, D. Blane, & G. Davey-Smith (Eds.), *The sociology of health inequalities.* Oxford: Blackwells.

Neeleman, J., Wilson-Jones, C., & Wessely, S. (2005). Ethnic density and deliberate self harm; A small area study in south east London. *Journal of Epidemiology and Community Health, 55*, 85–90.

Noble, M., Wright, G., Dibben, C., Smith, G. A. N., McLennan, D., Anttila, C., et al. (2004). *The English indices of deprivation 2004.* West Yorkshire: ODPM Publications.

Oakes, J. (2004). The (mis)estimation of neighbourhood effects: Causal inference for a practicable epidemiology. *Social Science & Medicine, 58*, 1929–1952.

Parslow, R., El-Shimy, N., Cundall, D., & McKinney, P. (2001). Tuberculosis, deprivation, and ethnicity in Leeds, UK, 1982–1997. *Archives of Disease in Childhood, 84*(2), 109–113.

Pascutto, C., Wakefield, J., Best, N. G., Richardson, S., Bernardinelli, L., Staines, A., et al. (2000). Statistical issues in the analysis of disease mapping data. *Statistics in Medicine, 19*(1718), 2493–2519

Petticrew, M., Cummins, S., Ferrell, C., Finday, A., Higgins, C., Hoy, C., et al. (2005). Natural experiments: An underused tool for public health. *Public Health, 119*(9), 751–757.

Potvin, L., Gendron, S., Bilodeau, A., & Chabot, P. (2005). Integrating social theory into public health practice. *American Journal of Public Health, 95*, 591–595

Ricketts, T. (2003). Geographic information systems and public health. *Annual Review of Public Health, 24,* 1–6.

Rogerson, P., & Han, D. (2002). The effects of migration on the detection of geographic differences in disease risk. *Social Science & Medicine, 55,* 1817–1828.

Rose, G. (1992). *The strategy of preventive medicine.* Oxford: Oxford University Press.

Ross, N. A., Tremblay, S., & Graham, K. (2004). Neighbourhood influences on health in Montreal, Canada. *Social Science & Medicine, 59*(7), 1485–1494.

Schwartz, S. (1994). The fallacy of the ecological fallacy: The potential misuse of a concept and the consequences. *American Journal of Public Health, 84*(5), 819–824.

Shkolnikov, L., McKee, M., & Leon, D. (2001). Changes in life expectancy in Russia in the mid-1990s. *Lancet, 357*(9260), 917–921.

Stern, H., & Cressie, N. (1999). Inference for extremes in disease mapping, in A. Lawson, A. Biggeri, D. Böhning, E. Lasaffre, J. F. Viel, & R. Bertollini (Eds.), *Disease mapping and risk assessment for public health.* Chichester: Wiley.

Stafford, M., Cummins, S., Sacker, A., Wiggins, D., & Macintyre, S. (in press). Pathways to obesity: Identifying local, modifiable determinants of physical activity and diet. *Social Science & Medicine.*

Subramanian, S., Acevedo-Garcia, D., & Osypuk, T. (2005). Racial residential segregation and geographic heterogeneity in black/white disparity in poor self-rated health in the US: A multilevel statistical analysis. *Social Science & Medicine, 60,* 1667–1679.

Subramanian, S. V., Lochner, K. A., & Kawachi, I. (2003). Neighborhood differences in social capital: A compositional artifact or a contextual construct? *Health & Place, 9*(1), 33–44.

Susser, M. (1994). The logic in Ecological 1: The logic of analysis. *American Journal of Public Health, 84*(5), 825–829.

Taylor, P., & Derudder, B. (2004). Porous Europe: European cities in global urban arenas. *Tijdschrift voor Economische en Sociale Geografie, 95*(5), 527–538.

Thomas, R., Evans, S., Huxley, P., Gately, C., & Rogers, A. (2005). Housing improvement and self-reported mental distress among council estate residents. *Social Science & Medicine, 60*(12), 2773–2783.

Torsheim, T., Currie, C. Boyce, W, Kalnins, I., Overpeck, M., & Haugland, S. (2004). Material deprivation and self-rated health: A multi-level study of adolescents from 22 European and North American countries. *Social Science & Medicine, 59*(1), 1–12.

Trevelyan, B., Smallman-Raynor M., & Cliff. A. (2005). The spatial structure of epidemic emergence: Geographical aspects of poliomyelitis in north-eastern USA, July–October 1916. *Journal of the Royal Statistical Society: Series A, 168*(4), 701–722.

Veenstra, G. (2000). Social capital, SES and health: An individual-level analysis. *Social Science & Medicine, 50,* 619–629.

Wakefield, J. (2004). A critique of statistical aspects of ecological studies in spatial epidemiology. *Environmental and Ecological Statistics, 11,* 31–54.

Weitzman, E. R., & Kawachi, I. (2000). Giving means receiving: The protective effect of social capital on binge drinking on college campuses. *American Journal of Public Health, 90*(12), 1936–1939.

Wilkinson, R.G. (1996). *Unhealthy societies: The afflictions of inequality.* London: Routledge.

Chapter 17
Making Causal Inferences About Macrosocial Factors as a Basis for Public Health Policies

Jay S. Kaufman

1. Introduction

Things happen. A common colloquial phrase expresses this same sentiment in more scatological terms. For those who aspire to affect change in the world, the central question is always about making one thing happen rather than another. Therefore, in order to plan an effective series of policies or actions toward a desired outcome, we require some scientific knowledge about causation. That is, we need an understanding of how actions are connected to outcomes so that we can act in ways that will further our goals (Woodward, 2003).

Causal relations may be described as explanations for series of events that occurred in the past. For example, Packard (1989) suggested that the organization of migrant labor policies in South Africa during the first half of the 20th century exacerbated the spread of tuberculosis. The implication is that an alternate set of labor policies would have resulted in a different historical distribution of tuberculosis incidence and mortality. Specifically, Packard argued that Apartheid-era racial segregation necessitated labor migrancy, which spread disease more rapidly than if workers and their families had been allowed to live together near places of employment.

Alternatively, causal relations may be expressed as theories about future actions and their consequences. For example, Ahmad (2004) suggested that a 20 percent increase in the price of cigarettes in the state of California would lead to 14 million fewer years of life lost to premature death over the next 75 years, as well as a savings of $188 billion in smoking-related medical costs. Again, a manipulative interpretation of such a claim suggests that various alternative actions (e.g., increases in cigarette price of 0 percent or 100 percent) would yield different outcome distributions, as functions of the mechanistic relation between cigarette price and smoking behavior.

Causal relations may be inferred from extant knowledge, estimated by observational or experimental studies or by some combination of these approaches. The identification of causal relations is necessarily subject to uncertainty, but virtually all policy discussions are premised on causal theories, whether articulated formally or not. For example, some suggest that vaccination of all US women against human papillomavirus using current bivalent or quadrivalent vaccine formulations would prevent up to 70 percent of all cervical, anal, and genital cancers (Steinbrook, 2005). Others argue against such a vaccination policy, however, because they assert that it would alter adolescent sexual behavior, leading to increases in other adverse outcomes, such as sexually transmitted diseases and unwanted pregnancies. The policy debate revolves around the costs and benefits of the various outcomes, but in every case it requires causal theories for tying past or future actions to their respective consequences.

Oftentimes our causal models are in fact horrendously wrong, leading to policy disasters. For example, city leaders in Hamburg, Germany, faced an epidemic of cholera in 1892. They rejected John Snow's causal theory for the propagation of cholera, published decades earlier, in favor of Max von Pettenkofer's miasma theory, which asserted that cholera arose from toxic contamination of the ground. Thus, the well-intentioned people of Hamburg ignored the water supply and instead expended their resources digging up and carting away the soil underneath slaughterhouses (Evans, 1987). The causal theory being completely misguided, this did not turn out to be a successful intervention.

Just as we cannot escape the necessity of causal models as a basis for policy formation, likewise we must also embrace the necessity of values. Actions generally have multiple and incommensurable consequences. For example, increasing the price of cigarettes may reduce smoking deaths, but it may also increase the prevalence of obesity and its sequelae (Chou, Grossman, & Saffer, 2004). Vaccination against human papillomavirus may decrease cervical cancer incidence, but it could adversely affect teen pregnancy rates. The magnitudes and directions of the causal relations implied in these statements are subject to debate, but regardless of the final consensus on the theory, no policy is possible unless one is able to adjudicate between the competing outcome considerations. Epidemiologists sometimes may prefer a single commensurable outcome, such as mortality, whereas economists may prefer to express everything in terms of monetary costs. In order to even agree upon a metric and then convert all other relevant outcomes into this metric (for example, what is the monetary value of a human life?), there is no way to avoid the imposition of some set of value judgments. Any consideration of values is necessarily extra-scientific, meaning that no policy can ultimately be described as strictly rational.

This chapter explores the relations between causal effect estimation and formation of policies at the macrosocial level. Following this introduction, Section 2 describes how potential outcome contrasts can be used to describe the predicted impacts of various policy regimes. Section 3 highlights some considerations that result from focusing on the aggregate behavior of a population rather than on contrasts between individual units. Section 4 describes the crucial distinction between policies, events, and conditions in public health research and how attention to this distinction affects analytic choices and interpretations. Section 5 shows how specification of population level summaries for contrasting potential policy options requires the imposition of values and an accounting for uncertainty.

2. Formal Models for Causal Effects

2.1. Potential Outcomes

Because public health policy decisions relate to potential actions, it is fitting in this context to consider theories of causality that are based on intervention (Woodward, 2003). This is not the only possible foundation for causal theories (Pratt & Schlaifer, 1988), but it is a formulation that is advantageous because it explicitly links information from experiments and observational research with predictions for the outcome distribution that will pertain under the various intervention regimes.

A key concept in manipulative theories of causation is the idea of a potential outcome distribution. The idea is that for every action, often referred to as a "treatment" (making an analogy with experiments), there exists a potentially counterfactual value of the outcome measure that would be observed in a specific target population and in a specified time period, were that action to be realized. For example, consider manipulating the average sale price of a pack of cigarettes in California through taxation; for every potential sale price, there exists some value for the proportion of Californians who will smoke at the designated follow-up time. This value is not observed unless or until we enact the specific policy, and so it must be estimated in some way from existing data or theory. Prior to enacting a policy, therefore, all potential outcomes are latent, in the sense of being unobserved. Once an intervention is made, the value of the outcome corresponding to that specific treatment becomes observable, whereas all the other potential outcome values remain latent.

Theoretically, potential responses exist even if never observed and may be considered as "missing data". For example, even if we never act to raise the average sale price of a pack of cigarettes in California by 100 percent, there does exist an unobserved value for the proportion of Californians who will smoke under this treatment policy. In the simplest case, the outcome vector has as many elements as there are levels of treatment. Thus, for a binary treatment with levels 0 and 1, a population parameter, such as the proportion P of Californians who will smoke at the specified follow-up time, is a vector with two elements, $[P_0, P_1]$, only one element of which is ever observed at a particular time. Observation of both elements can be made indirectly by switching the policy over time, but this requires several assumptions, such as that values are invariant to time periods and order of treatment assignments. The model becomes exceedingly more complicated if the potential outcome values for units are not mutually independent. For example, if state cigarette tax rates vary, then smoking prevalence in each state at follow-up time may depend not only on the price set in a given state, but also on the price set in neighboring states from which residents may smuggle cheaper cigarettes (see Section 3.2 below).

2.2. Effects as Contrasts

Manipulative formulations of causality define effects as contrasts between the outcome parameters under various treatments. For example, consider the proportion of Californians who will smoke at the designated follow-up time under a policy raising the average sale price of a pack of cigarettes in California by 20 percent in contrast to the proportion under a policy raising the average price by 0 percent. This contrast, $P_{20} - P_0$, is the causal effect of a new policy in relation to taking no action. When estimated from the data via some causal model, it is a causal effect measure (or estimate). Any other algebraic contrast, such as P_{20}/P_0, is a similarly well-defined casual effect for these two defined policy options (as long as $P_0 > 0$) (Maldonado & Greenland, 2002). For difference contrasts such as $P_{20} - P_0$, the null value (i.e., no causal effect) is 0, whereas for ratio measure of effect, such as P_{20} / P_0, the null value is 1. Often in popular discourse, we carelessly omit the referent value for this contrast, speaking loosely of "the effect of raising the average sale price of a pack of cigarettes in California by 20 percent." However, the denominator need not be the status quo; we could just as readily consider causal effects of contrasting interventions such as $P_{20} - P_{10}$ or $P_{40} - P_{20}$.

2.3. Estimating Causal Effects from Observational Data

Because most potential outcomes remain latent, we most often use subject matter knowledge, statistical models, or both to estimate the unobserved values. For example, suppose that a new policy is enacted that raises the average price of a pack of cigarettes in California by 20 percent, and the proportion of Californians who smoke at the designated follow-up time is 0.15. The value P_0 will not be observed at the follow-up time if the invention is enacted, and yet researchers assuming stability of smoking behavior over some short period of follow-up time may believe that this quantity is close to its value before the intervention, say 0.20. Note that in the presence of some true secular trend, the value of P_0 might not truly be 0.20 at the follow-up time, and so the causal effect estimate is only identifiable by imposition of a stability assumption (which is often not stated overtly). Researchers might further assume some simple functional form in order to extrapolate to other unobserved potential outcomes. For example, if $P_{20} - P_0 = -0.05$, it might be assumed, on the basis of a linear extrapolation, that $P_{40} - P_0 = -0.10$, even though both of the component potential outcomes in that contrast remain unobserved. For near-continuous or multilevel treatments, such as in this example, the number of "missing" values is necessarily large compared to the number of observed values, so estimation of the latent values is often heavily dependent on the choice of functional form.

When values for potential outcomes are observed passively (as opposed to experimentally), an additional problem arises because the values that are contrasted to obtain an effect estimate may be confounded by unobserved covariates (Greenland & Morgenstern, 2001). For example, suppose that a team of policy makers would like to consider the effect on the proportion of Californians who will smoke at the designated follow-up time under a policy raising the average sale price of a pack of cigarettes by 20 percent in contrast to keeping the average price constant. Without the capacity to engage in experimental manipulation of state-level cigarette prices as a strategy for estimating the necessary potential outcome values P_{20} and $P0$, suppose that the researchers are forced to instead rely on regional variations in cigarette pricing within the state. Further, suppose they identify a county (Sacramento) in which the average price of a pack of cigarettes is equal to the overall state average, and they identify a county (Orange) in which the average price of a pack of cigarettes is 20 percent higher than the state average. The investigators might then contrast the observed proportions of smokers in these two counties $P^*_{20} - P^*_0$ as a means to estimate the contrast of unobservable values $P_{20} - P_0$ for the entire state.

Disregarding sampling variability, the estimate formed by contrasting passively observed values $P^*_{20} - P^*_0$ may not equal the true potential outcomes contrast $P_{20} - P_0$ if there are unmeasured differences between the two counties that correlate with both cigarette pricing and smoking behavior (e.g., socio-economic level of the county, proportion foreign born, age-structure of the population, etc). The same problem could occur even if researchers instead used fluctuating state-level prices over time in order to estimate the potential outcome values, since the smoking prevalence obtained through specific historical process might differ from that which would occur under the legislative intervention (Greenland, 2005). The contrast of observed values, $P^*_{20} - P^*_0$, is generally called a measure of association, rather than a measure of effect. If a measure of association is confounded, this bias in the estimation of the causal effect estimate can often be reduced by conditioning on measured covariates that are 1) associated with (but not affected by) treatment and 2) independently predictive of the outcome (Greenland & Morgenstern, 2001).

2.4. Graphs, Structural Equations Models, and Other Representations of Causal Theory

Although causal knowledge is necessary for estimating the effects that are the basis for setting policies, there are numerous traditions for the representation of this knowledge. Historically, sociology and economics have focused on path analysis, structural equations models, and simultaneous equations models as representations of causal structure and as tools for the estimation of causal effects (Sobel, 1995). Recently, however, several authors have linked these traditions to graphical methods to show that the approaches are isomorphic (Greenland & Brumback, 2002). The graphical language of Pearl (2000) can be considered a non-parametric form of structural equations models, and this graphical language can also be translated directly into the potential outcomes model. The different representations have subtle advantages and disadvantages for highlighting or obscuring assumptions, but all information in a causal graph can be represented algebraically. The primary strength of graphs is their transparency in revealing causal structure and independence assumptions succinctly.

2.5. Permissible Causes and Policy-Relevant Causal Statements

A long-standing debate in the causality literature focuses on the implications of the manipulative interpretation of causality for poorly specified interventions. The potential outcomes model has a clear experimental analogy that gives a ready interpretation for causal effects, which is a primary strength of this model. For example, to say that vaccination of all US women against human papillomavirus (HPV) would prevent up to 70 percent of all cervical, anal, and genital cancers is to compare this intervention against the alternative of doing nothing and to contrast the potential outcome for the population summary measure under each of these treatment policies. The potential outcomes are specific to the intervention, however, so we need to be unambiguous about the nature of that intervention: the age range and geographic range of women to be vaccinated, the range of HPV subtypes covered by the vaccine, the dose of vaccine, and so forth. We need to be specific because the potential outcome under a slightly different intervention could take a different value.

In a linear regression or structural equations model, it is simple to estimate a slope parameter for a variable and describe that slope in causal language as the expected change in the outcome for a unit change in the exposure. To do so requires no specific information on how the exposure would be changed by one unit, and yet the exact nature of the intervention could clearly be consequential for determining the value of the potential outcome. For example, in a logistic regression model predicting preterm delivery (< 37 weeks gestational age) as a function of mothers' achieved educational level, one might obtain a fitted estimate for the logistic slope of -0.04, leading to an estimated odds ratio contrast comparing women reporting 8 years of formal education with those that have a high school diploma of $\exp(-0.04 \times 4 \text{ years}) = 0.85$. A causal interpretation of this parameter would be that intervening on pregnant women with 8 years of completed education to bring them to the point of high school graduation would reduce their odds of experiencing a preterm birth by 15 percent. But surely handing these women a piece of paper declaring them to be high school graduates would not affect this change. Nor is it even clear that forcing these women to stay in school for an additional four years would give them the same risk as those observed to have completed high school in the absence of an intervention.

This example clearly shows that casual effect estimates can only be directly relevant to policy if the intervention strategy is unambiguously defined. For immutable variables such as year of birth and ethnicity, a regression coefficient may be estimated, but it has no obvious causal interpretation in the sense defined above (Kaufman & Cooper, 1999). Even for manipulable variables, a causal interpretation that could be relevant for policy considerations requires an explicit statement about the intervention mechanism (Hernan, 2005). It may be seen as an advantage of the potential outcomes model that this problem is made explicit, although it sometimes conflicts with common-sense notions of cause and effect. For example, to say that 739 deaths were due to the Chicago heat wave of 1995 is to assert that had climatic history been different, this number of "excess" deaths would not have occurred (Whitman, Good, Donoghue, Benbow, Shou, & Mou, 1997). This statement conforms reasonably well with causal thinking in the informal sense, as well as to some alternative theories of causality such as that of Granger in economics (Sobel, 1995). Nonetheless, this statement provides no relevant information for making policy decisions, as would, for example, a statement about the effect of providing air conditioned shelters for the elderly on heat related mortality.

3. Applications to Populations

3.1. An Aggregate Model of Causal Effects

Although many expositions of causal theory in public health focus on outcomes that would occur at the individual level, it is entirely reasonable to define potential outcomes for aggregate parameters as well, such as a population death rate, a proportion affected, or the mean of some quantitative measure such as birth weight. Note, however, that this formulation masks the individual-level behavior that gives rise to the aggregate measure. For example, the anticoagulation therapy rt-PA can prevent death in those with an ischemic stroke, and yet it can hasten death in those with a hemorrhagic stroke. Under the policy of approving this therapy for use in hospital emergency rooms, there exists a potential outcome value for a population summary such as "stroke case fatality proportion", and this may be contrasted with the similar potential outcome corresponding to a policy of withholding rt-PA from use. The use of the population summary, however, obscures the fact that some individuals who are treated with rt-PA would have died if untreated, yet other individuals died only because they were treated and would have lived had they been untreated. Therefore, it is possible, for example, that a true summary causal effect that is null (e.g., a causal risk difference equal to 0) could arise because half of the population is harmed and half the population is benefited (Greenland, Robins, & Pearl, 1999). There is no obvious solution to this problem except to recognize that causal effects for sub-categories of the outcome summary may take very different values. The additive scale causal effect of the rt-PA therapy on the summary outcome "ischemic stroke case fatality proportion" is likely larger in magnitude, for example, than on the broader summary outcome "stroke case fatality proportion".

Another characteristic of the aggregate potential outcomes model for population effects is that a particular exposure intervention level will not always unambiguously define a unique potential outcome value. Consider the case of only two levels of exposure, exposed and unexposed, and two levels of response, disease and no disease. Furthermore, define policy 1 as exposing all members of the population and policy 0 as exposing none of the members of the population, and define the potential outcomes of interest as the numbers of new cases under these policies, A1 and A0, respectively. These summary potential outcomes are determined unambiguously by the proportions of individuals in the population who have the individual response types "will always get the disease" and "will get the disease if exposed" (for A1) or "will get the disease if unexposed" (for A0). On the other hand, define policy 1* as exposing 75% of the members of the population and policy 0* as exposing 25% of the members of the population, and consider once more the potential outcomes of interest as the numbers of new cases under these policies, A1* and A0*, respectively. In this latter scenario, the summary outcome measure under each policy is no longer determined by the individual response type proportions in the population because now it matters *which* 75% is exposed and *which* 25% is exposed. For example, some individuals may be immune from getting the disease regardless of their exposure status, and if these individuals are differentially assigned the treatment, then the casual effect magnitude is reduced. One solution to this problem is to assign treatment in a manner independent of the individual potential outcome, as would be accomplished, for example, through randomization (Kaufman & Kaufman, 2002).

3.2. Direct and Indirect Effects of Policy Interventions

Another consequence of using an aggregate model for causal effects is that the mechanism of action may involve both direct and indirect elements. This is especially relevant to infectious processes where units affect one another. A classic example of this phenomenon is "herd immunity" in vaccination interventions. In this setting, one needn't vaccinate 100 percent of the population in order to eliminate disease. It is only necessary to vaccinate a sufficient number of individuals so that the average number of new cases generated by each existing infection falls below 1.0 (Garnett, 2005). In economic interventions, such as the previous example of raising the average price of a pack of cigarettes in California in order to reduce smoking prevalence, compensatory behavior often emerges at extreme values of the policy regime. For instance, individuals may smuggle cigarettes from neighboring states if the sale price is too high. A potential result is that even while per capita cigarette consumption appears to fall in California under some substantial price increase, it may appear to rise in Nevada (Gruber, Sen, & Stabile, 2003).

A hallmark of the concept of indirect effects in public health policy evaluation is that the outcome is affected not by the direct action of the intervention on individuals, but through interactions between individuals (Halloran & Struchiner, 1995). For example, smoking interventions not only influence the health of the smokers who quit, but also the exposure of their spouses to second-hand smoke. Likewise, anti-retroviral therapy for HIV positive individuals not only lowers risk of progression to AIDS, but also lowers the risk of incident infection in their sex partners. These kinds of indirect effects often make identification of potential outcomes for summary measures difficult because the full range of indirect effects is not always anticipated or adequately modeled. For example, in the Moving to Opportunity (MTO) Study, individuals in poverty were randomly assigned to receive vouchers that would allow them to move out of high poverty neighborhoods into low poverty neighborhoods. An unintended consequence of this intervention, however, was to change the composition of both the old and the new neighborhoods (Sobel, 2006). Finally, it should be noted that the use of the words "direct" and "indirect" to describe types of effects in this section differs from their use in the structural equations or effect decomposition contexts, in which the question is about causal pathways between variables, not between individuals within the population.

3.3. Competing Risks

Interactions between units are an important source of indirect effects, but another source is interactions between outcomes. A paradigmatic example arises from policies of health outcome reduction or elimination. For an intervention such as syphilis eradication, the situation is relatively simple in the sense that an individual who would have acquired syphilis prior to the intervention will have a different outcome if syphilis is eradicated, but the absence of syphilis probably has no important deleterious effects on risk of other health outcomes. The situation is quite different, however, if one considers a health outcome defined as "cause of death". Being mortal, people are constrained to die of something, and if one disease is reduced or eliminated as a cause of death, then another must logically take its place.

This once again emphasizes the central importance of the specific intervention mechanism. There are many ways to reduce the burden of a disease, and these have very different implications. For example, the age-standardized death rate for coronary heart disease has declined by about 50 percent in the US over the last 30 years (Jemal, Ward, Hao, & Thun, 2005). Although vital statistics are not as complete, it is likely that a similar change occurred in South Africa during this period, as the proportion of adult deaths due to HIV/AIDS changed from 0 percent to 25 percent over this same time interval. Obviously, therefore, either increasing or decreasing age-specific overall death rates can reduce or eliminate a cause of death. Another way to state this is that the reduction of an important risk factor for one disease (e.g., cigarette smoking in relation to lung cancer mortality) is itself a risk factor for some alternate outcome (e.g., heart disease mortality). Thus, a target outcome distribution is not an ideal basis for policy decisions because it is causally ambiguous. Rather, the relevant choice is between specific intervention policy regimes, each of which implies a multi-dimensional potential outcome distribution that must be estimated and then weighed against alternatives (Greenland, 2005).

4. Macrosocial Factors as Causes

4.1. Policies, Events, and Conditions

The potential outcomes model makes it clear why we are interested in causal effects of potential actions, rather than contrasts of health outcome summaries under various conditions that arise through historical or natural processes not subject to human intervention (see Section 2.5 above). Nonetheless, it can often be useful to make contrasts between groups strictly for purposes of surveillance, without any casual inference. For example, to say that the prevalence of diabetes at some specified point in time is higher in adult African Americans than in US adult whites is a statement about the real world as it exists. Such a statement involves no contrast between outcomes under alternative interventions and therefore is not directly relevant for policy decisions. Surveillance data certainly could inform policies for resource provision, for example if diabetes screening and treatment facilities were to be concentrated in areas of high population risk. However, any attempt to define the impact of these policies would require posing a very different question, a question of pursuing one resource provision policy versus another.

4.2. Implications for Statistical Modeling and Interpretation

In much of the epidemiologic literature on macrosocial determinants of health, the important distinction between policies, events and conditions is often lost, and this can make sensible interpretation of data analysis very difficult. In particular, this distinction has profound implications for model selection because conditioning on covariates is premised on a causal interpretation and therefore on manipulable exposures. Consider the diabetes example described above. To say that the prevalence ratio for diabetes in adult African-American versus white Americans is 1.5 in 2005 is to make a statement about reality, not about how reality would change under some potential intervention. As such (assuming representative sampling from the population and no misclassification of ethnicity or disease status), it simply is what it is, and no further adjustment is necessary or appropriate. In fact, conditioning on any other variable provides a summary measure that is no longer a valid depiction of reality.

In practice, such contrasts are often standardized to some distribution of 10-year age categories whenever the condition is a function of age, as it is for diabetes. This is often justified on the grounds that it removes the imbalance associated with different population age structures. For example, African-Americans have a higher proportion of the population in younger age categories, in which diabetes risk is lower. Taking age category-specific diabetes risks and weighting them to some common population age standard, such as the US population in 2000, inflates the prevalence ratio for the black-white contrast to 1.8. This adjusted estimate is not a description of any real world populations, however it is the value that would pertain if both populations had the same age distribution as the standard. Since they do not, it is a fiction, albeit one that is considered attractive for revealing how populations would compare conditional on age. A value above the null for the unstratified summary does not imply, however, that within any given age category, African-Americans have higher diabetes prevalence than whites. Rather, there can be heterogeneity in the contrast measure across groups, so no particularly unambiguous interpretation can be granted to the summary, other than the one premised on the fiction of the two groups having age structures equal to the standard.

Without a homogeneity assumption of stratum-specific contrasts, the link to policy may therefore be quite obscure.

Further statistical adjustment only serves to make the surveillance activity even more opaque, as it removes the summary measure even further from linkage to real world populations or policies. Multivariable adjustment can only be sensible, therefore, when one wishes to engage not in surveillance, but in causal inference. As described above, this requires a statement about alternative actions or policies, which must be specified. For example, one might be interested in the ratio of the prevalence of diabetes that pertains in US adults now to the prevalence that would pertain if we were to replace all sugared soft-drinks with artificially sweetened soft-drinks (Schulze, Manson, Ludwig, Colditz, Stampfer, Willett, & Hu, 2004). The purpose of covariate adjustment is to make statements about the consequences of potential actions on the basis of passively observed data (Pearl, 2000). Once these potential actions are well-defined, background knowledge determines which variables need to be conditioned on so that the frequency measure contrast will have a causal interpretation (Robins, 2001).

Consider an example from House et al (House, Lepkowski, Williams, Mero, Lantz, Robert, & Chen, 2000), a stratified multi-stage probability sample of 3617 US adults. Among many other findings, the authors reported that the estimated all-cause mortality hazard rate in 1986–1994 in the US for urban black males ages 65 years and older was 3.18 times higher than for rural non-black females of the same age range, adjusted for education, income, marital status and "health". Because the contrast estimate is adjusted for a number of covariates, it does not describe any real populations. This must therefore be a causal estimate, yet there is no policy or action specified, nor is it remotely conceivable that any potential action could turn urban black males into rural non-black females. However, even if there were some action, however hypothetical, it would presumably also affect the variables that are held constant in this model: education, income, marital status and "health". Indeed, it would be rather to absurd to imagine an intervention that would impact mortality risk without affecting "health". For these reasons, the estimate fails to have interpretability as either a surveillance measure or as a causal effect estimate, and therefore its utility is questionable. Examples like this one, in which confusion between policies, events and conditions makes the estimate essentially uninterpretable, are unfortunately the norm in contemporary public health research.

4.3. Examples

4.3.1. Race and Racism

As many authors have noted, racial categorization is inadmissible as a cause in the sense of contrasting actions or policies because it is not generally a mutable characteristic of individuals (Kaufman & Cooper, 2001). For this reason, it has a legitimate role in public health surveillance and as a confounder or effect measure modifier when examining the causal effects of other factors, but it is not itself an exposure in any definable causal contrast (Holland, 2001). However, while the race of an individual may generally be fixed in his or her identity and consciousness, it is malleable in the perceptions of others. Several experimental study designs demonstrate how racial categorizations can be manipulated in decision-making contexts and therefore have causal effects external to the individuals whose race is recorded (e.g., Schulman, Berlin, Harless, Kerner, Sistrunk, Gersh, Dube, Taleghani, Burke, Williams, Eisenberg, & Escarce, 1999). This gives race a valid interpretation as an exposure in etiologic studies based on observational data only when the casual effect operates through the mechanism of discrimination on the part of some decision maker (i.e., "racism").

For example, Loring and Powell (1988) estimated the causal effect of race on making psychiatric diagnoses. Because their study was actually an experiment, as opposed to an observational analysis, the specific intervention is defined unambiguously. Similar experiments have identified causal effects of race in other kinds of decision-making, such as medical referral, employment and housing decisions (e.g., Bertrand & Mullainathan, 2004). This contrasts with biomedical studies of physiologic processes within the individuals whose race is categorized. In these latter studies, which are more common in the epidemiologic and public health literature, adjusted effect parameters for race in multivariate models have no obvious interpretation or relevance to policy (Kaufman, in press).

4.3.2. Education and Training

Another classic example where the distinction between policies, events and conditions is neglected in public health research is the use of years of achieved education as an exposure (Yen & Moss, 1999). In economics, by contrast, education and training as causal effects of interest are generally tied to specific policy interventions (e.g., Sakellariou, 2006). The failure to do so in public health research is evidenced by model selection decisions that defy existing background knowledge. For example, adjusted regression coefficients for achieved education are generally given a causal interpretation, suggesting some intervention that would encourage or compel students to remain in school longer than they would without the intervention (e.g., Elo & Preston, 1996). However, the models are usually conditioned on income or other measures of socioeconomic status that would presumably be directly affected by educational achievement and which would therefore be affected if education were to be modified by the imposition of the policy (Kaufman & Kaufman, 2001). The implications of this example are similar to those stated above. There is no well-defined causal effect of years of completed education. Rather, what is estimable is a causal effect of modifying educational achievement by, for example, a policy of providing low-cost student loans, or by modifying admissions policies for public universities, or by more generous funding of remedial programs for potential drop-outs.

4.4. Macrosocial Factors Beyond Human Control

As noted in Section 2.5 above, the causal model described in this chapter does not directly address macrosocial factors that are outside of human agency because it focuses instead on our policy actions in anticipation of, or in response to, these events or conditions. For example, given our current state of knowledge and technology, we can't yet set a policy of having earthquakes or not, or even of affecting their timing or magnitude. Nonetheless, we can have various policies about where and how we construct our dwellings in relation to the threat of earthquakes. To the extent that earthquake mortality is a function of policies around zoning and construction practices, we can affect the health outcome distribution in predictable ways. Therefore, the relevant scientific task is to estimate these potential outcomes distributions and assess the costs and benefits of various policies in order to act appropriately with respect to our values and priorities.

For example, the estimated cost per year of life saved to strengthen buildings in earthquake prone areas is 18 million dollars. This contrasts with many potential alternative interventions, such as $140 per year of life saved for universal influenza vaccination (Tengs, Adams, Pliskin, Safran, Siegel, Weinstein, & Graham, 1995). Therefore, with respect to policy formation, the "cause" of a death when a building collapses in an earthquake is not the natural event itself but rather the policy decision to forgo potentially protective engineering of the building. At the same time, the policy of providing resources to reinforce buildings in order to affect the mortality outcome of earthquakes is one that necessarily prevents the allocation of those resources to any number of other potential purposes.

5. Summarizing Outcomes

5.1. Why Summary Measures of Health Depend on Values

As mentioned briefly in Section 1, all policy decisions must involve values because alternative actions precipitate numerous consequences, and any statement about the optimal configuration of these multiple outcomes requires a framework for weighing one kind of event against another. The situation is further complicated in the case of policies that change the distributions of more than a single risk factor (Murray, Ezzati, Lopez, Rodgers, & Vander Hoorn, 2003). For example, a policy of taxing cigarettes more heavily may have the relatively atomistic impact of reducing the quantity of cigarettes consumed. However, a policy of income supplementation for the poor will potentially affect myriad health behaviors, including diet quality, use of medical services, and consumption of alcohol. Thus, estimating the outcome distribution under contrasting complex policies requires some joint effects model for the various exposure distributions that are simultaneously modified, and this can be both prohibitively difficult and assumption-laden.

Even in the best case scenario of a simple intervention that affects a single risk factor one must summarize across diverse consequences. For example, a policy such as requiring air bags in every automobile sold in the US results in reduced overall mortality from automobile crashes, compared to the absence of such a policy. At the same time, however, many who would have died in crashes previously will, in the presence of air bags, survive head-on crashes with significant life-long disabilities (especially to lower extremities, which are not protected by the air bags) and with astronomical costs for medical treatment and long-term disability care (Graham, Thompson, Goldie, Segui-Gomez, & Weinstein, 1997). Furthermore, some individuals are actually killed by airbags, especially children, and the death of a child may be considered more consequential, if gauged in terms of years of potential life lost, for example. Even ignoring additional behavioral consequences of the intervention (e.g., if people who feel protected by airbags are less likely to utilize seat-belts), a summary metric is needed in order to weigh the reduced mortality against the increased morbidity, or the saving of adult lives against the loss of children's lives, or the cost of a life saved against the cost of manufacturing more expensive cars, the vast majority of which will never experience a head-on crash.

A wide variety of summary measures have been proposed in the literature, including disability-adjusted life expectancy (DALE), quality adjusted life expectancy (QALY), and disability-adjusted life-years (DALY) (Murray, Salomon, & Mathers, 2002). A central feature of such summaries is the relative valuation of health states. For example, if an intervention were to save the lives of some people but leave many others blind or disabled, how does one value the loss of a life against the loss of some vital component of a life? The answer depends on some relative valuation of the disabled state as a discounted healthy life. The basic logic is that if being blind discounts a healthy life by 50 percent, then an intervention that saves ten lives but blinds twenty people is an equal trade-off, whereas a higher or lower number of blindings in relation to the ten lives saved motivates a preference for one policy or the other. These valuations may be highly context dependent. For example, being unable to walk in an urban U.S. setting that includes access ramps and elevators may discount a life less heavily than being unable to walk in a rural agricultural society. Being rendered infertile may discount a life more heavily for a 15 year old with no children than for a 35 year old with two children.

5.2. How Summary Measures Create Winners and Losers

How we value the various incommensurate outcomes under consideration will determine which policy is deemed preferable, and these valuations can be functions of culture, class status and other characteristics. It is therefore not surprising that many valuations tend to favor in some way groups of people in power. A clear example of this phenomenon is conveyed by the famous Lawrence Summers memo of December 12, 1991, a document signed by Summers when he was Chief Economist of the World Bank but actually written by an aide (Rosenberg, 2001). The memo advocates a policy of dumping more pollution from industrialized nations into less-developed countries on the basis of several arguments about health valuation. First, the memo states that the cost of morbidity and mortality due to toxic pollution is in foregone earnings, so the cost is minimized in low-income countries. Second, the memo suggests that the health impacts of pollution are likely to be non-linear, so nations with low levels of industrialization can accommodate additional pollution with lower absolute levels of attributable morbidity and mortality. Finally, the memo notes that since health effects may take decades to become evident, populations with lower life expectancy will have lower absolute numbers of attributable cases because individuals will be less likely to survive to experience the long-term health consequences.

Another example in which the necessity of a relative valuation favored advantaged versus disadvantaged groups arose in the conduct of the World Health Organization and World Bank funded Global Burden of Disease Study, for which DALYs (disability adjusted life-years) were calculated in order to provide valuations for various health states (Nord, 2002). The investigators used several techniques to quantify alternative health states from carefully selected panels of respondents. The investigators then used these valuations in order to conclude that the most important health problems facing the world were ischemic heart disease and cerebrovascular disease. Critics of this approach noted that it is agnostic to socioeconomic context and therefore gives the same weight to outcomes for all income groups. The non-communicable diseases identified by this process as having the highest impact are in fact much more consequential for the rich than for the poor. For example, among the richest fifth of the world, 85 percent of deaths are due to non-communicable diseases and 8 percent to communicable diseases. Conversely, among the poorest fifth of the planet, non-communicable and communicable diseases account for 34 percent and 56 percent of deaths, respectively (Gwatkin, 1997).

5.3. Incommensurability and Uncertainty as Limitations in Policy Formation

It may be clear from the preceding discussion that a fundamental problem in the evaluation of alternative macrosocial actions or policies is that the definition of an optimal outcome distribution is inherently subjective. Furthermore, the comparison of health states is only the tip of this philosophical iceberg. How does one value loss of freedom when considering prohibition of some behaviors as a policy option, or the weighing of some individuals rights against others, as in the example of policies for second-hand smoke? Ultimately, these are scientific decisions for which extra-scientific inputs are required.

Another important limitation in the process of identifying optimal macrosocial policies for reducing poor health is that the evidentiary basis for such decisions also necessarily involves some uncertainty. For example, in a study cited above, Ahmad (2004) estimated that a 20 percent increase in the price of cigarettes in the state of California would lead to 14 million fewer years of life lost to premature death over the next 75 years. This estimate is sensitive to a large number of model parameters, but in this case, as in many others, the author provides no sensitivity analysis nor uncertainty bounds for the estimates, remarking only that "estimates of input variables were based on the best available data, and where there was uncertainty, [he] tried to err toward figures that would produce in the model more conservative estimates of the health and economic benefits." No argument is made for why it may be advantageous to base policy decisions on the most conservative scenario, and in general, most policy makers would prefer to have uncertainty intervals available so that the plausible outcomes that will be realized under a potential set of actions can be more realistically appraised. A better approach might be to express model parameters as probability distributions rather than as point estimates and then generate outcome distributions as functions of these joint distributions. Regardless, even when outcome distributions are provided with uncertainty intervals, the translation of this information into policy still requires applications of extra-scientific judgments in the form of values. For example, when considering macrosocial policies, should the goal be to maximize the expected outcome for the whole population? Or to minimize the worst possible harm to any sub-group?

6. Conclusion and Summary

Public health is not a passive observational science like astronomy or paleontology. While describing the natural world (i.e., surveillance) is an important component of public health research, the focus of the field is on interventions and policy choices that improve the health of populations. There is little doubt that changes at the societal level affect the health of populations for good or for ill, but planning such changes rationally in order to maximize some health outcome distribution is a complex and formidable task. First, we need to conduct and interpret etiologic studies to develop an increasingly refined casual understanding; next models must be developed based on this causal understanding to predict the expected outcome distributions under various potential intervention regimes. Ideally, these models also involve sensitivity analysis to account for systematic and random sources of error in estimating the relevant outcome distributions. The policy decision-making process also requires a set of values for deciding on the priorities for the desired outcome distribution, for example, whether the goal is to maximize the average outcome, minimize the gap between advantaged and disadvantaged sub-groups, or avoid worsening the outcome for any sub-group (e.g., "first do no harm"). Moreover, some set of values is required for summarizing multiple health endpoints into a single metric so that it may be maximized as desired.

This process of forming policy on the basis of anticipated population level health effects is therefore fraught with error and controversy. For public health researchers and activists, however, there is no alternative. Countless choices are made every second at the individual and the macrosocial levels, often with only the haziest sense of their consequences for health and other outcomes. A diligent and honest quantification of these expected outcomes is therefore a minimum expectation of good public health science. At the end of the day, however, this information is necessary but not sufficient for adoption of progressive policy formation, as it also requires relentless agitation for the values and principles of equity and justice.

References

Ahmad, S. (2004). Increasing excise taxes on cigarettes in California: A dynamic simulation of health and economic impacts. *Preventive Medicine, 41*(1), 276–283.

Bertrand, M., & Mullainathan, S. (2004). Are Emily and Greg more employable than Lakisha and Jamal? A field experiment on labor market discrimination. *American Economic Review, 94*(4), 991–1013.

Chou, S. Y., Grossman, M., & Saffer, H. (2004). An economic analysis of adult obesity: Results from the Behavioral Risk Factor Surveillance System. *Journal of Health Economics, 23*(3), 565–587.

Elo, I. T., & Preston, S.H. (1996). Educational differentials in mortality: United States, 1979–85. *Social Science & Medicine, 42*(1), 47–57.

Evans, R. J. (1987). *Death in Hamburg: Society and politics in the cholera years, 1830–1910.* New York: Oxford University Press.

Garnett, G. P. (2005). Role of herd immunity in determining the effect of vaccines against sexually transmitted disease. *Journal of Infectious Diseases, 191*(Supplement 1), S97–S106.

Graham, J. D., Thompson, K., Goldie, S., Segui-Gomez, M., & Weinstein, M. C. (1997). The cost-effectiveness of airbags by seating position. *Journal of the American Medical Association, 278,* 1418–1425.

Greenland, S. (2005). Epidemiologic measures and policy formulation: Lessons from potential outcomes. *Emerging Themes in Epidemiology, 2*(5).

Greenland, S., & Brumback, B. (2002). An overview of relations among causal modeling methods. *International Journal of Epidemiology, 31,* 1030–1037.

Greenland, S., & Morgenstern, H. (2001). Confounding in health research. *Annual Review of Public Health, 22,* 189–212.

Greenland, S., Robins, J. M., & Pearl, J. (1999). Confounding and collapsibility in causal inference. *Statistical Science, 14,* 29–46.

Gruber, J., Sen, A., & Stabile, M. (2003). Estimating price elasticities when there is smuggling: The sensitivity of smoking to price in Canada. *Journal of Health Economics, 22*(5), 821–842.

Gwatkin, D. R. (1997). Global burden of disease. *Lancet, 350*(9071), 141.

Halloran, M. E., & Struchiner, C. J. (1995). Causal inference in infectious diseases. *Epidemiology, 6*(2), 142–151.

Hernan, M. A. (2005). Invited commentary: Hypothetical interventions to define causal effects—afterthought or prerequisite? *American Journal of Epidemiology, 162*(7), 618–620.

Holland, P. W. (2001). The false linking of race and causality: Lessons from standardized testing. *Race & Society, 4,* 219–233.

House, J. S., Lepkowski, J. M., Williams, D. R., Mero, R. P., Lantz, P. M., Robert, S. A., et al. (2000). Excess mortality among urban residents: How much, for whom, and why? *American Journal of Epidemiology, 90*(12), 1898–1904.

Jemal, A., Ward, E., Hao, Y., & Thun, M. (2005). Trends in the leading causes of death in the United States, 1970–2002. *Journal of the American Medical Association, 294,* 1255–1259.

Kaufman, J. S. (in press). Epidemiologic analysis of racial/ethnic disparities: Some fundamental issues and a cautionary example. *Social Science & Medicine.*

Kaufman, J. S., & Cooper, R. S. (1999). Seeking causal explanations in social epidemiology. *American Journal of Epidemiology, 150*(2), 113–120.

Kaufman, J. S., & Cooper, R. S. (2001). Commentary: Considerations for use of racial/ethnic classification in etiologic research. *American Journal of Epidemiology, 154*(4), 291–298.

Kaufman, J.S., & Kaufman, S. (2001). Assessment of structured socio economic effects on health. *Epidemiology, 12*(2), 157–167.

Kaufman, J. S., & Kaufman, S. (2002). Estimating causal effects. *International Journal of Epidemiology, 31*(2), 431–432.

Loring, M., Powell, B. (1988). Gender, race, and DSM-III: A study of the objectivity of psychiatric diagnostic behavior. *Journal of Health & Social Behavior, 29*(1), 1–22.

Maldonado, G., & Greenland, S. (2002). Estimating causal effects (with discussion). *International Journal of Epidemiology, 31,* 422–429.

Murray, C. J. L., Ezzati, M., Lopez, A. D., Rodgers, A., & Vander Hoorn, S. (2003). Comparative quantification of health risks: Conceptual framework and methodological issues. *Population Health Metrics, 1*(1).

Murray, C. J. L., Salomon, J. A., & Mathers, C. D. (2002). A critical examination of summary measures of population health. In C. J. L. Murray, J. A. Salomon, C. D. Mathers, & A. D. Lopez (Eds.), *Summary measures of population health: Concepts, ethics, measurement and applications. Collections of papers on summary measures of population health.* Geneva: World Health Organization.

Nord, E. (2002). My goodness—and yours: A history, and some possible futures, of DALY meanings and valuation procedures. In C. J. L. Murray, J. A. Salomon, C. D. Mathers, & A. D. Lopez (Eds.), *Summary measures of population health: Concepts, ethics, measurement and applications. Collections of papers on summary measures of population health.* Geneva: World Health Organization.

Packard, R. M. (1989). *White plague, black labor: The political economy of health and diseases in South Africa.* Berkeley: University of California Press.

Pearl, J. (2000). *Causality: Models, reasoning and inference.* Cambridge: Cambridge University Press.

Pratt, J., & Schlaifer, R. (1988). On the interpretation and observation of laws. *Journal of Econometrics, 39,* 23–52.

Robins, J. M. (2001). Data, design, and background knowledge in etiologic inference. *Epidemiology, 12*(3), 313–320.

Rosenberg, J. S. (2001). A worldly professor: Economist and former U.S. Secretary of the Treasury Lawrence H. Summers returns to Harvard as the university's twenty-seventh president. *Harvard Magazine, 103*(5), 30–38.

Sakellariou, C. (2006). Education policy reform, local average treatment effect and returns to schooling from instrumental variables in the Philippines. *Applied Economics, 38*(4), 473–481.

Schulman, K. A., Berlin, J. A., Harless, W., Kerner, J. F., Sistrunk, S., Gersh, B. J., et al. (1999). The effect of race and sex on physicians' recommendations for cardiac catheterization. *New England Journal of Medicine, 340*(8), 618–626.

Schulze, M. B., Manson, J. E., Ludwig, D. S., Colditz, G. A., Stampfer, M. J., Willett, W. C., et al. (2004). Sugar-sweetened beverages, weight gain, and incidence of type 2 diabetes in young and middle-aged women. *Journal of the American Medical Association, 292*, 927–934.

Sobel, M. E. (1995). Causal inference in the social and behavioral sciences. In G. Arminger, C. Clogg, & M. E. Sobel (Eds.), *Handbook of statistical modeling for the social and behavioral sciences. New York:* Plenum.

Sobel, M. E. (2006). Spatial concentration and social stratification: Does the clustering of disadvantage "beget" bad outcomes? In S. Bowles, S. N. Durlauf, & K. Hoff (Eds.), *Poverty traps.* Princeton, NJ: Princeton University Press.

Steinbrook, R. (2005). The potential of human papillomavirus vaccines. *New England Journal of Medicine, 354,* 1109–1112.

Tengs, T. O., Adams, M. E., Pliskin, J. S., Safran, D. G., Siegel, J. E., Weinstein, M. C., et al. (1995). Five-hundred life-saving interventions and their cost-effectiveness. *Risk Analysis, 15*, 369–390.

Whitman, S. Good, G., Donoghue, E. R., Benbow, N., Shou, W., & Mou, S. (1997). Mortality in Chicago attributed to the July 1995 heat wave. *American Journal of Public Health, 87*(9), 1515–1518.

Woodward, J. (2003). *Making things happen: A theory of causal explanation.* New York: Oxford University Press.

Yen, I. H., & Moss, N. (1999). Unbundling education: A critical discussion of what education confers and how it lowers risk for disease and death. *Annals of the New York Academy of Sciences, 896,* 350–351.

Chapter 18
Estimating the Health Effects of Macrosocial Shocks: A Collaborative Approach

Ralph Catalano, Jennifer Ahern, and Tim Bruckner

1. Introduction

The empirical literature concerned with macrosocial determinants of health has emerged from so many disciplines, each with its favored methodological approach, that a meeting of contributors evokes the Tower of Babel construction site. Contributors concerned with how, if at all, macrosocial shocks to the population affect the incidence of illness appear to have a particularly difficult time communicating across disciplinary boundaries.

We define macrosocial shocks as changes in the environment to which many, if not most, individuals in a population must simultaneously adapt. The literature has explored the health effects of such shocks as economic recessions (Brenner, 1983; Catalano, Hansen, & Hartig, 1999; Ruhm, 1995), extreme weather (Vandentorren, Suzan, Medina, Pascal, Maulpoix, Cohen, & Ledrans, 2004), air pollution (Lyster, 1974), ecological disasters (Mangano, 2006), and terrorist attacks (Galea, Ahern, Resnick, Kilpatrick, Bucuvalas, Gold, & Vlahov, 2002). Much of the work examines individual data, typically in the form of serial cross-sections (i.e., panel data) using generalized linear models, while other contributions examine ecological data using time-series methods. In this chapter, we provide a non-technical summary of these approaches, offer a simple scheme for determining when to use one or the other, and describe their strengths and weaknesses. More important, we propose a combined method that uses the strength of each method to compensate for the weakness of the other. Although this approach seems intuitive and employs widely disseminated statistical routines, we have not seen it used in studies of population health, probably because few researchers regularly analyze both time-series and panel data. We argue that the combined method could be implemented through the collaboration of panel and time-series analysts, as we have done in this chapter.

Finally, we demonstrate the combined method by applying it to a question of great interest to us and likely of general interest to researchers who would consult this volume. Did the events of September 11, 2001, sufficiently perturb the physiology of Americans living in the most involved states (i.e., New York, New Jersey, Pennsylvania, Virginia and Maryland/Washington DC) to reduce the secondary sex ratio (i.e., ratio of male to female live births)?

2. Strategies for Controlling "Third Variables" in Observational Studies

Ethical and practical constraints preclude researchers from experimentally manipulating the dose of macrosocial shocks to populations assembled through random assignment. Work in our field, therefore, typically uses observational data measuring health and risk factors for illness in populations more or less exposed to macrosocial shocks. Much of the work takes advantage *post hoc* of opportunities in which nature or society varied the dose of a macrosocial stressor over time and, optimally, across space.

Approaches to analyzing data from these opportunities typically strive to statistically rule out rival hypotheses arising from confounders, or "third variables," that may either induce a spurious association between exposure and outcome or mask a true association. The two most frequently used approaches, those that examine either panel or time-series data, have complementary strengths and weaknesses in controlling third variables. We argue that the methods can be combined such that the strengths of one compensate for the weaknesses of the other. To help make this argument, we separate third variables into categories defined by three dichotomous attributes, as shown in Figure 18.1.

The first attribute separates third variables into those available and unavailable for an empirical test. Variables suspected of confounding a theorized association may be unavailable for a test because they were not measured in the populations exposed to a macrosocial shock. Other third variables, however, may be unavailable simply because no one suspects them.

The second attribute divides third variables into those that affect only one test population and those that affect many or all. Geography commonly defines test populations in the literature. We refer to third variables that affect only one test population or a subset of test populations as "local" and those that affect all populations as "general".

A third attribute separates third variables into those that exhibit patterns over time and those that do not. These patterns, typically referred to as "autocorrelation", can take the form of secular trends, cycles, or the propensity to remain elevated or depressed or to oscillate after high or low values.

We believe that any third variable can be located in one of the eight cells formed by these three dichotomies. Each cell, moreover, implies a control strategy for the variables it contains (see Figure 18.1). All available third variables, for example, should be specified in a test equation. A researcher can control unavailable, generally occurring (i.e., those that affect all test populations) third variables by removing the variance in the dependent variable shared over time by the test populations. Any association between the residuals and the macrosocial stressor, therefore, could not result from the effect of any generally occurring unavailable third variable. Researchers can control unavailable, local, patterned third variables by identifying and removing any

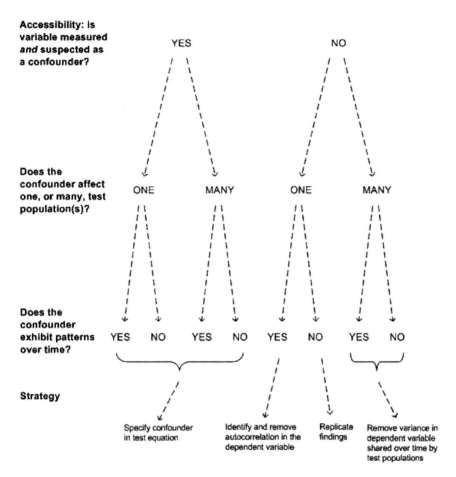

FIGURE 18.1. Strategies for controlling third variables in observational studies.

autocorrelation in the dependent variable measured in the population exhibiting such patterns.

As we discuss below, controlling the effects of available third variables would appear as a strength of panel and a weakness of times-series analysis. The two strategies differ on how they remove variance in the dependent variable shared over time among test populations, and removing patterns poses a more difficult challenge for panel than for time-series analyses. Neither panel nor times-series methods, nor any other that we know of, can statistically control unavailable, local, unpatterned third variables. However, replication of an association in two or more test populations reduces the threat of such variables. The argument that each test population in which an association appears has a unique unavailable, local, unpatterned variable that coincides in time and dose with a macrosocial shock strikes us, at least, as less parsimonious than strong theory.

3. Implementing Control Strategies

Panel and time-series approaches differ in how well they implement the strategies described above. Knowing the strengths and weaknesses of each approach not only allows a researcher to calibrate the confidence he or she should have in reported associations between macrosocial stressors and population health, but also illuminates how the approaches might be combined into a more compelling method.

3.1. How Panel Studies Implement Control Strategies

Most panel analyses use some form of a generalized linear model encompassing both normal linear regression as well as logistic, Poisson, and log-linear models (Fitzmaurice, Laird, & Ware, 2002; Kutner, Nachtsheim, Neter, & Li, 2004). Generalized linear models share the following characteristics:

1. $Y_1 \ldots Y_n$ are n response variables that follow a particular probability distribution, with expected value $E\{Y_i\} = \mu_i$.
2. A linear predictor based on the independent variables $X_{i1}, \ldots, X_{ip}$ is used, where X_{ip} denotes the pth covariate for the ith subject, indicated by $X'_i\beta$:

$$X'_i\beta = \beta_0 + \beta_1 X_{i1} + \ldots + \beta_p X_{ip}$$

3. A link function g that relates the linear predictor to the mean response:

$$X'_i\beta = g(\mu_i)$$

Logistic regression methods are especially popular in our field because the response variable usually divides individuals into dichotomies, such as meeting diagnostic criteria or not, or in case, male or female births. The logistic model used in our approach(described in section **7.6.**), requires the following transformation to link the linear predictor to the mean response μ_i, the probability of the event:

$$g(\mu_i) = g(\pi_i) = \log_e(\pi_i / 1-\pi_i) = X'_i\beta$$

This link function represents the familiar "logit", or "effect on log-odds," response metric.

The macrosocial stressor, as well as covariates that comprise $X'_i\beta$, may take any form (dichotomous, polytomous, or continuous). In logistic regression, the dependent variable for each individual is the odds of the outcome (e.g., being male) for the combination of the independent variables in which he or she falls. As described above, the dependent variable is transformed to its natural logarithm (i.e., logit) to allow the multiplicative relationship expressed by a contingency table to be estimated with additive models.

Controlling available third variables in a generalized linear model simply involves specifying them in the test model. Controlling unavailable third variables poses a greater challenge. Researchers typically reduce the threat of unavailable, generally occurring third variables, whether patterned or not, by adding dichotomous indicator variables for each time, less one, at which the test populations were measured. Unavailable, generally occurring third variables could include, for example, an administrative change in data collection rules that affects all the observed populations or population growth due to illegal immigration into all the populations. To add such an indicator, all the measurements at time t would be scored 1 on this variable, and those taken at other times would be scored 0. The coefficients of each of these $T-1$ time-of-measurement variables would be the average logit of the dependent variable, adjusted for other independent variables, for the individuals measured at the time scored 1 for the variable.

Researchers typically add another group of indicator variables to reduce the threat of locally occurring, unpatterned third variables that can cause the mean of the dependent variable for all individuals at a place to be different from the mean of individuals at other places. This circumstance could induce a type I error if the place coincidentally experiences greater than average doses of the macrosocial stressor. The added variables are scored 1 for all individuals in a given place and 0 otherwise. The number of dichotomous place variables equals one less than the total number of populations defined by place.

Reducing the threat of unavailable, locally occurring, patterned third variables (e.g., unmeasured ambient air pollution), whether or not they affect the mean of dependent scores, most challenges panel designs. The time-of-measurement dichotomous variables will not reduce the threat because they adjust only for generally occurring third variables. Nor will the place dichotomous variables reduce the threat because they only ensure that the mean of the residuals of each place equals 0. The residuals could have a mean of 0 but also exhibit, for example, a secular trend (i.e., half the trend has negative values while the other half has symmetric positive values). The circumstance in which a macrosocial stressor occurs late in a place exhibiting a secular trend could induce a type I error because scores late in the series for that place will, by axiom, be disproportionately represented among the high residuals of the model. The same problem arises from locally occurring cycles or oscillations in residuals because the shock may occur when the series routinely exhibits high values.

Researchers using panel designs have often dealt with the secular trend problem by adding a surrogate "sequence number" variable. All measurements of the dependent variable at time 1 are scored 1 on the variable, while all those at time 2 are scored 2, and so on. Adding interactions of this secular trend variable and all the dichotomous place variables could remove trends from places that would otherwise exhibit them. The surrogate variable approach could be applied to cycles as well, if the researcher ventures an accurate guess as to when these would exhibit peaks and troughs. He or she could construct a surrogate cycle variable scored 0 for trough and 1 for peak phases and estimate the interaction terms of this variable and all the dichotomous place variables. The coefficient would estimate the average difference between presumed peaks and troughs in each test population.

We believe that using this type of surrogate variable reduces the confidence a researcher can have in the panel approach in testing the hypothesized effect of a macrosocial stressor on health. Fitting a sequence number variable can leave much autocorrelation in data that trend in other than a straight line. Further, guessing where the troughs and peaks of cycles occur is, after all, guessing. Autocorrelation, moreover, can take forms (e.g., tendency to remain elevated or depressed or to oscillate after high or low values) other than cycles or secular trends.

A researcher could, of course, inspect the time-series of the dependent variable for each place and inform his or her choice of a surrogate variable intended to control locally occurring, patterned third variables. Researchers have, for example, used "spline regression" to control linear trends that shift in slope over a time-series. This approach yields a segmented line with slope shifts at nodes determined by rules based on the number and size of shifts allowed (Greenland, 1998). The fitted values of these models can be assigned to individuals and added to test equations in the manner that simple sequence number values have been added.

Spline regression inspects time-series only for segmented lines, but its underlying logic of empirically identifying and modeling autocorrelation, rather than guessing *a priori*, can be extended to identify and model all forms of autocorrelation. Conventions for the detection and modeling of autocorrelation in time-series have been developed over three decades and can be implemented with widely disseminated computational programs. After describing how the time-series approach has been used to estimate the effect of macrosocial shocks on population health and pointing out the weaknesses of the approach, we suggest that its strength (i.e., the detection and modeling of autocorrelation) can help overcome the panel approach's difficulty in controlling locally occurring, patterned third variables when they are employed as a combined method.

3.2. How Time-Series Approaches Implement Control Strategies

As in logistic regression, the dependent variable in time-series analyses can be expressed as logits. Each population defined, for example, by geographic space will exhibit odds of the outcome occurring in each measured period, and these odds can be transformed to their natural logarithms. Unlike logistic regression, the time-series test will not assign these logits back to individuals from whom they were derived and to whom we can link covariates. The unit of analysis becomes ecological (i.e., the time period for a specific population).

In the time-series method, researchers specify an available third variable as a characteristic of a group, not an individual. Available continuous third variables could appear in test equations as the mean value for all the individuals measured in each period. Available dichotomous third variables could appear as the proportion of one condition's occurrence in the population for each period. This treatment of available covariates weakens the appeal of the approach to most researchers because it does not allow for control of confounders at the individual level, nor does it allow the researcher to examine interactions of individual covariates with macrosocial shocks. The time-series approach to testing such interactions requires creating a separate series for a hypothesized vulnerable subset of the population and repeating the test for that group.

Researchers using time-series analyses typically reduce the threat of unavailable, generally occurring third variables, whether patterned or not, by using comparison populations in places subjected to low or no doses of the macrosocial shock (Catalano & Serxner, 1987). In other words, time-series test equations include independent variables that are logits of the outcome variable measured in comparison groups. The estimated coefficients of these variables measure the shared variance over time in the test and comparison community. The residuals from these estimates would be free of the effect of any generally occurring third variables. The hypothesis that a macrosocial shock to the test population at a particular time increased the likelihood of an outcome in that population and not the comparison populations implies that the residuals of the estimation at the time of the shock appear above the upper bound of the appropriate confidence interval.

The fact that time-series methods can effectively reduce the threat of locally occurring, patterned third variables has been among its principal attractions. Time-series analysts have developed highly effective and widely accepted methods for identifying and modeling autocorrelation. The methods, based on the work of Box and Jenkins (Box, Jenkins, & Reinsel, 1994) and commonly referred to as Auto Regressive, Integrated, Moving Average (i.e., ARIMA) modeling, have been described in detail elsewhere (Box et al., 1994; Chatfield, 2004; McCleary & Hay, 1980). The Box-Jenkins approach identifies which of a very large family of possible models best fits a time-series. ARIMA models mathematically express various filters through which a series without patterns can pass; each filter imposes a unique pattern. The Box-Jenkins approach uses a model-building process by which the researcher infers the filter that imposed the observed pattern (Box et al., 1994).

The general form of our ARIMA model (as used in Section 7.0) appears as follows:

$$\nabla_d Z_t^e = c + \frac{\left(1 - \theta B^q\right)}{\left(1 - \Phi B^p\right)} a_t \qquad (1)$$

∇_d is the difference operator that indicates a series was differenced at order d (i.e., Z at time t subtracted from Z at time t-d) to remove secular trends or cycles (i.e., to render the series stationary in its mean). Z_t^e is the logit of sex ratio for a given population at time t.

c is the mean of the series.

Φ is an autoregressive parameter. Autoregressive parameters measure a series' tendency to remain above or below or to oscillate around its means after a perturbation.

θ is the "moving average" parameter. Moving average parameters measure the tendency of perturbations to be present for more than one time.

B is the "backshift operator", or value of the conditioned variable at time t − q or t − p.

a_t is the error term at year t.

A typical application of Box-Jenkins routines in a time-series test of the effect of a macrosocial shock would proceed through the following steps: The dependent variable would be regressed on any available third variables specified as noted above and on the dependent variable measured in comparison populations to control for any generally occurring third variables. The researcher would then use Box-Jenkins methods to detect any autocorrelation in the residuals of the regression; this step discovers autocorrelation peculiar to the test population because the regression would have removed any shared with the comparison populations. The researcher assumes the remaining autocorrelation, if any, reflects the influence of unavailable, local, patterned third variables. Adding the appropriate ARIMA parameters to the original model leaves its residuals free of the effect of all available third variables, generally occurring third variables, and patterned local third variables. If the hypothesis stated that a macrosocial shock increased the odds of the outcome, then the residuals at the time of the shock, or those after a delay expected from *a priori* considerations, would appear above the upper bound of the set confidence interval.

The possibility that a locally occurring, unpatterned third variable induced a spurious association between the shock and the outcome remains in this test as it did in the panel test. Replication of the test in different populations, however, can reduce the threat of such a third variable because finding the association in another community weakens the argument that a locally occurring variable (i.e., one peculiar to the test community) induced the original result.

4. Is Choosing Between the Approaches Still Necessary?

The quantity and quality of data available *post hoc* from opportunities to study macrosocial shocks would logically guide the choice between time-series and panel designs (see Figure 18.2). Devising a rule for choosing between the methods requires organizing research opportunities in a conceptual space defined by three dimensions. The first dimension separates research opportunities dichotomously into whether or not the data allow linking covariates with outcomes in individuals. The second ranks the opportunities by how many times someone measured the outcome and covariates in the population, whether or not the covariates can be linked with individuals. The third dimension ranks the opportunities by how many measured populations experienced a different dose and/or timing of the shock.

As a general rule, research opportunities falling in cells characterized by more test populations, fewer measurements over time, and availability of covariates linkable to individuals will favor panel analysis (Hsiao, 1989). The benefits of this approach include the familiar estimation of covariate-by-shock interaction effects, as well as good estimation of generally occurring third variables. The unavoidable costs include poor control of locally occurring, patterned third variables.

The above rule implies the complement, that time-series approaches better apply to opportunities falling in cells characterized by few test populations,

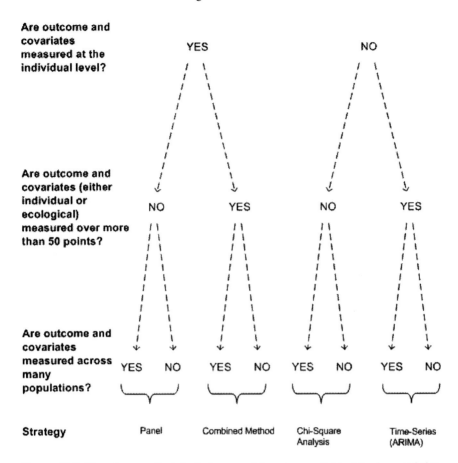

Are outcome and covariates measured at the individual level?

YES   NO

Are outcome and covariates (either individual or ecological) measured over more than 50 points?

NO   YES   NO   YES

Are outcome and covariates measured across many populations?

YES   NO   YES   NO   YES   NO   YES   NO

Strategy   Panel   Combined Method   Chi-Square Analysis   Time-Series (ARIMA)

FIGURE 18.2. Choosing a methodological approach based on available data characteristics.

ecologically measured covariates and outcomes, and relatively many measurements in time. Though this approach improves control of any unavailable, patterned third variables, researchers will be unable to characterize the role of individual level covariates in mediating or inducing any association between the macrosocial shock and outcome.

Based on the rules described above, opportunities with no covariates linkable to individuals, with data from only one population, and with relatively few measurements in time cannot be analyzed with either approach we described. Conversely, where covariates have been measured relatively many times in individuals from relatively many places exposed to varying doses of a macrosocial shock, a researcher could choose, based on his or her skills, either approach to these data sets. We suspect that the growing emphasis on health surveillance across the developed world will increasingly yield such opportunities, but the limitations of each approach would still apply. However, a collaboration of researchers skilled in each approach could allow combining panel analyses with

ARIMA modeling to arrive at more compelling results than those provided by the separate approaches. We suggest such a combination for review and criticism.

5. A Combined Approach

Our proposed approach requires ARIMA modeling of time-series of the odds of the outcome in each test population. The fitted values of these models gauge the propensity, conditional on time (hereafter referred to as propensity), of the population exhibiting the outcome at each measurement. As such, these fitted values can be assigned back to each individual measured in each time period and can then be used as a covariate in the panel analysis to control for locally occurring, patterned third variables. This method uses the strength of the time-series approach to shore up the weakness of the panel approach. Researchers can estimate and express the effect of macrosocial shocks on individuals in ways familiar to most contributors to the field. The shocks can be understood as ambient phenomena that interact with specified individual level characteristics to affect the risk of an outcome. Results cannot be attributed to available (i.e., specified) third variables, to unavailable, generally occurring third variables, or to unavailable, local third variables that exhibit autocorrelation. Findings, furthermore, cannot be attributed to unavailable, local, unpatterned third variables if the dose-response among the test populations supports the theory (i.e., the effect cannot be local because it appears as predicted in more than one population).

Implementing the approach we suggest will likely require collaboration among researchers with different methodological backgrounds because few, if any, among us has invested the time to become proficient at both panel and time-series analyses. Indeed, doing so would probably distract us from the substantive controversies that attracted us to the field. It makes sense, therefore, to form teams of researchers who share interests in a given macrosocial stressor (e.g., economic recessions) or in a population response (e.g., substance abuse) and who have among them those who can implement time-series and panel analyses. Such teams could experiment with our proposed approach and others to determine if any convey the benefits in certainty and transparency we anticipate.

6. The Secondary Sex Ratio as an Indicator of Macrosocial Shocks

Research reports that the ratio of male to female live births (i.e., the human secondary sex ratio) varies over time with the frequency or virulence of environmental insults to the population. The sex ratio reportedly falls following natural (Fukuda, Fukuda, Shimizu, & Moller, 1998) and human-made disasters (Lyster, 1974; Mocarelli, Brambilla, Gerthoux, Patterson, & Needham, 1996), terrorist attacks (Catalano, Bruckner, Gould, Eskenazi, & Anderson, 2005), and disruptions of regional economies (Catalano, 2003; Catalano & Bruckner, 2005). Consistent with theory, moreover, the sex ratio varies inversely with the dispensing of antidepressants among women in Sweden (Catalano, Bruckner, Hartig, & Ong, 2005). Understanding the mechanisms that induce these associations would contribute not only to the basic literature concerned with human reproduction, but also, for reasons explained below, to the applied literature concerned with population health.

The literature offers two groups of explanations for the observed associations. The first group hypothesizes that stressful environments reduced the likelihood of conceiving males by reducing the frequency of coitus and by reducing sperm motility (Fukuda, Fukuda, Shimizu, Yomura, & Shimizu, 1996; James, 1999; Lazarus, 2002; Martin, 1997). The second group posits that maternal adaptation to stressful environments threatens gestation, especially of males. These explanations assume that natural selection conserved any mutation by which gravid women increased their yield of grandchildren (Trivers & Willard, 1973). This yield presumably fell when mothers invested time and energy in bearing and raising offspring with relatively low odds of reaching or of surviving through reproductive age. For reasons as yet unclear, males more likely die than females until well past reproductive age (Kraemer, 2000). The dose response of male fetuses to maternal stress supposedly increases more steeply than that for females (Owen & Matthews, 2003), implying that the liability of weak sons increases during relatively stressful times (Byrne & Warburton, 1987; Forchhammer, 2000; Mizuno, 2000; Moller, 1996). This difference suggests that natural selection conserved mutations that allowed women's bodies to detect and terminate the gestation of weak males when environmental stressors increased in frequency or virulence. These mutations presumably remain at work in contemporary populations even though culture and medical advances may have voided their benefit to mothers in the yield of grandchildren. All the theories in this family of explanations assume that some mechanism continues to gauge the reproductive potential of fetuses and to terminate the gestations of those who fall below some critical value.

Consistent with the male fetal loss hypothesis, sex ratios appear to drop 3, 4, or 5 months after shocks to the population rather than 8, 9, or 10 months later, as predicted by theories assuming reduced conception of males (Catalano, Bruckner, Gould et al., 2005; Catalano, Bruckner, Marks, & Eskenazi, 2006). The sex ratio of fetal deaths, moreover, reportedly increases shortly after population shocks (Catalano, Bruckner, Anderson, & Gould, 2005).

Testing the fetal loss mechanism holds implications for population health because, unlike the reduced male conception theory, fetal deaths induce somatic and psychological pain in parents as well as sympathetic pain in families and the community. Fetal death also affects the timing of future pregnancies. Women in the Western world increasingly delay childbearing, want fewer children, and desire to become pregnant over a shorter interval (Abma, Chandra, Mosher, Peterson, & Piccinino, 1997; Hall, 1999). A poorly timed pregnancy may impose a social and economic burden on the parents and increase the risk of late initiation of prenatal care (Kost, Landry, & Darroch, 1998; Piccinino, 1994). An increase in the incidence of male fetal deaths, moreover, suggests that the biology of women of childbearing age can be altered by macrosocial shocks. The public health community should be concerned with mechanisms that induce such change.

In sum, the research to date supports the notion that macrosocial shocks to the population lead to spontaneous abortion of males. If true, this scenario necessitates additional attention to gravid mothers following macrosocial shocks. Naturally, we need more empirical testing of the key links in this suspected chain before acting on implications. Thus, we apply the combined method described in Section 5.0 to test the link between macrosocial shocks and the sex ratio. More specifically, we use data from 13 American states to the test the hypothesis that the secondary sex ratio among birth cohorts in New York, New Jersey, Pennsylvania, Virginia, and Maryland/Washington DC in the second trimester of gestation during the events of September 11, 2001, fell below levels expected from the birth cohorts in other states and from historical trends. We selected these states because of their geographic proximity to the events on September 11, 2001, considering them more exposed than other states to the events of September 11, 2001. The World Trade Center towers were located in New York City, which is across the Hudson River from New Jersey. Flight 93 crashed in a field in Pennsylvania. The Attack on the Pentagon occurred in Virginia, across the Potomac River from Washington, DC, and Maryland.

7. A Demonstration of the Combined Method

To incorporate the strengths of time-series analysis with the strengths of generalized linear models, we propose a combined method. This method requires individual level serial cross-sectional data from multiple places with at least fifty consecutive time periods. To summarize, we first apply the Box-Jenkins methods to the dependent variable for each test population to identify autocorrelation. We build ARIMA models to predict values of the time-series from autocorrelation. These predicted values gauge the population's propensity of exhibiting the outcome based solely on time.

Next, we build the generalized linear model, including typical "right side" indicator variables for time and place to control for generally occurring confounders and differences in mean values, as described above in Section 1.2. We also add the predicted outcome values from the time-series routines. Places in which we detect no autocorrelation in the outcome receive a propensity score of zero. We create interactions of the place (i.e., state) indicators and these propensity variables to adjust for local, patterned third variables (i.e., the propensity toward the outcome in each state due solely to autocorrelation). In addition, we include individual level covariates to control confounding in the form deemed most appropriate given the available data and the topic of study. Finally, we examine the impact of the macrosocial shock of interest by inserting interaction terms between the time of expected impact of the shock with the places expected to be most affected.

7.1. Data

To illustrate this combined approach, we used data from the National Center for Health Statistics Natality Files for the United States from 1996 to 2002 (2004). The Natality Files contain data from birth certificates for all births in the United States, including the place and time of the birth as well as demographic characteristics of the mother and infant. We grouped the births geographically by state and temporally by month. For this illustrative analysis, we included the ten largest states (based on the greatest number of births over the time period), as they would have the most stable sex ratio estimates for each month given their large populations of births. Based on this criterion, we analyzed California, Texas, New York, Florida, Illinois, Ohio, Pennsylvania, Georgia, Michigan, and North Carolina. We also included New Jersey, Virginia, and Maryland/Washington DC in the analysis because, in addition to New York and Pennsylvania, these states may have been more affected by the population shock of interest—the events of September 11, 2001.

7.2. Specifying Available Third Variables

Potential confounders of interest include characteristics of the mother potentially associated with the exposure (i.e., the September 11, 2001 attacks) in terms of time or place as well as the outcome under study (i.e., the sex of an infant). While we would not expect the events on September 11, 2001 to have been temporally associated with large demographic shifts in characteristics that may be associated infant sex, we were concerned about the possibility of a demographic shift, by chance, coinciding with the period of expected influence of the September 11 attacks. Moreover, states we considered more exposed to the September 11, 2001 terrorist attacks differ demographically from the less exposed states; those differences might have been associated with infant sex. As a conservative approach, we adjusted for individual level characteristics that reportedly influence the sex of an infant (Erickson, 1976; James, 1984, 1985, 1987; James & Rostron, 1985; Teitelbaum & Mantel, 1971). These characteristics included the race/ethnicity of the mother classified as White, Black, Hispanic, or other; mother's age classified as less than 18 years, 18–34 years, and 35 years or older; mother's parity classified as first birth, second to fifth birth, and sixth or greater birth; and mother's education classified as less than high school, or greater than or equal to high school.

7.3. Constructing the Place and Time Indicators

We created indicator variables for each of the 84 months spanning 1996 to 2002 except one, leaving the first month (January 1996) as the reference category. As noted above, we included 13 States in this analysis. We used indicator variables for each state except one leaving Texas as the reference category. We selected Texas as the reference state because it exhibited sex ratio values closest to the overall median across all times and states.

7.4. Defining the Exposure, Proximity to the Events of September 11, 2001

We hypothesized that the events of September 11, 2001 would induce a lower than expected sex ratio, particularly in New York, New Jersey, Pennsylvania, Virginia and Maryland/Washington DC, which were more exposed to the events. Based on our theory of male fetal loss, as well as extensive research in maternal stress hormones (Giannakoulopoulos, Sepulveda, Kourtis, Glover, & Fisk, 1994; Gitau, Fisk, Teixeira, Cameron, & Glover, 2001; Hobel, Dunkel-Schetter, Roesch, Castro, & Arora, 1999; Lou, Hansen, Nordentoft, Pryds, Jensen, Nim, & Hemmingsen, 1994; Owen & Matthews, 2003), we posit that the shock would affect pregnancies in the second trimester (i.e., fourth through sixth month of gestation). We therefore test our hypothesis by examining the sex ratio in November 2001, December 2001, and January 2002, the time when fetuses in the second-trimester in gestation at the time of the attacks were scheduled to be born. We created interaction terms between each of the five exposed states and each of the three months of interest, for a total of 15 interaction terms, treating all of the other states and months as the reference category.

7.5. ARIMA Modeling of the State Specific Sex Ratios

Applying Box-Jenkins routines to our data detected autocorrelation in Florida, Illinois, Michigan, Virginia and New Jersey. Table 18.1 shows the best fitting models. The fact that none of the series required differencing implies that none of the sex ratios exhibited trends or strong cycles. Five states exhibited autoregressive parameters implying that unusually large or small values were "echoed" by similar, but diminishing, outlying values at delays ranging from 2 months in New Jersey to 11 in Illinois and Michigan. Using these ARIMA models, we estimated

TABLE 18.1. Best fitting ARIMA models of the monthly secondary sex ratio, transformed to natural logarithms, in states exhibiting autocorrelation.

State	ARIMA Model
Florida	$z_t = .0484 + \dfrac{1}{\left(1 + .2373B^3\right)} a_t$
Illinois	$z_t = .0454 + \dfrac{1}{\left(1 - .2402B^{11}\right)} a_t$
Michigan	$z_t = .0486 + \dfrac{1}{\left(1 - .3164B^{11}\right)} a_t$
New Jersey	$z_t = .0500 + \dfrac{1}{\left(1 - .2583B^2\right)} a_t$
Virginia	$z_t = .0613 + \dfrac{1}{\left(1 - .3503B^4\right)} a_t$

the sex ratio (on the $\log_e$ scale) that would be expected for each month in those states. These sex ratio propensities were included as a covariate in the final model, along with interactions between the sex ratio propensity and the state to allow this propensity variable to have a different strength of association with the actual sex ratio depending on the state. This inclusion precludes an unavailable patterned third variable inducing a type I error.

We set all values of the propensity variable to zero for states with no autocorrelation. We could not predict early values of the sex ratios in the states with autocorrelation because all five models included autoregressive parameters that required at least two months to pass before making predictions. Models with a delay of 11 months (i.e., Illinois and Michigan), for example, required 11 months to pass before they predicted an initial value. We set these early values to zero.

7.6. Final Generalized Linear Model

The final model takes a logistic form:

$$\log_e(\pi_{ijk}/\,1\text{-}\pi_{ijk}) = \beta_0 + \beta_1 ST_{1j} + \ldots + \beta_{12} ST_{12j} + \beta_{13} MO_{1k} + \ldots$$

$$+\beta_{95} MO_{83k} + \beta_{96} ST^* MO_{1jk} + \ldots + \beta_{110} ST^* MO_{15jk} + \beta_{111} SRP_{jk}$$

$$+ \beta_{112} SRP^* ST_{1j} + \beta_{115} SRP^* ST_{4j} + \beta' IND'_{ijk} + e_{ijk}$$

where:

π_{ijk} = probability of a male infant
β = a fixed effect coefficient
i = individual
j = state
k = time
ST = state indicator variables
MO = month indicator variables
SRP = sex ratio propensity – from the ARIMA models
IND' = vector of individual level covariates

8. Results

There were 17,341,852 births over the years 1996–2002 in the 13 states under study. The demographic characteristics of the births are described in Table 18.2. Fifty one point nine percent of the mothers were White, 16.3% were Black, 25.0% were Hispanic, and 5.6% were of other race/ethnicity. The majority of mothers were aged 18–34 years (81.7%). Forty percent of infants were first born, and 57.7% were the second through fifth births. Seventy six percent of mothers had at least a high school degree. The state with the most births was California (21.3% of total), followed by Texas (14.2%) and New York (10.4%).

The results of the final model using the combined method are presented in Table 18.3. All coefficients (betas) in the model represent changes in the log odds

TABLE 18.2. Sample description: Births 1996–2002 in 13 states.

	N	%
Total	17341852	100
Infant Sex		
Male	8868281	51.14
Female	8473571	48.86
Maternal Race/Ethnicity		
White	8998570	51.89
Black	2831496	16.33
Hispanic	4342848	25.05
Other	972357	5.61
Unknown	196581	1.13
Maternal Age		
< 18 years	743116	4.29
18–34 years	14170198	81.72
≥ 35 years	2428538	14.01
Parity		
1	6942107	40.03
2–5	10007286	57.7
≥6	329641	1.9
Unknown	62818	0.36
Education		
≥ High School	13102908	75.56
< High School	3991806	23.02
Unknown	247138	1.43
State		
CA	3693517	21.3
FL	1389932	8.01
GA	880819	5.08
IL	1278361	7.37
MD	560858	3.23
MI	933939	5.39
NC	792799	4.57
NJ	802418	4.63
NY	1799198	10.37
OH	1064865	6.14
PA	1016434	5.86
TX	2457182	14.17
VA	671530	3.87

of a male birth, or equivalently, changes in the log sex ratio. For the sake of brevity, we have not included the coefficients for the indicator variables from all of the months, as they are neither central to our hypothesis nor critical for interpreting the results. We present only coefficients for November 2001, December 2001 and January 2002, the months in which we tested our hypothesis.

The interaction terms for New York, New Jersey, and Pennsylvania in January of 2002 suggest lower than expected sex ratio values in that month, compared to the other states and times that we considered unexposed. In New York, the effect was most dramatic (beta $= - 0.0388$, p $= 0.01$). To illustrate the magnitude of

TABLE 18.3. Logistic regression model predicting log odds of a male birth, 1996–2002, in 13 states.

Parameter	Beta	SE	95% CI		P-value
Intercept	0.0598	0.0049	(0.0503,	0.0694)	<0.01
Month[a]					
November 2001	−0.0075	0.007	(−0.0212,	0.0061)	0.28
December 2001	−0.0164	0.007	(−0.03,	−0.0027)	0.02
January 2002	0.005	0.0069	(−0.0086,	0.0186)	0.47
State					
TX	–	–			–
CA	−0.001	0.0017	(−0.0042,	0.0023)	0.57
FL	−0.0096	0.0091	(−0.0274,	0.0082)	0.29
GA	−0.0049	0.0025	(−0.0098,	0.0001)	0.05
IL	−0.0067	0.0052	(−0.0169,	0.0034)	0.19
MD	−0.0032	0.0031	(−0.0092,	0.0028)	0.30
MI	−0.0046	0.0057	(−0.0159,	0.0066)	0.42
NC	−0.0003	0.0026	(−0.0054,	0.0048)	0.91
NJ	−0.0245	0.0128	(−0.0496,	0.0006)	0.06
NY	0.0039	0.002	(0, 0.0079)		0.05
OH	−0.0033	0.0024	(−0.0079,	0.0014)	0.17
PA	−0.0019	0.0024	(−0.0067,	0.0029)	0.44
VA	−0.0142	0.0093	(−0.0324,	0.004)	0.13
State by Month Interactions					
NY*Nov01	0.0006	0.0151	(−0.0289,	0.0301)	0.97
NJ*Nov01	−0.0067	0.0218	(−0.0494,	0.0359)	0.76
PA*Nov01	0.0219	0.0198	(−0.017,	0.0607)	0.27
VA*Nov01	0.0508	0.0229	(0.0059,	0.0957)	0.03
MD*Nov01	−0.0169	0.0255	(−0.0669,	0.0331)	0.51
NY*Dec01	0.0091	0.0151	(−0.0205,	0.0387)	0.55
NJ*Dec01	0.0444	0.0219	(0.0014,	0.0873)	0.04
PA*Dec01	0.0247	0.0197	(−0.0139,	0.0632)	0.21
VA*Dec01	0.0206	0.0232	(−0.0248,	0.066)	0.37
MD*Dec01	−0.0052	0.0253	(−0.0548,	0.0444)	0.84
NY*Jan02	−0.0388	0.015	(−0.0681,	−0.0095)	0.01
NJ*Jan02	−0.0348	0.0215	(−0.0768,	0.0073)	0.11
PA*Jan02	−0.034	0.0194	(−0.0721,	0.0041)	0.08
VA*Jan02	0.0111	0.0228	(−0.0335,	0.0558)	0.63
MD*Jan02	0.0523	0.0253	(0.0027,	0.1019)	0.04
Sex Ratio Propensity	0.2744	0.2074	(−0.1322,	0.6809)	0.19
Sex Ratio Propensity					
by State Interactions					
SRprop*VA	–	–	–		–
SRprop*FL	0.0064	0.2747	(−0.532,	0.5449)	0.98
SRprop*IL	−0.1339	0.2361	(−0.5966,	0.3288)	0.57
SRprop*MI	−0.1481	0.2382	(−0.6149,	0.3187)	0.53
SRprop*NJ	0.2884	0.3261	(−0.3507,	0.9276)	0.38
Maternal Race/Ethnicity					
White	–	–	–		–
Black	−0.0207	0.0014	(−0.0234,	−0.0179)	<0.01
Hispanic	−0.0113	0.0014	(−0.0139,	−0.0086)	<0.01
Other	0.0107	0.0022	(0.0065,	0.015)	<0.01
Unknown	−0.0068	0.0047	(−0.016,	0.0024)	0.15

(*Continued*)

TABLE 18.3. (*Continued*)

Parameter	Beta	SE	95% CI	P-value
Maternal Age				
< 18 years	0.0106	0.0026	(0.0055, 0.0157)	<0.01
18−34 years	−	−	−	−
≥ 35 years	−0.0038	0.0014	(−0.0066, −0.001)	0.01
Parity				
1	−	−	−	−
2−5	−0.0058	0.001	(−0.0078, −0.0038)	<0.01
≥6	−0.011	0.0036	(−0.0182, −0.0039)	<0.01
Unknown	−0.0063	0.0081	(−0.0221, 0.0096)	0.44
Education				
≥ High School	−	−	−	−
< High School	−0.004	0.0013	(−0.0066, −0.0014)	<0.01
Unknown	0.0062	0.0041	(−0.0019, 0.0143)	0.13

[a] only coefficients for the indicator variables from November 2001, December 2001 and January 2002 are presented because these are the months in which we tested our hypothesis. January 1996 is the reference month.

the effect, additive combinations of the intercept, time, place and individual covariates can be created to estimate predicted sex ratios for particular strata in the model. Based on the model and holding the individual level covariates constant at their reference levels, in January 2002 the predicted sex ratio for the reference state (Texas) was 1.067[i], while the predicted sex ratio in New York was 1.030[ii]. The interaction for New York was the only negative one with a p-value below the traditional cut point for statistical significance ($p < 0.05$), however New Jersey and Pennsylvania had interaction terms of similar magnitude that met the usual criterion for interaction of $p < 0.2$ (New Jersey beta $= -0.0348$ $p = 0.1$, Pennsylvania beta $= -0.0340$ $p = 0.08$). The predicted sex ratios for New Jersey and Pennsylvania in January 2002 were 1.029[iii] and 1.029[iv] respectively.

Consistent with the literature, individual level demographic covariates were associated with infant sex (James, 1984; James & Rostron, 1985; Teitelbaum & Mantel, 1971). Compared with White mothers, Black and Hispanic mothers had somewhat lower odds of delivering a male infant (Black beta $= -0.0207$, $p < 0.01$, Hispanic beta $= -0.0113$, $p < 0.01$). Younger mothers had increased odds of a male infant, while older mothers had decreased odds of a male infant (<18 years beta $= 0.0106$, $p < 0.01$, ≥35 years beta $= -0.0038$, $p < 0.01$). First born infants were the most likely to be male compared with those born second through fifth (beta $= -0.0058$, $p < 0.01$), and those born sixth or higher (beta $= -0.011$, $p < 0.01$).

9. Understanding the Results

The secondary sex ratio fell below its expected value in New York, New Jersey, and Pennsylvania after the terrorist attacks of September 11, 2001. The New York findings converge with prior time-series research that examined the sex ratio after September 11, 2001 in New York City (Catalano, Bruckner, Marks, & Eskenazi, 2006). Our results, however, do not support the notion of a geographic "dose response" associated with a state's distance from the attacks for all of the states we tested.

By combining the panel approach with the time-series approach, we believe that we have improved upon more conventional methods used to reduce the chance of Type I or II errors due to confounding. Returning to the concepts introduced in Section 2, we have adjusted for all available third variables with the inclusion of individual level covariates. These specified third variables included maternal race/ethnicity, age, and educational attainment, as well as parity of the birth. We have also adjusted for all generally occurring, unavailable third variables by the inclusion of month of birth dichotomous variables. We then accounted for locally occurring, unavailable, patterned third variables with the inclusion of the sex ratio propensities derived from time-series. Last, by estimating the association in several states thought to be at uniquely high risk of a response, we provided evidence against the argument that the a relationship discovered in one state could have been induced by a locally occurring, unavailable, unpatterned third variable.

The predicted sex ratios are produced holding constant the individual level covariates. Therefore, the results indicate sex ratios of infants born to mothers who are white, aged 18–34, primiparous, and have at least a high school education (the reference groups from the model). We note this important caveat that generalized linear models require this conditional interpretation; to predict any particular sex ratio value from the model, the reader must specify the combination of covariates of interest.

We include the sex ratio time-series propensities and interactions by state in the model to account for unavailable, locally occurring patterned third variables. Before adding the interactions by state, the overall sex ratio propensity coefficient was statistically significant, and as expected was positively associated with the actual sex ratio (beta = 0.20, p<0.01, model not shown). The interactions were included to allow the strength of autocorrelation to differ depending on the state. While these interaction terms were not statistically significant, their inclusion ensures that autocorrelation has been fully adjusted in the model. It is also notable that the final model results remained essentially the same whether or not the sex ratio propensities were included in the model. This suggests that autocorrelation did not appreciably distort the final results.

One challenge of integrating these propensities into the model is that a value must be included for those states and time periods where there is no autocorrelation. We have included the propensities on the log scale and used 0 as the reference value. However, other reasonable choices could have been made in this regard. Future explorations might consider the implications of entering these propensities and the reference value in different forms.

We did not pose any hypotheses related to unusually high values of the sex ratio in any of the months under study, however a few interactions suggested significantly greater than expected sex ratios (Virginia in November 2001, New Jersey in December 2001, Maryland/Washington DC in January 2002). We hesitate to interpret these values given our original "one tailed" hypothesis, but the findings may merit more consideration.

In this analysis, we tested the hypothesis that the sex ratio decreased more after September 11, 2001 in states directly affected by the terrorist attacks compared with other reference states. As a result, the reader should not interpret the results as a test of the more global hypothesis about whether the sex ratio declined after September 11, 2001 across all of the states under study. However, subsequent examination of the global test suggests that the 13 states, in aggregate, did not experience a statistically significant decrease in the sex ratio following September 11, 2001 (results not shown).

While our hypotheses pertained to specific states that we expected to be more affected by the September 11, 2001 attacks, we conducted a follow-up exploratory analysis that looked at interactions for all of the states in November 2001, December 2001, and January 2002. The results of that analysis appear consistent with those presented here for New York, New Jersey and Pennsylvania in January 2002. Interestingly, they also suggested lower than expected sex ratios for California and Florida in December 2001. While these states are not geographically proximate to the September 11, 2001 terrorist attacks, they may have been affected for other reasons. The decline in travel after September 11, 2001 may have been particularly detrimental to their economies as California and Florida are the first and second largest domestic tourism destinations in the United States (Bigano, Hamilton, Lau, To, & Zhou, 2004). In addition, these states also have many residents with family and other ties to the places of the attacks. For example, 9.3% of Florida residents were born in New York (U. S. Census Bureau, 2005). The lower than expected sex ratio for California in December 2001, moreover, converges with previous research that used time-series methods (Catalano, Bruckner, Gould, et al., 2005).

10. Summary and Conclusions

The heightened focus on surveillance in the developed world has led to greater availability of individual-level data measured over relatively many times and places. As a result, researchers concerned with population health consequences of macrosocial shocks are increasingly faced with the dilemma of choosing appropriate statistical methodology for their investigations. This choice, we presume, will be made in part by which strategy best rules out Type I and II errors due to confounding.

This chapter illustrates a method that we believe combines the strengths of both panel and time-series analyses. This combined approach, which uses already widely disseminated statistical routines, reduces bias due to confounding of both individual and ecological "third" variables. By implementing this approach, we believe that researchers concerned with macrosocial shocks may arrive at more compelling results than those provided by separate panel or time-series analyses. Results of the combined method, moreover, allow for an interpretation of coefficients familiar to epidemiologists and social scientists.

Although the combined method does not employ a novel statistical approach, we have not seen it used in the literature. We recommend that researchers form collaborative teams with expertise in both panel and time-series analysis, as we have done in this chapter. Through inter-disciplinary approaches we may better quantify the spatial and temporal population responses to macrosocial shocks.

Endnotes

i. $1.067 = e^{\wedge}(0.0598$ (intercept) $+ 0.005$ (Jan02)

ii. $1.030 = e^{\wedge}(0.0598$ (intercept) $+ 0.005$ (Jan02) $+ 0.0039$ (NY) $- 0.0388$ (NY*Jan02)

iii. $1.029 = e^{\wedge}(0.0598$ (intercept) $+ 0.005$ (Jan02) $- 0.0245$ (NJ) $- 0.0348$ (NJ*Jan02) $+ 0.2744^{*}0.047$ (propensity coefficient * sex ratio NJ Jan02) $+ 0.2884^{*}0.047$ (propensity coefficient *NJ coefficient*sex ratio NJ Jan02)

iv. $1.029 = e^{\wedge}(0.0598$ (intercept) $+ 0.005$ (Jan02) $- 0.0019$ (PA) $- 0.0340$ (PA*Jan02)

Acknowledgements.   Support for the preparation of this chapter provided by the Robert Wood Johnson Health and Society Scholars Program.

References

Abma, J., Chandra, A., Mosher, W., Peterson, L., & Piccinino, L. (1997). Fertility, family planning, and women's health: New data from the 1995 National Survey of Family Growth. *Vital Health Statistics, 23*(19), 1–114.

Bigano, A., Hamilton, J. M., Lau, M., To, R. S., & Zhou, Y. (2004). A global database of domestic and international tourist numbers at national and subnational level. Hamburg (November 2, 2004); http://www.uni-hamburg.de/Wiss/FB/15/Sustainability/tourismdata.pdf

Box, G., Jenkins, G., & Reinsel, G. (1994). *Time series analysis: Forecasting and control.* 3rd edition. London: Prentice Hall.

Brenner, M. H. (1983). Mortality and economic instability: Detailed analyses for Britain and comparative analyses for selected industrialized countries. *International Journal of Health Services, 13,* 563–620.

Byrne, J., & Warburton, D. (1987). Male excess among anatomically normal fetuses in spontaneous abortions. *American Journal of Medical Genetics, 26,* 605–611.

Catalano, R. A. (2003). Sex ratios in the two Germanies: A test of the economic stress hypothesis. *Human Reproduction, 18,* 1972–1975.

Catalano, R. A., & Bruckner, T. (2005). Economic antecedents of the Swedish sex ratio. *Social Science & Medicine, 60,* 537–543.

Catalano, R., Bruckner, T., Anderson, E., & Gould, J. B. (2005). Fetal death sex ratios: A test of the economic stress hypothesis. *International Journal of Epidemiology, 34,* 944–948.

Catalano, R., Bruckner, T., Gould, J., Eskenazi, B., & Anderson, E. (2005). Sex ratios in California following the terrorist attacks of September 11, 2001. *Human Reproduction, 20,* 1221–1227.

Catalano, R., Bruckner, T., Hartig, T., & Ong, M. (2005). Population stress and the Swedish sex ratio. *Paediatric and Perinatal Epidemiology, 19,* 413–420.

Catalano, R., Bruckner, T., Marks, A. R., & Eskenazi, B. (2006). Exogenous shocks to the human sex ratio: The case of September 11, 2001 in New York City. *Human Reproduction, 21*(12), 3127–3131.

Catalano, R., Hansen, H. T., & Hartig, T. (1999). The ecological effect of unemployment on the incidence of very low birthweight in Norway and Sweden. *Journal of Health and Social Behavior, 40,* 422–428.

Catalano, R., & Serxner, S. (1987). Time series designs of potential interest to epidemiologists. *American Journal of Epidemiology, 126,* 724–731.

Chatfield, C. (2004). *The analysis of time series: An introduction.* 6th edition. New York: Chapman and Hall.

Erickson, J. D. (1976). The secondary sex ratio in the United States 1969–71: Association with race, parental ages, birth order, paternal education and legitimacy. *Annals of Human Genetics, 40,* 205–212.

Fitzmaurice, G. M., Laird, N. M., & Ware, J. H. (2002). Review of generalized linear models. In G. M. Fitzmaurice, N. M. Laird, & J. H. Ware (Eds.), *Applied longitudinal analysis.* Hoboken, NJ: Wiley-Interscience.

Forchhammer, M. C. (2000). Timing of foetal growth spurts can explain sex ratio variation in polygynous mammals. *Ecology Letters, 3,* 1–4.

Fukuda, M., Fukuda, K., Shimizu, T., & Moller, H. (1998). Decline in sex ratio at birth after Kobe earthquake. *Human Reproduction, 13,* 2321–2322.

Fukuda, M., Fukuda, K., Shimizu, T., Yomura, W., & Shimizu, S. (1996). Kobe earthquake and reduced sperm motility. *Human Reproduction, 11,* 1244–1246.

Galea, S., Ahern, J., Resnick, H., Kilpatrick, D., Bucuvalas, M., Gold, J., et al. (2002). Psychological sequelae of the September 11 terrorist attacks in New York City. *New England Journal of Medicine, 346,* 982–987.

Giannakoulopoulos, X., Sepulveda, W., Kourtis, P., Glover, V., & Fisk, N. M. (1994). Fetal plasma cortisol and beta-endorphin response to intrauterine needling. *Lancet, 344,* 77–81.

Gitau, R., Fisk, N. M., Teixeira, J. M., Cameron, A., & Glover, V. (2001). Fetal hypothalamic-pituitary-adrenal stress responses to invasive procedures are independent of maternal responses. *Journal of Clinical Endocrinology and Metabolism, 86,* 104–109.

Greenland, S. (1998). Introduction to regression models. In S. Greenland & K. J. Rothman (Eds.), *Modern epidemiology.* 2nd edition. Philadelphia: Lippincott-Raven.

Hall, D. M. (1999). Children in an ageing society. *British Medical Journal, 319,* 1356–1358.

Hobel, C. J., Dunkel-Schetter, C., Roesch, S. C., Castro, L. C., & Arora, C. P. (1999). Maternal plasma corticotropin-releasing hormone associated with stress at 20 weeks' gestation in pregnancies ending in preterm delivery. *American Journal of Obstetrics and Gynecology, 180,* S257–S263.

Hsiao, C. (1989) *Analysis of panel data.* Cambridge: Cambridge University Press.

James, W. H. (1984). The sex ratios of black births. *Annals of Human Biology, 11,* 39–44.

James, W. H. (1985). The sex ratio of Oriental births. *Annals of Human Biology, 12,* 485–487.

James, W. H. (1987). The human sex ratio. Part 1: A review of the literature. *Human Biology, 59,* 721–752.

James, W. H. (1999). The status of the hypothesis that the human sex ratio at birth is associated with the cycle day of conception. *Human Reproduction, 14,* 2177–2178.

James, W. H., & Rostron, J. (1985). Parental age, parity and sex ratio in births in England and Wales, 1968–77. *Journal of Biosocial Science, 17,* 47–56.

Kost, K., Landry, D. J., & Darroch, J. E. (1998). Predicting maternal behaviors during pregnancy: Does intention status matter? *Family Planning Perspectives, 30,* 79–88.

Kraemer, S. (2000). The fragile male. *British Medical Journal, 321,* 1609–1612.

Kutner, M. H., Nachtsheim, C. J., Neter, J., & Li, W. (2004). Logistic regression, Poisson regression, and generalized linear models. In M. H. Kutner, C. J. Nachtsheim, J. Neter, & W. Li (Eds.), *Applied linear statistical methods.* 5th edition. Boston: McGraw-Hill.

Lazarus, J. (2002). Human sex ratios: Adaptations and mechanisms, problems and prospects. In I. Hardy (Ed.), *Sex ratios: Concepts and research methods.* Cambridge: Cambridge University Press.

Lou, H. C., Hansen, D., Nordentoft, M., Pryds, O., Jensen, F., Nim, J., et al. (1994). Prenatal stressors of human life affect fetal brain development. *Developmental Medicine and Child Neurology, 36,* 826–832.

Lyster, W. R. (1974). Altered sex ratio after the London smog of 1952 and the Brisbane flood of 1965. *British Journal of Obstetrics and Gynecology, 81,* 626–631.

Mangano, J. J. (2006). A short latency between radiation exposure from nuclear plants and cancer in young children. *International Journal of Health Services, 36,* 113–135.

Martin, J. F. (1997). Length of the follicular phase, time of insemination, coital rate and the sex of offspring. *Human Reproduction, 12,* 611–616.

McCleary, R., & Hay, R. A. (1980). *Applied time series analysis for the social sciences.* London: Sage.

Mizuno, R. (2000). The male/female ratio of fetal deaths and births in Japan. *Lancet, 356,* 738–739.

Mocarelli, P., Brambilla, P., Gerthoux, P. M., Patterson Jr., D. G., & Needham, L. L. (1996). Change in sex ratio with exposure to dioxin. *Lancet, 348,* 409.

Moller, H. (1996). Change in male:female ratio among newborn infants in Denmark. *Lancet, 348,* 828–829.

National Center for Health Statistics Natality Files, 1996 to 2002. (2004). CD-Rom Series 21. Hyattsville, MD: U.S. Department of Health and Human Services.

Owen, D., & Matthews, S. G. (2003). Glucocorticoids and sex-dependent development of brain glucocorticoid and mineralocorticoid receptors. *Endocrinology, 144,* 2775–2784.

Piccinino, L. J. (1994). Unintended pregnancy and childbearing. In L. S. Wilcox & J. S. Marks (Eds.), *From data to action: CDC's public health surveillance for women, infants, and children.* Hyattsville, MD: US Department of Health and Human Services, Public Health Service.

Ruhm, C. J. (1995). Economic conditions and alcohol problems. *Journal of Health Economics 14,* 583–603.

Teitelbaum, M. S., & Mantel, N. (1971). Socio-economic factors and the sex ratio at birth. *Journal of Biosocial Science, 3,* 23–41.

Trivers, R. L., & Willard, D. E. (1973). Natural selection of parental ability to vary the sex ratio of offspring. *Science, 179,* 90–92.

U.S. Census Bureau. (2005) State Population. (Dec. 31, 2005); http://www.census.gov/population/cen2000/phc-t38/phc-t38.xls

Vandentorren, S., Suzan, F., Medina, S., Pascal, M., Maulpoix, A., Cohen, J. C., et al. (2004). Mortality in 13 French cities during the August 2003 heat wave. *American Journal of Public Health, 94,* 1518–1520.

Chapter 19
What Level Macro? Choosing Appropriate Levels to Assess How Place Influences Population Health

Theresa L. Osypuk and Sandro Galea

1. Introduction

I should venture to assert that the most pervasive fallacy of philosophic thinking goes back to neglect of context.

John Dewey

Although it has strong historical roots (Davey Smith, Dorling, & Shaw, 2001; Krieger, 2001), the focus on area or contextual causes of health has only recently resurged in epidemiologic studies (Diez Roux, 2001). Most current epidemiologic inquiry continues to be concerned with studying determinants of health or disease that are proximal to the disease process (compared to causes that are more distal) and causes that are individual-level (compared to those at the population level) (McMichael, 1999). Although higher level causes must be mediated through individual-level and more proximal causes (Diez Roux, 2004b), certain disease causes may not be entirely operationalized at the individual level (Morgenstern, 1985). Increasingly we are recognizing that distal causes manifesting at higher spatial levels (e.g., neighborhoods, states) may present greater potential for health prevention than more proximal causes and, as such, are more fundamental causes of health (Link & Phelan, 1996; Schwartz & Diez Roux, 2001). As discussed throughout this book, studying macro-level causes of health and disease above and beyond individual causes may suggest avenues for disease prevention, intervention, and treatment that would not be evident from inquiry restricted to individual-level determinants.

Despite our growing appreciation that macro- or higher-levels of causes are fundamental for population health and health disparities, it is often unclear at what level to conceptualize and operationalize these macro-level causes. This chapter seeks to address this gap. In this chapter, we are concerned with issues pertaining to "macro-level" factors that exist at levels[i] of spatial aggregation above the individual and that may pertain to social and physical context as related to health.

We begin by discussing historical examples of different spatial levels that have been utilized for examination of health. We next review criteria for choosing what macro level to study, we provide examples of justifications for using various spatial levels and we present practical issues that must be considered when choosing a level including defining boundaries, data availability, validity, and inference. We focus our discussion on US-based research, informed both by our experience and by the dominant body of work. However, our observations may also be germane to other countries and other levels of analysis. We additionally restrict our focus to examine macro levels pertaining to geography or space, leaving aside institutional contexts (e.g., schools, hospitals, workplaces) which merit separate discussion. We focus principally on a view of space or place that is useful for quantitative statistical analysis, e.g., for multilevel modeling[ii] or ecologic analysis.

2. Historical Operationalizations of Place for Health Inquiry

The idea that place matters for health is not new (Kawachi & Berkman, 2003a, b), and historical examinations of place and health have invoked numerous alternative definitions of "place." By the mid-19th century, data on geographic health patterns (including mapping of these patterns) had been produced in Britain and other parts of Europe (Macintyre & Ellaway, 2003). We discuss some of these historic examinations with an eye towards what level macro they examined.

In 1826, Louise Rene Villermé documented with census data that variations in annual mortality rates across Parisian neighborhoods (arrondissements) were patterned by poverty and wealth (Krieger, 2001; Macintyre & Ellaway, 2003). In 1837, Farr documented the geographic health variability and social class patterns of mortality in Britain with life-tables by district, observing,

" . . . the health of all parts of the kingdom is not equally bad. Some districts are infested by epidemics constantly recurring; the people are immersed in an atmosphere that weakens their powers, troubles their functions, and shortens their lives. Other localities are so favourably circumstanced that great numbers attain old age in the enjoyment of all their faculties, and suffer rarely from epidemics." (Farr, 2001)

Farr thus highlighted healthy and unhealthy districts, noting the excess age and sex adjusted mortality rates in London and other urban towns (Liverpool, Manchester). He discussed several contemporary reports that summarized health variability at different levels of geography, including districts, villages, streets, parishes, towns, cities, and counties (Farr, 2001).

In *The Condition of the Working Class in England* (1845), Engels cited geographic variability in mortality and disease among towns in the mid-19th century, noting the particularly high rates in the largest factory towns (Manchester, Liverpool). Engels reproduced the mortality rate variability by social class of streets and houses originally reported by Holland and discussed variations in epidemic rates, epidemic mortality, and childhood accident mortality by comparing large towns (Manchester, Liverpool, and London) to country districts (Engels, 1845).

In 1902, Charles Booth utilized school board subdivisions, or "blocks", within districts as his units of inquiry to examine spatial patterns of poverty in London.

Booth implied that districts corresponded to areas of the city (e.g., "the huge district of East London") and were of a size conducive for school board employees to gain "extensive knowledge of the people" (Booth, 2001):

"The inhabitants of every street, and court, and block of buildings in the whole of London, have been estimated in proportion to the numbers of the children ... The streets have been grouped together according to the School Board subdivisions or "blocks", and for each of these blocks full particulars are given ... The numbers included in each block vary from less than 2,000 to more than 30,000, and to make a more satisfactory unit of comparison I have arranged them in contiguous groups, 2, 3, or 4 together, as to make areas having each about 30,000 inhabitants, these areas adding up into the large divisions of the School Board administration. The population is then classified by Registration districts, which are likewise grouped into School Board divisions, each method finally leading up to the total for all London" (Booth, 2001).

Thus, Booth's analysis examined place units of several sizes. Booth preserved the school board block unit, but he also created an alternate unit of comparable population size – "a more satisfactory unit of comparison" – by aggregating blocks. Moreover, he superimposed another administrative unit in addition to blocks: the Registration district. It appears that Booth used School Board data as the method for collecting poverty data on the population because the School Board kept extensive records; he noted, "every house in every street is in their books, and details are given of every family with children of school age" and because school board employees ("visitors") had "very considerable knowledge of the parents of the school children, especially of the poorest among them, and of the conditions under which they live." Indeed, parents and school board visitors were in daily contact. The results of Booth's analysis culminated in a map of poverty by blocks (Booth, 2001).

Even among these few historical examples, researchers used many different sizes of "place" to document geographic health patterns, although the justification for the unit of place (even as today) is not often transparent.

3. How Does Spatial Frame Matter?

Central to our concern is the question of what level macro should be examined. Just as the topic of place has not received sufficient attention for health, so too, conceptualizations of what constitutes a place, of what is the appropriate level of analysis, and of how to model space have not occupied much space in epidemiologic writings. Harvey (2006) wonders:

"Are there rules for deciding when and where one spatial frame is preferable to another? Or is the choice arbitrary, subject to the whims of human practice? The decision to use one or the other conception certainly depends on the nature of the phenomena under investigation." (Harvey, 2006).

As a geographer, Harvey eloquently suggests there is no "one" spatial level that matters (Harvey, 2006); rather, the choice of which specific geographic level to model must be derived from theoretical models for the specific research question at hand (Diez Roux, 2000; Leyland & Groenewegen, 2003). This theoretical specification of relevant levels must precede data collection and statistical analysis (Diez Roux, 2004b). Generically, this requires defining what it is about a place that may provide adverse or protective exposures that affect health (O'Campo & Kogan, 2005). One must identify the exact hypothesis for examination and the hypothesized pathway by which the exposure translates to the outcome, i.e., via social and biological pathways (O'Campo & Schempf, 2005). Since different processes operate at different scales, issues of spatial scale naturally must be considered when choosing the level or unit of analysis (Macintyre, Ellaway, & Cummins, 2002). For example, the scale at which food availability affects diet may vary depending on the scale of human activity through which people come into contact with food stores. The spatial range of impoverished individuals may be more limited because of access to transportation, as compared with the spatial range of higher income individuals.

Few theories of area influences have been articulated in the health sciences literature, and one of the most vital issues impeding progress in place and health research may be lack of theory articulating the mechanisms of how place affects health (Diez Roux, 2000; O'Campo, 2003; O'Campo & Kogan, 2005). Indeed, since investigators fail to conceptualize, operationalize, and measure place effects with sufficient theory, selection of area variables becomes driven by available data (Macintyre et al., 2002). To advance the field, investigators must rigorously test alternate theories about why place matters for health. It is important not only to frame one's specific hypothesis with appropriate theoretical grounding, but also to test unifying explanations for empirical observations by contrasting one's theory against alternate theories.

Although researchers in epidemiology and public health have largely failed to ground place-health research in relevant theory, researchers in disciplines such as geography, sociology, criminology, and urban planning have articulated theories as to why place matters, and these conceptualizations can be applied to health studies. For instance, geographers have long struggled with what makes a place a place and with the defintion of "space". One prominent geographer presents a model of three conceptualizations of space: absolute, relative, and relational (Harvey, 2006). Absolute space is bounded and fixed, symbolized as preexisting and immovable or as the space of Euclid in geometric terms. Through a social lens, absolute space encompasses boundaries of private property or territorial boundaries such as administrative units or states.

Relative space is defined by one thing in relation to another. Relationally, places may be conceived as "nodes in relational settings" or as "articulated moments in networks" (Castree, 2004). In application to health, a relational perspective would examine how people move through space from one destination to another and how the context along these specific routes or nodes may affect health. As an example, a relational perspective of how place affects health may operationalize neighborhood as the path one takes to walk or drive from one point to another – e.g., from home to work. The relational investigator may then model aspects of the neighborhood that one might encounter *on that path* as influencing health. Thus, instead of a spatial area that would be modeled in an absolute framework, the investigator models individual paths through space. The third conceptualization of relational space is experiential, how people experience space and how a person internalizes information related to a space, including what memories or emotions people bring to or take from a space to construct meaning. This experiential notion of space may be very relevant for mental health outcomes, e.g., where the meaning of place reactivates trauma. Tension exists inherently among these three conceptualizations, and the particular spatial conceptualization to adopt is contingent on the circumstances (Harvey, 1973, 2006). For a relational understanding of place in health research, including a discussion of a relational contrasted with an absolute (Euclidean) viewpoint, we point the reader to other sources (Cummins, Curtis, Diez Roux, & Macintyre, In Press).

From a different tradition, American sociologists concern themselves with understanding how macro-level factors have inhibited and influenced individual behavior and social structure. For instance, many early sociologists argued that neighborhoods were fundamental building blocks of the larger system of stratification in the US and that social relations became manifested in spatial relations (Anderson & Massey, 2001). Illustrating this sociological perspective in his 1987 book *The Truly Disadvantaged*, William Julius Wilson argued that urban poverty was not only perpetuated through individual and family level pathways, but also through structural pathways, including within and between neighborhoods characterized by concentrated poverty (Anderson & Massey, 2001; Wilson, 1987). In a similar vein, some criminologists emphasize the importance of social disorganization theory – a community level explanation for crime that highlights the role of community structures and cultures that cause differential crime rates. This theory is often spatially expressed. For instance, structural features of neighborhoods, including economic status, ethnic homogeneity, and residential mobility, disrupt the social organization of communities, which in turn causes differential crime and delinquency rates across neighborhoods (Sampson & Wilson, 1995). However, the conception of community does not have to be strictly geographic or spatial, since social and organizational networks of residents may transcend smaller levels of geography (Sampson & Wilson 1995).

Transportation, urban design and planning disciplines focus on the importance of neighborhood design and land use development for understanding how and why people make transportation choices, for instance, whether people walk, use public transportation, and/or drive cars. This transportation/urban planning literature discusses how urban form or the built environment may influence physical activity (walking, cycling), for instance, through the layout of the street network or placement of buildings, proximity of residential to retail land uses, and detail of urban design features (Frank & Engelke, 2005, 2001; Saelens, Sallis, & Frank, 2003; Sallis, Frank, Saelens, & Kraft, 2004).

In sum, theory is specific to the phenomena under study and is necessary for choosing the appropriate macro-level unit and variables of interest for one's analysis. Although epidemiology offers few population theories of disease distribution, we add to the writings that have encouraged researchers to draw from the rich theory cultivated in other disciplines, as well as to voice explicitly how these exposures link to the disease outcome of interest through biologic plausibility and prior evidence.

4. Different Spatial Levels Relevant to the Study of Population Health

Researchers have considered many different units or levels in exploring why place matters for health, including neighborhoods, counties, states, nations. Decisions about what level of space may be appropriate for analysis should follow from a theoretic appreciation of what characteristic of a particular space may matter for what health indicator. Assumptions and hypotheses that may be valid at one level may not be valid at others. For example, while census tract-level analyses may be appropriate to consider the relation between characteristics of the built environment and mental health, the role of factors such as employment markets, residential segregation, or state policies governing alcohol sales to minors may not be studied meaningfully at the neighborhood level, since those constructs operate at higher levels like metropolitan areas or states. And although an investigator may be able to operationalize variables at the census tract level (e.g. tract-level unemployment rate, tract-level percent black), these variables may capture only part of a process that operates at higher levels (e.g. regional unemployment trends or racial segregation at the metropolitan level).

In the following section, we discuss the historical meaning or definition of different spatial units as originally conceived in the US, why research at such a level is relevant for health, and some limitations involved with considering how characteristics at that level may influence population health. Many of the drawbacks inherent in choosing any one unit of analysis may also be relevant to other levels of analysis. We will address different units working from smallest to largest geographic areas.

4.1. Neighborhoods

4.1.1. Historical Roots and Why the Level May Matter for Health

Some historians posit that the American neighborhood structure emerged in the mid- to late-19th century, as American cities transitioned from small "walking cities" into more segmented, larger urban units. American cities before 1860 were small, compact, and generally integrated. Before technological advances in travel (e.g., the omnibus and the horsecar), settlement sizes were small enough that the city was virtually entirely walkable; the size of cities rarely extended beyond a 2 mile radius from the city center. In the mid-19th century, however, technological innovations allowed the elite to escape the overcrowded conditions of the walking city. The exodus of the elite sorted populations by residence, a sorting which was accelerated by additional transportation innovations, large-scale immigration, and internal migration to American cities in the late 19th century. As the cities grew, their internal structure became characterized by distinct areas, and the residential housing areas came to be known as neighborhoods (Melvin, 1985).

Neighborhoods are a common level for conceptualizing the importance of place (National Research Council, 2002) and are often what is meant by "place" in the contemporary population health literature (Diez Roux, 2001; Macintyre et al., 2002; National Research Council, 2002). A neighborhood effects literature has developed over the past decade, of which health forms one part; neighborhood effects are defined as outcomes from a causal process of an exposure of living in a particular neighborhood (Altshuler, Morrill, Wolman, Mitchell, & Committee on Improving the Future of U.S. Cities Through Improved Metropolitan Area Governance, 1999).

Several theoretical models discuss why neighborhoods may matter for well-being, highlighting material and social pathways. For example, criminologists have emphasized the role of community social organization and disorganization for producing crime, particularly at the level of neighborhoods. Sociologists have discussed how individuals are embedded within the ecology of neighborhoods, and particularly harmful ecologic contexts for outcomes (e.g., health, education, or employment) include concentrated poverty neighborhoods. The neighborhoods and health literature has been burgeoning lately, so there is no shortage of conceptual frameworks on how neighborhoods may affect health. For an overview on neighborhoods and health, see Kawachi & Berkman 2003a or Ellen, Mijanovich, & Dillman, 2001. As one example of a conceptual framework, from a review of the literature, Ellen et al. (2001) present four mechanisms describing how neighborhoods may matter for health: (1) neighborhood institutions and resources (e.g., food environment, opportunities to promote exercise), (2) stressors in the physical environment (e.g., polluting factories, older housing structures, quality of municipal services), (3) stressors in the social environment (e.g., crime victimization, witnessing crime, noise), and (4) neighborhood-based networks and norms (e.g., for transmitting information, norms, and social support) (Ellen et al., 2001). These pathways may be very important for health, especially if neighborhoods are the dominant social context for an individual or group.

4.1.2. Drawbacks

Chief among the limitations to considering neighborhoods as the key macro-level unit of analysis is the problem of selection in observational studies, whereby individuals with particular characteristics migrate to neighborhoods characterized by the features of analytic interest (Diez Roux, 2002a, 2004a). Selection of individuals into neighborhoods threatens causal inference about neighborhood characteristics and their role in shaping health (Kawachi & Berkman, 2003b). Migration-related selection may be a greater threat to validity in observational studies using neighborhoods than in studies using higher-level spatial units. Residential mobility *between* neighborhoods *within* counties, metropolitan areas (MAs), or states is much more common than mobility *between* counties or MAs or states. The forces operating to sort people into certain locations (e.g., discrimination in housing markets, employment opportunities) are more prominent *within* metropolitan areas *between* neighborhoods than *between* metropolitan areas, states, or counties (Ellen, 2000; Osypuk, 2005). Related to the issue of migration is the relevance of the size and meaning of the neighborhood unit with respect to relevant exposures of interest. Residents often travel beyond the boundaries of their neighborhood daily, so neighborhood-focused studies will not allow modeling of other aspects of their context (e.g., workplaces, schools, travel routes, social spaces) that may impact their health.

Because of the powerful racial and socioeconomic sorting mechanisms operating in metropolitan housing markets, people of different racial and socioeconomic backgrounds often live in different neighborhoods in the metropolitan area (Acevedo-Garcia, Lochner, Osypuk, & Subramanian, 2003; Massey & Denton, 1993). While this is a complex sociological phenomenon, one implication of this sorting is that it becomes difficult to consider all racial and social class groups together in one neighborhood analysis because such empiric models often violate exchangeability assumptions (Diez Roux, 2004a)(Diez Roux, 2005). A related but distinct concern is non-overlap of populations within neighborhoods with respect to confounders, which can lead to off-support inference (Diez Roux, 2004a; Oakes, 2006). When members of different racial groups live in starkly separate neighborhoods, which is the case in many U.S. metropolitan areas given patterns of racial residential segregation (see (Morenoff, Diez Roux, Osypuk, & Hansen, 2006) for an empiric example with Chicago neighborhoods), stratifying on race may reduce these validity threats (of lack of exchangeability or non-overlap) in neighborhoods analysis. However, residual confounding may remain even after stratification.

Another challenge pertains to ensuring that the sampling scheme that was used to obtain the analytic sample for a particular study appropriately lends itself to the analysis in question. Often neighborhood health studies derive from one of two sampling plans: from national probability samples of individuals or from neighborhood studies within a city or metropolitan area. In the former sampling scheme, the study was typically conceived with individual-level hypotheses in mind, so individuals are typically sampled as the unit of interest and then geocoded to their neighborhood tract. As a result, the application of multilevel modeling to such analysis may be improper; multilevel modeling assumes that the higher-level units are randomly drawn from a larger source population (Duncan, Jones, & Moon, 1998), while in the case of national sampling plans, the assumption is that individuals, not the neighborhoods, are drawn from the larger source population. In addition, this approach plucks neighborhoods from their metropolitan areas and thus models neighborhoods absent their metropolitan context (Diez Roux, 2001); again, this may not be proper if the characteristic of interest is most meaningful relative to its own metropolitan area rather than in an absolute sense compared to the rest of the country. Even if multilevel modeling were used, this design likely precludes complex covariance structures (e.g., random effects models) given the limited analytic power dictated by the small sample size in each neighborhood (Duncan et al., 1998). Therefore, investigators using this design often employ marginal models (or population average models), which allow the modeling of the average effect of a type of neighborhood (characterizing neighborhoods by variables of interest) without modeling the variance attributable to each level (Diez Roux, 2002b).

The second type of neighborhood sampling plan typically involves sampling a sufficient number of neighborhoods within one metropolitan area or city and then sampling persons within these neighborhoods. This type of sample design may be more appropriate for assessing how the neighborhood matters and more generalizable regarding neighborhood effects or associations, at least for that city/MA. Examples of studies that have used such a design include the Project for Human Development in Chicago Neighborhoods (PHDCN) (Raudenbush & Sampson, 1999) and the Los Angeles Family and Neighborhood Study (L.A. FANS, 2006). Since these studies are designed to examine hypotheses about the influence of neighborhood characteristics on population health, they wield sufficient power for analyzing random effects and are appropriate for multilevel statistical analysis. A limitation of this approach is the restriction of the study to only one site or metropolitan area; this hampers generalizability if comparable features of neighborhoods produce different health effects in different places throughout the country.

The spatial autocorrelations of observations within neighborhoods requires special methods to either adjust for or model statistical dependency (e.g. multilevel models). Analyzing neighborhoods may have limited policy relevance unless resources are allocated along these neighborhood boundaries. Adopting administrative definitions that cities use for neighborhoods may be one solution to enhance policy relevance (e.g., the 59 New York City community districts (New York City Department of City Planning, 2006) or the 77 Chicago community areas).

A last important limitation to using neighborhoods regards their definition. Although typically neighborhoods are defined as one's immediate residential environment (Diez Roux, 2001), operationalizing neighborhood boundaries is a challenge. We will discuss these challenges of operationalizing levels in the next section, and in Section 4.3.

4.1.3.1. Historical Roots of Operationalizing Neighborhoods as Census Tracts

The relevant definition of neighborhoods has garnered much attention in neighborhood health research since it is not clear how to bound or define neighborhoods. Neighborhoods have been defined using geographical criteria, historical criteria, administrative boundaries, characteristics of residents, and resident perceptions (Diez Roux, 2001; Diez Roux, 2003). For the purposes of this chapter we discuss the two administrative units most commonly used as proxies for neighborhoods: Census Tracts and ZIP Code postal areas.

Many quantitative researchers have used administrative units defined by the US Census, i.e., census tracts, interchangeably with "neighborhoods", despite the fact that census tracts are only one particular operationalization of neighborhood. The principal reason why census tracts have been adopted enthusiastically as proxies for neighborhoods within the neighborhoods and health literature is that US Census data exists at the census tract level, hence providing readily available administrative data that may be used to characterize these "neighborhoods".

The idea of census tracts originated with Walter Laidlaw, who first divided New York City into tracts for the 1910 Census. Census tracts are artificial units created only for analyzing the population distribution by different geographies, at a smaller and more consistent scale than political jurisdictions afford. To define census tracts, committees of local data users are asked to create units that follow recognizable boundaries and encompass areas of between 2500 and 8000 population. The Census and community groups draw boundaries based on homogeneity of population in terms of economic status and housing conditions. Once the geographic units of tracts have been established, the Census permits only splits or recombinations of tracts from a previous census. One of the main goals of tracting the population is to provide continuity across time. Therefore, the Census Bureau prioritizes preserving the fixed boundaries over preserving the within-tract homogeneity (Plane, 2004). Hence, the main strength of using tracts relates to the availability of data and the stability of the units' boundaries across time.

4.1.3.2. Drawbacks of Operationalizing Neighborhoods as Census Tracts.

Despite the advantages of census tracts, residents rarely conceive of neighborhoods along census tract boundaries (O'Campo & Kogan, 2005). Local areas like neighborhoods may not be simple places around which one can draw a line (Massey, 1991). Rather, the line to capture a certain exposure perfectly at the neighborhood level may not be fixed for any one person or population but may be contingent on different purposes, processes, or health outcomes (Diez Roux, 2003; Diez Roux & Aiello, 2005; O'Campo & Kogan, 2005). Therefore, the use of census tracts as proxies for neighborhoods is necessarily crude. However, modeling variables at arbitrarily-defined administrative units may still capture some notion of context even if it is not capturing the construct as accurately as possible (Duncan et al., 1998). Since census tracts are artificial units created for administrative purposes, they are probably relevant units for health because their boundaries crudely approximate social and physical phenomena that affect health but that operate at other, unspecified spatial scales. The implications of using census tracts to proxy the neighborhood construct involve measurement error, internal validity, and the Modifiable Areal Unit Problem (MAUP), which we will discuss in Section 5.3. For example, since measurement of groups and of group-level constructs affecting health remains in its infancy, tract-level variables capturing neighborhood-level phenomena likely contain a great deal of measurement error (Diez Roux & Aiello, 2005).

An additional drawback to using census tracts for operationalizing neighborhoods relates to one of the strengths: use of available data. The most common variables investigated in neighborhood health research to date have been indicators of aggregate socioeconomic position derived from administrative (e.g., Census) data (Diez Roux, 2001). Although census tracts allow one to access and model Census data, the variables one is able to model with Census data (e.g., tract-level, census defined economic and demographic variables) are not themselves the literal cause of health or disease patterns. Census variables are likely crude proxies for other more direct social or physical characteristics, resources, services, or hazards of a place which affect health (Diez Roux, 2007). Choosing tracts and tract-level census data might be important for initial descriptive analysis, for replicating prior findings, or for monitoring place-based disease patterns; however, an important direction for neighborhood health studies at this stage includes utilizing data sources and variables that are not derived from the census. Non-census based variables may capture better the specific social and physical features of the neighborhood that cause health and illness, thereby informing the mechanisms by which neighborhood is relevant for health and informing interventions to improve health (Diez Roux, In press). We note that although we discuss this issue with respect to census tracts, the issue is equally relevant to other units (e.g., ZIP codes, discussed below) and other census-based units, such as block groups, that have also been used in some studies as proxies for neighborhoods.

4.1.4.1. Historical Roots of Operationalizing Neighborhood as ZIP Code Postal Areas

Between 1863 and 1963, individuals in the U.S. addressed letters by the street address of the recipient, including the city and state, or by denoting the rural delivery route. When thousands of postal employees left the U.S. Postal Service (USPS) to serve with the military during World War II, the USPS created a zoning address system in 124 of the largest Post Offices to facilitate mail sorting. For this system, 1 or 2 numbers were placed between the city and state in the addressing of a letter – e.g., Birmingham 7 Alabama. In 1963, the Post Office improved upon this rudimentary coding system by implementing the Zoning Improvement Plan (ZIP) code. Beginning on July 1, 1963, every address in the US was assigned a 5-digit ZIP code:

"The first digit designated a broad geographical area of the United States, ranging from zero for the Northeast to nine for the far West. This number was followed by two digits that more closely pinpointed population concentrations and those sectional centers accessible to common transportation networks. The final two digits designated small Post Offices or postal zones in larger zoned cities." (U.S. Postal Service, 2003)

In 1983, the USPS introduced the ZIP + 4 code, with a hyphen and four digits added to the existing 5-digit ZIP code:

"The first five numbers continued to identify an area of the country and delivery office to which mail is directed. The sixth and seventh numbers denoted a delivery sector, which may be several blocks, a group of streets, a group of Post Office boxes, several office buildings, a single high-rise office building, a large apartment building, or a small geographic area. The last two numbers denoted a delivery segment, which might be one floor of an office building, one side of a street between intersecting streets, specific departments in a firm, or specific Post Office boxes. This ZIP + 4 code again improved the efficiency of mail delivery by reducing the number of times a piece of mail is handled, and by reducing the amount of time letter carriers spent organizing the mail for delivery." (U.S. Postal Service, 2003)

A good deal of data is collected and available at the ZIP code level, also making this level a convenient candidate for considering the influence of space on health. As the USPS notes, "Today's use of a ZIP Code extends far beyond the mailing industry. ZIP Code numbers are embedded into the way that businesses work and have become an integral element of the 911 emergency system that uses ZIP code mailing codes as an aid in saving lives"(U.S. Postal Service, 2006a). For instance, businesses collect customer ZIP codes for establishing new store locations and for direct mail marketing (where businesses target products and services to certain addresses). The Census released population data based on ZIP codes in 1990 (Summary Tape File 3) (U.S. Census Bureau, 2002, 2006b), and the US Economic Census releases data on American businesses by ZIP code (U.S. Census Bureau, 2006a). ZIP codes may be a rough proxy of a person's location of residence for research purposes, and with the inclusion of " + 4", the precision increased substantially. Therefore, ZIP codes may approximate neighborhood of residence.

Since the public has requested statistics at the ZIP code level, the Census Bureau has created a new statistical area called the ZIP Code Tabulation Area (ZCTA) for Census 2000 data. This statistical geographic entity approximates the area defined by a 3 or 5-digit postal service ZIP code (U.S. Census Bureau, no year).

"ZCTAs were designed to overcome the operational difficulties of creating a well-defined ZIP Code area by using Census blocks (and the addresses found in them) as the basis for the ZCTAs." (U.S. Census Bureau, 2005b).

For the most part, ZCTAs coincide with ZIP codes (U.S. Census Bureau, 2001a). We refer the reader to the US Census (U.S. Census Bureau, 2000) for further detail about the ZCTA methodology.

One potential benefit of the ZIP code relates to how it is defined: ZIP code boundaries are conceptually related to how people (postal employees) move through space. For a given scale at which ZIP codes operate, ZIP code delineations may be more relevant than Census geography because of people's routes through them. Since ZIP code boundaries were defined with a mail carrier's route in mind (and this is often by foot in densely settled areas), the ZIP code's rear property boundaries indicate that people living across a street from each other share the same "neighborhood". With Census geography, streets are often boundaries, thus dividing people across the street from one another into separate blocks or tracts.

The USPS has several sources of data that might be relevant for historical study. Postal routes, post office locations, or postal employees that existed before ZIP codes may inform historical health questions involving population settlement or geography. The USPS has cultivated sources for archival research on aspects of historical postal service, post offices, postal routes, mail contracts/contractors, and personnel (e.g., postmasters, salaries) (U.S. Postal Service, 2006b). For instance, historical post route maps, available for the 1830s to the 1940s at the National Archives and the Library of Congress (U.S. Postal Service, 2006b), may indicate settlement patterns related to population density and shipping patterns (U.S. Postal Service, 2006b).

4.1.4.2. Drawbacks of Operationalizing Neighborhoods as ZIP Code Postal Areas

Unfortunately, the key drawback to the use of ZIP codes for the purposes of defining characteristics of space that may influence population health is that ZIP codes are very heterogeneous in terms of area and population size and population composition. ZIP code addresses correspond to historical post office locations, which may not correspond to current political nomenclature (e.g., names of places for the purposes of mailing addresses may differ from the name of the political unit). Historically, "Post Office names were typically suggested by prospective patrons; there are no postal records that explain their origin"(U.S. Postal Service, 2006b). Moreover, given that some ZIP codes refer to points or routes of delivery, it may be difficult to model spatial effects of ZIP codes. Although in some areas ZIP codes conform neatly to polygons (urban areas especially), in other areas (e.g., rural areas) polygons cannot be created accurately (U.S. Census Bureau, 2006b). Therefore, they are primarily a collection of linear or point features (e.g., carrier routes).

Although the system was geographically derived, the US Postal Service had created ZIP codes to facilitate efficient mail delivery, as groupings of mailing addresses or delivery nodes. According to the Census, "ZIP codes do not respect political or census statistical area boundaries. ZIP codes usually do not have clearly identifiable boundaries, often serve a continually changing area, are changed periodically to meet postal requirements, and do not cover all the land area of the United States" (US Census Bureau). ZIP code "boundaries do not necessarily follow clearly identifiable visible or invisible map features; also, the carrier routes for one ZIP code may intertwine with those of one or more other ZIP codes, and therefore this area is more conceptual than geographic" (US Census Bureau, 2001b). ZIP code boundaries often cross state, place, county, census tract, block group, and census block boundaries (US Census Bureau, 2006a). Although the geographic units by which the Census Bureau tabulates data are relatively stable across time, ZIP codes are altered periodically to meet day-to-day operational needs of the US Postal Service; thus, continuity across time may be a problem (U.S. Census Bureau, 2006a).

ZIP codes may approximate neighborhoods or cities, although that representation varies considerably. ZIP codes cover large geographic areas, including upwards of 30,000 people (Krieger, Williams, & Moss, 1997), though ZIP + 4 codes certainly improve precision. We recently documented that the median ZCTA in US metropolitan areas in year 2000 contained about 15,000 people. Ordering ZCTAs by population, the 1st quartile was at 6,723 people and 3rd quartile at 28,146. However, these sample sizes per ZCTA varied considerably (Osypuk, 2006).

4.2. Cities

4.2.1. Historical Roots and Why the Level May Matter for Health

Cities or townships are Minor Civil Divisions in the US and are considered tertiary political subdivisions (with states as primary political units below the federal government and counties as secondary political units). As such, this municipal level comprises one of the lower political units in the United States. Reporting data for the municipal level dates back to the first Census in 1790, with data provided for local governmental units (Plane, 2004). In 2002, there were 35,933 municipal or town/township general-purpose governments in the United States (US Census Bureau, 2004a). The largest cities in America house a good proportion of the US population. For instance, in the year 2000, 8.5 percent of the US population lived in the largest 10 cities, and 16 percent of the population lived in the largest 50 cities (U.S. Census Bureau, 2001c). Twenty-seven percent of the U.S. population lived in incorporated places (e.g., cities) of over 100,000 population (Katz & Lang, 2003).

The city or municipality is a politically relevant unit for education and service distribution, local public health regulation, and other domains of local control (e.g., zoning). Cities matter for health because of the immediate physical and social environments and the range of available services that they provide for residents, as well as economic and political factors (Galea, Freudenberg, & Vlahov, 2006). For instance, Galea and colleagues posit that three broad municipal-level determinants influence health, including government (policies and practices implemented in cities), markets (food, housing, labor), and civil society (community organizations, community capacity, social movements) (Freudenberg, Galea, & Vlahov, 2006; Galea et al., 2006).

Government influences population health via provision of municipal services, regulation of health activities, and dictation of parameters for urban development. Municipal services include education, social services, policing, courts/jails, fire services, housing, parks and recreation, sanitation, transit, environment protection/water supply, economic development, and zoning and urban planning (Freudenberg et al., 2006). As depicted in Figure 19.1, governmental expenditures at the city level accounted for 25 percent of all expenditures at the city, county, and state levels. Cities spend more on average than counties (comprising 16 percent of total expenditures) and spend less than half as much as states (comprising 59 percent of total expenditures). Three of the main expenditure categories for cities are for public utilities (water, electric, gas, transit), public safety (police protection, fire protection, corrections, protective inspection and regulation), and environment/housing (natural resources, parks and recreation, housing and community development, sewerage, solid waste management). As Figure 19.2 shows, cities spend more in these three categories than counties or even states (U.S. Census Bureau, 2004b). Therefore, the city level might be relevant for studying determinants of health in these or other domains where cities dominate governmental spending relative to other governmental levels. If one's research hypothesis relates to governmental provision of services or resources, then comparing governmental expenditures at different levels of government might be one criterion for deciding on an appropriate unit of analysis.

The network of cities comprising the core of every current major US region except Las Vegas was established in the 19th century (Katz & Lang, 2003), so historical factors certainly played a role in the evolution of US urban form. Freudenberg et al. (2006) emphasize four social trends that contributed to historical geographic explanations for health patterns: migration, suburbanization,

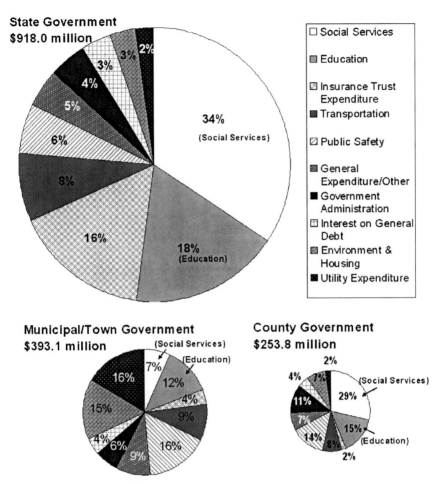

FIGURE 19.1.   Expenditure categories for state, county, and local governments, proportional to size of total expenditures, 2002 Census of Governments Social services (public welfare including cash assistance payments, vendor payments and other public welfare; hospitals; health; social insurance administration; veteran's services); education (higher, elementary, and secondary education; other education; libraries); insurance trust expenditure (unemployment compensation, employee retirement, workers' compensation, other); public safety (police protection, fire protection, correction, protective inspection and regulation); transportation (highways, airports, parking facilities, sea/inland port facilities, transit subsidies,); environment and housing (natural resources, parks and recreation, housing and community development, sewerage, solid waste management); general expenditure (miscellaneous commercial activities, other and unallocable); governmental administration (financial administration, judicial and legal, general public buildings, other); utility expenditure (water supply, electric supply, gas supply, transit); interest on general debt.

Source: U.S. Census Bureau, 2004b.

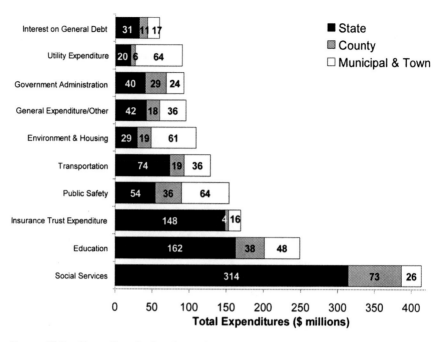

FIGURE 19.2.   Expenditure by function and government level for state, county, and local governments, Census of Government Expenditures 2001–2002. Social services (public welfare including cash assistance payments, vendor payments and other public welfare; hospitals; health; social insurance administration; veteran's services); education (higher, elementary, and secondary education; other education; libraries); insurance trust expenditure (unemployment compensation, employee retirement, workers' compensation, other); public safety (police protection, fire protection, correction, protective inspection and regulation); transportation (highways, airports, parking facilities, sea/inland port facilities, transit subsidies,); environment and housing (natural resources, parks and recreation, housing and community development, sewerage, solid waste management); general expenditure (miscellaneous commercial activities, other and unallocable); governmental administration (financial administration, judicial and legal, general public buildings, other); utility expenditure (water supply, electric supply, gas supply, transit); interest on general debt.

Source: U.S. Census Bureau, 2004b.

changes in the role of government, and changes in the global economy. Finally, Cities hold significant historical and non-historical meaning, which might be integral for the identity or pride of residents.

4.2.2. Drawbacks

Some residents in the US are not served by a municipal government because they live outside of incorporated areas. Therefore, examination of cities will exclude some portions of the population. A related drawback of choosing cities as a unit of analysis relates to truncation of the population distribution, leading to reduced variance or limited generalizability. For instance, choosing the city as the unit of analysis for a nationwide study of the largest US cities omits suburban populations. If one is interested in assessing the macrosocial determinants of racial or socioeconomic inequality, excluding suburban populations means omitting the most privileged group from the analysis, since development patterns and policies promoting suburban development have facilitated migration of higher social class, white populations to the suburbs.

Another central limitation to the use of cities as an analytic spatial unit of interest is the tremendous heterogeneity among cities and in their definitions; this is a drawback for other spatial units of analysis as well (counties, states, nations). Cities are complex communities of heterogeneous individuals, and although multiple factors are important determinants of population health, some of these factors may be unique to a specific city. Assessing how urban living may affect health raises issues often not easily addressed through the application of simple analytic methods. Empiric inquiry in health presupposes that there are identifiable factors that influence average levels of health. Although certain aspects of city living may be universal (e.g., population density) and relevant for the health of populations in different cities, other urban characteristics that are important in one city (e.g., local transportation patterns and air pollution) may not be important in others, limiting the generalizations that can be drawn about how urban living influences health.

Further complicating this task is the fact that the populations of cities change over time due to migration, which has implications for the relative contribution of different factors in affecting population health. For example, municipal taxation of alcohol and cigarettes may be an important determinant of alcohol and cigarette consumption in a particular city at one point in time (Grossman, 1989). However, changing social norms around smoking and alcohol use may either obviate or reinforce the influence of taxation. Therefore, when considering urban characteristics that affect health, it is important to note both the prevailing context within which such characteristics operate and that the role of these characteristics may change over time.

Finally, definitions of cities may vary. Particularly with regard to cross-national analysis, investigators must ensure consistent definition of cities. As discussed elsewhere in this book, the US Bureau of the Census (2006c) defines an urbanized area as "an area consisting of a central place(s) and adjacent territory with a general population density of at least 1,000 people per square mile of land area that together have a minimum residential population of at least 50,000 people." (US Census Bureau, 2006c) However, this definition, as all other possible definitions of "city", has inherent limitations. Most cities are actually far-reaching densely populated areas, containing peri-urban and suburban areas, which continue relatively uninterrupted for miles beyond the municipal city boundaries and the city center. Therefore, any empiric analysis that considers how characteristics of cities may influence population health must consider an appropriate definition of city that is relevant for all the urban units under consideration or cross-nationally.

4.3. Counties

4.3.1. Historical Roots and Why the Level May Matter for Health.

Counties are the primary divisions of US states. The United States has 3,066 counties, and 48 of the 50 US states maintain operational county governments[iii] (US Census Bureau, 2004a). Historically, the county is rooted in the function of English shires, which served a dual function as both an administrative body of the national government and the residents' local government. The framers of the US Constitution relegated local government to the power of states and thus did not call for local governments. State constitutions created the counties as an extension of state government. (National Association of Counties, 2006b)

Historically, the state mandated that counties perform tasks such as keeping property and vital statistics records, assessing property, administering elections and judicial functions, maintaining rural roads, and directing poverty programs. For instance, counties continue to handle responsibility for elections at all levels, including voter registration, education, and ensuring integrity of the voting process. Currently, counties also run programs including economic development, child welfare, consumer protection, zoning and planning, water quality, and training/employment. According to the 2002 US Census of Governments (depicted in Figure 19.1), county expenditures are allocated mostly to social services and health services – 29 percent for public welfare (e.g., cash assistance, hospitals, health, social insurance administration, and veteran's services), 15 percent for education services, 14 percent for public safety (e.g., police protection, fire protection, corrections), and 11 percent for governmental administration (financial administration, judicial and legal, general public buildings) (U.S. Census Bureau, 2004b). Relevant to analyses that consider the role of county-level characteristics that may influence population health, the majority of county employees have jobs in education, hospitals, and police protection, but other large job categories include streets/highways, corrections, public welfare, fire protection, health, justice/legal system, and financial administration (National Association of Counties, 2003, 2006b). Relative to state and city expenditures, however, county governmental expenditures budgets are small.

4.3.2. Drawbacks

As we discussed with regard to cities, counties vary greatly in their functions and service delivery, in terms of both infrastructure (utilities, water, roads) and social service responsibility. For instance, although most counties build and maintain roads as a core function, North Carolina counties have no responsibility to do so. In terms of service delivery, certain states entirely administer Medicaid (e.g., Alabama), alleviating counties of fiscal and administrative responsibility. However in Iowa, counties play a much larger fiscal role with Medicaid, e.g., funding 100 percent for certain waiver services not covered by the federal government and half of the case management funding not covered by the federal government. (National Association of Counties, 2003, 2006b)

The number and size of counties varies substantially throughout the states. For instance, Texas has the most counties (254), while Delaware and Hawaii have the least (3). County areal size ranges from 26 square miles in Arlington, VA, to 87,860 square miles in North Slope Borough, AL. County population size ranges from 67 residents in Loving County, TX, to 9.5 million residents in Los Angeles County, CA. (National Association of Counties, 2006a).

There are many differences among the states and counties in the form of their political areas. For instance, not all geographic areas called counties have county governments. In some places, like New York City and Philadelphia, municipal and county governments have merged or have been consolidated and are therefore counted as municipal governments for the purposes of government statistics. Some cities are outside areas of adjacent counties, and these independent cities are considered county equivalents – e.g., Baltimore, MD, Carson City, NV, St. Louis, MO, and 40 cities in Virginia (Plane, 2004). Therefore, almost 10 percent of the US population is not served by a county government, although in these cases they are served by a large municipal government (U.S. Census Bureau, 2004a). The majority of counties are sparsely populated; nearly three quarters of all county governments in 2000 were comprised of counties with populations under 50,000 (National Association of Counties, 2006b). Thus, an unweighted county-level analysis will overemphasize rural areas.

As noted in Figures 19.1 and 19.2, among sub-national government levels, counties expend fewer dollars than either cities or states, at least in the aggregate. Counties comprise only 28 percent of the size of state expenditures, but this may vary substantially in certain places or by expenditure category.

4.4. Metropolitan areas

4.4.1. Historical Roots and Why the Level May Matter for Health.

A metropolitan area is defined by the United States Office of Management and Budget (OMB) as a core area with a large population nucleus (an area containing at least one urbanized area with a population of at least 50,000) combined with adjacent communities that share a high degree of economic and social integration with that core (Office of Management and Budget & Spotila, 2000). The 1910 Census first officially recognized the metropolitan concept and designated metropolitan districts for cities with populations over 100,000. By 1930, the government expanded metropolitan district definitions to cities with populations of more than 50,000, creating 140 recognized metropolitan districts in 1940. Population density was the basis of metropolitan district boundaries from 1910 to 1940, and minor civil divisions (municipalities/cities/townships) were used as the building blocks. However, since 1950, counties have been the building blocks for delineating metropolitan units, except in New England, where towns are more powerful governmental units. Therefore, although they are not political units themselves, Metropolitan areas are defined using standard political areas (counties or towns) as their building blocks (Plane, 2004). Metropolitan areas are therefore much larger than cities and counties but smaller than states.

The Census defines three different types of metropolitan areas: Metropolitan Statistical Areas (MSAs), Consolidated Metropolitan Statistical Areas (CMSAs), and Primary Metropolitan Statistical Areas (PMSAs). CMSAs are large regions with a population size over 1 million, comprised of several smaller component parts (called PMSAs). MSAs are stand-alone metro areas that are not part of CMSAs. Since CMSAs are so much larger than typical employment markets, often metropolitan-level analyses include PMSAs and MSAs, not CMSAs (Jargowsky, 2003; Osypuk, 2005; Subramanian, Acevedo-Garcia, & Osypuk, 2005).

Over 80 percent of the US population resides in one of the 331 metropolitan areas defined in 1999 for the 2000 Census (Orfield, 2002). As such, the metropolitan area level captures how the majority of US residents interact with the housing market, job market, and educational systems, which operate beyond one city, county, and sometimes state boundary but usually within a regional area proxied by the metropolitan area spatial unit. Metropolitan areas may therefore be an appropriate level of analysis for racial inequality related to the housing market (including racial residential segregation, housing, lending) or to employment markets that may operate outside of any local jurisdiction.

The sociology literature suggests that the metropolitan area is a conceptually relevant unit for studying racial inequality (and links between racial inequality and health) because the significance of race may be powerful in terms of local race relations, residential housing and neighborhood processes, and labor market outcomes – processes that operate beyond individual-level attitudes or acts of discrimination. Metropolitan areas are the context within which geographic inequalities in the housing and education markets developed during the 20th century along a central city-suburban spatial divide (Frey, 2001; Jargowsky, 1997). Residential suburbanization and deconcentration of industry has transformed the geography of urban settlement, shifting new housing development and new jobs toward suburban areas – changes that have disproportionately harmed minorities (O'Connor, 2001). The concentration of minorities, especially African Americans, in impoverished neighborhoods of metropolitan areas embodies the spatial distribution of metropolitan racial inequality (Altshuler et al., 1999).

Metropolitan areas are frequently referred to as geographic regions; since much advertising is purchased locally, the metropolitan area may be a meaningful unit for analyzing advertising, marketing campaigns, and other media related health effects. Metropolitan areas may also be relevant for analyzing the built environment, given regional development patterns across the 20th century, e.g., suburban sprawl. Transportation infrastructure is often something that transcends one municipality to affect neighboring regional areas, as is sewage infrastructure or pollution.

4.4.2. Drawbacks

Unfortunately, metropolitan areas are often redefined at every Census, which complicates temporal comparisons. For instance, after the 2000 Census, the Census Bureau defined a new system for 2003, the Core Based Statistical Area (CBSA) classification, and this system is not entirely comparable to prior definitions of metropolitan areas. MA definition changes have chiefly occurred due to (1) recognition of new areas reaching the minimum required city area population and (2) addition of counties (or cities and towns in the case of New England) to existing areas as a result of new decennial Census data (U.S. Census Bureau, 2005a).

Americans often view the two components of metropolitan areas, suburbs and central city areas, as separate types of places; however, the interests and future of both places are intertwined, financially and otherwise (Orfield, 2002). Some problems require regional solutions, for instance transportation, water infrastructure, real estate prices. However, metropolitan areas are not very politically relevant units. A metropolitan area is not a legal or political entity but a statistical entity. There is rarely a political body corresponding to their boundaries. Indeed, state government deference to local governments with respect to land use, incorporation of municipalities, and fiscal systems has resulted in fragmented, decentralized structures that have exacerbated socioeconomic and racial inequality (Altshuler et al., 1999). Despite the current political limitations to metropolitan governance, some advocate political strategies to pursue a common regional agenda, e.g., "Metropolitics" and regionalism for community growth (Orfield, 2002). Some places have developed regional governance bodies to share the cost burdens of transportation or to contain growth patterns (e.g., Minneapolis, MN, Portland, OR), but they remain the exception. For researchers positing political hypotheses for health, this suggests that MAs are unlikely to be the most relevant unit of analysis.

Additional drawbacks of the metropolitan unit include exclusion of the rural population, and as with other units discussed here, there is vast heterogeneity in the physical size and population composition of MAs across the US.

4.5. States

4.5.1. Historical Roots and Why the Level May Matter for Health

States are the primary political units in the US. There are 50 states in the United States proper, although the District of Columbia is treated equivalently to states by the Census Bureau (Plane, 2004). Since states are responsible for service provision to their populations, they are a relevant level for many public health programs. The majority of public health statutes in the US are found at the state level, including the missions, functions, structures, and powers of public health agencies (Gostin, Koplan, & Grad, 2003). Indeed, many responsibilities not set forth explicitly for the (relatively weak) federal government by the US Constitution fall to states. As a result, judicial case law often reinforces the realm of states to exert power in areas of health and public health.

Government at any level, although especially the state level, has several tools to promote public health, including tax and spend policy; the power to shape the informational environment; direct regulation of individuals (e.g., behavior such as seatbelt use), professionals (licensing), or businesses (restaurant health codes); indirect regulation through tort litigation (to incite businesses to engage in less risky activities, e.g., the tobacco Master Settlement Agreement, litigation to restrict tobacco advertising and promotion); and deregulation (Gostin et al., 2003). For instance, states are relevant for health because elected officials as part of state legislatures or regulatory bodies pass numerous laws and regulations (Osypuk, Kawachi, Subramanian, & Acevedo-Garcia, 2006). States are therefore particularly relevant units for statistical analyses because of the policies they enact.

States also directly implement and evaluate health programs to ensure the health of their populations. To that end, states routinely collect information for monitoring, planning, and evaluation of programs. States also use health data to inform program eligibility (e.g., Medicaid, SCHIP). Identifying geographic patterns in health at the state level allows the prioritizing of programs and allocating of resources for high-risk populations, as well as planning for future disease treatment programs (Osypuk et al., 2006). As Figure 19.1 and Figure 19.2 demonstrate, the state expenditures far outweigh those of county and local governments, at over twice the size of local governments and 4 times the size of county government expenditures (US Census Bureau, 2004b). States spend the majority of their budget on social service and insurance trust provision, including for welfare cash assistance payments, hospitals, health, social insurance administration, veteran's services, unemployment compensation, employee retirement, and workers' compensation (US Census Bureau, 2004b).

4.5.2. Drawbacks

As with other political levels we have discussed here, the size, form, and function of states and their governments differ considerably across the United States. Some states are almost entirely rural, while others are dominated by very large urban areas. States differ along many dimensions aside from size, including the composition of the population, economic activity, urban/rural residence, and climate – all of which likely affect health. For instance, some states are destination points for large numbers of immigrants (New York, California, Texas), while others contain practically no immigrants. Some states house large numbers of so-called "snow-birds" – retired persons migrating from northern states to warmer states, e.g., Florida or Arizona. As such, Florida has the highest average population age. Therefore, without standardizing the population by age, Florida and other snowbird states would appear to contain an excess of disease, since age is a strong individual-level predictor of morbidity and mortality.

Some phenomena under study are less relevant for state level analysis because the state has failed to step in with policy or action. For instance, land use policies are typically localized, and although states theoretically could regulate this area, they typically do not. Therefore, in this instance, state would be the less appropriate level for analysis, and localities or municipalities would be the more appropriate level. Further, although states may be attractive and appropriate for some types of policy analysis, if the responsibility for funding programs or enforcing the laws falls to lower governmental units (e.g., counties), then modeling these lower units is more fitting. Lastly, many state laws or regulations (e.g., state health codes) are quite fragmented because they evolved independently, resulting in profound differences among states in the structure, content, and procedures of regulations for disease monitoring, control, and prevention (Gostin et al., 2003).

4.6. Nations

4.6.1. Historical Roots and Why the Level May Matter for Health

Countries are clearly the relevant spatial unit of interest when we are concerned with the influence of macro-level social and economic factors that relate to national governmental decisions and actions. Nations are appropriate units because of the power of federal governments to create policies, to tax and spend, and to regulate activities in all sectors of life. For instance, some countries have passed comprehensive social policies to aid their populations, and these policies likely affect health through their influence on socioeconomic position or provision of concrete resources to the population (e.g., subsidies to buy housing or health care). Since they are financed by federal government dollars (raised by taxation), these social policies are redistributive in domains such as education, child care/maternity policy, unemployment, and health care. Taxation is largely controlled at the national level, although variation within any nation may exist (e.g., in the US there is variation in state and local income tax rates), and taxation is one main income redistribution mechanism. Because the nation is such a relevant level for income distribution (e.g., minimum wage policy) and redistribution (e.g., taxation, payroll deductions for social programs), some investigators have found the unit appropriate for examining how income inequality between countries may affect population health (Wilkinson, 1992b, 1992a; Wilkinson & Pickett, 2006). Health economists have studied national factors such as economic development, political economy, and employment structure in relation to health. For instance, capitalism (Cereseto & Waitzkin, 1986a, 1986b) or the degree of political freedom (e.g., democracy) (Franco, Alvarez-Dardet, & Ruiz, 2004; Martyn, 2004) may be associated with population health.

The federal government plays a key role in ensuring quality of consumer products and of the food supply in the US by regulating corporate practices. For example, some impacts on food supply relate to the nutritional content of nationally distributed packaged goods. Therefore, the inclusion of harmful or less nutritionally beneficial ingredients in this food supply (e.g., trans fats) may only be regulated at the federal level. Federal governments can also add nutrient additives to the food supply to prevent disease, for instance, fortification of bread with folic acid to prevent neural tube defects or fortification of water with fluoride to prevent tooth decay (Grosse, Waitzman, Romano, & Mulinare, 2005). Government at this level also can regulate the safety of products, for example, standardizing automobile design, mandating lower vehicle emissions, mandating flame-retardant children's clothing, or regulating firearms (Hahn, et al., 2005). Economic development is beneficial for population health and economic cycles may operate at the national level (or above – e.g., the Great Depression). Some have researched how between-country differences in diet, family structure, social custom, or distribution of income within a society may influence health (Kawachi, Wilkinson, & Kennedy, 1999; Rose, 1992). The national level may also be meaningful for examining between-country corporate practices that may affect health but are not adequately regulated by government – e.g., tobacco marketing, product design, or advertising (Ballin, 1994; Freudenberg, 2005; Gilmore & McKee, 2004). It will be interesting to observe whether national boundaries may decline in importance in places where international migration is easier (e.g., the European Union).

4.6.2. Drawbacks

One of the primary drawbacks of cross-national studies is the availability of data. Although data is more often available for ecologic studies, multilevel studies require individual-level data to examine contributions to individual health. Cross-national comparisons are difficult given the variations in the fundamental geographic units for which data is gathered in different countries (variations in name, function, power of primary and secondary political units) (Plane, 2004). International comparisons are additionally complicated by the many other factors by which nations differ from each other; issues such as the meaning and measurement of constructs may be complicated by multiplicities of language and cultural differences. As discussed in relation to other levels, countries are incredibly heterogeneous and impart different historical meaning and identities to their residents.

4.7. Other Administrative Units

4.7.1. Historical Roots and Why the Level May Matter for Health

Spatial areas delineated for administrative purposes may be appropriate for studying health if the causal processes are related to that unit. Examples include Congressional districts (the districts with an elected representative in the U.S. House of Representatives), legislative districts (those represented by lawmakers in the state legislature), school districts, traffic zones, and neighborhood planning districts (Plane, 2004). For instance, Congressional districts may be relevant for examining policy making, voting districts may be relevant for measuring political empowerment or disenfranchisement, and police precincts are relevant if police monitor these areas and provide crime statistics at that level.

There were 34,683 specialized-function governments (aside from school districts) according to the 1997 Census of Governments (Plane, 2004). Special district governments provide a single service or one group of related specific services not supplied by general purpose governments, for instance, hospitals, fire protection, mosquito abatement, or cemetery maintenance (U.S. Census Bureau, 2004a). Analyzing special district governmental units would therefore be relevant when examining such purposes as they relate to public health (e.g., mosquito abatement related to vector-born infectious disease). Once again, use of an administrative unit makes sense if the exposure or the outcome is conceptually patterned at this level.

4.7.2. Drawbacks

Since specialized governmental entities are very specific, the causal pathways must be conceptually relevant. Further, depending on the unit and its usage by administrative bodies, these units may or may not be stable across time; for instance, in some western states, election precincts may be altered after each election based on the number of votes cast (Plane, 2004).

5. Practical Issues: Operationalizing Constructs and Units

Choice of unit or level for analysis affects all aspects of one's study. Many of these issues overlap, so although we organize them here in certain categories, they should not be considered mutually exclusive. We recommend that a number of factors be taken under consideration when an investigator chooses the levels and units of analysis in his/her study. The spatial level at which an exposure of interest is measured may influence the construct validity of the exposure measure, the internal validity and external validity of the study, and the potential threats to statistical conclusion validity due to data availability and power. We will discuss each of these topics in turn below. Ultimately, as discussed, one must refer to theory to explicate constructs of interest and to specify the causal model.

5.1. Validity

First, choice of level affects construct validity, which is defined as whether the measured variable accurately represents the higher order construct (Shadish, Cook, & Campbell, 2002). The two issues involved with construct validity include initially conceptualizing a construct and then operationalizing or measuring it (Shadish et al., 2002). The first is theoretical, the second empirical. If the construct is operationalized or estimated with error, a biased estimation results. An important, and perhaps the primary, threat to construct validity here is measurement error; this is discussed below as it relates to threats to validity arising from how one operationalizes levels and boundaries.

Second, choice of level affects internal validity. Internal validity refers to inferences about whether the covariation between two variables reflects an unbiased causal relationship (Shadish et al., 2002). Serious threats to internal validity include selection and confounding, which we will discuss below. Another issue with regard to internal validity is the validity of inferences that derive from the data and study design, since the study design (including level of data) bears greatly here.

Third, external validity will be affected by one's choice of unit, defined as the inferences of whether a presumed causal effect is maintained across variations in persons, settings, treatment variables, and measurement variables (Shadish et al., 2002). Fourth, statistical conclusion validity concerns the use of statistics for inferring covariation of two variables, including whether the observed covariation of two variables is likely due to chance (Shadish et al., 2002). Statistical conclusion validity concerns power, sample size, and effect sizes.

5.2. Data Availability and Power

Even if one identifies the ideal level, definition of units at that level, or spatial range of exposure, the availability of data at that level may be limited (Macintyre et al., 2002). Else, if primary data collection is desired, cost may be limiting. Secondary data may be helpful. Some secondary data is not released as individual-level units or at units small enough to be manipulated in the way researchers may want; often data is aggregated into larger units, e.g., for confidentiality protections, so the researcher may have to manage with the unit available to him/her.

Data used by researchers is often collected for other purposes (e.g., administrative purposes) (Diez Roux, 2005). Therefore, it is important to examine whether the data is etiologically relevant for the health outcome or exposure process under study. If not, construct validity is threatened. If cost required for primary data collection limits data availability, one solution may be to collaborate efforts across studies in the same area for shared data collection efforts (O'Campo, 2003).

Power may be limited in studies where data was intended for only individual-level analysis, and this threatens statistical conclusion validity. In multilevel analysis, power is determined by the number of groups and by the number of observations per group (Diez Roux, 2005). The former determines the power to assess between-context associations; the latter determines power for within-context associations (Duncan et al., 1998). Sparse data means analyses are possible only at higher levels (e.g., cities, counties) rather than at lower levels (census tracts). Power is also influenced by the variability or homogeneity of the sample. The same techniques that increase power in an individual-level study will also generally improve power in a multilevel study, including larger heterogeneity and range of units on the independent variable; matching, stratifying or blocking; multivariate analysis; using larger sample sizes; using equal cell sample sizes; improving measurement; reducing random setting irrelevancies; and ensuring that assumptions are met for powerful statistical tests (Shadish et al., 2002). For instance, one will have more power to detect area socioeconomic effects on health with homogeneous socioeconomic areas, and areas tend to be more internally homogeneous at smaller levels (Greenland, 2002).

5.3. Operationalizing Levels and Boundaries

Although operationalizing or defining the relevant unit of analysis is straightforward in some cases, such as institutional settings (e.g. schools) or political boundaries, it can be more challenging in other cases – especially with regard to neighborhoods. The bounding or definition of neighborhoods in neighborhood health research is a topic of contention (O'Campo, 2003). As with any exposure, bias can result if the neighborhood construct of interest does not map onto the units chosen for operationalizing neighborhoods and their constructs. Defining neighborhoods (or any relevant unit) mainly threatens construct validity, although it threatens internal validity as well (e.g., non-differential exposure misclassification tends to bias the effect estimate towards the null).

One important methodologic problem for operationalizing neighborhood boundaries and interpreting the conclusions in spatial studies is the Modifiable Areal Unit Problem, commonly known as MAUP. MAUP is defined as "a problem resulting from the imposition of artificial units of spatial reporting on continuous geographical phenomenon resulting in the generation of artificial spatial patterns" (Heywood, 1998). MAUP is a concern in spatial analyses when the definitions of boundaries may be unclear, and as a result, differences in how one draws spatial boundaries may lead to artificial statistical spatial patterns – an issue of exposure misclassification. Two issues are at play with MAUP – scale and aggregation. First, the scale problem results in different statistical answers when the same data is aggregated at different scales (corresponding to different sizes of areal units). If one does not have a clear idea about the level at which a certain phenomenon is operating, one might choose a certain unit of analysis because it minimizes aggregation bias. For example, Bailey and Peterson (1995) chose cities instead of metro areas or states in an analysis of how gender socioeconomic inequality affects female homicide victimization because cities minimized aggregation bias; as crime statistics are collected at the city level, modeling crime statistics at higher levels (metro areas or states) would have required aggregating data collected at the city level.

The second MAUP issue is the aggregation problem or zoning effect, which occurs when one receives a different answer when drawing the line differently at a particular scale (Yang, 2005). For instance, a neighborhood social phenomenon that may affect health (for instance, social capital) is not likely bounded by the edges defined by tract boundaries. In other words, social capital may not be sharply higher or lower as one crosses the arbitrary census tract boundaries. *Some* census tract boundaries may coincide with sharp breaks in the true construct of social capital, e.g., breaks that occur across a busy street or highway that is difficult to traverse or across a river or ravine, because this geographic boundary meaningfully separates different people from these places, and there may be little social mingling across the barrier. However, social capital in other places may gradually decrease or increase across space, despite the fact that our methods model the construct as abruptly decreasing or increasing across these boundaries.

The issue of how to define neighborhoods may also be a conceptual one. For instance, how an outsider defines neighborhood boundaries might be different from how a resident him/herself does. There is also likely heterogeneity within a certain neighborhood as to how residents define their neighborhood. It is difficult to claim that these differences are simply a result of measurement error; it is more likely that the underlying construct of neighborhood varies for different people. If one is interested in social exposures that affect health (e.g., social interactions), then resident perceptions or definitions of neighborhood might be more relevant for that examination than for, say, resource distribution, which may occur according to administrative boundaries (Diez Roux, 2001). It is also important to keep in mind that some processes occurring in neighborhoods that an investigator hypothesizes to affect health (e.g., social networks) are not necessarily contained within any given spatial boundary (O'Campo, 2003).

Although the challenges for operationalizing relevant neighborhoods are important to consider as one weighs level of analyses, they should not paralyze one's empiric investigation (Diez Roux, 2001). Since different phenomena may operate at different scales to affect health, multiple appropriate neighborhood units may be defined to accommodate inclusion in one's study of multiple processes that operate in the neighborhood environment, including institutional, political, economic, or cultural phenomena (O'Campo, 2003). Indeed, a multitude of different groups/units may be relevant for a specific research question (Diez Roux, 2004b).

One satisfactory solution for bounding neighborhoods is to define them according to how the city planners define them, which may also relate to resource or service distribution (e.g., public utilities, public safety services like policing). For instance, some neighborhood health studies have identified neighborhoods by how cities identify them for administrative purposes – e.g., the 59 New York City community districts (New York City Department of City Planning, 2006) or the 77 Chicago community areas.

Finally, although neighborhoods have dominated the discussion in the literature with regard to proper bounding of areas, it is certainly not the only level featuring challenges to operationalization. For example, another level that might be difficult to operationalize is media markets, which may be relevant for health-related communications messages – e.g., the reach of television stations in a metropolitan area. There may be difficulties in defining a market based on topography that dictates signal strength or on individual subscription to cable versus satellite providers.

5.4. Measurement and Measurement Error

Although epidemiologists have become sophisticated at measuring individual-level phenomena, measuring group-level phenomena related to health remains in its infancy (Diez Roux, 2004b; Diez Roux et al., 2005; Oakes & Kaufman, 2006). As a result, existing studies have measured group-level effects with much measurement error, and these exposures may be grossly misspecified, either because of error in defining the group or in operationalizing the group-level variable (Diez Roux et al., 2005). Many population-level causes of health are irreducible to individual level analogs and are thus constitutive properties of only populations. Examples of such causes are income inequality and herd immunity, two determinants of population health that have no individual analog. Although some group-level variables have analogs at the individual level or at multiple higher-levels, their meaning and theoretical connection to health likely differs at each level (Diez Roux, 2000). We refer the reader to other sources for further discussion of group-level factors in epidemiologic study (Diez Roux, 2001, 2004b).

Measurement reliability and study replicability are affected by choice of macro-level units, since both refer to the reproducibility of measurement or results across different variables or studies. For instance, one reason to employ a certain level of analysis may be because the rest of the literature does it that way. Replicating analytic approaches from prior studies improves the comparability of results across studies and communicates transparency of methods. Thus, one might choose cities as the unit of analysis because all other studies in the extant literature do so as well (Bailey & Peterson, 1995). Types of reliability include interrater (how different people define the same construct in the same way) and test-retest reliability (the stability of the construct and its measure across time). These dimensions of reliability relate to measurement of the construct of interest (construct validity); while the issues involved with macro-level constructs may be extended from the individual-level psychometric literature, there are other reliability issues specific to the ecometrics of context. Consider an example where we assess the reliability of a measure of school context derived from a scale reported by individual teachers. Psychometric principles suggest that the reliability of a measure can be increased by adding more items to a scale; more important for improving the reliability of the school level measure is increasing the degree of rater agreement within a school and increasing the number of raters per school (Raudenbush & Sampson, 1999). While some investigators have proposed statistical methods to assess the validity and reliability of group-level measures (e.g., Raudenbush et al., 1999), creation of valid and reliable measures of context as they relate to health remains a need in the public health literature (Diez Roux, 2001, 2004b; Raudenbush et al., 1999).

5.5. Inference

The level of data aggregation for the variable affects the inference and meaning of the variable. For instance, the unemployment variable at census tract-level seems to indicate the relative deprivation or affluence of the tract population; however, tract-level unemployment would not represent employment markets since people travel well beyond their own tract of residence for work. An unemployment rate at the city, metro, or state level is more likely representative of structurally-patterned employment opportunities since employment markets operate at these levels; moreover, unemployment rates at these levels seem orthogonal to other aspects of relative affluence or deprivation levels at these levels (Land, Cantor, & Russell, 1995). At the national level, unemployment rates fluctuate with business cycles (Land et al., 1995) and would not be appropriate measures of relative affluence or deprivation.

The level of variable operationalization holds implications for the level at which one may derive inferences about study effects. False inferences arise when there is a mismatch between the level at which one has data and the level at which one wants to infer effects; these errors have been classified as the ecologic fallacy, atomistic fallacy, psychologistic fallacy, or sociologistic fallacy, depending on the mismatch. Ecologic fallacy is committed when one uses group level data to draw inferences about relationships at the individual level. Conversely, the atomistic fallacy may be present when one makes inferences about groups or group-level variables based on individual-level data (or more generally, drawing inferences about units at a higher level based on data collected for units at a lower level).

Fallacies arising from mismatch between data and inferences have received considerable attention in epidemiology; however, other more substantive problems regarding ignoring variables at different levels have not been as much discussed (Diez Roux, 2000). For instance, the psychologistic fallacy derives from failing to consider group characteristics when drawing inferences about causes of variability among individuals. In other words, this fallacy arises when one assumes that exclusively individual-level characteristics explain individual-level outcomes. Conversely, the sociologistic fallacy arises when one fails to consider individual level characteristics when making inferences about the causes of variability among groups (Diez Roux, 2002b). Ultimately, to avoid incorrect inferences, the researcher needs to use the right level of data as well as appropriate methods to ask the right question (Schwartz & Carpenter, 1999). Further, although this discussion has focused on choosing one level of analysis for study, disease processes related to social structure invariably concern multiple levels of constructs that may operate independently, successively, or simultaneously to affect health. As discussed in other chapters of this book, a more comprehensive understanding of disease processes will be gained by considering these multiple levels of causes and understanding their causal associations with health.

Generalizability, or external validity, is another relevant inferential issue to consider when choosing one's macro-level data. External validity is determined by the structure and execution of the sampling frame/plan with respect to the theoretical study population. For example, if data are based on a survey, then that data might not be representative at smaller levels than the specified sampling frame. In the same vein, the sampling frame must be examined closely to guide methodologic issues regarding how certain levels should be represented in a multilevel model. For example, in a multistage sample design it is unclear whether a level that was not part of the sampling frame should be used as a level in the analyses. If it is used, certain variance correction techniques may need to be undertaken to adjust properly for clustering (e.g., in the outcome); investigators of multistage samples often view clustering as a necessary nuisance for more efficient survey execution instead of as an inherent piece of information that may relate to common causes. However, the capacity is currently limited for common multilevel statistical programs to adjust for multistage survey designs and simultaneously model variance at different levels, particularly if the primary sampling units are masked for confidentiality (Osypuk et al., 2006).

5.6. Policy or Intervention Relevance

Other criteria that might guide decisions about level of analysis may relate to the purpose of the analysis in terms of the salience of one level for action versus another (O'Campo & Kogan, 2005). From this perspective, policy actionability is constrained by political or administrative boundaries, since political boundaries are relevant for distribution or exclusion of rights, services, and resources. For instance, one drawback to examining the city level concerns the ability of policy at the city level to address regional issues – issues that transcend one city – e.g., sprawl or transportation infrastructure. Even if cities represent a conceptually-relevant unit, cities have fewer resources to address public health problems and their antecedents, including a declining local tax base, declining federal financial support, and limited national leadership to advance an urban agenda (Freudenberg et al., 2006). Alternately, as we have discussed, examining neighborhoods has limited policy relevance, although it may be related to administrative distribution of resources (e.g., targeting of programs for the elderly based on the population distribution of elders by neighborhood).

6. Conclusion

The goal of this chapter was to provide conceptual and practical guidance for choosing a macro-level unit that is relevant for examining how place affects population health. We aim to stimulate investigation of multiple systems, including various structural, political, physical, social, or organizational attributes of place, as potential upstream determinants of population health (Diez Roux, 2001). By articulating theoretical and empirical justifications for using alternate definitions of place, including neighborhoods, cities, counties, metropolitan areas, states, and nations, we strive to broaden the conceptualization of how place affects health in a way that may be useful for future research. We hope that research that considers the potential influence of factors at multiple and different levels of space can contribute to a more complete understanding of the macrosocial determination of the health of populations.

Endnotes

i. For the purposes of this chapter, levels are composed of spatial units that can be observed, sampled, and analyzed (Leyland & Groenewegen, 2003).

ii. Multilevel modeling, or hierarchical linear modeling, refers to a method whereby variables are statistically modeled at 2 or more levels, the outcome variance is partitioned into 2 or more levels, and units are often nested (e.g. individuals within neighborhoods). Multilevel modeling allows examination of group level and individual level variables on individual-level outcomes and accounts for the dependence of observations within groups (Diez Roux, 2002b).

iii. Although Rhode Island and Connecticut are divided into counties, the counties do not employ functioning governments as defined by the Census Bureau. Certain other areas in the US may also be called counties but lack county governments. Alaska calls its county government a borough, and Louisiana a parish, and both are classified as counties for the purposes of the census statistics of US governments (U.S. Census Bureau, 2004a).

Aknowledgments.   The authors would like to thank M. Maria Glymour, Steve Cummins, and the anonymous reviewer for their helpful comments. We also thank the Robert Wood Johnson Foundation for their financial support of this work via the Health and Society Scholars Program.

References

Acevedo-Garcia, D., Lochner, K. A., Osypuk, T. L., & Subramanian, S. V. (2003). Future directions in residential segregation and health research: A multilevel approach. *American Journal of Public Health, 93*(2), 215–221.

Altshuler, A., Morrill, W., Wolman, H., Mitchell, F., & Committee on Improving the Future of U.S. Cities Through Improved Metropolitan Area Governance (1999). *Governance and opportunity in metropolitan America.* Washington, DC: National Academy Press.

Anderson, E., & Massey, D. S. (2001). The sociology of race in the United States. In E. Anderson & D. S. Massey (Eds.), *Problem of the century: Racial stratification in the United States.* New York: Russell Sage Foundation.

Bailey, W. C., & Peterson, R. D. (1995). Gender inequality and violence against women. In J. Hagan & R. D. Peterson (Eds.), *Crime and inequality.* Stanford, CA: Stanford University Press.

Ballin, S. D. (1994). Thirty years of tobacco industry domination of tobacco control efforts in the federal government. *Circulation, 89*(2), 543–544.

Booth, C. (2001). On the city: Physical pattern and social structure. Introduction. In G. Davey Smith, D. Dorling, & M. Shaw (Eds.), *Poverty, inequality, and health in Britain 1800–2000: A reader.* Bristol, UK: The Policy Press.

Castree, N. (2004). Differential geographies: Place, indigenous rights, and "local" resources. *Political Geography, 23*, 133–167.

Cereseto, S., & Waitzkin, H. (1986a). Capitalism, socialism, and the physical quality of life. *International Journal of Health Services, 16*(4), 643–658.

Cereseto, S., & Waitzkin, H. (1986b). Economic development, political-economic system, and the physical quality of life. *American Journal of Public Health, 76*(6), 661–666.

Cummins, S., Curtis, S., Diez Roux, A. V., & Macintyre, S. (In press). Understanding and representing "place" in health research: a relational approach. *Social Science & Medicine.*

Davey Smith, G., Dorling, D., & Shaw, M. (2001). *Poverty, inequality, and health in Britain 1800–2000: A reader.* Bristol, UK: The Policy Press

Diez Roux, A. V. (2007). Neighborhoods and health: where are we and where do we go from here? *Revue d'Epidemiologie et de Sante Publique, 55*(1), 13–21.

Diez Roux, A. V. (2000). Multilevel analysis in public health research. *Annual Review of Public Health, 21*, 171–192.

Diez Roux, A. V. (2001). Investigating neighborhood and area effects on health. *American Journal of Public Health, 91*(11), 1783–1789.

Diez Roux, A. V. (2002a). Invited commentary: Places, people, and health. *American Journal of Epidemiology, 155*(6), 516–519.

Diez Roux, A. V. (2002b). A glossary for multilevel analysis. *Journal of Epidemiology and Community Health, 56*(8), 588–594.

Diez Roux, A. V. (2003). Issues related to multiple levels of organization. In I. Kawachi & L. F. Berkman (Eds.), *Neighborhoods and health.* New York: Oxford University Press.

Diez Roux, A. V. (2004a). Estimating neighborhood health effects: The challenges of causal inference in a complex world. *Social Science & Medicine, 58*(10), 1953–1960.

Diez Roux, A. V. (2004b). The study of group-level factors in epidemiology: Rethinking variables, study designs, and analytical approaches. *Epidemiologic Reviews, 26*(1), 104–111.

Diez Roux, A. V. (2005). Commentary: Estimating and understanding area health effects. *International Journal of Epidemiology, 34*(2), 284–285.

Diez Roux, A. V., & Aiello, A. E. (2005). Multilevel analysis of infectious diseases. *Journal of Infectious Disease, 191*(Supplement 1), S25–S33.

Duncan, C., Jones, K., & Moon, G. (1998). Context, composition, and heterogeneity: Using multilevel models in health research. *Social Science & Medicine, 46*(1), 97–117.

Ellen, I. G. (2000). Is segregation bad for your health? The case of low birth weight. In W. G. Gale & J. R. Pack (Eds.), *Brookings-Wharton papers on urban affairs 2000.* Washington, DC: Brookings Institution Press.

Ellen, I. G., Mijanovich, T., & Dillman, K. N. (2001). Neighborhood effects on health: Exploring the links and assessing the evidence. *Journal of Urban Affairs, 23*(3–4), 391–408.

Engels, F. (1845). The condition of the working class in England. The great towns. In G. Davey Smith, D. Dorling, & M. Shaw (Eds.), *Poverty, inequality, and health in Britain 1800–2000: A reader.* Bristol, UK: The Policy Press.

FANS, L. A. (2006). The Los Angeles Family and Neighborhood Survey: Overview of L.A. FANS Survey Design. RAND. (August 2, 2006); http://www.lasurvey.rand.org/thesurvey.htm.

Farr, W. (2001). Vital statistics: A memorial volume of selections from the reports and writings of William Farr. In G. Davey Smith, D. Dorling, & M. Shaw (Eds.), *Poverty, inequality, and health in Britain 1800–2000: A reader.* Bristol, UK: The Policy Press.

Franco, A., Alvarez-Dardet, C., & Ruiz, M. (2004). Effect of democracy on health: Ecological study. *British Medical Journal, 329*(7480), 1421–1423.

Frank, L. D., & Engelke, P. O. (2001). The built environment and human activity patterns: Exploring the impacts of urban form on public health. *Journal of Planning Literature, 16*(2), 202–218.

Frank, L. D., & Engelke, P. (2005). Multiple impacts of the built environment on public health: Walkable places and the exposure to air pollution. *International Regional Science Review, 28*(2), 193–216.

Freudenberg, N. (2005). Public health advocacy to change corporate practices: Implications for health education practice and research. *Health Education and Behavior, 32*(3), 298–319.

Freudenberg, N., Galea, S., & Vlahov, D. (2006). Changing living conditions; changing health: US cities since World War II. In N. Freudenberg, S. Galea, & D. Vlahov (Eds.), *Cities and the health of the public.* Nashville, TN: Vanderbilt.

Frey, W. H. (2001). *Melting pot suburbs: A census 2000 study of suburban diversity. Census 2000 Series.* Washington, DC: The Brookings Institution Center on Urban & Metropolitan Policy.

Galea, S., Freudenberg, N., & Vlahov, D. (2006). A framework for the study of urban health. In N. Freudenberg, S. Galea, & D. Vlahov (Eds.), *Cities and the health of the public.* Nashville, TN: Vanderbilt.

Gilmore, A., & McKee, M. (2004). Tobacco and transition: An overview of industry investments, impact and influence in the former Soviet Union. *Tobacco Control, 13,* 136–142.

Gostin, L. O., Koplan, J. P., & Grad, F. P. (2003). The law and the public's health: The foundation. In R. A. Goodman, M. A. Rothstein, R. E. Hoffman, W. Lopez, & G. W. Matthews (Eds.), *Law in public health practice.* New York: Oxford University Press.

Greenland, S. (2002). A review of multilevel theory for ecologic analyses. *Statistics in Medicine, 21*, 389–395.

Grosse, S. D., Waitzman, N. J., Romano, P. S., & Mulinare, J. (2005). Reevaluating the benefits of folic acid fortification in the United States: Economic analysis, regulation, and public health. *American Journal of Public Health, 95*(11), 1917–1922.

Grossman, M. (1989). Health benefits of increases in alcohol and cigarette taxes. *British Journal of Addiction, 84*, 1193–1204.

Hahn, R., Bilukha, O., Crosby, A., Fullilove, M., Liberman, A., Moscicki, E., et al. (2005). Firearms laws and the reduction of violence: A systematic review. *American Journal of Preventive Medicine, 28*(2 Supplement 1), 40–71.

Harvey, D. (1973). *Social justice and the city.* London: Edward Arnold Publishers Ltd.

Harvey, D. (2006). Space as a keyword. In N. Castree & D. Gregory (Eds.), *David Harvey: A critical reader.* Malden, MA: Blackwell Publishing.

Heywood, D. I. (1998). *Introduction to geographical information systems.* New York: Addison Wesley Longman

Jargowsky, P. A. (1997). *Poverty and place: Ghettos, barrios, and the American city.* New York: Russell Sage Foundation

Jargowsky, P. A. (2003). Stunning progress, hidden problems: The dramatic decline of concentrated poverty in the 1990s. In Center on Urban and Metropolitan Policy (Ed.), Washington, DC: Brookings Institution.

Katz, B., & Lang, R. E. (2003). Introduction. In B. Katz & R. E. Lang (Eds.), *Redefining urban & suburban America: Evidence from census 2000.* Washington, DC: Brookings Institution

Kawachi, I., Wilkinson, R. G., & Kennedy, B. P. (1999). Introduction. In I. Kawachi, B. P. Kennedy, & R. G. Wilkinson (Eds.), *The society and population health reader: Income inequality and health.* New York: The New Press.

Kawachi, I., & Berkman, L. F. (2003a). *Neighborhoods and health.* New York, NY: Oxford University Press

Kawachi, I., & Berkman, L. F. (2003b). Introduction. In I. Kawachi & L. F. Berkman (Eds.), *Neighborhoods and health.* New York: Oxford University Press.

Krieger, N. (2001). Historical roots of social epidemiology: Socioeconomic gradients in health and contextual analysis (letter to the editor). *International Journal of Epidemiology, 30*, 899–900.

Krieger, N., Williams, D. R., & Moss, N. E. (1997). Measuring social class in US public health research: Concepts, methodologies, and guidelines. *Annual Review of Public Health, 18*(1), 341–378.

Land, K. C., Cantor, D., & Russell, S. T. (1995). Unemployment and crime rate fluctuations. In J. Hagan & R.D. Peterson (Eds.), *Crime and inequality.* Stanford, CA: Stanford University Press.

Leyland, A. H., & Groenewegen, P. P. (2003). Multilevel modeling and public health policy. *Scandinavian Journal of Public Health, 31*, 267–274.

Link, B. G., & Phelan, J. C. (1996). Editorial: Understanding sociodemographic differences in health — The role of fundamental social causes. *American Journal of Public Health, 86*(4), 471–473.

Macintyre, S., & Ellaway, A. (2003). Neighborhoods and health: An overview. In I. Kawachi & L.F. Berkman (Eds.), *Neighborhoods and health.* New York: Oxford University Press.

Macintyre, S., Ellaway, A., & Cummins, S. (2002). Place effects on health: How can we conceptualise, operationalise, and measure them? *Social Science & Medicine, 55*, 125–139.

Martyn, C. (2004). Politics as a determinant of health. *British Medical Journal, 329*(7480), 1423–1424.

Massey, D. (1991). The political place of locality studies. *Environment and Planning Series A, 23*, 267–281.

Massey, D. S., & Denton, N. A. (1993). *American apartheid: Segregation and the making of the underclass.* Cambridge, MA: Harvard University Press

McMichael, A. J. (1999). Prisoners of the proximate: Loosening the constraints on epidemiology in an age of change. *American Journal of Epidemiology, 149*(10), 887–897.

Melvin, P. M. (1985). Changing contexts: Neighborhood definition and urban organization. *American Quarterly, 37*(3), 357–367.

Morenoff, J. D., Diez Roux, A. V., Osypuk, T., & Hansen, B. (2006). *Residential environments and obesity: What can we learn about policy interventions from observational studies? National Poverty Center Working Paper.* Ann Arbor, MI: University of Michigan.

Morgenstern, H. (1985). Socioeconomic factors: Concepts, measurement, and health effects. In A. M. Ostfeld & E. D. Eaker (Eds.), *Measuring psychosocial variables in epidemiologic studies of cardiovascular disease: Proceedings of a workshop.* Washington, DC: National Institutes of Health.

National Association of Counties (2003). A brief overview of county government. Washington DC: NACO.

National Association of Counties (2006a). About counties. July 8, 2006; http://www.naco.org/Template.cfm?Section = About_Counties.

National Association of Counties (2006b). An overview of county government. (July 8, 2006); http://www.naco.org/Content/NavigationMenu/About_Counties/County_Government/Default271.htm.

National Research Council (2002). *Equality of opportunity and the importance of place: Summary of a workshop.* Washington DC: National Academy Press

New York City Department of City Planning (2006). New York: A city of neighborhoods. New York (2006); http://www.nyc.gov/html/dcp/html/neighbor/neigh.shtml.

Oakes, J. M. (2006). Commentary: Advancing neighbourhood-effects research—selection, inferential support, and structural confounding. *International Journal of Epidemiology, 35*, 643–647.

Oakes, J. M., & Kaufman, J. S. (2006). Introduction: Advancing methods in social epidemiology. In J. M. Oakes & J. S. Kaufman (Eds.), *Methods in social epidemiology.* San Francisco: Jossey Bass.

O'Campo, P. (2003). Invited commentary: Advancing theory and methods for multilevel models of residential neighborhoods and health. *American Journal of Epidemiology, 157*(1), 9–13.

O'Campo, P., & Kogan, M. D. (2005). Multilevel modeling in perinatal research. (February 2, 2005); http://www.uic.edu/sph/cade/mchepi/meetings/feb2005/index.htm.

O'Campo, P., & Schempf, A. (2005). Racial inequalities in preterm delivery: Issues in the measurement of psychosocial constructs. *American Journal of Obstetrics and Gynecology, 192*, S56–63.

O'Connor, A. (2001). Understanding inequality in the late twentieth-century metropolis: New perspectives on the enduring racial divide. In A. O'Connor, C. Tilly, & L. D. Bobo (Eds.), *Urban inequality: Evidence from four cities.* New York: Russell Sage Foundation.

Office of Management and Budget, & Spotila, J. T. (2000). Part IX, Office of Management and Budget, standards for defining metropolitan and micropolitan statistical areas; notice. *Federal Register*, *65*(249), 82228–82238.

Orfield, M. (2002). *American metropolitics: The new suburban reality*. Washington, DC: Brookings Institution Press

Osypuk, T. L. (2005). *Demographic and place dimensions of racial/ethnic health disparities. Unpublished dissertation.* Boston, MA: Harvard University School of Public Health, Department of Society, Human Development, and Health.

Osypuk, T. L. (2006). Inequality in exposure to fast food outlets by race/ethnicity & social class across 325 US metropolitan areas. *American Journal of Epidemiology*, *163*(11 Supplement), S144.

Osypuk, T. L., Kawachi, I., Subramanian, S. V., & Acevedo-Garcia, D. (2006). Are state patterns of smoking different for different racial/ethnic groups? An application of multi-level analysis. *Public Health Reports*, *121*(5), 563–577.

Plane, D. A. (2004). Population distribution: Geographic areas. In J. S. Siegel & D. A. Swanson (Eds.), *The methods and materials of demography*. 2nd edition. San Diego, CA: Elsevier Academic Press.

Raudenbush, S. W., & Sampson, R. J. (1999). Ecometrics: Toward a science of assessing ecological settings, with application to the systematic social observation of neighborhoods. *Sociological Methodology*, *29*, 1–41.

Rose, G. (1992). *The strategy of preventive medicine*. New York, NY: Oxford University Press

Saelens, B. E., Sallis, J. F., & Frank, L. D. (2003). Environmental correlates of walking and cycling: Findings from the transportation, urban design, and planning literatures. *Annals of Behavioral Medicine*, *25*(2), 80–91.

Sallis, J. F., Frank, L. D., Saelens, B. E., & Kraft, M. K. (2004). Active transportation and physical activity: Opportunities for collaboration on transportation and public health research. *Transportation Research Part A: Policy and Practice*, *38*(4), 249–268.

Sampson, R. J., & Wilson, W. J. (1995). Race, crime, and urban inequality. In J. Hagan & R.D. Peterson (Eds.), *Crime and inequality*. Stanford, CA: Stanford University Press.

Schwartz, S., & Carpenter, K. M. (1999). The right answer for the wrong question: Consequences of type III error for public health research. *American Journal of Public Health*, *89*(8), 1175–1180.

Schwartz, S., & Diez Roux, A. V. (2001). Commentary: Causes of incidence and causes of cases — a Durkheimian perspective on Rose. *International Journal of Epidemiology*, *30*(3), 435–439.

Shadish, W. R., Cook, T. D., & Campbell, D. T. (2002). *Experimental and quasi-experimental designs for generalized causal inference*. New York: Houghton Mifflin.

Subramanian, S. V., Acevedo-Garcia, D., & Osypuk, T. L. (2005). Racial residential segregation and geographic heterogeneity in black/white disparity in poor self-rated health in the U.S.: A multilevel statistical analysis. *Social Science & Medicine*, *60*(8), 1667–1679.

U.S. Census Bureau. (2000). Census 2000 ZCTAs ZIP code tabulation areas technical documentation. Washington, DC: U.S. Census Bureau.

U.S. Census Bureau. (2001a). ZIP code tabulation areas (ZCTAs). U.S. Census Bureau. Washington, DC (April 13, 2001); http://www.census.gov/geo/ZCTA/zcta.html.

U.S. Census Bureau. (2001b). Geographic changes for Census 2000 + glossary. Washington, DC (September 20, 2001); http://www.census.gov/geo/www/tiger/glossary.html.

U.S. Census Bureau. (2001c). Ranking tables for incorporated places of 100,000 or more: Population in 2000 and population change from 1990 to 2000 (PHC-T-5). Table 2: incorporated places of 100,000 or more ranked by population: 2000. Washington, DC (July 31, 2002); http://www.census.gov/population/www/cen2000/phc-t5.html.

U.S. Census Bureau. (2002). U.S. Gazetteer: 2000 and 1990: 1990 Census gazetteer files. Washington, DC (May 3, 2005); http://www.census.gov/geo/www/gazetteer/gazette.html.

U.S. Census Bureau. (2004a). 2002 Census of Governments, Volume 3, Number 1, employment of major local governments GC02(3)-1. Washington, DC: U.S. Government Printing Office.

U.S. Census Bureau (2004b). Federal, state, and local governments, state and local government finances, 2002 census of governments: Viewable data: State and local summary tables by level of government and by type of government. U.S. Census Bureau. Washington, DC (October 14, 2004); http://www.census.gov/govs/www/estimate02.html.

U.S. Census Bureau (2005a). About metropolitan and micropolitan statistical areas. U.S. Census Bureau. Washington, DC (June 7, 2005); http://www.census.gov/population/www/estimates/aboutmetro.html.

U.S. Census Bureau (2005b). Answers to frequently asked questions about census bureau geography, maps and mapping engines: ZIP code information. Washington, DC (August 19, 2005); http://www.census.gov/geo/www/tiger/tigermap.html#ZIP.

U.S. Census Bureau (2006a). ZIP Code Statistics. July 10, 2006. http://www.census.gov/epcd/www/zipstats.html.

U.S. Census Bureau (2006b). TIGER Frequently Asked Questions. July 10, 2006. http://www.census.gov/geo/www/tiger/faq-index.html.

U.S. Census Bureau (2006c). American factfinder. Urbanized area. U.S. Census Bureau. October 8, 2006.

U.S. Census Bureau (no year). Appendix A: Census 2000 geographic terms and concepts.

U.S. Postal Service (2003). The United States Postal Service: An American history 1775 – 2002. Publication 100. U.S. Postal Service. (September, 2003); http://www.usps.com/cpim/ftp/pubs/pub100/pub100.htm#thepostalrole.

U.S. Postal Service (2006a). Mr ZIP: The nation's original "digital" icon. July 10, 2006. http://www.usps.com/postalhistory/mrzip.htm.

U.S. Postal Service (2006b). Sources of historical information on post offices, postal employees, mail routes, and mail contractors: Publication 119. U.S. Postal Service. (October, 2006); http://www.usps.com/cpim/ftp/pubs/pub119/welcome.htm.

Wilkinson, R. G. (1992a). National mortality rates: The impact of inequality? *American Journal of Public Health*, *82*(8), 1082–1084.

Wilkinson, R. G. (1992b). Income distribution and life expectancy. *British Medical Journal*, *304*(6820), 165–168.

Wilkinson, R. G., & Pickett, K. E. (2006). Income inequality and population health: A review and explanation of the evidence. *Social Science & Medicine*, *62*, 1768–1784.

Wilson, W. J. (1987). *The truly disadvantaged: The inner city, the underclass, and public policy*. Chicago: University of Chicago Press

Yang, T. C. (2005). Modifiable areal unit problem. GIS resource document 05–65 (GIS_RD_05–65). (February, 2005); http://www.pop.psu.edu/gia-core/pdfs/gis_rd_05–65.pdf.

Chapter 20
Integrative Chapter: Methodologic Considerations in the Study of the Macrosocial Determination of Population Health

Sandro Galea

The second section of this book includes five chapters each of which considers particular issues pertinent to those interested in the study of how macrosocial factors influence the health of populations. These chapters primarily adopt an epidemiologic methodologic perspective but all borrow freely from methods that are much more common in other disciplines and all advocate, implicitly or explicitly, the use of methods from diverse disciplines to aid in understanding the determination of the health of populations. While these chapters, as might be expected, are quite diverse I highlight some common themes that arise.

These chapters clearly suggest that the study of how macrosocial determinants influence the health of populations is not easy. All five methodologic chapters in this section discuss both the daunting complexity inherent in some of the methods discussed and how these methods fall short in several respects when applied to some of the questions of population health etiology articulated in the first part of this book. There is no doubt that understanding how macrosocial determinants shape the health of populations will be challenging. As the chapters in the first part of this book make eminently clear, the relations between macrosocial factors and population health are complicated and characterized by multiple and overlapping pathways. Elucidating the pathways linking, for example, culture and population health will require not only conceptual clarity, as discussed in the book's first section, but also imaginative and rigorous methodologic applications, as discussed in this section. Even further, a clear and compelling empiric argument for the role that macrosocial factors play in *causing* adverse or favorable health indicators will require methodologic ingenuity that will probably depend not only on extant methods, but on future methodologic developments.

Perhaps this latter point is best illustrated by the overwhelming emphasis in these chapters, very much reflecting the state of the extant peer-reviewed literature, on neighborhood factors that may influence health. While neighborhoods and factors at the neighborhood level indeed represent an important area of social epidemiologic inquiry and likely represent a level of group aggregation at which health is importantly determined, they clearly are only one of many levels whose characteristics influence health. The chapters in the first part of this book focused primarily on factors that manifest at state or at national levels. Analyses at these levels would undoubtedly be necessary to do justice to some of the questions raised in those chapters and would clearly stretch the available methods as ably summarized by the authors of chapters in this second section.

These chapters all raise key methodologic challenges that we face in trying to understand macrosocial production of health and disease. Three key challenges emerge. First, extant analytic modeling strategies are limited in their ability to account both for the cross-level inference that is necessary to satisfactorily consider how macrosocial factors at different levels of influence shape population health and also for factors that mediate the relations between macrosocial factors and health. Analytic strategies also are limited in accounting for reciprocal relations and discontinuous effects, both characteristics of the complex systems that likely characterize the macrosocial production of population health. Second, our analytic methods are predicated on a need for greater measurement precision and specificity, both with respect to the key constructs of interest and with respect to the levels at which we are interested in understanding the role of these constructs. This is clearly brought home both in Chapter 19 and its discussion of the different levels of spatial analysis in US-based research, and in Chapter 17, which discusses the challenges that bedevil causal inference that may be useful for the purposes of policy interventions. Achieving specificity of constructs to be measured, of course, is not a methodologic issue alone but rather requires both conceptual (as outlined in many of the chapters in Section I) and methodologic (as outlined in Section II) clarity. Third, fundamentally, the application of empiric methods to questions of interest to the study of the macrosocial determination of health is predicated on formulating clear questions and using the right methods to answer the right questions. Therefore, conceptual differences in the determination of group rates and individual risks are important both from the point of view of theoretical clarity, and also from the point of view of guiding the choice of analytic strategy and the application, or development, of methods to address clearly specified and articulated research questions.

While the empiric study of the relations between macrosocial factors and population health indeed may be challenging, these chapters all suggest, in different ways, that such study is *possible*, and that while future developments likely will help us in the particular quest of interest here, we can do quite well with the methods we already have in hand. A particularly interesting example in this regard is provided in Chapter 18 which considers the application of methods that are typically used in different disciplines to address one particular question that concerns the authors. Similarly, other chapters show how ecologic analyses can be applied to questions concerned with the determination of population rates of health and disease and how multilevel analyses can be applied to the study of social factors at multiple levels of influence. It emerges from these chapters that there is no one simple methodologic approach that can be applied to the study of macrosocial determinants of population health. Indeed, given the complexity of the task, as outlined in the chapters in the first section of this book, it would have been surprising if there were any one simple methodologic approach. Rather, testing hypotheses that pertain to the macrosocial determination of health will require the creative and deliberate application of different empiric methods and that careful and judicious inference be drawn from the application of these same methods.

A final point to emerge from these chapters pertains not only to the creative applications of analytic strategies that is necessary to satisfactorily tackle the questions of interest here, but also to the creative collaborations between researchers adept at the use of different methods that will be needed to tackle the questions that emerge in this book. In the first chapter of this book we suggested that while we adopt an epidemiologic perspective, we mean that only insofar as epidemiology is concerned with the determination of health and disease. Clearly, the epidemiologic methodologic armamentarium, left to its own devices, is unlikely to provide adequate solutions for all the methodologic challenges relevant to addressing the questions posed by many chapters in the first part of this book. And neither should it, particularly when we recognize that fields as diverse as economics, sociology, and engineering have developed methods that may fruitfully and creatively be applied to the study of the determination of population health. Therefore, the task at hand here is not so much the wholesale absorption of methodologic capacity into any one discipline, but rather the application of methods from across disciplines to questions of cross-disciplinary concern.

Section III
Improving population health

Chapter 21
Acting Upon the Macrosocial Environment to Improve Health: A Framework for Intervention

Jan C. Semenza and Siobhan C. Maty

1. Introduction

Societal health inequalities are ubiquitous. Today, across populations, substantial differences in health outcomes are found on every continent and in every country. Macrosocial factors within society cause the inequitable distribution of resources and provide more opportunity to some but less to others. These factors are large-scale determinants, such as health policy, taxation, or urbanization, which can be modified and improved. Experts no longer dispute the claim that the poor suffer disproportionately from stressful life events and have lower levels of self-determination and greater demands from work and family than their wealthier counterparts. Such taxing circumstances undoubtedly increase harmful exposures – whether they be smoking, drinking, poor diet, or lack of exercise – and, more often than not, are found in combination with a lack of access to health-promoting incentives. Unfavorable residential and occupational exposures can also contribute to such health inequalities. Thus, social stratification results in an uneven distribution of risk factors and health endpoints.

These inequalities manifest as systematic differences in mortality and morbidity, in which individuals with lower levels of education, income, or a lower occupational class die at earlier ages and suffer more illnesses. Mortality differences can be observed in the young but persist in elderly populations as well. Differences are found for both sexes, although more so for men, and for almost all causes of death. Morbidity follows a similar pattern, in which indicators of class, educational attainment, or social exclusion are associated with poor self-rated health, chronic diseases, mental health problems, or disabilities. The premise of Section III of this book is that, despite the fact that disparities are very widespread, they are entirely preventable. Individuals at the margins of society do not have to live shorter and sicker lives.

Even though health inequalities caused by socioeconomic status have proven to be remarkably resilient to intervention, encouraging successes have been documented, as will be seen in the next chapter. Nevertheless, creative and coordinated action will be required to close the widening health gap between the advantaged and disadvantaged. In order to design and implement effective health interventions to improve health for both the individual and the general population, the connection between individual risk and the larger social context must be considered. Health authorities must move beyond the current myopic focus on the individual as the unit of intervention to determine what environmental and social factors put individuals at risk in the first place (Rose, 1985). Unless the fundamental causes of disease, such as socioeconomic status and social support, are addressed, interventions will be inefficacious and short-lived because they do not alter the underlying causes – lack of access to resources and opportunities (Link & Phelan, 1995). Interventions must be based on a comprehensive understanding of how macrosocial forces influence health outcomes, and this chapter builds on the sophisticated description of the macrosocial determinants of health in the previous chapters to develop a framework for action.

Individual behavioral changes may be necessary, but if not accompanied by environmental interventions, they will not be sufficient. Moreover, barriers to unhealthy options should be institutionalized (limiting access), while financial incentives for healthy options should be put in place (promoting use). Implementation must occur simultaneously and sustainably. However, this requires a greater understanding of the role of society, economics, and politics in influencing the development of health at multiple levels; as articulated by the great German public health pioneer of the last century, Rudolf Virchow (1821–1902), "Medicine is a social science, and politics is nothing but medicine on a larger scale. Medicine as a social science, as the science of human beings, has the obligation to point out problems and to attempt their theoretical solution; the politician, the practical anthropologist, must find the means for their actual solution." (Ackerknecht, 1957)

Interventions into the macrosocial determinants of health must build upon a social and ecological framework integrating ecosocial theory, which describes the social inequalities and population health resulting from the dynamic interaction between biological processes and social, material, and ecological conditions over time and across classes (Krieger, 2001a). As with the social-ecological model, ecosocial theory implies that individuals and the populations that they comprise are dependent on and influenced by multiple environments (Grzywacz & Fuqua, 2000). Interventions based upon the social-ecological framework and ecosocial theory, therefore, require consideration of the connections among multiple systems over time: the microsystem (individual), the mesosystem (interrelation among individuals and higher social contexts) (Bronfenbrenner, 1979), the exosystem (settings and events that influence individuals but do not directly involve them as active participants), and the macrosystem (correlates of lower systems as they are expressed in belief systems, cultural ideology, social policy, and the global environment) (Grzywacz & Fuqua, 2000).

Interventions improve health by eliminating the origins of poor health outcomes and disparities. The next chapter builds on this idea and discusses the prerequisites to implementation (Figure 21.1). Consideration is given to: 1) the socio-political context of the country where the program will be

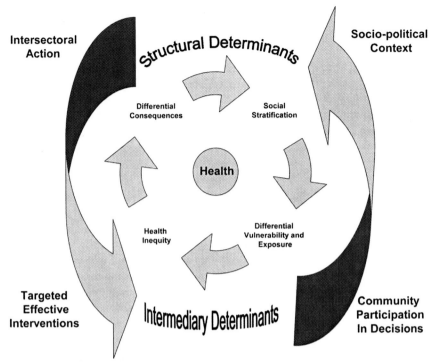

FIGURE 21.1. Framework of action on macrosocial determinants of health according to the World Health Organization Commission on Social Determinants of Health.

implemented; 2) intersectoral participation and collaboration; 3) specific, cost-effective, and evidence-based interventions, as well as 4) community participation in the decision-making process. By engaging a community in its own program design, implementation, and evaluation, intervention components become integrated into the community, thereby enhancing stability and redistributing power to the group in question. Additional, yet essential, actions include changing the values and customs of the culture that lead to the increased risk in the first place (Altman, 1995; Brown, 1991; Wallack & Winkleby, 1987).

This chapter uses the social-ecological/ecosocial approach and builds on the interventional framework that the World Health Organization's (WHO) Commission on Social Determinants of Health is currently developing (World Health Organization, 2005). The structural determinants of health (income, education, race/ethnicity, sexual orientation, etc.) set the process of social stratification in motion, while the intermediary determinants (living and working conditions) determine the differences in exposure and vulnerability. Specific examples will help to demonstrate the important place of each determinant in the development of highly effective interventions.

2. Framework

2.1. Synthesis of a Conceptual Model

The World Health Organization created the Commission on Social Determinants of Health in March 2005 to focus international efforts on the social determinants of health. Commissioners from a wide range of disciplines have synthesized the existing knowledge on social determinants and have developed a framework for analysis and action. The synthesis is based on two reports commissioned by the European Regional Office of the World Health Organization (Dahlgren & Whitehead, 1992; Whitehead, 1990), and the model is based on reports from Acheson (1998) and the King's Fund (Benzeval, Judge, & Whitehead, 1995), as well as other research (Diderichsen, Evans, & Whitehead, 2001; Diderichsen & Hallqvist, 1998; Mackenbach, van de Mheen, & Stronks, 1994).

The purpose of this literature synthesis is to unravel and explain the macrosocial causes of health inequalities. For example, in the debate over the source of socioeconomic health inequalities, some argue that sick individuals descend in social position due to an inability to work. While this mechanism is undeniable, its contribution to large-scale inequalities is likely to be small. In contrast, longitudinal cohort studies of groups with different socioeconomic status clearly show a higher disease incidence in the lower socioeconomic groups. Based on this research, "causation" has prevailed over "selection" as the guiding philosophy in the design of large-scale public health interventions. Another example is the "life course" concept, which stresses the significance of a susceptible biological or social period early in life. Early life events are particularly important, with long-lasting, even life-long, consequences.

According to the conceptual model, the social, political, cultural, and economic contexts constitute the structural determinants of health (Figure 21.1). These give rise to the distribution of income, education, and professional success among certain groups, as defined by specific social, gender, or race/ethnicity norms. The result is social stratification. One's socioeconomic position, in turn, defines the intermediary determinants of health, such as living and working conditions, food availability, social success, psychological outlook, and behavioral factors (e.g. smoking and drinking), which in turn generate potentially harmful exposures. Structural and intermediary determinants influence each other in a self-perpetuating cycle. Thus, inequity drives a "vicious cycle," wherein social stratification leads to different exposures that undermine or promote health to varying degrees. Disadvantaged groups suffer disproportionately the consequences of ill health, since healthcare costs and loss of work can result in impoverishment and a descent down the socioeconomic ladder.

2.2. Framework for Action

The Commission asserts that strategies must address those inequalities that generate health disparities or other factors that place people and communities at risk of poor health (Petticrew & Macintyre, 2001; Rose, 1985; World Health Organization, 2005). The social-ecological/ecosocial model identifies various levels and types of social determinants and the mechanisms or pathways by which they affect health risks and outcomes. Thus, the Commission's strategy builds upon the social-ecological/ecosocial model by incorporating those political structures, opportunities, and processes that interact with social determinants to influence health outcomes and through which interventions must operate. Rather than focusing exclusively on individual behaviors, this approach analyzes the underlying mechanisms of a society's responsibility for the inequitable distribution of health in its population. The framework allows identification both of potential causes of health problems at the societal level and appropriate, politically feasible solutions (World Health Organization, 2005).

This strategy is based upon three models that were created to aid in the development of interventions into and policies on the social determinants of health: Stronks (2002), Dahlgren and Whitehead (1995), and Diderichsen et al. (2001). These models inform on the various levels for intervention and specify the principles within which interventions can take place. Thus, according to the Commission, interventions into the social determinants of health must be implemented with the following principles and methods: Interventions 1) are responsive to the local or national socio-political context; 2) are inclusive of other sectors, such as education, housing, and transportation; 3) engage communities in the decision-making process; and 4) have been tested and validated for their effectiveness (WHO, 2005). With these principles in mind, intervention entry points can range from the macro to micro level and be both challenging and efficacious at the same time. The model proposed by Diderichsen et al. identifies four relevant entry points or levels of action: social stratification, differential exposure, differential vulnerability, and differential consequences. The Commission's framework adopts these four entry points and adds a fifth, the equitable provision of health services (World Health Organization, 2005). Each of these pathways is discussed below in detail, and accompanied by examples of action.

2.3. Social Stratification

The rich and the poor differ by more than just wealth because wealth shapes health. For every country examined, average life expectancy is consistently shorter among the socioeconomically disadvantaged (Huisman et al., 2004). Premature mortality among those with lower levels of education, occupation, or income is particularly pronounced in men but is also present, although to a lesser extent, in women (Mackenbach et al., 1999). Such mortality inequalities are found for many causes of death, including cardiovascular disease, cancers, and injury (Mackenbach, Cavelaars, Kunst, & Groenhof, 2000). The widening gap between the rich and the poor is a growing health hazard, as reflected in the increasing mortality gradient, both within and between countries (Mackenbach et al., 2003). Even in egalitarian Sweden, which has very low absolute mortality rates, the relative difference in mortality persists (see Chapter 22). Nevertheless, societies that suffer from wide economic and social divides are less healthy than those that have reduced such disparities (Leinsalu, Vagero, & Kunst, 2003). Morbidity also displays an inequality gradient, whereby individuals with lower income, less education, or a lower occupational class suffer from a higher prevalence of specific diseases, such as mental illness and disability (Dalstra et al., 2005).

The persistent correlation between socioeconomic groups and health outcomes across countries is compelling and poses a considerable challenge to public health practitioners. Some argue that reducing health inequalities may augment the average health of the general population (Mackenbach, Bakker, Sihto, & Diderichsen, 2002). Moreover, discrepancies between social strata are incompatible with the ideals of social justice and fairness and ought to be attenuated, if not abolished. Absolute differences in health inequalities can be reduced, although relative differences have proven to be remarkably unrelenting.

2.4. Intervention Strategies to Decrease Social Stratification

Albeit challenging, interventions that address socioeconomic inequalities are critical now more than ever. Thus, a rational approach to reducing social stratification requires a comprehensive plan combining both social inclusion and health equalization policies. Innovative and unconventional policies ought to be devised to lessen health inequalities. Social justice, activism, child development programs, the institutionalization of labor rights, and progressive taxation are all examples of remedies for social hierarchy.

The integration of different policies requires a multifaceted strategy. One facet aims directly at equalizing the distribution of resources and opportunities across social strata through progressive taxation, education, entitlement programs, antidiscrimination laws, etc. (Diderichsen, et al., 2001), while the other aims at alleviating the negative consequences of stratification (Mackenbach, et al., 1994). Through health promotion among high-risk groups, harmful exposures to tobacco smoke, alcohol, or poor diet can be prevented. Such efforts are supported at environmental entry points (housing and working conditions) and social entry points (social integration, social support, etc). Furthermore, access to high-quality healthcare can prevent the socioeconomic decline from illness into disability. Environmental and legislative changes support and sustain behavioral changes (Link & Phelan, 1995).

A detailed case study of Sweden's new public health policy to promote socioeconomic equality can be found in Chapter 22. Another example is Sir Donald Acheson's 1998 United Kingdom Policy Brief, which recommended addressing health inequalities through one of the fundamental causes: poverty (Acheson, 1998). In 1999, the Department of Health launched one of the most comprehensive programs to address health inequalities, entitled *Reducing Health Inequalities: an Action Report*. The proposed agenda focused on reducing the causes, rather than the symptoms, of poverty and social exclusion. It included improving social benefits by raising living standards and tackling low earnings by promoting employment, increasing wages, and improving benefit levels. Under this initiative, Britain introduced its "first-ever" national minimum wage in April 1999 (Benzeval, 2002).

The combined effect of this legislation and other measures (tax credits, welfare-to-work schemes, reform of the insurance system, etc.) has helped redistribute income toward low-income families. By 2000, disposable income had increased by an average of 9 percent in the poorest deciles, while it decreased by 1 percent in the richest (Benzeval, Dilnot, Judge, & Taylor, 2000). In absolute terms, the average income-per-week had increased by over £5.00 for both men and women. As a result of the effort to lift children out of poverty, a real increase was observed among pensioners and in families with children, compared to singles or childless couples.

"Health Action Zones" were also created in disadvantaged neighborhoods with the greatest need for advances in public health. By eliminating the root cause of ill health and social deprivation, Health Action Zones build and regenerate healthy communities. Preliminary assessment of the initiative has been positive, with a recommendation for funding through 2008, at which point the program will be fully evaluated.

2.5. Differential Exposure

Individuals in lower socioeconomic positions are at increased risk of exposure to various harmful factors. Compared to their socioeconomically advantaged peers, they are more likely to live in potentially dangerous environments, where they may develop unhealthy behaviors or illness. For example, compared to wealthy neighborhoods, many low-income urban neighborhoods have a higher concentration of liquor stores (Gorman & Speer, 1997; LaVeist & Wallace, 2000), more violence and health-related social problems (Escobedo & Ortiz, 2002; Tatlow, Clapp, & Hohman, 2000), an unbalanced distribution of fast food outlets (Reidpath, Burns, Garrard, Mahoney, & Townsend, 2002; Cummins, McKay, & MacIntyre, 2005; Laranjeira & Hinkly, 2002), and insufficient fresh food outlets, recreational areas for exercise, or community centers (Cradock et al., 2005).

Both men and women from lower socioeconomic groups are less likely to eat fruits and vegetables and are more likely to be overweight (Cavelaars, Kunst, & Mackenbach, 1997). Although custom or tradition may be partially responsible for these differences, the environmental and financial forces in poor neighborhoods nevertheless tend to make foods that are high in calories and low in nutrients easier to obtain than balanced, nutritious foods. Furthermore, individuals from lower socioeconomic groups are often limited to working in low-paying occupations that can be hazardous. They are also regularly segregated into unhealthy, crowded, dilapidated housing. Environmental justice research has documented disproportional exposure of low socioeconomic groups to toxic substances (Soliman, Derosa, Mielke, & Bota, 1993). Consequently, the high morbidity and mortality rates associated with unhealthy lifestyles plague the members of poor communities (Bostrom, 2006).

2.6. Intervention Strategies to Decrease Differential Exposures

Intervention programs that do not differentiate between the rich and poor have been shown to be ineffective in lower socioeconomic groups (Beaglehole, 1990). For example, interventions that call for participants to eat healthy foods without regard for environmental factors or physical activity are inefficacious (Dansinger, Gleason, Griffith, Selker, & Schaefer, 2005). Therefore, in order for an intervention to be successful and sustainable, designers and implementers must acknowledge the differential impact of social position on risk behaviors and potential for change.

Public health practitioners have long used zoning and other land-use tools to protect the public from environmental hazards (Ashe, Jernigan, Kline, & Galaz, 2003). These traditional strategies now offer new opportunities to control the proliferation of alcohol, gun dealers, and fast food outlets in inner cities and to limit sales of tobacco products. Such legislative interventions can be employed to limit differential exposure among the most susceptible populations of society. Since relatively small increases in the availability of alcohol increase consumption and related problems (Scribner, MacKinnon, & Dwyer, 1995), communities in California in the 1980s began to implement innovative local ordinances restricting the location and operation of alcohol outlets. The conditional use permits were challenged in court, but they were affirmed under the notion that governments may enact land-use laws in the interests of public health. A decade later, over half of California's cities had ordinances regulating the sale of alcohol (Ashe et al., 2003).

The higher rates of crime and delinquency among youth in poor inner cities are a consequence of differential exposures to dangerous environments (Molnar, Miller, Azrael, & Buka, 2004). In the early 1990s in response to escalating gun violence in California, the California Wellness Foundation established its Youth Violence Prevention Initiative, which focused on two policy goals: 1) limiting the availability of handguns to youth, and 2) increasing the state's investment in youth resources. This initiative was successful due its clear delineation of policy objectives, strategic issue framing, use of advantageous political events, and effective mobilization of resources. As a result, over 110 communities passed more than 300 ordinances over a 10-year period, which restricted gun accessibility and enhanced gun safety. State legislators passed 24 gun control laws and increased financial support for youth programs. Consequently, California experienced a decrease in gun-related violence in the late 1990s (Wallack, Winett, & Lee, 2005), although the degree of contribution of the new policies needs to be assessed in greater detail.

From these examples, urban planning can be a public health tool to limit differential exposure among socioeconomically deprived groups by informing the placement of fast food outlets, toxic waste dumps, and other health hazards.

2.7. Differential Vulnerability

Reducing individual exposures will undoubtedly have beneficial consequences for at-risk populations. However, eliminating one or even several harmful exposures does not address the underlying vulnerability of susceptible populations. Thus, increasing the general knowledge base of the individual or community through education and outreach is a more comprehensive strategy. Indeed, education, a strong predictor of social position, is also a significant determinant of adult health (Whalley, 2006). Through education and training, social conditions improve such that synergistic exposures can be simultaneously avoided (Diderichsen et al., 2001).

2.8. Intervention Strategies to Decrease Differential Vulnerability

The Mexican "Oportunidades" (Progresa) anti-poverty initiative, established by the Federal government in 1997, allocates cash payments to poor and rural parents to encourage them to send their children to school. The substantial monetary incentives are intended to offset lost wages from child labor, to increase household incomes, and to lead to improvements in the health and education of children. The payments, however, are contingent upon all family members accepting preventive health services, including family planning, pre- and postnatal care, sanitation, and injury prevention (Skoufias, Davis, & de la Vaga, 2001). An evaluation of the intervention thus far has found remarkable health improvements in both the children and adults who have participated in the program (Gertler & Boyce, 2001).

The Baraka School, an experimental boarding school located in Laikipia, Kenya, East Africa, in partnership with the Baltimore City Public School System and the Abell Foundation, provides a second example. The program, now closed due to security concerns in Kenya, brought disadvantaged junior high school students from inner-city Baltimore, MD, to attend a school situated in an idyllic locale and noted for its strict academic and disciplinary standards. During the two year program, the African-American youth developed their academic skills while experiencing what it meant to be a "normal" teenager. The objectives of the program stated that students who completed the program would be academically prepared and have a significant social and emotional foundation, which would increase their ability to succeed in high school and beyond. A recent evaluation demonstrated that the students who attended the Baraka school were indeed academically successful and prepared to enter Baltimore City high schools (Chief of Educational Accountability, 2002).

Both of these programs seek to improve the lives of disadvantaged social groups through education. Each program affects multiple determinants of social inequality and health, such as education, income, self-esteem, and access to health services. It is likely, though not yet proven, that in addition to improving social and physical health for program participants, the multi-tiered intervention may also reduce the vulnerability of the subject groups to future social disadvantage and health-damaging exposures.

2.9. Differential Consequences

Sickness and disease often result in rapid social decline. If ill health cannot be prevented or treated, sick individuals may lose their jobs and related social opportunities. An inability to pay for health services may further reduce one's ability to return to a state of optimal health. Thus, inequalities in health outcomes are partially due to the impact of negative health on socioeconomic opportunities, i.e., when someone loses his job after an injury, he loses the income necessary to get well and get another job. Inequitable access to health services and the financial repercussions of emergency care, if passed on to individuals of all socioeconomic levels, will ultimately strain the ability of the poor to afford healthier lifestyles. Differences across social groups in health-seeking behavior and experience with the health system result in differential economic and health consequences (Doherty & Gilson, 2006).

2.10. Intervention Strategies to Decrease Differential Consequences

The sick are less socially mobile than the healthy (World Health Organization, 2005). Therefore, interventions that attempt to decrease differential consequences from illness should focus their attention on the healthcare of socially disenfranchised individuals by providing material and psychosocial support to assure that they can return to and/or maintain full employment. Health services delivered to all persons, regardless of ability-to-pay, would alleviate some socioeconomic strain resulting from the cost of medical treatment, and reintegrate the sick back into the workforce. Rehabilitation programs for high-risk groups can attenuate the effects of disability on wage earners and thus prevent the socioeconomic decline of entire families (World Health Organization, 2005).

The US National Breast and Cervical Cancer Early Detection Program (NBC-CEDP) is an example of a national strategy that reduces the differential consequences of breast and cervical cancer observed among medically underserved and socially disadvantaged women. The early detection of breast and cervical cancer improves cancer patients' survival and reduces mortality. However, uninsured or underinsured US women are more likely to die from breast and cervical cancer than insured women, despite the availability of screening tests. Women who are older, have less than a high school education, live below the poverty level, or are members of certain racial and ethnic minority groups do not use preventive mammography and Papanicolaou (Pap) tests at recommended screening intervals, if at all (Anderson & May, 1995; Swan, Breen, Coates, Rimer, & Lee, 2003).

To address the disparity, the US Congress passed the Breast and Cervical Cancer Mortality Prevention Act of 1990, which created the National Breast and Cervical Cancer Early Detection Program. The NBCCEDP is a comprehensive public health program that helps underserved women nationwide gain access to breast and cervical cancer screening. The Centers for Disease Control and Prevention (CDC) administers the NBCCEDP, which is implemented through cooperative agreements with state and territorial health departments and American Indian/Alaska Native tribal organizations. The program provides mammograms, clinical breast examinations, Pap tests, and diagnoses in the case of abnormal result to low-income, uninsured women aged 18 to 64 from priority populations. Although the majority of providers identify external resources for treatment through the program, the US Congress allotted additional money for treatment. The legislation also provided for additional services, such as education, quality assurance, and monitoring of program activities (Centers for Disease Control, 2005).

The program now serves all 50 states, the District of Columbia, four US territories, and 13 American Indian/Alaska Native tribes. Since its inception, the NBCCEDP has provided more than 4 million screening and diagnostic tests to almost 1.75 million low-income, uninsured women. As a result, approximately 10,000 cases of breast cancer, 12,000 cases of precancerous cervical lesions, and 832 cases of invasive cervical cancer have been diagnosed. Most important, the program has reduced some of the differential consequences that result from breast and cervical cancer, such as early mortality, that underinsured, low-income US women often experience. As a result of early detection, the women are more likely to survive their cancer (Centers for Disease Control, 2005).

2.11. Access to Health Services

Unlike most other conceptual models of the social determinants of health, the Commission's model specifically includes the healthcare system and its differential impact on health outcomes. Having access to health services can affect health in several ways. Access can improve the likelihood of early diagnosis and treatment of disability and disease. Illness, especially chronic conditions, can also negatively affect social standing, as described in the previous section. Finally, the healthcare industry, especially powerful in the US, plays a significant role in developing and implementing health policy (World Health Organization, 2005).

In the US, access to healthcare services is not equitably distributed. In 2004, 45.8 million Americans (approximately 15.7 percent of the total population) did not have health insurance, a necessary condition for receiving regular, routine medical care (DeNavas-Walt, Proctor, & Lee, 2005). Unfortunately, as the number of uninsured people increases, everyone in the US, regardless of individual health insurance coverage, becomes subject to reduced access to hospital-based care, specialty services, and emergency room care (Institute of Medicine, 2003). Also when the number of the uninsured increases, health and related sectors are more likely to reduce or restrict services, a consequence that stems from community-level policy decisions that divert public resources and tax money away from health promotion and disease prevention programs and toward the large healthcare systems, in order to reimburse them for the uncompensated costs (Institute of Medicine, 2003).

Given the health crisis in the US, it is understandable that policymakers focus on programs that will contain medical costs. However, policies that efficiently, effectively, and equitably finance and deliver medical services and health promotion programs to the entire population would be likely to affect, and interact with, other social determinants, in order to improve overall national health (World Health Organization, 2005). Interventions that hope to improve population health, therefore, must engage key players in the health sector in improving access to and quality of health services for all individuals and, in collaboration with other social systems, develop public health policies and programs that are effective and available to all who could benefit from them (Mackenbach & Gunning-Schepers, 1997).

2.12. Strategies to Improve Access to Health Services

One way to provide health services equitably is to adopt a government-financed and government-managed healthcare system for the entire population. All industrialized countries have some sort of healthcare system that provides for the basic health needs of the entire population. Additional services often require payment of premiums and longer wait times; however, data has shown that countries where basic healthcare services are provided free-of-cost at time of service have better health outcomes than the fee-for-service form of delivery typical in the US. For example, in a recent assessment by the Joint Canada/US Survey of Health, US residents, compared to Canadians, were less likely to have regular access to a healthcare provider and more likely to have health needs that had gone unmet. The authors concluded that the universal healthcare coverage afforded to Canadians removed most disparities attributable to access (Lasser, Himmelstein, & Woolhandler, 2006).

The US Medicare program is an example of a government-subsidized health insurance program. The Medicare program was signed into law in 1965 as a mechanism for alleviating the health costs of what was, at the time, a significant, impoverished segment of the US population: the elderly. Financing is provided primarily through contributions from employee payroll taxes. Currently, Medicare's services are restricted to legal citizens aged 65 years or older, some disabled persons under age 65, and people of all ages with End-Stage Renal Disease (Centers for Medicare, 2006). Over the last thirty years, the program has alleviated the problem of access to healthcare for a significant portion of the US population. However, the future of the program is uncertain, given the aging of the "baby boomers" (a significant percentage of the population), their relative wealth, and the limited number of employed persons under age 65, whose payroll taxes fund the program.

3. Challenges to and Limitations of Interventions at the Macrosocial Level

The challenges to advancing the macrosocial determinants of heath on a global scale are considerable. Currently, the Millennium Development Goals (MDGs) determine the agenda for the elimination of the societal roots of health inequalities. These goals include: 1) eradicate extreme poverty and hunger; 2) achieve universal primary education by 2015; 3) promote gender equality and empower women; 4) reduce child mortality; 5) improve maternal health; 6) combat HIV/AIDS, malaria, and other diseases; 7) ensure environmental sustainability; and 8) forge a global partnership for development (United Nations Development Program, 2003). Interestingly, only three of these goals are related directly to health; the others are related only indirectly. It is increasingly apparent that, without specifically addressing poverty reduction, food security, education, women's empowerment, and housing, health disparities will escalate. The international development policies of the United Nations support the agenda and are in harmony with the thrust of the macrosocial determinants of health. Other international authorities, such as the Group of Eight (G-8), recognize the importance of global hunger reduction and debt cancellation in improving the prosperity and quality of life of several African countries.

The WHO's Commission on Social Determinants of Health desires to synchronize worldwide efforts to improve public health and support institutional change through cross-sectoral partnerships and advocacy (World Health Organization, 2005). To do so, potential and willing allies and opponents must be identified within medical institutions, governments, businesses, non-governmental organizations, and civil society. The use of scientific evidence will help create successful policies and intervention programs, and compelling social marketing tools. Health interventions are most effective when change occurs at many levels (Green & Krueter, 1999; Stokols, 1996), and the social/ecological framework and ecosocial theory dictate that any action on the social determinants of health must take into consideration the connections between multiple social levels. Unfortunately, few countries have the political capacity to implement over time the comprehensive social changes that would lead to improvements in public health. Nevertheless, the Commission endeavors to work with such societies to develop national policies on the social determinants of health and advocates the implementation of any resultant interventions or programs.

To create social or health policies but fail to ground them in scientific fact is a recipe for failure, but it is equally futile to continue generating scientific evidence only to ignore its implications for policy. For example, despite ample proof of the significance to public health of physical injuries, strategies for injury-control, both national and international, remain inadequate. If public health experts are to entertain any hope that policymakers will adopt their recommendations, they must base them on accurate analyses of their cost-effectiveness and make them easily adaptable to different cultures. Furthermore, policy recommendations must be acceptable to vulnerable populations and, if necessary, tailored to different contexts. Thus, it is essential for scientists to collaborate with public health practitioners and policymakers to translate research findings into specific programs. Moreover, scientists must also advise public health officials as to a policy's likelihood of success in a particular setting or with a particular population. Such information is also essential to effective policy development (Koplan & McPheeters, 2004). Without such recommendations, public health achievements are impossible.

Nevertheless, even when in possession of scientific evidence and clear policy recommendations, there is no guarantee that policymakers will implement effective macrosocial interventions. Other factors can still stall effective action. When those most affected are poor and disenfranchised, a lack of political resolve may be particularly pronounced. Religious, political, social, and economic ideologies can also block public health policies.

Persistent activism is essential to drive public health policy through the maze of political interest groups. Advocacy on behalf of the vulnerable is the hallmark of public health practice. Such advocacy entails scientific skill, political talent, and luck. To ensure that relevant issues are discussed or that established policies or programs are successfully implemented, some advocacy campaigns join certain public health "stars" in partnership with key political stakeholders or decision-makers. Recall the great public health interventions of the 20th century, which have been credited with adding 25 years to the life expectancy of residents of the United States (Centers for Disease Control, 1999a). These efforts tackled mainly macrosocial determinants of health and relied on powerful alliances between non-government organizations, public health advocates, activists, and other stakeholders to push back entrenched interest groups that wished to maintain the harmful *status quo*. For example, death rates from motor vehicle accidents per 100 million vehicle miles traveled have decreased by 90 percent over the last century, due in large part to legislation for and litigation over safer vehicles with head rests, energy-absorbing steering wheels, shatter-resistant windshields, safety belts, and airbags, as well as safer roads (Centers for Disease Control, 1999b). Dental caries and tooth decay declined in the second part of the 20th century because of the fluoridation of community drinking water (Centers for Disease Control, 1999c), and both maternal and infant mortality rates have declined more than 90 percent over the last century as a result of environmental interventions, improved nutrition, and access to pre-natal care (Centers for Disease Control, 1999d; 1999e). Public health practitioners have successfully controlled many infectious diseases (Centers for Disease Control, 1999f), vaccinated children (Centers for Disease Control, 1999g), increased workplace safety (Centers for Disease Control, 1999h), improved food safety (Centers for Disease Control, 1999i), and reduced smoking (Centers for Disease Control, 1999j), to mention only a few of the triumphs.

4. Conclusions

Macrosocial factors are the fundamental causes of disease worldwide. If we are to reduce systemic health inequities and eradicate disease, we must intervene in these macro-level causes. Acting upon the macrosocial environment entails the age-old predicament of public health: how to take decisive action despite the lack of definite data. More often than not, public health practitioners are forced to act even in the absence of solid evidence in order to protect the health of the public. Many governments throughout the world feel both the urgency of the situation and a responsibility to act. An analysis of national interventions in the macrosocial determinants of health within Europe has revealed different approaches to the challenge (Judge, Platt, Costongs, & Jurczak, 2006). Countries can be grouped into four categories, according to their national policy: 1) countries with well-articulated and integrated plans to diminish health inequalities specifically; 2) countries with a general public health policy that promotes equity but no specific inequality plan; 3) countries acting upon health inequalities, with or without a plan; and 4) countries that lack any particular focus on the macrosocial determinants of health (though they often have taken at least some action on these determinants at the national or local level). The variety of tactics reflects the many different possible approaches to tackling the macrosocial determinants within each country's own historic, cultural, and social situation.

The responsibility for action usually resides with the local department of health but, as illustrated in this and the next chapter, considerable advantages accrue from engaging other departments. Intersectoral integration of a wide range of stakeholders that collaborate around a focused and specific action plan will move health indicators toward a country's desired targets. Monitoring progress in all phases of an intervention and a realistic timetable are also essential for success. The key to effective macrosocial interventions is that fiscal and regulatory incentives must simultaneously and sustainably support behavior change so that the healthiest option is also the cheapest and easiest. By undertaking to change our macrosocial conditions, we aspire to advance the health of all.

References

Acheson, D. (1998). *The report of the independent inquiry into the inequalities in health.* London: The Stationery Office.

Ackerknecht, E. H. (1957). *Rudolf Virchow: Arzt, politiker, anthropologe.* Stuttgart: Enke.

Altman, D. (1995). The market and regulation: Where community forces fit. *Frontiers of Health Services Management, 11*(4), 49–51.

Anderson, L. M., & May, D. S. (1995). Has the use of cervical, breast, and colorectal cancer screening increased in the United States? *American Journal of Public Health, 85*(6), 840–842.

Ashe, M., Jernigan, D., Kline, R., & Galaz, R. (2003). Land use planning and the control of alcohol, tobacco, firearms, and fast food restaurants. *American Journal of Public Health, 93*(9), 1404–1408.

Beaglehole, R. (1990). International trends in coronary heart disease mortality, morbidity, and risk factors. *Epidemiological Review, 12,* 1–15.

Benzeval, M. (2002). England. In J. Mackenbach & M. Bakker (Eds.), *Reducing inequalities in health: A European perspective.* London: Routledge.

Benzeval, M., Dilnot, A., Judge, K., & Taylor, J. (2000). Income and health over the life-course: Evidence and policy implications. In H. Graham (Ed.), *Understanding health inequalities.* Berkshire: Open University Press.

Benzeval, M., Judge, K., & Whitehead, M. (1995). *Tackling Inequalities in health; An agenda for action.* London: King's Fund.

Bostrom, G. (2006). Habits of life and health. *Scandinavian Journal of Public Health, 67,* 199–228.

Bronfenbrenner, U. (1979). *The ecology of human development: Experiments by nature and design.* Cambridge, MA: Harvard University Press.

Brown, E. R. (1991). Community action for health promotion: A strategy to empower individuals and communities. *International Journal of Health Services, 21,* 441–456.

Cavelaars, A. E., Kunst, A. E., & Mackenbach, J. P. (1997). socioeconomic differences in risk factors for morbidity and mortality in the European Community. *Journal of Health Psychology, 2*(3), 353–372.

Centers for Disease Control (CDC). (1999a). Ten great public health achievements—United States, 1900–1999. *Mortality and Morbidity Weekly Report (MMWR), 48*(12), 241–243.

Centers for Disease Control (CDC). (1999b). Achievements in public health, 1900–1999: Motor-vehicle safety: A 20th century public health achievement. *Mortality and Morbidity Weekly Report (MMWR), 48*(18), 369–374.

Centers for Disease Control (CDC). (1999c). Achievements in public health, 1900–1999: Fluoridation of drinking water to prevent dental caries. *Mortality and Morbidity Weekly Report (MMWR), 48*(41), 933–940.

Centers for Disease Control (CDC). (1999d). Achievements in public health, 1900–1999: Family planning. *Mortality and Morbidity Weekly Report (MMWR), 48*(47), 1073–1080.

Centers for Disease Control (CDC). (1999e). Achievements in public health, 1900–1999: Healthier mothers and babies. *Mortality and Morbidity Weekly Report (MMWR), 48*(38), 849–858.

Centers for Disease Control (CDC). (1999f). Achievements in public health, 1900–1999: Control of infectious diseases. *Mortality and Morbidity Weekly Report (MMWR), 48*(29), 621–629.

Centers for Disease Control (CDC). (1999g). Achievements in public health, 1900–1999: Impact of vaccines universally recommended for children—United States, 1990–1998. *Mortality and Morbidity Weekly Report (MMWR), 48*(12), 243–248.

Centers for Disease Control (CDC). (1999h). Achievements in public health, 1900–1999: Improvements in workplace safety—United States, 1900–1999. *Mortality and Morbidity Weekly Report (MMWR), 48*(22), 461–469.

Centers for Disease Control (CDC). (1999i). Achievements in public health, 1900–1999: Safer and healthier foods. *Mortality and Morbidity Weekly Report (MMWR), 48*(40), 905–913.

Centers for Disease Control (CDC). (1999j). Achievements in public health, 1900–1999: Tobacco use—United States, 1900–1999. *Mortality and Morbidity Weekly Report (MMWR), 48*(43), 986–993.

Centers for Disease Control and Prevention (CDC). (2005). *The national breast and cervical cancer early detection program, 1991–2002: National report.* Atlanta, GA: United States Department of Health and Human Services.

Centers for Medicare and Medicaid Services, U.S. Department of Health and Human Services. (2006). Medicare. Washington, DC (2006); http://www.cms.hhs.gov/home/medicare.asp.

Chief of Educational Accountability; Division of Research, Evaluation, and Accountability. (2002). *An evaluation of the Baraka School: A program evaluation prepared for the Board of School Commissioners.* Baltimore, MA: Baltimore City Public School System.

Cradock, A. L., Kawachi, I., Colditz, G. A., Hannon, C., Melly, S. J., Wiecha, J. L., et al. (2005). Playground safety and access in Boston neighborhoods. *American Journal of Preventive Medicine, 28*(4), 357–363.

Cummins, S. C., McKay, L., & MacIntyre, S. (2005). McDonald's restaurants and neighborhood deprivation in Scotland and England. *American Journal of Preventive Medicine, 29*(4), 308–310.

Dahlgren, G., & Whitehead, M. (1992). *Policies and strategies to promote equality in health.* Copenhagen: World Health Organization.

Dahlgren, G., & Whitehead, M. (1993). *Tackling inequalities in health: what can we learn from what has been tried?* Background paper for The King's Fund International Seminar on Tackling Health inequalities. Ditchely Park, Oxford: King's Fund.

Dalstra, J. A., Kunst, A. E., Borrell, C., Breeze, E., Cambois, E., Costa, G., et al. (2005). Socioeconomic differences in the prevalence of common chronic diseases: An overview of eight European countries. *International Journal of Epidemiology, 34*(2), 316–326.

Dansinger, M. L., Gleason, J. A., Griffith, J. L., Selker, H. P., & Schaefer, E. J. (2005). Comparison of the Atkins, Ornish, Weight Watchers, and Zone diets for weight loss and heart disease risk reduction: A randomized trial. *Journal of the American Medical Association, 293*(1), 43–53.

DeNavas-Walt, C., Proctor, B. D., & Lee, C. H. (2005). *U.S. Census Bureau, Current population reports: Income, poverty, and health insurance coverage in the United States: 2004.* Washington, DC: U.S. Government Printing Office.

Diderichsen, F., Evans, T., & Whitehead, M. (2001). The social basis of disparities in health. In T. Evans, M. Whitehead, F. Diderichsen, A. Bhuiya, & M. Wirth (Eds.), *Challenging inequalities in health: From ethics to action.* New York: Oxford University Press.

Diderichsen, F., & Hallqvist, J. (1998). Social inequalities in health: Some methodological considerations for the study of social position and social context. In B. Arve-Parés (Ed.), *Inequality in health—a Swedish perspective.* Stockholm: Swedish Council for Social Research.

Doherty, J., & Gilson, L. (2006). *Health system knowledge network discussion document no. 1; Proposed areas of investigation for the KN: An initial scoping of the literature.* Geneva: World Health Organization.

Escobedo, L. G., & Ortiz, M. (2002). The relationship between liquor outlet density and injury and violence in New Mexico. *Accident Analysis and Prevention, 34*(5), 689–694.

Gertler, P., & Boyce, S. (2001). *An experiment in incentive-based welfare: The impact of PROGRESA on health in Mexico.* Washington, D.C.: World Bank.

Gorman, D. M., & Speer, P. W. (1997). The concentration of liquor outlets in an economically disadvantaged city in the northeastern United States. *Substance Use and Misuse, 32*(14), 2033–2046.

Green, L. W., & Krueter, M. W. (1999). *Health promotion planning: An educational and ecological approach.* 3rd edition. Mountain View, CA: Mayfield.

Grzywacz, J. G., & Fuqua, J. (2000). The social ecology of health: Leverage points and linkages. *Behavioral Medicine, 26,* 101–115.

Huisman, M., Kunst, A. E., Andersen, O., Bopp, M., Borgan, J. K., Borrell, C., et al. (2004). Socioeconomic inequalities in mortality among elderly people in 11 European populations. *Journal of Epidemiology and Community Health, 58*(6), 468–475.

Institute of Medicine (IOM). (2003). *A shared destiny: Community effects of uninsurance.* Washington, DC: National Academies Press.

Judge, K., Platt, S., Costongs, C., & Jurczak, K. (2006). *Health inequities: A challenge for Europe.* London: Central Office of Information (COI).

Koplan, J. P., & McPheeters, M. (2004). Plagues, public health, and politics. *Emerging Infectious Diseases, 10*(11), 2039–2043.

Krieger, N. (2001a). Theories for social epidemiology in the 21st century: An ecosocial perspective. *International Journal of Epidemiology, 30*, 668–677.

Laranjeira, R., & Hinkly, D. (2002). Evaluation of alcohol outlet density and its relation with violence. *Revista de Saúde Pública, 36*(4), 455–461.

Lasser, K. E., Himmelstein, D. U., & Woolhandler, S. (2006). Access to care, health status and health disparities in the United States and Canada: Results of a cross-national population-based survey. *American Journal of Public Health. 96*(7), 1300–1307.

LaVeist, T. A., & Wallace, J. M., Jr. (2000). Health risk and inequitable distribution of liquor stores in African American neighborhoods. *Social Science & Medicine, 51*(4), 613–617.

Leinsalu, M., Vagero, D., & Kunst, A. E. (2003). Estonia 1989–2000: Enormous increase in mortality differences by education. *International Journal of Epidemiology, 32*(6), 1081–1087.

Link, B. G., & Phelan, J. (1995). Social conditions as fundamental causes of disease. *Journal of Health and Social Behavior, 35*(Extra issue), 80–94.

Mackenbach, J. P., Bakker, M. J., Sihto, M., & Diderichsen, F. (2002). Strategies to reduce socioeconomic inequalities in health. In J. Mackenbach, & M. J. Bakker (Eds.), *Reducing inequalities in health: A European perspective.* London: Routledge.

Mackenbach, J. P., Bos, V., Andersen, O., Cardano, M., Costa, G., Harding, S., et al. (2003). Widening socioeconomic inequalities in mortality in six Western European countries. *International Journal of Epidemiology, 32*(5), 830–837.

Mackenbach, J. P., Cavelaars, A. E., Kunst, A. E., & Groenhof, F. (2000). Socioeconomic inequalities in cardiovascular disease mortality: An international study. *European Heart Journal, 21*(14), 1141–1151.

Mackenbach, J. P., & Gunning-Schepers, L. J. (1997). How should interventions to reduce inequalities in health be evaluated? *Journal of Epidemiology and Community Health, 51*(4), 359–364.

Mackenbach, J. P., Kunst, A. E., Groenhof, F., Borgan, J. K., Costa, G., Faggiano, F., et al. (1999). Socioeconomic inequalities in mortality among women and among men: An international study. *American Journal of Public Health, 89*(12), 1800–1806.

Mackenbach, J. P., van de Mheen, H., & Stronks, K. (1994). A prospective cohort study investigating the explanation of socioeconomic inequalities in health in The Netherlands. *Social Science & Medicine, 38*, 299–308.

Molnar, B. E., Miller, M. J., Azrael, D., & Buka, S. L. (2004). Neighborhood predictors of concealed firearm carrying among children and adolescents: Results from the project on human development in Chicago neighborhoods. *Archives of Pediatrics and Adolescent Medicine, 158*(7), 657–664.

Petticrew, M., & Macintyre, S. (2001). What do we know about the effectiveness and cost-effectiveness of measures to reduce inequalities in health? *Proceedings from the HEN Conference 2001*, University of Glasgow.

Reidpath, D. D., Burns, C., Garrard, J., Mahoney, M., & Townsend, M. (2002). An ecological study of the relationship between social and environmental determinants of obesity. *Health & Place*, *8*(2), 141–145.

Rose, G. (1985). Sick individuals and sick populations. *International Journal of Epidemiology*, *14*, 32–38.

Scribner, R. A., MacKinnon, D. P., & Dwyer, J.H. (1995). The risk of assaultive violence and alcohol availability in Los Angeles County. *American Journal of Public Health*, *85*(3), 335–340.

Skoufias, E., Davis, B., & de la Vaga, S. (2001). Targeting the poor in Mexico: An evaluation of the selection of households into PROGRESA. *World Development*, *29*(10), 1769–1784.

Soliman, M. R., Derosa, C. T., Mielke, H. W., & Bota, K. (1993). Hazardous wastes, hazardous materials and environmental health inequity. *Toxicology & Industrial Health*, *9*(5), 901–912.

Stokols, D. (1996). Translating social ecological theory into guidelines for community health promotion. *American Journal of Health Promotion*, *10*, 282–298.

Stronks, K. (2002). Generating evidence on interventions to reduce inequalities in health: The Dutch case. *Scandinavian Journal of Public Health*, *30*(supplement 59), 20–25.

Swan, J., Breen, N., Coates, R. J., Rimer, B. K., & Lee, N. C. (2003). Progress in cancer screening practices in the United States: Results from the 2000 National Health Interview Survey. *Cancer*, *97*, 1528–1540.

Tatlow, J. R., Clapp, J. D., & Hohman, M. M. (2000). The relationship between the geographic density of alcohol outlets and alcohol-related hospital admissions in San Diego County. *Journal of Community Health*, *25*(1), 79–88.

United Nations Development Program (UNDP). (2003). *Human Development Report 2003: Millennium Development Goals: A compact among nations to end human poverty*. New York: United Nations Development Program.

Wallack, L., Winett, L., & Lee, A. (2005). Successful public policy change in California: Firearms and youth resources. *Journal of Public Health Policy*, *26*(2), 206–226.

Wallack, L., & Winkleby, M. (1987). Primary prevention: A new look at basic concepts. *Social Science & Medicine*, *25*(8), 923–930.

Whalley, L. J. (2006). Commentary: Childhood education and disparities in adult health—the need for improved theories and better data. *International Journal of Epidemiology*, *35*, 466–467.

Whitehead, M. (1990). *The concepts and principles of equality in health*. Copenhagen: World Health Organization.

World Health Organization Commission on Social Determinants of Health. (2005). Towards a conceptual framework for analysis and action on the social determinants of health. Geneva (2005, July 1); http://www.who.int/social_determinants/resources/framework.pdf

Chapter 22
Case Studies: Improving the Macrosocial Environment

Jan C. Semenza

1. Introduction

Health is a function of individual and ecological risk factors (Lloyd, 1978). High-risk behavior, such as smoking, drug abuse, unsafe sex, overeating, or physical inactivity, can negatively affect personal health, and health promotion advocates have long stressed the importance of behavioral change to ameliorate adverse health outcomes. The benefits of changing personal health behaviors seem intuitive, tangible, and direct. A preponderance of interventions that address individual behavioral changes have already been studied; regrettably, well-designed evaluations of behavior-change interventions have consistently revealed disappointing results. Upon extended follow-up, the interventions have not met their health targets (Dansinger, Gleason, Griffith, Selker & Schaefer, 2005).

Health-behavior interventions have been particularly inefficacious in populations with a lower socioeconomic status (Beaglehole, 1990). How then, can personal health outcomes be improved, and from an epidemiological perspective, how can population health be advanced? Needless to say, individual behavioral change is necessary, but not sufficient, for successful health interventions (Link & Phelan, 1995). Interventions addressing behavioral changes must be embedded in a framework addressing several aspects of risky behavior, as discussed in the previous chapter. Behavioral change interventions must also be accompanied with fiscal and legislative incentives that make healthy behavior the cheapest and easiest option. Furthermore, the various aspects of a health intervention have to be implemented simultaneously and in a sustainable manner. This chapter focuses on macrosocial approaches to health interventions that encompasses multiple levels simultaneously, where the focus is not on individual health, *per se*, but on promoting health opportunities for all.

While it can be challenging to modify personal risk factors (Syme, 1996), it seems even more daunting to tackle the larger societal, political, economic, and environmental determinants of public health. The most pragmatic approach to health inequities would be ameliorate the unfavorable circumstances of the disadvantaged. This chapter will discuss the inadequacy of such a limited strategy from a public health perspective, without questioning its value for the individual.

Further, this chapter illustrates four different successful macrosocial intervention strategies that have improved the macrosocial environment at the global, national, regional, or community level and documents their benefits to public health. The theoretical underpinning of the interventions described here is based on work synthesized by the World Health Organization (WHO) Commission on Social Determinants of Health (2006) (see Chapter 21 for a comprehensive treatment). The interventions also serve to illustrate the four policy principles that the WHO Commission on Social Determinants of Health has proposed for interventions (2005). First, effective interventions should be evidence-based and prioritized according to strategies with a high probability of success, reflecting the most promising and state-of-the-art approaches. Second, community participation is an essential component of the decision-making process. Community capacity has to be built into the protocol to assure a participatory process. Third, interventions ought to integrate a variety of sectors besides healthcare, drawing from civil engineering, urban planning, education, non-governmental organizations, and other stakeholders to assure a comprehensive approach. Fourth, interventions should consider each particular socio-political situation and alter project goals accordingly. Each country has its own socio-political circumstances requiring special attention and adjustment.

All four policy principles must be considered simultaneously, prior to implementation. The four case studies described below are, in fact, successful examples of integration of all four policy principles. However, since the interventions gave different weights to each principle, each case study is presented in terms of a single principle as a way of illustrating the importance of that particular approach. It may seem that macrosocial determinants are more abstract, impersonal and indirect than individual determinants; however, as will be shown, their efficacy is actually quite remarkable and far-reaching.

2. Case Studies

2.1. Targeted, Effective Intervention: A City Government Intervention to Provide Social Support

Heat waves are sporadic, but recurrent. Because they are invisible, silent, and underrated, they tend to be insidious killers. On average in the United States, heat kills 1,700 individuals during a typical heat wave year. Early in the summer of 1995, Chicago, Illinois, experienced a heat wave of historic proportions. Over the course of a few days in early July, maximum and minimum temperatures reached unprecedented highs, accompanied by extreme relative humidity. Only a few days after the heat wave began, the Cook County Medical Examiner's Office noticed a sharp increase in the number of heat-related deaths (Centers for Disease Control and Prevention, 1995). Politicians and public health officials alike were taken aback by the unexpected toll of over 700 deaths.

Immediately afterwards, the Centers for Disease Control and Prevention (CDC) conducted a large epidemiological investigation with the goal of identifying risk-factors for heat-related mortality (Semenza et al., 1996). The primary objective was to identify the public health strategies that would be most effective in reaching people at risk and preventing future heat-related mortality. The extensive field investigation, comprised of over 700 interviews with the relatives of the victims and survivors, exposed the vulnerability to heat-related mortality of socially and economically deprived individuals. The elderly and the isolated were found to be at increased risk, particularly if they suffered from underlying medical conditions, such as cardiovascular or mental diseases (Semenza, McCullough, Flanders, McGeehin & Lumpkin, 1999). Being confined to bed or unable to care for oneself also increased one's risk of death during the heat wave. Risk was particularly pro-nounced among the urban poor (Semenza, 1996), those not leaving home at least once a day, or those living on the top floor of an apartment building. Conversely, having access to any air-conditioned area, even an air-conditioned lobby, reduced the risk for heat-related mortality.

Nevertheless, isolation and poverty remained overarching risk-factors, even beyond personal cooling behaviors, such as drinking sufficient fluids and air-conditioning. For example, individuals who lived alone were twice as likely to die during the hot weather, while those who participated in group activities, such as churches, clubs, or support groups, were protected. Individuals with friends in the city were one-third as likely to die as individuals without friends. The most dra-matic consequence of isolation was the large number of unclaimed bodies brought to the Cook County morgue for mass burial. Thus, the Chicago case exemplifies the importance of social networks, above and beyond individual behavior, in the prevention of heat-related mortality.

The 1995 experience has resulted in a proactive approach to attenuating the impact of excessive heat through a comprehensive heat emergency response plan that incorporates the findings from the CDC study (Ebi, Teisberg, Kalkstein, Robinson, & Weiher, 2004; Palecki, Changnon, & Kunkel, 2001; Weisskopf et al., 2002). Results from the field investigation identified political, mass media, environmental, societal, and behavioral risk factors for heat-related mortality. Based on the epidemiologic evidence, a macrosocial intervention was developed with a number of specific steps, including meteorologic monitoring of weather conditions; defining the roles of agencies and organizations; preparing for a heat emergency; initiating emergency procedures during the heat wave; and media advocacy, outreach, and evaluation (Bernard & McGeehin, 2004).

The plan was tested during a heat wave in 1999 in Milwaukee, Wisconsin. Early dissemination of information and regular status checks of family members, particularly the socially isolated, proved to be crucial in saving lives. Twenty-four hour hotlines were established to provide information on the nearest cooling shel-ter, transportation, and recommended treatment for heat stroke. Established data-bases (Heat Outlook) were used to contact at-risk individuals, such as the elderly and the very isolated, either by phone or in person. Health officials and politicians disseminated behavioral messages through a variety of media. The improved public health response resulted in fewer heat-related deaths than expected (Weisskopf et al., 2002). There was a 17 percent and 51 percent reduction in heat-related deaths and emergency medical service runs, respectively, compared to 1995, and those adverse health outcomes that did arise were not the result of heat levels alone.

In contrast, the absence of extreme temperature alert systems and prevention measures became painfully apparent during the landmark European heat wave of 2003 that resulted in over 50,000 excess deaths (Conti et al., 2005; Johnson et al., 2005; Vandentorren et al., 2004). At the time, only two cities in Europe, Rome and Lisbon, had sophisticated heat wave alert plans (World Health Organization, 2004); however, virtually all European cities now have prevention plans in place for high-risk populations during hot weather and for directing prevention messages through the most effective channels.

While sporadic and recurrent heat waves cannot be avoided, the public health consequences of such extreme weather are entirely preventable. Simple individual behavioral changes can prevent heat-related mortality; however, prevention efforts that are tailored to populations at risk have been more effective. Although Chicago's public health calamity was the turning point in the development and execution of heat preparedness plans, which proved to be effective at reducing heat-related deaths, it did not address the underlying determinants of isolation. The next case study examines how promotion of civic engagement within several urban communities counteracted the negative health effects of isolation.

2.2. Community Participation in Decisions: A Community Intervention to Reverse Social Isolation

The previous example and other published reports illustrate how isolation can have life-threatening consequences (Berkman & Syme, 1979; Kawachi, Kennedy, Lochner & Prothrow-Stith, 1997; Semenza et al., 1996). Is it possible to design interventions that augment social support and thus the health of a community?

The majority of Americans live in cities, where the social glue that holds people together is declining. A weakening of communal ties and relationships and alienation from collective norms and shared values in urban neighborhoods is leading to the progressive erosion of social capital (Putnam, 2000). A macrosocial approach to the problem seems next to impossible, due to entrenched interest groups (such as developers) and legal frameworks (such as local land-use authorities) that are not amenable to solving it (Buzbee, 2003).

In an attempt to reverse the trend, The City Repair Project, a non-profit organization in Portland, Oregon, has committed itself to engaging residents in an urban revitalization that promotes cohesion and generates a sense of belonging and community (City Repair, 2006). In 2003, as part of an asset-mapping process involving a situation analysis, an extensive outreach to community members and other stakeholders was undertaken (Green & Kreuter, 2005). Through a number of informal meetings between a core group of residents and representatives of The City Repair Project, a common vision for the neighborhood was developed, with specific plans to build interactive art features. The plans included large outdoor street murals, benches, trellises for hanging gardens, and traffic-calming planters in the streets (Semenza, 2005).

Through a cycle of successive improvements in its structures, the community increased its capacity to address external stressors. For example, through the discussions and informal meetings, the residents built friendships and social networks that ultimately increased localized social capital, which is the capacity within social groups to address issues collectively (Figure 22.1) (Semenza & Krishnasamy, in press). The localized capital inherent in existing social or religious groups is essential, but not sufficient, for neighborhood problem-solving because it may produce superfluous information not relevant to improving inner-city neighborhoods (Granovetter, 1973). Because they are too homogeneous, such local groups may not reach beyond the limits of the subculture or ethnicity and thus do not infuse the problem-solving effort with new ideas and expertise,

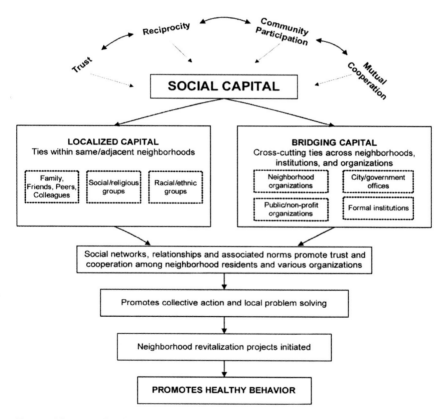

FIGURE 22.1. Localized and bridging social capital to advance community competence.
Source: Semenza, J. C., & Krishnasamy, P. V. (in press).

despite the members' strong social ties. Nevertheless, the informal meetings play a key role in bringing people together and promoting discussions about neighborhood issues.

The capacity to establish cross-cutting ties outside the immediate neighborhood increased bridging social capital, which connected various groups, divulging new information for problem-solving and generating new opportunities (Figure 22.1). For example, City Repair staff, project organizers, architects, and natural builders assisted neighborhood groups in developing designs for projects implemented during a ten day building workshop that attracted thousands of volunteers and builders. The organizers helped the groups to acquire building materials for the projects and assisted them in the completion of construction permits. Applying for permits was an important component as it introduced residents to interfacing with city and government officials, neighborhood associations, and businesses.

The shared building experience during the implementation of the projects in turn improved and expanded both established and newly formed social ties in a continuous social capital sustainability cycle (Figure 22.2). Numerous projects have since been implemented in Portland, Oregon. Diverse populations have

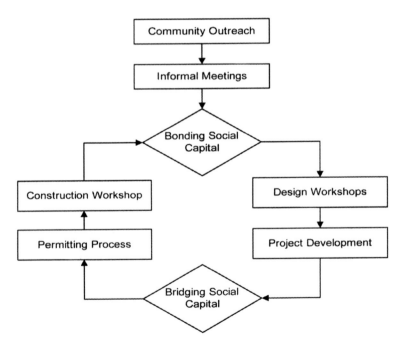

FIGURE 22.2. Social capital sustainability cycle, Portland, Oregon.

Source: Semenza, J. C., & Krishnasamy, P.V. (in press).

provided the community with an opportunity to develop a common ground and allowed people to rise above differences, develop deeper relationships with each other and their neighborhoods, and create vibrant communities (Semenza, 2003). Interactive art features have enhanced the urban experience and become a catalyst for interactions and conversations. For example, in April 2003, 507 pedestrians were observed passing through one of the projects sites, and 164 (32 percent) of passers-by interacted with a stranger about the art, read the signs about the project, or took a photograph, compared with 7 percent (p<0.01) at a similar, unimproved intersection (Semenza, 2003). An epidemiological panel study surveyed residents within a two-block radius before (N = 325) and after (N = 349) the macrosocial intervention at three different sites in Portland (Semenza, March, & Bontempo, 2007). Of these, 265 participants responded to both surveys, and revealed an increased sense of community (p<0.01) and an overall expansion of social capital (p = 0.04). Improvements in mental health (p = 0.03) were also documented.

Through such macrosocial interventions at the community level, it has become apparent that the individual leadership capacity of the core group must be sufficiently developed (Semenza & Krishnasamy, in press). Outreach should be expanded to a broad base of residents and should engage important stakeholders, such as neighborhood associations, community centers, and businesses. Participation in politics is based on consensus decision-making, and has been known to obstruct the implementation of projects. Thus ample time should be devoted to outreach in order to allow the process to take its natural course, so outreach efforts must begin early.

Insofar as the residents worked collectively to strengthen localized social capital and communicated with various government organizations and professionals beyond the immediate neighborhood to build bridging social capital, the strategy vindicated the merits of community participation in urban design (Semenza et al., 2007). Urban planners and public health practitioners must facilitate dialogue and collaboration with residents, developers, and politicians to create livable and healthy cities. The next macrosocial case study illustrates such collaboration across multiple sectors on an international scale.

2.3. Intersectorial Action: Global Interventions to Improve the Macrosocial Determinants of Health

Uzbekistan is a conflict-ridden country under authoritarian rule in Central Asia with a population of over 26 million. One of the main exports is ginned cotton, grown in the desert plains. As a result of excessive cotton production and poor water management, the Aral Sea, a landlocked, endorheic sea, has become the biggest ecological disaster of our time. Since 1960, the Aral Sea has decreased 60 percent by size and 80 percent by volume due to the diversion of river water for irrigation into poorly built canals. Salinity has increased by a factor of four, extinguishing what had once been a thriving fishing industry. Numerous fishing vessels now lie abandoned in the desert, miles from the retreating shore. By the twilight of the Soviet Union, the lake's rich biodiversity in flora and fauna had utterly collapsed.

Nukus, the administrative capital of the region, with a population of 200,000, is located on the Amudar'ya River, one of the tributaries of the Aral Sea. Water mismanagement has resulted in reductions in water quality and availability, with direct health consequences for the inhabitants. In 1996, the Public Water Works of Nukus, with funding from the United States Agency for International Development (USAID), installed a water chlorination system to ameliorate the water quality. In order to improve the salinity of the water, reverse osmosis, a process of removing salt from drinking water, was considered, but was deemed to have prohibitively high operating costs. After consultation with an engineering firm (Environmental Policy and Technology Project) and various non-profit organizations, the CDC was requested to evaluate the benefits of a chlorination upgrade and the usefulness of reverse osmosis technology for the city of Nukus.

In collaboration with the public health department (Sanitary-Epidemiologic Services), CDC researchers examined the surveillance data for unusual trends. The data did not reflect any benefits of the water chlorination system, although the passive surveillance system might have lacked sensitivity; however, evaluation of regional health indicators revealed excessive rates of diarrheal diseases in Nukus, particularly in the summer months. Thus, a goal was set to reduce diarrheal rates in the population by identifying the source of infections and eliminating exposure. A baseline for diarrheal rates was established through a randomized community intervention. Nukus residents were divided into two populations: those with access to municipal water piped into their house or yard and those without (Semenza, Roberts, Henderson, Bogan & Rubin, 1998). In each group, 120 households were selected and the residents interviewed. Households without access to piped water were randomized so that one group was provided with a plastic water container and a chlorine dispenser for home chlorination; the data from these households served as the baseline for diarrheal rates.

A team of physicians and health professionals monitored the three groups (with piped water; without piped water or home chlorination; without piped water but with home chlorination) (Figure 22.3) for diarrheal illness over a period of nine weeks. Active diarrheal surveillance during the period revealed that individuals with home chlorination had fewer episodes of diarrhea than individuals in households with piped water, despite lower socioeconomic status and poorer sanitation and hygiene. The diarrheal rate in the home chlorination group was 38 percent that of the households with piped water, and one-sixth that of the control group with no piped water. Furthermore, one-third of the households with piped water had no detectable levels of chlorine residue in their drinking water. Nevertheless, having piped water was associated with approximately half the incidence of diarrhea when compared to households with no piped water. Moreover, chlorination of piped drinking water was an important determinant of diarrheal episodes.

Observations indicated that summertime diarrhea was predominantly waterborne, and the water distribution system was the source of the disease. Further, since intermittent lack of chlorine in the piped drinking water predicted the risk of

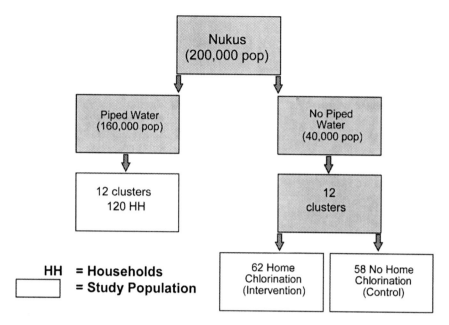

FIGURE 22.3. Study design of community intervention in Uzbekistan, 1996.

diarrhea, the distribution system must have been contaminated with diarrheal pathogens. Thus, investigators determined that though the water supply was chlorinated twice at the plant, it was subsequently contaminated in the distribution system through cross-contamination with the sewage lines when water pressure dropped and contaminants were siphoned into the drinking water lines from surrounding sewage lines (Figure 22.4). Findings from the study were immediately translated into policy recommendations to augment water availability to maintain pressure, decreasing cross-contamination with sewage lines. The recommendations were provided to the government, non-governmental agencies, and to USAID, and engineers were instructed to increase the water supply and reduce losses and/or over-consumption. Assuring proper chlorination levels at booster stations and conducting regular monitoring for chlorine residue in household tap water maintained chlorine levels.

The randomized community trial in Nukus illustrates how epidemiological methods can be used to identify structural limitations in an underlying infrastructure for population-wide health benefits (Semenza, 2004). The intervention was not used to modify personal high-risk behavior but rather to provide epidemiological information to an interdisciplinary team for an "upstream" public health solution. Through improvements to the infrastructure, the intervention minimized

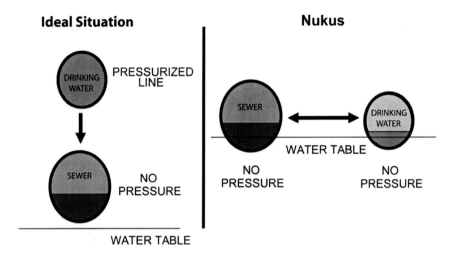

FIGURE 22.4. Cross-connection of water distribution systems with sewer lines in Nukus, Uzbekistan, 1996.

harmful exposure, not only among disadvantaged populations, but for all the residents of Nukus.

However, had the intervention not taken place, the poor would most likely have suffered disproportionately, due to lack of access to healthcare and resources. Given the political situation in Uzbekistan, with a relatively unresponsive government, sweeping changes to the socio-political conditions would have been unrealistic. Concrete changes to the infrastructure proved to be much more feasible. By contrast, the next case study illustrates how policies that reduce inequality can be institutionalized on a national level.

2.4. Socio-Political Context: A National Intervention for Optimal Public Health

Sweden's public health policy has grown out of a cultural tradition of solidarity and evidence-based decision-making dating back to the 18th century (Statens Folkhälsoinstitut, 2006). In 1748, Sweden was the first country in the world to implement compulsory civil registrations of all births, deaths, and cause of death. The reasons for the policy were to gain better understanding of birth and death rates and, specifically, to address the high mortality rates among the young. The population statistics were used to describe the health disparities between rural and urban populations, and to intervene appropriately.

As democracy emerged, political assemblies began to view public health as a social issue and to address healthcare needs and other health determinants. In contrast to many other countries, including the US, the federal and local governments were perceived as allies in the struggle for social justice. In the first half of the 20th century, the Swedish Welfare Society was established, with progressive taxation policies for children's healthcare, school food programs, housing policies, and labor laws, all of which would have direct implications for life expectancy and infant mortality. Public health was valued and strengthened in the coming years, while discrepancies between the rich and the poor diminished through the egalitarian distribution of disposable income and high public expenditure (Mahler & Jesuit, 2006). Specific objectives were established for tobacco and alcohol consumption, traffic, environment, and disease prevention. In 1987, the government appointed a commission to direct public health policy, with the establishment of a National Institute of Public Health in 1992. In 2003, it resolved "to create social conditions that will ensure good health on equal terms for the entire population" (Persson, 2006).

The Institute was charged with monitoring 18 national public health objectives that contribute to poor health outcomes and with intervening on related societal factors or living conditions (Statens folkhälsoinstitut, 2006). The explicit strategy was to include many facets of society, such as different political parties, government sectors, trade unions, non-government organizations, healthcare providers, municipalities, and researchers. Through a survey of different sectors of society, feedback was solicited concerning the health consequences of various activities, which was then incorporated into the new policy.

Of the 18 national public health objectives, 11 pertain to public health works, whereas the remainder specify the need for public health research or training, provisions for health information, or organizational needs for public health practice. The 11 Swedish national public health objectives are broad-based societal interventions on macrosocial determinants with considerable health benefits for Swedish citizens. The first six objectives are structural interventions that aim to create the basic conditions of optimal health, including social, cultural and economic factors that frame the context of disease risk-factors and create the circumstances that shape peoples' exposures. By definition, such factors are distal causes of disease, in that they are removed from the actual disease process. Nevertheless, they are important determinants of disease. The remaining five objectives center on proximal causes of disease, such as infectious diseases, physical activity, nutrition, or tobacco and alcohol use, that can be controlled at the individual level. However, the objectives not only focus on individual-level interventions aimed at behavioral changes, they also address the social context that frames health behaviors. Indeed, interventions to change high-risk health behavior are destined to fail in the absence of contextual modifications, such as fiscal or environmental barriers. The 11 objectives and their corresponding policy interventions are discussed below in more detail.

2.4.1. Participation and Influence in Society

Cooperation and participation in democracy advances common goals for the public good. However, the benefits of public participation extend to the individual; a sense of control over the world around us confers significant health benefits (Kelly, Hertzman, & Daniels, 1997; Kristenson et al., 1998; Wilkinson, 2005).

Sweden has specifically tackled the challenge through labor market policies, gender equality, integration, and disability policies, in order to facilitate the democratic process. Of great importance are media policies that stress the significance of access to information, particularly among marginalized groups. Cities with populations at risk have experimented with cultural initiatives, popular movements, and youth policy efforts. Empirical data indicate that membership in associations, interpersonal trust, informal interactions, and other social capital indicators score at high levels in Sweden (Rothstein, 2001; Rothstein & Stolle, 2003). Meanwhile, in other countries, such as the US, social capital has been in steady decline (Putnam, 2000).

2.4.2. Economic and Social Security

Wealth affects health. Researchers have connected inequalities in income and wealth with poor health statistics (Kawachi & Kennedy, 2002). Insecurity and lack of access to healthcare and resources may contribute to the discrepancy. One of the cornerstones of Swedish welfare policy is an emphasis on sustainable economic growth. Without economic prosperity, little economic or social security is possible. Sweden's strong judicial system and law enforcement are important, not only for economic productivity, but also for marginalized groups. Education policies and labor laws are equally vital social services. The social security system supports families with children and the elderly and facilitates access to health insurance.

Since 1984, infant mortality in Sweden has been cut in half, with 3.1 deaths during the first year of life per 1,000 infants born alive (Persson et al., 2005). Since 1970, life expectancy has increased and has been the highest in Europe for the greater part of the modern period (Lindberg & Persson, 2006). A Swedish girl born in 2004 can expect to live 82.7 years and a boy 78.4 years. In 2003, an analysis of Swedish mortality rates found that income inequality has little impact on mortality at the municipal level, in contrast to most other countries (Gerdtham & Johannesson, 2004). It is possible that Sweden's policies have created an even playing field, and attenuated the negative impact of inequalities in wealth and income.

2.4.3. Secure and Favorable Conditions During Childhood and Adolescence

The position of families with children has been addressed with economic family policies, a social insurance system, and social services. According to an international ranking of children's health (0–14 years) based on an aggregate assessment of major health problems for children (diseases of infancy, congenital malformations, accidental injuries, mental ill-health, infectious disease, cancer, and asthma), Sweden ranks number one (Hjern, 2006). Particular emphasis has been placed on risk reduction in smoking, physical inactivity, and alcohol abuse among adolescents. For example, the number of pregnant women who smoke has decreased consistently over the last 20 years to 11 percent (Hjern, 2006). The number of deaths during the first year of life has decreased from 16 per 1,000 live births to 4 over the last four decades, although discrepancies regarding the health of children and adolescents in different social classes persist (Bremberg, 2003). Fortunately, relative health inequalities have not worsened over the last few years, but regrettably, they can still be documented for obesity, neonatal death, mental health, abuse, accidental injuries, and asthma (Hjern, 2006).

2.4.4. Healthier Work Life

Higher mortality and morbidity rates are found among blue-collar workers compared to white-collar employees (Rosengren, Orth-Gomer, & Wilhelmsen, 1998). As a result, the Swedish Work Environment Authority has placed particular attention on the physical and psychosocial aspects of the workplace. An effort has been made to create healthier workplaces with good working conditions and a sense of control over the work situation. Based on national surveys, a continued decline during the 1990s in the psychosocial aspects of working conditions has been reversed over the last few years, (Stenbeck & Persson, 2006). Physical activity is incorporated into the working hours, and occupational and ergonomic principals are considered. Furthermore, women have been integrated into the workforce, with special emphasis on women's health. As a result of these comprehensive policies, many classic work-related diseases have decreased. Improvements have been documented for some physically hazardous factors, but not in all sectors (Stenbeck & Persson, 2006).

2.4.5. Healthy and Safe Environments and Products

With regard to modern technology, the Swedish government applies the precautionary principle in its decision-making process. If a reasonable suspicion of harm or scientific uncertainty exists, the precautionary principle advocates that one has a duty to take action to prevent harm. If alternatives to toxic products and procedures are available, they should be adopted to protect the environment and public health. The policy framework focuses on certain environmental quality objectives that have public health implications, including well-designed cities, limiting global warming, clean air, a non-toxic environment, a protective ozone layer, and safe radiation levels. Effective pedestrian safety policies decreased pedestrian fatalities by over 80 percent between 1975 and 2001 (Pucher & Dijkstra, 2003). In contrast, an American pedestrian is over 6 times more likely, per mile and per trip walked, to be killed by a car than his average European counterpart. American pedestrian injuries fare only slightly better.

2.4.6. Health and Medical Care that Actively Promotes Good Health

In Sweden, a transition to policies of active health-promotion and prevention that consider the entire person and his/her family and society has taken place. A prevention focus, as opposed to a treatment focus, stresses lifestyle factors, such as not smoking, physical activity, healthful eating habits, and avoidance of alcohol. Preventive medicine and protective measures are the guiding principles of maternity and child healthcare, youth guidance centers, and healthcare in schools and companies. Furthermore, medical professionals are trained in social medicine and public health. In 2004, almost half of Swedes (47 percent) between 18 and 84 lived healthy lives (Bostrom, 2006). They abstained from alcohol abuse, smoking, or physical inactivity, and did not suffer from obesity. They ate sufficient amounts of fruits and vegetables. Only 33 percent had one, and 20 percent had between two and five risky living habits. However, when it came to unhealthy lifestyles, differences by sex and socioeconomic status were revealed. Men, blue-collar workers, and poorly educated Swedes were all at increased risk.

2.4.7. Effective Protection Against Communicable Diseases

Past programs have been exceptionally effective at reducing the burden of infectious diseases through environmental interventions, high vaccination coverage, systematic testing, and contact tracing. For example, tuberculosis transmission among native-born Swedes has been almost completely interrupted (2 cases per 100,000 inhabitants per year). Control of antibiotic resistance, such as methicillin-resistant *Staphylococcus aureus* (MRSA), pneumococci; or *Mycobacterium tuberculosis*, fares better in Sweden than in Europe as a whole. Deterioration of vaccination coverage for children's diseases (e.g., MMR) was halted during the 1990s (Carlson, 2006).

2.4.8. Safe Sex and Good Reproductive Health

Sex education and teen-pregnancy prevention has been a cornerstone of public health work in Sweden, and it is part of a very long tradition of information campaigns about sexuality and partnership. For example, in the 1960s, the teenage birth rate was high, and the teenage abortion rate was low; by the 1970s, however, teenage births had declined and abortions had increased, due to a change in abortion laws and attitudes. In 1975, comprehensive health education led to a decline in teenage abortions and is today comparable to the Scandinavian average. An international comparison of sexuality and reproductive health in Sweden and the US revealed no differences in sexual behavior (e.g., age at first intercourse or number of partners) but did reveal a discrepancy in knowledge and access to contraceptives and in motivation to avoid teen childbirth. Each year in Sweden, there are 8 births and 25 abortions per 1,000 women aged 15–19 years, compared to 55 births and 84 abortions per 1,000 women aged 15–19 years in the US (Danielsson & Sundstrom, 2006). Contraceptives are readily available to teenagers in Sweden but not to those in the US, where "abstinence-only" programs promote abstinence from sexual activity without teaching the basic facts of contraception. Abstinence-only programs have been shown to be ineffective at protecting adolescents from sexually transmitted diseases (Bennett & Assefi, 2005); nevertheless, the US government currently endorses and heavily funds them (Waxman, 2004).

Behavioral changes might not be a very effective prescription for marginalized groups, however. For example, sexually transmitted diseases among men who have sex with men, namely chlamydia, syphilis, gonorrhea, and HIV, have increased. Behavioral interventions might not work well for drug addicts, either, since they often resort to prostitution to support their drug habits and thus may engage in unsafe sex practices despite knowledge of the risks. Effective addiction counseling, treatment, and societal integration have been recognized as effective communicable disease control strategies.

2.4.9. Increased Physical Activity

Physical activity is a prerequisite for optimal health. Outdoor recreation in Sweden is stimulated through outdoor facilities. School and pre-school programs provide opportunities for children to participate in sport and exercise. Exercise habits have improved since the eighties, when 47 percent of men and 43 percent of women exercised regularly, compared to 58 percent of men and 60 percent of women in 2003 (Bostrom, 2006). However, the general favorable trend of leisure-time physical activity is not uniform. Exercise rates differ by age, educational level, race/ethnicity, and socioeconomic level. The prevalence of sedentary lifestyles among children is also increasing. Successful policies include better facilities for walking, traffic-calming in residential neighborhoods, restrictions on motor vehicle use in cities, strict traffic safety education and enforcement for drivers and pedestrians, as well as urban structures that are designed with the pedestrian in mind. Through urban planning practices, physical activity, recreation, and recuperation are incorporated into the design of newly constructed buildings to assure that the young and the elderly, as well as the disabled, have access to parks for exercise. In Sweden, 29 percent of trips in cities are made by walking and 10 percent by biking, compared to 6 percent and 1 percent, respectively, in the US (Pucher & Dijkstra, 2003).

2.4.10. Good Eating Habits and Safe Food

Sweden's Public Health Bill considers food policy as a key entry point of interventions and calls for ecologically, economically, and socially sustainable food production. Health education and promotion is also advanced through nutrition education. In a comparison of Nordic countries, the Swedes, Swedish women in particular, ate the most fruits and green vegetables (Bostrom, 2006). Consumption of sweets is on the rise among the young, and while the obesity epidemic in Sweden has not reached American proportions, the trend is increasing (currently, 10 percent of the adult population is seriously overweight) (Kark & Rasmussen, 2005).

Scandinavia has one of the most advanced tracking systems for the contamination of meats by *E. Coli* and *Salmonella* bacteria (Molbak et al., 1999). Following a 1957 salmonella outbreak traced to a meat packing plant, Sweden was the first nation to implement strict government inspections and regulation of the meat processing and poultry industry to ensure safe food and minimize the risk of exposure to food-borne pathogens. As a result of this macrosocial intervention, the prevalence of salmonella in laying hen flocks has reached 0 percent, the lowest in the European Union (de Jong & Ekdahl, 2006a). Interestingly, a European comparison shows a high, linear correlation (correlation coefficient 0.91) between salmonella prevalence in egg laying hens and human illness (de Jong & Ekdahl, 2006b). Sanitation standards in the US meat packing industry were de-regulated in the 1980s in response to corporate pressures. In contrast, in Sweden the consumer is protected through government regulations, rather than having to rely on individual action, such as rinsing contaminated meat and thoroughly cooking it. While such behaviors undoubtedly work for the well-informed, they may not work as effectively for the unaware. It may be safer and more effective to intervene at the policy level.

2.4.11. Reduced Use of Tobacco and Alcohol, a Society Free from Illicit Drugs and Doping, and a Reduction in the Harmful Effects of Excessive Gambling

As part of the Tobacco Act, smoking is banned in public places, and a smoking ban in restaurants and bars is also under consideration. Smoking has declined across all socioeconomic groups in Sweden since the early 1980s (Persson et al., 2006). Indeed, throughout Europe, Sweden has the lowest rate of daily smokers among men (but not women), which continues to decline for men of all ages and for women under 45 years of age (Bostrom, 2006).

Alcohol has been taxed and is available only in certain stores (Systembolaget AB). Since 1980, mortality from alcohol-related diseases has steadily decreased for most age groups, except women between 45 and 74 and men over 65 (Bostrom, 2006). However, since acceptance into the European Union, regulations have changed, and between 1996 and 2003, alcohol consumption, particularly wine and beer, increased by 29 percent. Meanwhile, liquor consumption has decreased. In Sweden, narcotics abuse is relatively uncommon compared to other countries, with only 10 percent of the Swedish adult population having used cannabis at some time. However, drug use is increasing, and a special narcotics coordinator has been appointed to address the problem. Excessive gambling is a serious societal problem, and an action plan has been put in place to help gambling addicts.

Sweden's example of a national intervention is an illustration of a new kind of public health policy with specific objectives and guiding principles. The key concept of Sweden's macrosocial approach is to carry out the majority of public health work outside the narrow confines of traditional medical care services and to place it instead in the broader social and political realm. International comparisons of health indicators attest to the fact that Sweden's public health approach has worked well there. Average death or infant mortality rates are exceptionally low compared to other countries. Sweden has succeeded in reducing the absolute difference in health indicators between socioeconomic groups, although some relative differences still remain, as highlighted above. The challenge for the committed public health practitioner is to devise policy strategies that reduce the overall burden of disease in society, while simultaneously pushing back health inequalities.

3. Conclusion

From a macrosocial perspective, structural determinants give rise to social stratification while intermediary determinants determine differences in exposure that can influence health. Material and psychosocial conditions, including access to clean water and healthy food, sanitation and hygiene, safe living and working conditions, resources and information, self-determination and stature in society, social networks, and social capital, can decrease an individual's risk for disease, above and beyond personal risk-factors. Throughout the history of public health, numerous examples can be cited of regulations and interventions that have successfully addressed intermediate determinants of public health, often after serious struggles with entrenched interest groups, who benefit from a *status quo* that can foster and perpetuate poor health. For instance, advertisement of and access to tobacco products has been curtailed despite staunch opposition by the tobacco industry. Successful efforts have required the installation of catalytic converters on cars for emissions control, despite resistance from automobile manufacturers. The Food and Drug Administration (FDA) has passed legislation regulating testing and marketing of drugs, despite pharmaceutical industry lobbying. Milk is now pasteurized, despite initial objections from the dairy industry. Building codes are enforced in the face of opposition from developers, and so on (Centers for Disease Control, 1999).

One example of a macrosocial intervention addressing intermediate determinants is "Moving to Opportunity", a randomized, controlled trial and the first experimental study of neighborhood effects on mental health (Leventhal & Brooks-Gunn, 2003). The study randomized families from public housing in high-poverty neighborhoods in New York City into private housing in less poor neighborhoods and found striking mental health benefits, both for parents and children. The benefits were particularly pronounced in boys, who manifested fewer distress and depressive symptoms.

Some efforts have taken a different approach to tackling the structural determinants of health by pushing back inequalities through education, progressive taxation, and other policies. The reallocation of material wealth has been shown to be a key factor in ameliorating such health disparities (Heymann, Hertzman, Barer, & Evans, 2006). One example is a randomized control trial in Indiana that allocated financial assistance to low-income mothers at high risk for adverse pregnancy outcomes. The financial assistance included income support with guaranteed minimum wage, which was associated with increased infant body weight, compared to the non-intervention group (Kehrer & Wolin, 1979). Another randomized control trial assigned out-of-home daycare to disadvantaged children in the US and found positive effects on the children's cognitive development and academic performance (Zoritch, Roberts, & Oakley, 1998). The study documented that the intervention altered not only the current but also the future life circumstances of the children, with elevated socioeconomic status, increased employment, lower teenage pregnancy rates, and decreased criminal behavior during long-term follow-up.

Both medicine and public health can be separated into either a disease-focused or a comprehensive approach. For example, alternative medicine takes the entire person into consideration to understand the disease process, whereas traditional allopathic medicine dissects the natural history of disease in accordance with its reductionist methods. In public health, technology-driven interventions, which have been shown to be very cost-effective under certain circumstances, such as the eradication of smallpox, are one approach. The efficacy of such hierarchical programs, which are narrowly focused on single diseases, has also been shown to be very limited in certain public health predicaments, and the cost of the limitations has already been recognized. Examples include the failed hookworm eradication campaign of 1909, the unsuccessful, seventeen-year campaign against Yellow Fever that ended in 1932, and the fruitless eradication campaign against malaria in the fifties and sixties (Litsios, 1997).

In contrast, a comprehensive conception of public health, which has been discussed in this chapter, is based on the realization that individual behavioral change works best if societal conditions support it. Ecological interventions aim to sustain behavioral change through an integrated approach to interacting variables, including the personal, social, cultural, and physical environment (Sallins & Owen, 1997). Thus, comprehensive public health uses a structural approach to influence innovative policy and legislation that are health-affirming. In the example of the Swedish national health objectives discussed above, policy did not aim to reduce mortality or morbidity directly; rather, it aimed to intervene in the social and environmental determinants of disease. Sweden's approach is based on the fact that greater economic inequality is associated with poorer public health, and that the creation of an egalitarian society ensures superior health, on equal terms, for the total population (Wilkinson, 2005). Interestingly, Swedish public health objectives largely circumvent the contribution of the healthcare system and intervene outside the sphere of medical care.

Optimal public health action can be defined as a comprehensive approach to society by which public health decisions are made in municipal assemblies (rather than in public health departments) to address unemployment, labor conditions, social security, housing, segregation, or access to tobacco and alcohol. The benefits to public health of political decisions made at the municipal level far outweigh those made in the medical care sector. Societies should democratically decide that health equity is the explicit ambition of a national public health policy. Ultimately, the goal is to create healthy environments for healthy people by humanizing the physical, social, cultural, economic, and political environment of an egalitarian society.

References

Beaglehole, R. (1990). International trends in coronary heart disease mortality, morbidity, and risk factors. *Epidemiological Review, 12,* 1–15.

Bennett, S. E., & Assefi, N. P. (2005). School-based teenage pregnancy prevention programs: a systematic review of randomized controlled trials. *Journal of Adolescent Health, 36*(1), 72–81.

Berkman, L. F., & Syme, S. L. (1979). Social networks, host resistance, and mortality: A nine-year follow-up study of Alameda County residents. *American Journal of Epidemiology, 109*(2), 186–204.

Bernard, S. M., & McGeehin, M. A. (2004). Municipal heat wave response plans. *American Journal of Public Health, 94*(9), 1520–1522.

Bremberg, S. (2003). Does an increase of low-income families affect child health inequalities? A Swedish case study. *Journal of Epidemiology & Community Health, 57*(8), 584–588.

Bostrom, G. (2006). Chapter 9: Habits of life and health. *Scandinavian Journal of Public Health Supplemental, 67,* 199–228.

Buzbee, W. W. (2003). Urban form, health and the law's limits. *American Journal of Public Health, 93*(9), 1395–1398.

Carlson, J. (2006). Related Chapter 5.9: Major public health problems—infectious disease. *Scandinavian Journal of Public Health Supplemental, 67,* 132–138.

Centers for Disease Control. (1995). Heat-related mortality—Chicago, July 1995. *Mortality and Morbidity Weekly Report (MMWR), 44,* 577–579.

Centers for Disease Control. (1999). Ten great public health achievements—United States, 1900–1999. *Mortality and Morbidity Weekly Report (MMWR), 48*(12), 241–243.

The City Repair Project. (2006). Portland, OR (December 5, 2006); http://www.cityrepair.org.

Conti, S., Meli, P., Minelli, G., Solimini, R., Toccaceli, V., Vichi, M., et al. (2005). Epidemiologic study of mortality during the summer 2003 heat wave in Italy. *Environmental Research, 98*(3), 390–399.

Danielsson, M., & Sundstrom, K. (2006). Chapter 6: Reproductive health. *Scandinavian Journal of Public Health, 67,* 147–164.

Dansinger, M. L., Gleason, J. A., Griffith, J. L., Selker, H. P., & Schaefer, E. J. (2005). Comparison of the Atkins, Ornish, Weight Watchers, and Zone diets for weight loss and heart disease risk reduction: a randomized trial. *Journal of the American Medical Association, 293*(1), 43–53.

de Jong, B., & Ekdahl, K. (2006a). The comparative burden of salmonellosis in the European Union member states, associated and candidate countries. *BMC Public Health, 6*(4).

de Jong, B., & Ekdahl, K. (2006b). Human salmonellosis in travelers is highly correlated to the prevalence of salmonella in laying hen flocks. *Euro Surveillance, 11*(7).

Ebi, K. L., Teisberg, T. H., Kalkstein, L. S., Robinson, L., & Weiher, R. F. (2004). Health watch/warning systems save lives: Estimated costs and benefits from Philadelphia 1995–1998. *Bulletin of the American Meteorological Society, 85*(8), 1067–1073.

Gerdtham, U. G., & Johannesson, M. (2004). Absolute income, relative income, income inequality and mortality. *Journal of Human Resources, 39*(1), 228–247.

Granovetter, M. (1973). The strength of weak ties. *American Journal of Sociology, 78*(6), 1360–1380.

Green, L. W., & Kreuter, M. W. (2005). *Health program planning. An educational and ecological approach.* 4th edition. New York: McGraw-Hill.

Heymann, J., Hertzman, C., Barer, M., & Evans, R. G. (Eds.). (2006). *Healthier societies: From analysis to action.* New York: Oxford University Press.

Hjern, A. (2006). Related Chapter 7: Children's and young people's health. *Scandinavian Journal of Public Health, 67,* 165–183.

Johnson, H., Kovats, R. S., MacGregor, G., Stedman, J., Gibbs, M., Walton, H., et al. (2005). The impact of the 2003 heat wave on mortality and hospital admissions in England. *Health Statistics Quarterly, 25,* 6–11.

Kark, M., & Rasmussen, F. (2005). Growing social inequalities in the occurrence of overweight and obesity among young men in Sweden. *Scandinavian Journal of Public Health, 33*(6), 472–477.

Kawachi, I., & Kennedy, B. P. (2002). *The health of nations: Why inequality is harmful to your health.* New York: New Press.

Kawachi, I., Kennedy, B. P., Lochner, K., & Prothrow-Stith, D. (1997). Social capital, income inequality, and mortality. *American Journal of Public Health, 87*(9), 1491–1498.

Kehrer B., & Wolin, V. (1979). Impact of income maintenance of low birth weight: Evidence from the Gary experiment. *Journal of Human Resources, 14,* 434–462.

Kelly, S., Hertzman, C., & Daniels, M. (1997). Searching for the biological pathways between stress and health. *Annual Review of Public Health, 18,* 437–462.

Kristenson, M., Kucinskiene, Z., Bergdahl, B., Calkauskas, H., Urmonas, V., & Orth-Gomer, K. (1998). Increased psychosocial strain in Lithuanian versus Swedish men: The LiVicordia study. *Psychosomatic Medicine, 60*(3), 277–282.

Leventhal, T., & Brooks-Gunn, J. (2003) Moving to opportunity: An experimental study of neighborhood effects on mental health. *American Journal of Public Health, 93*(9), 1576–1582.

Lindberg, G., & Persson, G. (2006). Chapter 4: Public health in an international perspective. *Scandinavian Journal of Public Health, 67,* 43–49.

Link, B. G., & Phelan, J. (1995). Social conditions as fundamental causes of disease. *Journal of Health and Social Behavior, 35*(Extra issue), 80–94.

Litsios, S. (1997). Malaria control, the cold war, and the postwar reorganization of international assistance. *Medical Anthropology, 17*(3), 255–78.

Lloyd, G. E. R. (1978). Hippocratic medical corpus: Airs, water, places, 500 B. C. In *Hippocratic writings.* Harmondsworth, England: Penguin.

Mahler, V., & Jesuit, D. (2006). Fiscal distribution in the developed countries: New insights from the Luxembourg Income Study. *Socio-Economic Review, 4*(3), 483–511.

Molbak, K., Baggesen, D. L., Aarestrup, F. M., Ebbesen, J. M., Engberg, J., Frydendahl, K., et al. (1999). An outbreak of multidrug-resistant, quinolone-resistant salmonella enterica serotype typhimurium DT104. *New England Journal of Medicine, 341*(19), 1420–1425.

Palecki, M. A., Changnon, S. A., & Kunkel, K. E. (2001). The nature and impacts of the July 1999 heat wave in the Midwestern United States: Learning from the lessons of 1995. *Bulletin of the American Meteorological Society, 82*(7), 1353–1368.

Persson, G. (2006). Chapter 1: The National Public Health Report 2005. *Scandinavian Journal of Public Health, 67,* 11–18.

Persson, G., Danielsson, M., Rosen, M., Alexanderson, K., Lundberg, O., Lundgren, B., et al. (2006). Health in Sweden: The National Public Health Report 2005. *Scandinavian Journal of Public Health, 67,* 3–10.

Pucher, J., & Dijkstra, L. (2003). Promoting safe walking and cycling to improve public health: Lessons from The Netherlands and Germany. *American Journal of Public Health, 93*(9), 1509–1516.

Putnam, R. D. (2000). Bowling alone: The collapse and revival of American community. New York: Simon & Schuster.

Rosengren, A., Orth-Gomer, K., & Wilhelmsen, L. (1998). Socioeconomic differences in health indices, social networks, and mortality among Swedish men. A study of men born in 1933. *Scandinavian Journal of Social Medicine, 26*(4), 272–280.

Rothstein, B. (2001). Social capital in a social democratic state. The Swedish model and civil society. *Politics and Society, 29*(2), 209–240.

Rothstein, B., & Stolle, D. (2003). Introduction: Social capital in Scandinavia. *Scandinavian Political Studies, 26*(1), 1–26.

Sallins, J., & Owen, N. (1997). Ecological Models. In K. Ganz, B. Rimer, & F.M. Lewis (Eds.), *Health behavior and health education: Theory, research and practice.* 2nd edition. San Francisco: Jossey-Bass.

Semenza, J. C. (1996). Deaths in the Chicago heat wave. *New England Journal of Medicine, 335,* 1848–1849.

Semenza, J. C. (2003). The Intersection of urban planning, art, and public health: The Sunnyside Piazza. *American Journal of Public Health, 93*(9), 1439–1441.

Semenza, J. C. (2004). Contaminated water distribution: An intervention strategy to solve a public health problem. In J. Pronczuk (Ed.), *Children's health and the environment: A global perspective. A resource manual for the health sector.* Geneva: World Health Organization.

Semenza, J. C. (2005). Building healthy cities: A focus on interventions. In D. Vlahov & S. Galea (Eds.), *Handbook of urban health: Populations, methods and practice.* New York: Springer Science and Business Media.

Semenza, J. C., & Krishnasamy, P. V. (in press). Design of a health-promoting neighborhood intervention. *Health Promotion Practice.*

Semenza, J. C., March, T., & Bontempo, B. (2007) Community-initiated urban development: An ecological intervention. *Journal of Urban Health, 84*(1), 8–20.

Semenza, J. C., McCullough, J., Flanders, D. W., McGeehin, M. A., & Lumpkin, J. R. (1999). Excess hospital admissions during the 1995 heat wave in Chicago. *American Journal of Preventive Medicine, 16*(4), 269–277.

Semenza, J. C., Roberts, L., Henderson, A., Bogan, J., & Rubin, C. H. (1998). Water distribution system and diarrheal disease transmission: A case study in Uzbekistan. *American Journal of Tropical Medicine and Hygiene, 59*(6), 941–946.

Semenza, J. C., Rubin, H. C., Falter, K. H., Selanikio, J. D., Flanders, D. W. & Wilhelm, J. L. (1996). Risk factors for heat-related mortality during the July 1995 heat wave in Chicago. *New England Journal of Medicine, 335*(2), 84–90.

Statens folkhälsoinstitut (2006). Stockholm (April 17, 2006); www.fhi.se/shop/material_pdf/newpublic0401.pdf

Stenbeck, M., & Persson, G. (2006). Chapter 10: Working life, work environment and health. *Scandinavian Journal of Public Health, 67,* 229–245.

Syme, S. L. (1996). Rethinking disease: Where do we go from here? *Annals of Epidemiology, 6*(5), 463–468.

Vandentorren, S., Suzan, F., Medina, S., Pascal, M., Maulpoix, A., Cohen, J. C., et al. (2004). Mortality in 13 French cities during the August 2003 heat wave. *American Journal of Public Health, 94*(9), 1518–1520.

Waxman, H. A. (2004). *The content of federally funded abstinence-only education programs.* United States House of Representatives. Committee on Government Reform—Minority Staff Special Investigation Division.

Weisskopf, M. G., Anderson, H. A., Foldy, S., Hanrahan, L. P., Blair, K., Torok, T. J., et al. (2002). Heat wave morbidity and mortality, Milwaukee, Wisconsin, 1999 vs. 1995: An improved response? *American Journal of Public Health, 92*(5), 830–833.

Wilkinson, R. G. (2005). *The impact of inequality: How to make sick societies healthier.* New York: New Press.

World Health Organization. (2004). *Heat waves: Risks and responses.* Copenhagen: World Health Organization.

World Health Organization (2005). *Towards a conceptual framework for analysis and action.* Discussion paper for the Commission on Social Determinants of Health. Geneva: World Health Organization.

World Health Organization (2006). Commission on social determinants of health. Geneva (2006); http://www.who.int/social_determinants/en/

Zoritch, B., Roberts, I., & Oakley, A. (1998). The health and welfare effects of day-care: A systematic review of randomised controlled trials. *Social Science & Medicine, 47*(3), 317–327.

Chapter 23
Integrative Chapter: Modifying Macrosocial Factors to Improve Population Health

Sandro Galea

We conclude this book with two chapters that consider how we may apply some of the insights to emerge from Sections I and II in order to improve population health. Those interested in studying macrosocial determinants of population health are not infrequently faced with skepticism about the practical relevance of this line of inquiry. We can all envision public health interventions that, for example, attempt to reduce smoking, but can we envision how public health can do something about the influence of culture, of patent policies, or political systems? These preceding chapters suggest that indeed we can and that concern with the macrosocial determinants of population health need not be simply a study in abstraction, but rather inquiry that can guide tangible manipulations of these determinants with the aim of improving the health of populations.

Chapters 21 and 22 provide the reader not only with a framework within which we may consider action to act upon macrosocial determinants, but also with tangible examples of such action at multiple levels of macrosocial influence. However, although in reading these chapters the reader may well be impressed by achievements in particular circumstances, one may also harbor lingering skepticism about the extent to which these examples offer practical motivation in other contexts. Can other countries really emulate macrosocial changes implemented in Sweden, where a culture of health equity and health promotion has been dominant for hundreds of years? I conclude by suggesting that these chapters, building on the preceding chapters in the book, indeed show not only that macrosocial factors can be changed for the purposes of improving health, but that doing so is essential if we are serious about improving population health in a sustainable and equitable manner.

It appears that there are two primary limitations we face in considering how we may intervene on macrosocial determinants to improve health. First, in many respects we lack theory that suggests how macrosocial factors influence population health, and second, we frequently fall short in the practical imagination required to inform how we can manipulate macrosocial factors. The bulk of this book has been devoted to an effort to articulate why and how specific macrosocial factors may indeed shape the health of populations and how we can fruitfully apply methodology to provide robust data that describe macrosocial production of the health of populations. Insofar as we currently remain short on theory and data, it is hoped that this book will encourage other efforts that build on, confirm, or refute the observations herein.

However, our second limitation has little to do with a paucity of theory, data, or adequate research methods. Rather, public health has not infrequently succumbed to the belief that there may be little, or nothing, that we can do to tackle the role that the media, corporate practices, or taxation may play in shaping health. As these last two chapters suggest this is not only false but also suggests a timidity on our part that is constrained by recent decades of public health practice that have been informed primarily by a focus on individual exposures and behaviors that influence personal health and disease. The case studies in Chapter 22 can be buttressed by numerous other current examples where macrosocial factors have indeed been intervened upon, and effectively. At this writing, for example, New York City, by far the US's largest urban area, is near banning *trans*fats from all restaurants. This clearly is a bold move that acts directly on one of the corporate practices discussed in Chapter 4. It is also an action that, it is reasonable to say, may well have been considered "unachievable" just before it was actually achieved. This is but one example. Political systems can be changed, and do change. Taxation policies can be modified, and global processes such as climate change or globalization can be influenced. Changing macrosocial factors and processes is not an impossibility but rather a matter of imagination, political will, and priorities. It is one of the goals of this book to suggest why and how these macrosocial factors influence health, and of these last two chapters to offer a framework for, and examples of, macrosocial intervention. It is up to the reader, and future work, to extend this thinking well beyond the examples offered here to consider actions that may influence the other macrosocial factors discussed in part I, and many other factors that were not included in this book.

One insight that emerges from Chapters 21 and 22 that is frequently forgotten in discussions about macrosocial factors is that it is not only desirable to consider how macrosocial determinants influence health but it is *essential* if we are genuinely interested in achieving long-term and sustainable improvements in population health. This argument is fully and elegantly articulated in Chapter 21. Briefly, a useful way to think about the centrality of macrosocial determination of health arises naturally from the notion that macrosocial factors influence all aspects of the world within which we live including, for example, both the presence or absence of environmental exposures and the social environment that shapes individual risk behaviors. It is these exposures and risk behaviors that have been the traditional (individual or "proximal") determinants of health considered by public health research and practice. However, when we consider the central role of macrosocial determinants, it is not difficult to suggest that macrosocial factors are, if not direct causes of health conditions themselves, causes of causes. Within a view of the production of health that encompasses multiple component causes working together, considering only causes that are proximal to the individual is then clearly omitting component causes, albeit at a higher "macro" level of influence, without which our understanding of disease determination is incomplete at best, and wrong at worst. In addition, acting only on these proximal causes is a near inevitable recipe for our continually "chasing" changing proximal causes which are shaped and informed by more fundamental macrosocial determinants. It then matters quite a bit that we consider the role played by macrosocial determinants in the production of population health, and to apply our practical ingenuity to identifying ways to manipulate these determinants for the betterment of population health. It is hoped that these last two chapters in the book offer one approach in that direction that can stimulate both further work and inspire action.

Health is central to the achievement of individual and group potential in all human endeavors. As such, understanding the macrosocial factors that determine our health so that we may improve it should be a universal concern. This book has discussed the role that macrosocial factors may play in shaping population health, presented several such factors, considered methodologic approaches to the study of their role, and now suggested potential interventions. It is hoped that the ideas sown in this book, future work that builds upon it, and a grounding in principles of equity and justice can provide us with powerful motivation to make thinking about macrosocial determination central to public health research and practice and to engage in a broader policy discourse that can lead to creating a national and global environment that improves the health of populations.

Index

Printed in the United States
100618LV00001BA/85-90/A

9 780387 708119